# MAGNETIC RESONANCE ANGIOGRAPHY of the HEAD and NECK: *A Teaching File*

Volumes in the *Teaching File* Series

- IMAGING of CNS DISEASE: A CT and MR TEACHING FILE
  Douglas H. Yock, Jr.

- ALIMENTARY TRACT IMAGING: *A Teaching File*
  C. Daniel Johnson

- NUCLEAR MEDICINE: *A Teaching File*
  Frederick L. Datz
  Gregory G. Patch
  John M. Arias
  Kathyrn A. Morton

- RADIOLOGY of THORACIC DISEASES: *A Teaching File*
  Stephen J. Swensen

- MAGNETIC RESONANCE ANGIOGRAPHY of the HEAD and NECK: *A Teaching File*
  Jeffrey S. Ross

- MAGNETIC RESONANCE IMAGING of CNS DISEASE: *A Teaching File*
  Douglas H. Yock, Jr.

# MAGNETIC RESONANCE ANGIOGRAPHY of the HEAD and NECK: *A Teaching File*

**Jeffrey S. Ross, M.D.**
Head
Section of Magnetic Resonance Imaging
Department of Radiology
The Cleveland Clinic Foundation
Cleveland, Ohio

with 822 illustrations

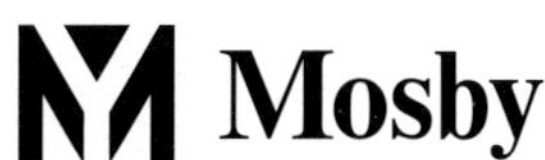


St. Louis Baltimore Berlin Boston Carlsbad Chicago London Madrid
Naples New York Philadelphia Sydney Tokyo Toronto

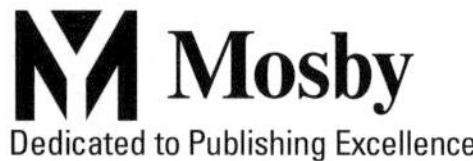
Dedicated to Publishing Excellence

*Executive Editor:* Susan M. Gay
*Project Manager:* Carol Sullivan Weis
*Senior Production Editor:* Pat Joiner
*Manufacturing Manager:* Kathy Grone
*Book Designer:* Sheilah Barrett



Printed in the United States of America
Composition by the Clarinda Company
Printing/binding by Maple-Vail Book Manufacturing Group

Mosby–Year Book, Inc.
11830 Westline Industrial Drive
St. Louis, MO 63146

**Library of Congress Cataloging in Publication Data**

Ross, Jeffrey S. (Jeffrey Stuart)
Magnetic resonance angiography of the head and neck: a teaching file / Jeffrey S. Ross.
p. cm.
Includes bibliographical references and index.
ISBN 0-8151-7409-8
1. Cerebrovascular disease—Magnetic resonance imaging. 2. Brain—Blood-vessels—Magnetic resonance imaging. I. Title.
[DNLM: 1. Magnetic Resonance Imaging—methods. 2. Angiography—methods—case studies. 3. Head—anatomy & histology. 4. Neck—anatomy & histology. 5. Cerebrovascular Disorders—diagnosis—case studies. WN 445 R824m 1994]
RC388.5.R686 1994
616.8′107548—dc20
DNLM/DLC
for Library of Congress 94-31810
CIP

94 95 96 97 98 / 9 8 7 6 5 4 3 2 1

**Where is the wise man? Where is the scholar? Where is the philosopher of this age? Has not God made foolish the wisdom of the world?**

***I Corinthians 1:20***

# PREFACE

Tremendous changes have taken place in hardware and software since my first involvement in the infant stages of MRA in 1987. Improvements such as shorter echo times, improved motion compensation, and faster and more user-friendly reconstructions have allowed MRA to become a mainstream, if not a prerequisite, part of the evaluation of a variety of neuropathologies. It is hard to imagine a complete evaluation of the cerebrovasculature without some element of MRA or the intracranial circulation or carotid bifurcation. However, MRA is not an easy modality to learn, since it requires the combined knowledge of MR, with its variety of artifacts, and neurovascular anatomy.

The purpose of this book is to try to help in that learning process of MRA by providing a variety of case material in a straightforward manner, with appropriate references and discussion of pathologic processes. The first chapter is an introduction to the concepts involved in MRA with a purposely "non-physics minded" approach. I apologize for the one equation that did slip in. The second chapter, which is supplemented with line drawings of the sequence setups, is devoted to the wide variety of techniques available and should be referred to if there is a question about individual case parameters in the other chapters. Each chapter covering specific pathologic processes begins with an introductory section, explaining the pathology or imaging considerations. The remainder of each chapter is a series of cases with illustrative MR imaging and MRA images and correlative conventional angiography or computed tomographic images. Because of the tremendous variety of hardware and software available, I have placed emphasis on different MRA techniques used by placing the parameters at the beginning of each case, along with a short history. The cases are set up so that, in general, the reader can first test his or her knowledge by evaluating the images, with the diagnosis, discussion, pertinent figures, and references available once the reader has arrived at the differential diagnosis. Although a wide variety of pathologies are certainly covered, I have also attempted to provide different views of the same pathologic process. This is particularly true of the chapter on the carotid bifurcation, which provides many variations on the theme of athersclerosis but with a variety of techniques, parameters, and views of this important MRA area. Although there is discussion of different pathologies presented in this series of teaching cases, this book is *not* meant as an all-encompassing primer on cerebrovascular disease, nor is it meant to supplant the current excellent textbooks on MR imaging. It is meant to serve as a complement to those works, with a particular emphasis on MRA and the unique problems MRA presents. Some of those problems are highlighted by the pitfall cases at the beginning of chapters. Since MR is such a dynamic technology, it is difficult to remain state of the art with the necessary production schedule of a book. Nevertheless, I have attempted to use mainstream or almost mainstream techniques in this series. The time-of-flight and phase-contrast techniques and underlying physical principle will remain the same regardless of the specific machine or field of strength used.


### Acknowledgments

I would like to extend thanks to the radiologists who so graciously gave me access to their case material and without whom this book could not have been completed.

John Huston, III, M.D.
Walter Kucharczyk, M.D.
John Sherman, M.D.
Alison S. Smith, M.D.

And, of course, a special thanks to my friends colleagues at the Cleveland Clinic who gave invaluable time and input into the substance of the text and images, and put up with my scavenging for cases.

Paul Ruggieri, M.D.
Micheal T. Modic, M.D.
Thomas J. Masaryk, M.D.
Jean Tkach, Ph.D.
Robert Wallace, M.D.
John Perl, M.D.

To Peg, Whitney and Tyler, my earthly foundation.


Jeffrey S. Ross

# INTRODUCTION

A similar convention regarding MRA techniques will be used throughout the book, with the following format as an example:

**Technique #1:** Carotid (1.0 T) / axial volume three-dimensional time-of-flight, 40/11/25, 256 × 256, 64 partitions, 80-mm slab, 20-cm field of view, 10:57. Echo time is prolonged relative to the usual 7-ms echo time at 1.5 T, since fat and water cycle inphase at 1.0 T with 7-ms echo time and opposed phase at echo time of 11. Prolonging the echo time to opposed phase improves background sufficiently to outweigh the increased dephasing that might occur.

**Technique #2:** Intracranial / axial volume, three-dimensional time-of-flight, 40/7/15, 256 × 256, 64 partitions, 80-mm slab, 20-cm field of view, 10:57.

## EXPLANATION

| | |
|---|---|
| **Carotid** | Cervical carotid artery protocol |
| **Intracranial** | Intracranial circulation protocol |
| **axial volume** | Orientation of individual partition (i.e., axial, sagittal, or coronal). |
| **40/11/25** | Repetition time / echo time / flip angle. |
| **256 x 256** | In-plane matrix size |
| **64 partitions** | Number of slices acquired for a two-dimensional sequence or in a three-dimensional data set |
| **80-mm slab** | Thickness of imaging volume; thickness ÷ number of partitions = slice thickness |
| **10:57** | Total imaging time (minutes:seconds). |

*All time-of-flight sequences have velocity compensation in read and slice and one excitation (acquisition) unless otherwise noted. Intracranial arterial MRAs uniformly have a superior saturation pulse.*

# CONTENTS


**1** BASIC PRINCIPLES, 1

**2** TECHNIQUES, 13

**3** NORMAL ANATOMY, VARIANTS, and CONGENITAL ANOMALIES, 41

**4** ANEURYSMS, 79

**5** VASCULAR MALFORMATIONS, 163

**6** INTRACRANIAL STENOSIS and OCCLUSION, 203

**7** TUMORS and VASCULAR LOOPS, 264

**8** VENOUS DISEASE (EXCLUDING VASCULAR MALFORMATIONS), 293

**9** CAROTID BIFURCATION, 313

**10** DISSECTION, 373

# CHAPTER 1

# Basic Principles

Magnetic resonance angiography (MRA) has been applied to several manifestations of cerebrovascular disease. Although these methods are powerful for demonstrating pathologic conditions, the clinician must keep their limitations in mind so that the appropriate method is applied to answer a specific clinical question and that the acquisition parameters are chosen to maximize the sensitivity and specificity of the study. After choosing the appropriate technique, the clinician must decide whether the conventional parenchymal MR imaging and MRA evaluation are sufficient in a particular clinical setting or whether a more traditional, invasive angiographic study is necessary. For the central nervous system, MRA studies and flow-measurement techniques compliment the more traditional spin-echo evaluation of patients with aneurysms, arterial and venous stenoses and occlusions, vascular malformations, and occasionally, neoplastic vascular invasions. When carefully defined protocols are used and attention to detail occurs, this new information and improved diagnostic sensitivity can be used routinely, with only minor increases in examination time.

## GENERAL TECHNIQUES

Before details of MRA sequences are discussed, some general terms must be defined. A generic spin-echo diagram is shown in Fig. 1-1, with Gz (slice-select), Gy (phase-encode), and Gx (frequency-encode or "read") gradients shown. A similar schematic for a generic gradient-echo sequence is shown in Fig. 1-2. It is assumed that the fundamentals of MR image production are known to the reader, and a detailed explanation is beyond the scope of this book.

### Three-Dimensional MR Imaging

In three-dimensional (3D) gradient-echo imaging, a thick slab of interest is defined by the initial radiofrequency (rf) excitation pulse rather than a thin slice, as in two-dimensional (2D) imaging. This volume of tissue is divided into thin, contiguous partitions (slices) by an additional direction of phase encoding along the slice-select direction. The in-plane phase and frequency-encoding gradients are applied as in 2D imaging. With phase encoding used in two different directions, the imaging time is proportionally increased by the number of slices selected (the additional phase-encoding steps) compared with the imaging time of 2D techniques. Imaging time is therefore equal to the following:

Repetition time (TR) × Number of excitations
× Number of in-plane phase-encoding steps
× Number of slices (slice-select phase encoding)

Although 3D Fourier transform imaging is possible with spin echo (SE) sequences, for all practical purposes, the short TRs achieved by gradient-echo imaging have allowed more widespread applications. Two types of 3D imaging can be used relative to the type of rf pulses utilized: The entire sensitive volume of the surface coil can be used (nonselective), or only a smaller specific volume of tissue can be imaged within the active area of the coil (selective).

There following are theoretical and practical advantages of 3D imaging:

1. There is an increase in the signal-to-noise ratio over 2D imaging, which is the square root of the number of partitions (slices) selected, because of reexcitation of the entire volume with each rf pulse or for every phase-encoding step in each of the two directions. This may be considered analogous to increasing the number of acquisitions in 2D imaging. It is therefore advantageous to increase the number of slices with this technique and increase the area covered.
2. Thin, contiguous slices can be obtained from the volume without the problem of cross-talk found in 2D imaging. (Cross-talk between adjacent 2D slices gives unwanted changes in image contrast from slice to slice and reduces the signal-to-noise ratio because of saturation of the peripheral spins in the slices.) Thinner and more accurate slices can be achieved with 3D techniques because slice thickness depends not on the fidelity of the rf profile but rather on the process of phase encoding. Minimum slice thickness is approximately 0.5 mm for 3D vs. 2.5 mm for 2D imaging.

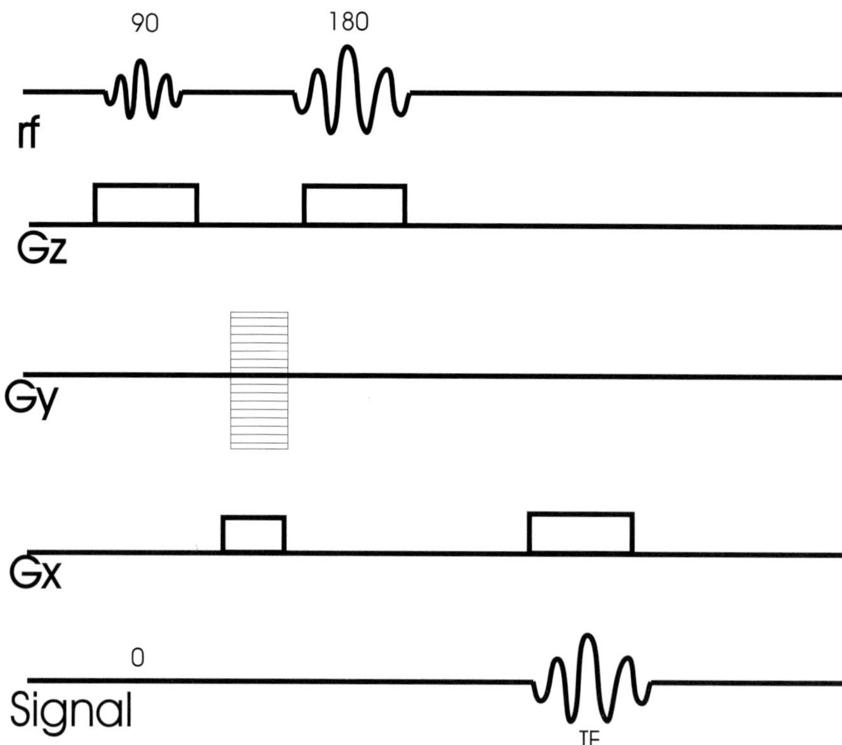


**Fig. 1-1** Diagram of conventional spin-echo sequence. The 90- and 180-degree rf pulses are followed by acquisition of the spin echo at the echo time *(TE)*. Three orthogonal magnetic field gradients are used in MR imaging to pinpoint the voxels in space (spatially encode). These gradients—frequency encoded *(Gx)*, phase encoded *(Gy)*, and slice select *(Gz)*—are produced by electromagnetic coils within the housing of the magnet. The frequency-encoded gradient is also called the *read gradient*.

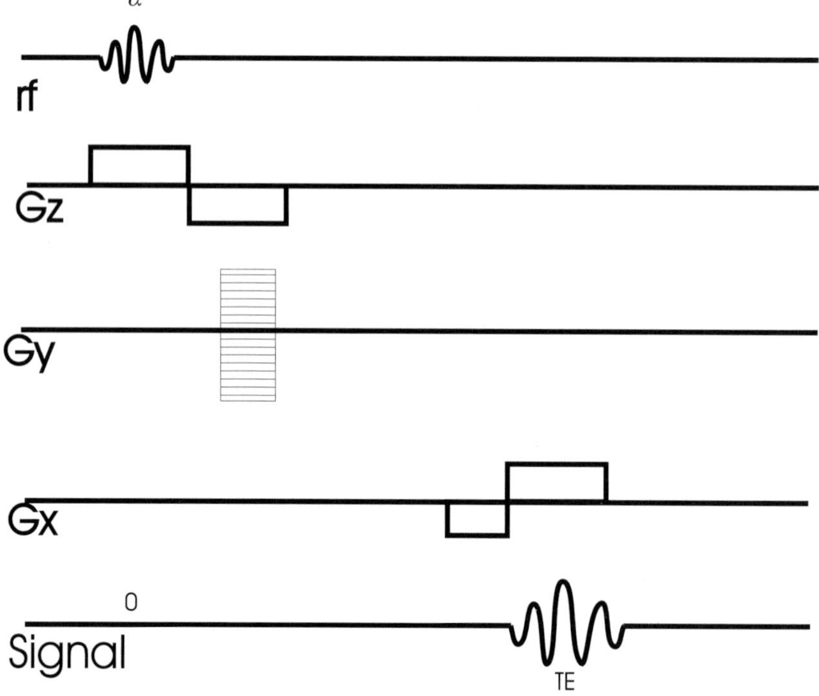


**Fig. 1-2** Gradient-echo diagram (2D). Note that the 180-degree rf pulse present in the spin-echo diagram is now missing, with the refocusing produced by the bipolar read gradient (the gradient is applied in one direction, followed by an inverted gradient). One of the advantages of this is a much quicker acquisition time because of shortened TRs in the absence of the necessity of a 180-degree rf pulse. α, Flip angle.

3. The 3D techniques have a reduction in susceptibility artifacts (i.e., T2* effects). Susceptibility artifacts can cause false "expansion" of bone at bone–soft tissue–air interfaces, which can result in loss of adjacent vascular signal. Susceptibiltiy artifacts occur when there is apposition of different tissues or air with different magnetic susceptibilities, resulting in the creation of local gradients that in turn produce spin dephasing and T2* signal loss. With smaller voxels, there is less tissue heterogeneity within the voxel and less signal loss.
4. Because a volume of data is collected, computer post-processing allows reformatting of the data along any desired imaging plane.

A problem with 3D imaging is truncation artifact (Gibbs artifact) in the in-plane direction (as in 2D) and in the slice-encoding direction because of finite sampling. Ghosting artifacts from motion are present not only along the in-plane phase-encoding directions (as in 2D imaging), but also along the additional direction of phase encoding in slice select. Gross motion artifacts are the most commonly encountered problems affecting the diagnostic quality of 3D techniques because of this sensitivity to motion and the longer acquisition times that make it more difficult for the patient to remain still throughout the examination. Magnetic susceptibility effects associated with the gradient-echo technique may also cause artifacts that are reduced or eliminated in spin-echo sequences. The rf profiles associated with selective and nonselective 3D sequences are not perfect. Although the individual slice thickness is preserved in 3D, the imperfect slice profile may result in excitation of matter outside the volume of interest, with subsequent aliasing of the information into the region of interest. The amount of slice-select aliasing for a fixed volume decreases as the number of partitions increases. The imperfect slice profile also causes nonuniform distribution of the flip angle across the volume and thus nonuniform contrast and signal-to-noise ratio from slice to slice. Although this may not be noticeable on one slice, it can degrade the quality of multiplanar reformats with a banding pattern.

## Blood Flow Signal

The signal of blood in MR imaging is roughly related to two aspects of the imaging process. The first is the pulse sequence itself, with variables such as slice orientation, repetition time, and flip angle. This is also called the *time-of-flight (TOF) effect*. TOF effects can increase or decrease vascular signal.[1-3] Spins (blood protons) must receive both the 90- and 180-degree rf pulses to be detected and included in the resultant image. TOF effects that decrease the signal of moving blood result from spins that do not remain within the selected imaging slice long enough to be acted on by *both* rf pulses used in conventional spin-echo imaging (see Figure 1-2). Blood that received a 90-degree pulse and then flowed out of the imaging plane before receiving the 180-degree pulse does not give a signal. Similarly, blood that flows into the imaging slice after the 90-degree pulse and thus receives only the 180-degree pulse does not give a signal and appears black on the MR image (a flow void).

TOF effects may also produce increased signal intensity of flowing blood, which is the basis for TOF MRA using gradient-echo imaging. Protons placed within a magnetic field tend to orient parallel to the magnetic lines. In routine gradient-echo MR imaging, an rf pulse that flips this vector of magnetization into the transverse plane is applied so that a signal can be detected. With time and if it is left undisturbed, the vector of magnetization grows back longitudinally parallel to the main magnetic field. If another rf pulse is delivered before this growth has occurred, the total detectable signal is decreased. An understanding of this concept is necessary to appreciate how flowing blood can give high signal on MR imaging. *Paradoxical enhancement*, *flow-related enhancement*, and *entry-slice phenomenon* are terms that generally refer to the same phenomenon: Blood moving into an imaging slice not previously exposed to rf energy can show high signal intensity. For conventional gradient-echo imaging with short repetition times, the stationary tissue within the imaging slice receives multiple rf pulses during image acquisition. The protons in this stationary tissue are called *partially saturated* because the repeated rf pulses have not allowed their longitudinal magnetization to recover completely. Spins that have recovered all their magnetization between rf pulses are called *unsaturated*, or *fully magnetized* or *fresh*. Unsaturated blood moving into the image slice can give a relative increase in signal intensity with subsequent applications of rf energy, which is flow-related enhancement.[4]

The second aspect of the imaging process that greatly influences the signal intensity of blood is the signal localizing gradients.[5-7] Blood flowing within an imaging plane demonstrates low signal intensity, since spins moving along a magnetic gradient rotate slower or faster depending on the gradient strength to which they are exposed (accumulate a phase change) with respect to stationary tissue. This phase change means that the spins do not rotate coherently. This loss of coherence causes loss of signal. Phase coherence might be compared to a rotating light. A tightly collimated light (such as a laser) has great intensity compared with the same light when it is allowed to disperse randomly around 360 degrees (like a regular light bulb). Phase change or loss of coherence may occur by blood motion along any of the three localizing gradient planes. This process is also called *spin dephasing* or *phase dispersion*.[8]

The factors that influence TOF angiography can therefore be grouped into two categories, each with three important components. The two main factors are *flow-related enhancement* and *phase dispersion*. Achieving the best possible MRA requires the maximization of flow-related enhancement and the minimization of phase dispersion. Factors that affect flow-related enhancement are geometry (slice or slab orientation with respect to the major direction of blood flow, TR, and flip angle. Vessel geometry is a very important consideration in TOF MRA so that high vascular signal can be maintained. In the ideal TOF geometry, the vessel is perpendicular to the imaging slice, which maximizes flow-related enhancement and minimizes saturation of blood. The main disadvantage of this technique is that it is difficult to cover large vessel lengths with axial 2D slices or 3D volumes. The TR should be long enough to allow full replacement of moving spins by unsaturated spins in the slice to give high vascular signal. The trade-off is that a longer TR allows regrowth of the longitudinal magnetization from the background tissue, which increases background signal intensity. Again, a balance must be struck between increased flow-related enhancement with a longer TR and potentially decreased vessel–soft tissue conspicuousness because background tissue also increases in signal. The appropriate flip angle is a compromise. A higher flip angle gives better signal-to-noise ratio and better suppression (saturation) of the background tissue. It also causes increased saturation of the blood flowing into the slice or slab; that is, the flowing spins become saturated with fewer rf pulses because of the higher flip angle used.

Factors that affect phase change (dispersion) are described later (echo time [TE], voxel, gradients). The phase change that occurs across a voxel is critical to understanding the methods used in MRA to increase vascular signal and may be approximately described by the following:

$$\text{Phase change} = \gamma\ TE^2 \bullet G \bullet \Delta\ V\ (X\rightarrow) \qquad 1\text{-}1$$

Where $\gamma$ is the gyromagnetic ratio, a constant specific for each nuclear species; G is the gradient magnetic field strength; $\Delta$ V is the velocity change across a voxel; and X is the directional vector.

This simplified equation describes the factors that can be manipulated to decrease the phase change of moving spins, which would increase vascular signal. All three of the parameters (G, V, TE) are usually manipulated together in MRA. For the sake of clarity, these factors are now be considered separately.

### Echo Time

The potential of MRA achieved widespread interest in 1982, when projection MRAs using short TE sequences with cardiac gating were demonstrated.[9-11] As shown in Equation 1-1, TE exerts a powerful effect on the phase change of a moving blood proton. Achieving as short as possible a TE reduces the signal loss associated with motion-induced loss of phase coherence of spins. With a short TE, there is less time for spins to dephase between the time of the excitation pulse and the application of the read gradient. However, depending on the individual hardware, there are physical limits on the shortest TE that can be used secondary to the available gradient strengths (given in mTesla/meter) and gradient rise and fall times (given in milliseconds).

Wedeen et al[9] were the first to use very short TEs to make projective (thick-slice) arteriograms. In their scheme, two separate sequences were performed, one with high vascular signal and the other with low vascular signal. The stationary soft tissues were the same on each scan, so when they were subtracted, only the vessels were apparent. The high-vascular-signal scan used short TEs coupled to cardiac gating in diastole. The slow blood flow in diastole allowed minimal phase change of spins, which gave high vascular signal. The low-vascular-signal images had the short TEs but were gated in systole, where the short TE by itself could not overcome the signal loss associated with high-velocity blood flow. In this way, they were able to manipulate TE and V in Equation 1.

### Effect of Echo Time on Fat Signal Intensity

It would seem that the shortest possible TE should always be used for MRA. This is not the case in routine clinical imaging for two reasons. A major reason is the interplay between TE and motion compensation gradients (discussed later). The other reason is related to chemical shift. The hydrogen nuclei of fat and water have different environments that cause different precessional frequencies (in fact, a 220-Hz difference at 1.5 Tesla [T]). In spin-echo imaging, the chemical shift effects and field inhomogeneities are mollified by the spin-echo 180-degree refocusing pulse. However, in gradient-echo imaging used in MRA, the spin echo is not present, so fat and water cycle in and out of phase related to the TE and field strength. This cycling from in to out of phase is 3.4 msec/T (every 2.26 msec at 1.5 T and every 3.4 msec at 1.0 T) (Table 1-1). In MRA the quality of images is improved with extraneous fat signal suppression, which is achieved by selecting an appropriately short TE. The shortest opposed phase echo should be used for MRA. For 1.5 T, a 6.5- to 7-msec TE is good, since it is very close to the precise opposed phase TE of 6.78 msec. Transferring this exact MRA sequence to a 1.0-T machine may give inferior image quality because the 7-msec TE would be close to the maximum in-phase echo of 6.8 msec. In this case, prolonging the TE to approximately 10 msec on a 1.0-T machine may improve image quality, since fat is then suppressed. In this example, the worsened phase dispersion present with the longer TE must be compared to the improved suppression of fat with improved postprocessed image quality (Fig. 1-3).

### Gradients

Some term definitions are also necessary before discussion of gradient-motion compensation schemes. The rate of change of a moving particle (blood) is its velocity (i.e., distance ÷ time), or first-order motion. The rate at which a spin's velocity changes is its acceleration, or second-order motion. Similarly, the rate at which a spin's acceleration changes is third-order motion, or jerk. Rates of motion

**TABLE 1-1 Timings for In-phase and Opposed Imaging at 1.0 and 1.5 T**

| T | TE(msec) | | | | | |
|---|---|---|---|---|---|---|
| 1.0 | 0 | 3.4 | **6.8** | 10.2 | 13.6 | 16.9 |
| 1.5 | 0 | 2.26 | 4.52 | **6.78** | 9 | 11.3 |
| | In phase | Out | In | Out | In | Out |

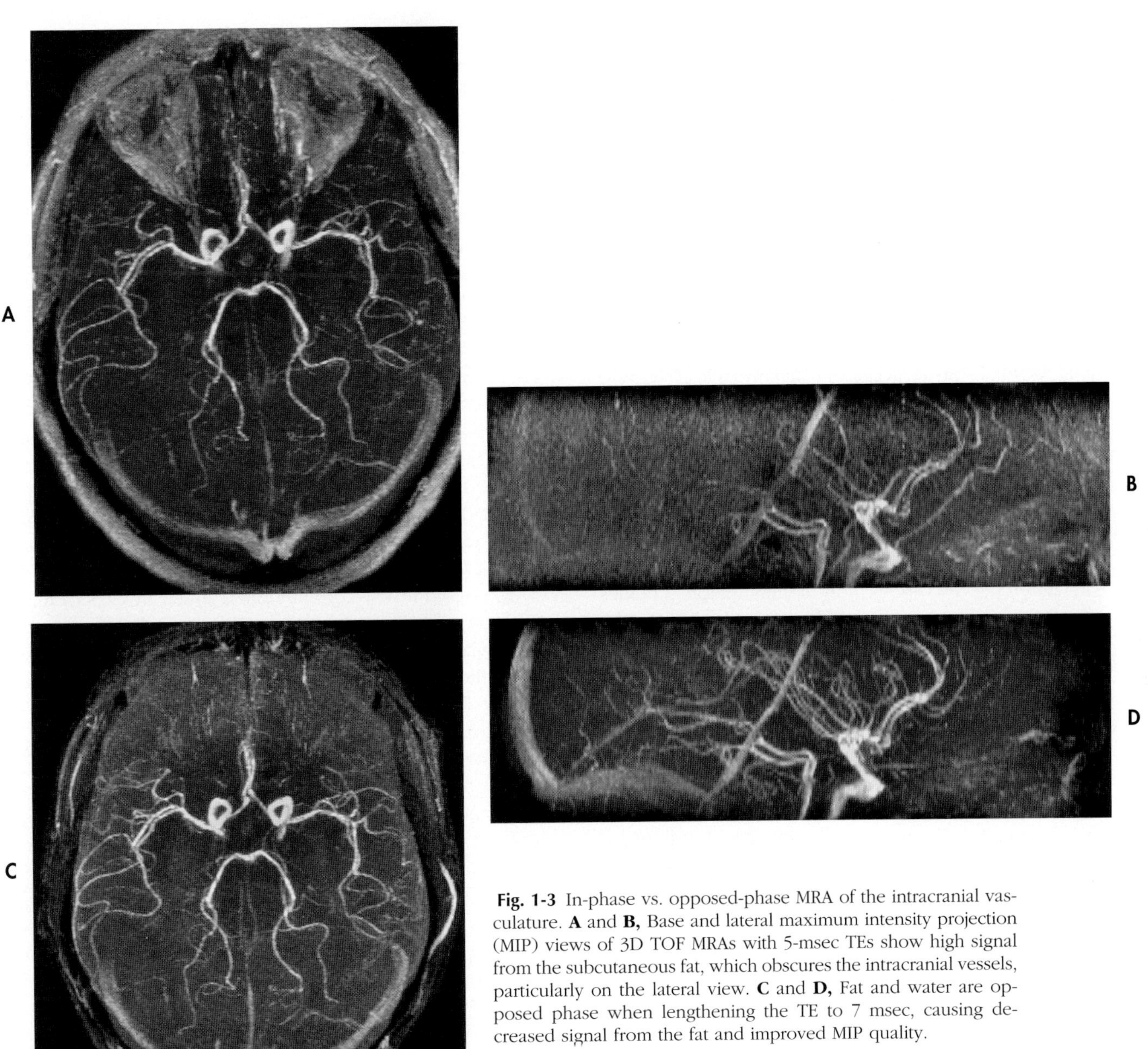


**Fig. 1-3** In-phase vs. opposed-phase MRA of the intracranial vasculature. **A** and **B,** Base and lateral maximum intensity projection (MIP) views of 3D TOF MRAs with 5-msec TEs show high signal from the subcutaneous fat, which obscures the intracranial vessels, particularly on the lateral view. **C** and **D,** Fat and water are opposed phase when lengthening the TE to 7 msec, causing decreased signal from the fat and improved MIP quality.

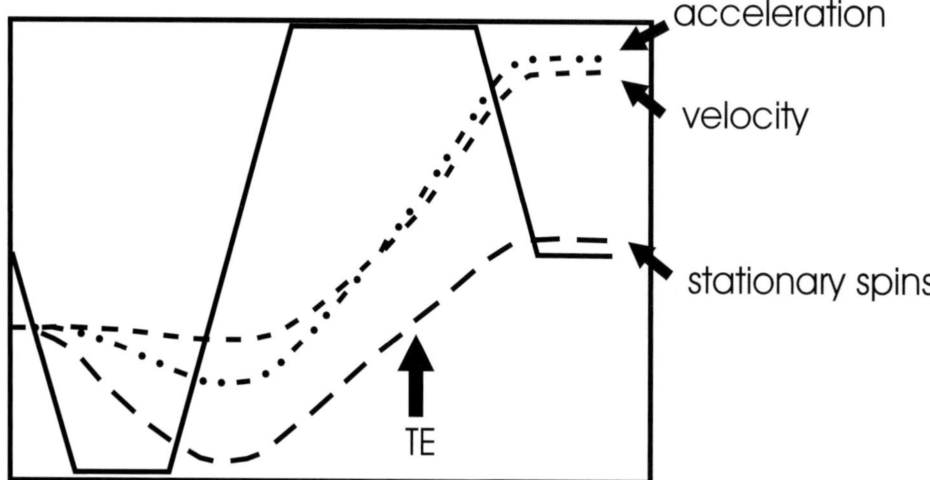


**Fig. 1-4** Zero-order compensation. Gradient waveform is shown in a solid line. Phase changes for stationary and moving spins are as follows: *Long, dashed line,* stationary spins; *short, dashed line,* constant velocity spins; *dashed and dotted line,* constant accelerated spins. Only stationary spins have zero phase change at the TE *(arrow).*

change beyond this order are generally referred to as *higher-order motion,* without specific names. Moran[12] first proposed the use of special gradients to modify the phase changes produced by blood moving along one of the three encoding gradients.[12-17] These compensations gradients (also called *gradient moment nulling, gradient motion refocusing,* and *flow compensation*) are most commonly used along the read and slice-select gradients.

The difference in various flow compensation schemes along the read direction for gradient-echo imaging is depicted in Figs. 1-4 through 1-6. The vertical axis displays the gradient magnitude *(solid line)* and the phase change of various spins *(dashed lines),* and the horizontal axis represents time. Fig. 1-4 depicts a simple bipolar gradient scheme, which will give zero phase change at the time of the echo for *only* stationary spins. Spins moving with a constant velocity or acceleration continue to have a net phase change at the TE, meaning signal loss. Fig. 1-5 shows a three-gradient scheme, which compensates for constant velocity spins. Stationary spins and spins moving with constant velocity have zero net phase change (all spins aligned with one another) at the time of the echo, meaning maximum vascular signal intensity. However, accelerated spins (e.g., those encountered in a tight carotid stenosis) continue to have a phase change at the echo. This phase change gives signal loss. In the negative sense, this has also been called *lack of spin rephasing.* This lack of spin rephasing may be related to at least the following factors:

1. The velocity compensation scheme has failed to sufficiently refocus the spins with higher-order motion such as acceleration, jerk (the derivative of acceleration), and turbulence.
2. The voxel size is finite.
3. The effects of flow are not compensated in the other two orthogonal planes.

The effect of voxel size is examined in more detail later.

With severe vessel stenosis, an acceleration of blood is required to maintain overall blood flow.[16] This acceleration along the localizing gradients leads to subsequent spin dephasing and signal loss. Further, turbulent flow distal to stenotic lesions results in randomly oriented spin motion along all three imaging planes, which cannot be rephased with gradient correction schemes in only one or two planes. For clinical MRA, turbulence can be thought of as disturbed or disordered flow where random changes in velocity and direction (in addition to the usual flow dynamics) occur. These changes are random or chaotic because the time in which they occur is shorter than the image acquisition time and the distances are shorter than the image resolution. To compensate for velocity and acceleration spin changes, a four-lobe gradient scheme may be implemented (Figure 1-6). With this sequence, spins moving with constant velocity and acceleration, as well as stationary spins, have zero net phase change at the time of the echo, meaning maximum signal intensity (at least theoretically). However, there is a significant drawback of increasing the complexity of the compensation schemes: the much longer TE necessary to provide time for the implementation of the gradient structure. With increasing TE comes increased spin dephasing and signal loss.

One might think that maximal vascular signal could be easily achieved by velocity- and acceleration-compensation gradients in all three orthogonal directions, as well as by a very short TE. However, there is a definite trade-off between TE and the use of compensation gradients. Ever more complex gradient refocusing places demands on the system hardware because gradients must be turned on and off many times within milliseconds of each other. Because these additional gradients must be applied between the rf pulse and the readout period, increasing the gradient compensation scheme also means increasing the TE. Therefore a balance must be struck between the rephasing gained by

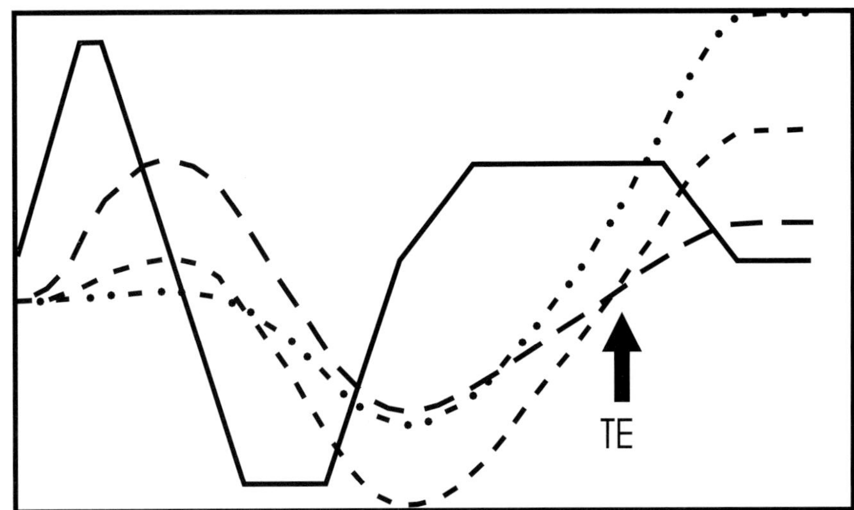


**Fig. 1-5** First-order compensation. At the TE *(arrow)* the stationary and constant-velocity spins have zero phase change while the accelerated spins are not refocused. *Long, dashed line,* stationary spins; *short, dashed line,* constant velocity spins; *dashed and dotted line,* constant accelerated spins.

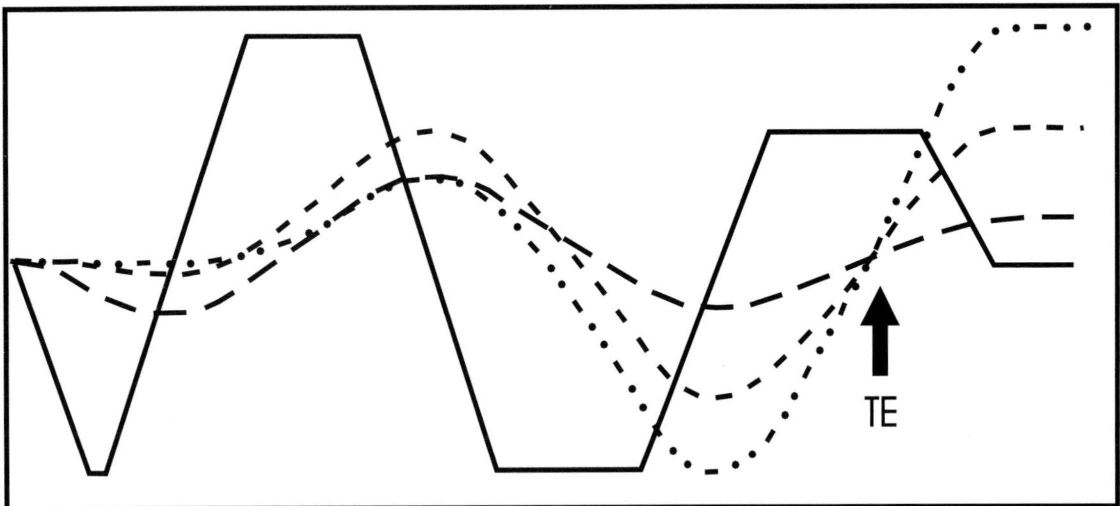


**Fig. 1-6** Second-order compensation. At the TE, stationary, constant-velocity, and accelerated spins have been refocused and have zero phase change. The overall length of the gradients must be increased to accommodate the complex gradient waveform, which necessarily increases the TE. (In these sequences, the TE is not in the center of the last gradient lobe by design.) *Long, dashed line,* stationary spins; *short, dashed line,* constant velocity spins; *dashed and dotted line,* constant accelerated spins.

the compensation gradients (increased vascular signal) and the dephasing occurring because of the increased TE (decreased vascular signal). For example, one comparison study of a three-gradient-lobe, velocity-compensated TE, 22-msec sequence with a four-gradient-lobe, velocity- and acceleration-compensated sequence (TE 34 msec) showed no discernible difference in images of the carotid bifurcations in healthy adults.[18] Although the TEs for this study are long compared with those in current sequences, the principle remains the same: The longer TE of the velocity- and acceleration-compensated sequence negates the advantage of the compensation gradients. This effect of TE should also be true for 2D and phase-contrast applications. Both of these 3D techniques had considerable drawbacks, including susceptibility to patient motion, overlap of the carotid image with the jugular vein, and inability to image carotid stenoses reliably. In 3D TOF angiography, the effect of TE becomes predominate, and it is more important to maintain a short TE with less complex motion refocusing. In general, velocity compensation in the frequency and slice-

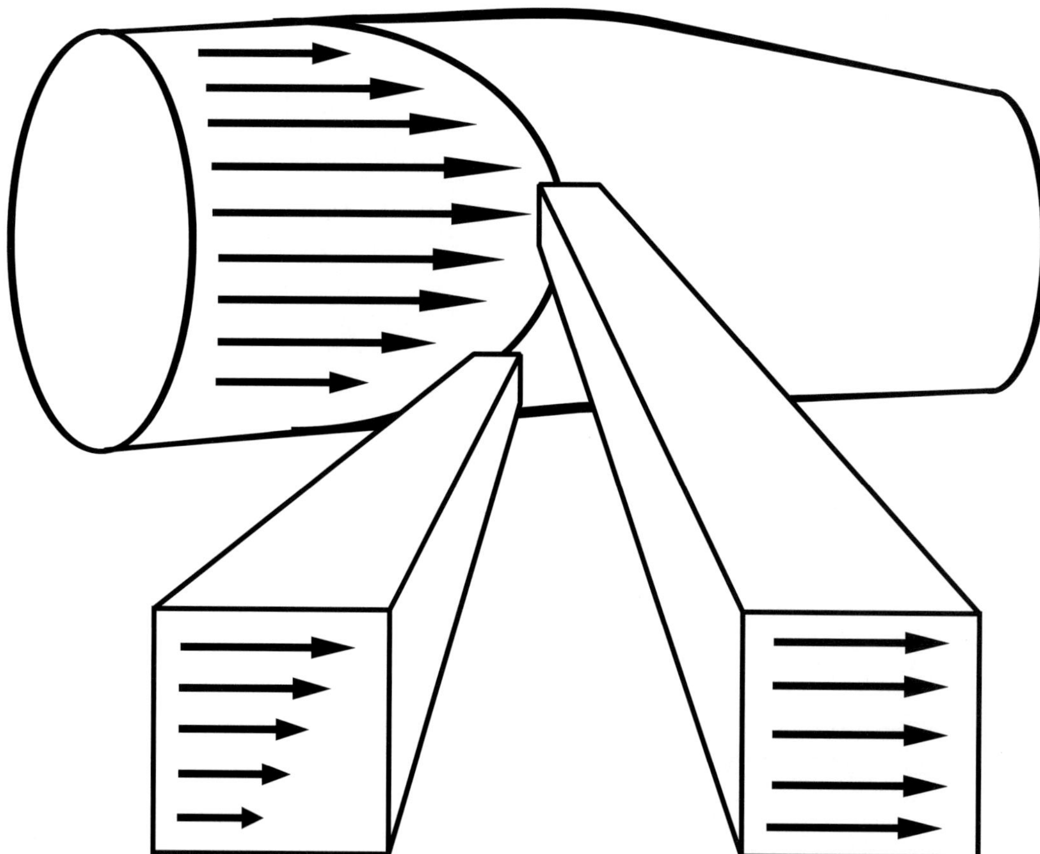

**Fig. 1-7** Velocity change across the voxel. Idealized laminar blood flow, with a parabolic flow profile across the vessel lumen (the highest velocity in the center) and decreasing velocities toward the vessel wall. An imaging slice that would encompass the whole vessel would be caused by a tremendous variety of velocities (i.e., a variety of phases), which decreases vascular signal. With decreasing slice thickness (voxel size) shown in the insets, there is a minimization of the velocity differences, which improves vascular signal.

select directions are sufficient for clinical imaging. The phase encode direction is not routinely compensated for motion. Because of the three spatially encoded directions, the least gradient amplitude is used in the phase-encode direction. Because of the small amplitude of the gradients, little phase dispersion occurs along this direction. Also, the duration of this gradient is very short, and it can be placed immediately before the readout period to minimize spatial misregistration. Again, the trade-off of making the gradients longer to accomplish motion correction defeats the purpose when the gradients do not contribute substantially to dephasing.

## Velocity Change Across the Imaging Voxel

Idealized blood flow in a vessel may be considered as laminar, with a parabolic flow profile across the vessel lumen and the highest velocity in the center. Any imaging voxel that spans the vessel will encounter a variety of velocities (i.e., a variety of phases). This variety tends to cancel vascular signal if not compensated. This is termed *intravoxel dephasing*. The spectrum of velocities occurring across an imaging voxel may be minimized by making the voxel smaller (Fig. 1-7). Minimizing the velocity change causes less phase cancellation and improved vascular signal. This concept—making the imaging slice thin to improve signal—is somewhat opposite to conventional digital imaging such as computed tomography (CT) or MR imaging of the brain parenchyma, in which thicker slices improve the signal-to-noise ratio. With vascular MR imaging, thinner slices are more effective in gaining signal from moving spins because of this decreased phase dispersion and may outweigh the decreased signal-to-noise ratio.[19] One way to decrease this voxel phase change is by using 3D volume imaging instead of the more conventional multislice imaging used for parenchymal imaging.

A practical application of the importance of this balance of TE, motion-compensation gradients, and hardware limitations can be found when smaller fields of view (FOVs) are used for intracranial MRA. Depending on the system hardware, reducing the FOV for intracranial MRA from 20 cm to 14 cm to improve resolution (while keeping the velocity compensation) may place such demands on the gradients that the TE must be increased. A typical TE for a 20-cm FOV might be 6.5 msec, but this may increase to 8 msec when the smaller 14-cm FOV is used. Again, the gradient "gas" is limited by the system hardware, and this gas can go toward a smaller FOV or a very short TE but not both. Even this seemingly small change of 1.5 msec can

**TABLE 1-2 Advantages and Disadvantages of Sequence Parameters**

| Technique | Advantages | Disadvantages |
|---|---|---|
| Perpendicular slice orientation | Maximal flow-related enhancement | Minimal length of vessel visualized |
| Long TR | Maximization of flow-related enhancement | Longer scan time<br>Increased background signal |
| High flip angle | Better S/N<br>Better suppression of background | Increased flow saturation |
| Short TE | Minimization of phase dispersion | Limitation because of hardware<br>Increase with use of compensation gradients<br>problem with in-phase bright fat |
| Compensation gradients | Minimization of phase dispersion | Increased TE<br>Possible limitation of minimal FOV |
| Small voxel size | Minimization of phase dispersion<br>Increased resolution<br>Decrease of partial volume effects | Reduced S/N<br>Increased scan time (phase encode direction)<br>Possible reduction of FOV |

have a profound effect on the quality of the MRA. Increasing the FOV to 18 cm in this instance may allow maintenance of the TE at 6.5 msec but achieve some measure of the increased resolution from the smaller FOV (smaller voxel size). These types of limitations will disappear as hardware becomes more available with increased gradient strengths (Table 1-2).

## PHASE-CONTRAST MRA

The relationships of Equation 1-1 also apply to phase-contrast imaging, the alternative method of MRA that is widely used.[20-31] Again, Equation 1-1 states that the phase shift of a spin moving through a gradient is proportional to its velocity. If a flow-sensitized gradient structure (bipolar) is used, stationary spins will have zero phase change, and moving spins will have some phase shift (Fig. 1-8). If a second sequence is then performed with reversed bipolar gradients, stationary spins will have zero phase change, and spins moving with a constant velocity will have some *different* phase shift. Complex subtraction of these two sequences eliminates signal from the stationary spins, leaving signal from moving spins. Velocity sensitization can be performed along any of the three orthogonal axes of imaging. For velocity encoding along a single axis, two image sets are acquired in an interleaved fashion, with the bipolar gradients reversed for the second sequence. Interleaving the sequence minimizes the effects of patient motion, which might degrade the image quality. In reconstruction, the two data sets are used to construct a phase-difference image that is multiplied by the average magnitude image to produce a weighted phase image in which brightness reflects velocity. Different methods of producing phase-contrast images are available. For 3D imaging, "balanced" techniques have opposed gradient pairs for each orthogonal direction, and "unbalanced" methods use three orthogonal gradients and an acquisition with no specific flow encoding (flow compensated).[32,33] From these three images in the unbalanced technique, each image is calculated for constructing the weighted phase image (Fig. 1-9).

Phase-contrast MRA differs in several important respects from TOF MRA. Because the image contrast depends on phase shifts instead of flow-related enhancement on T1-weighted images (as in TOF MRA), near-complete suppression of background signal intensity can be achieved without resorting to complex suppression schemes. (See Chapter 9 for discussion of background suppression schemes for TOF MRA.) Also, short T1 substances such as fat and methemoglobin are not high in signal intensity on phase-contrast, maximum-intensity-projection MRA images, since the phase-contrast technique sees these materials only as *stationary*, not with a short T1.

Phase contrast can be adjusted so that it is more sensitive to slow flow than 3D TOF imaging. Even 2D TOF imaging is limited in imaging slow flow resulting from saturation effects. With phase-contrast angiography, the ability to image slow flow relates only to the strength of the sensitizing gradient and the overall signal-to-noise ratio of the image. The ability to vary the flow-sensitizing gradient strength is used in phase-contrast imaging to selectively image different flow rates via the velocity-encoding setting, the number representing the maximum velocity encompassed by that particular sequence. In clinical practice, there is generally a "venous" setting around 10 to 20 cm/s and an "arterial" type image with a velocity encoding anywhere from 30 to 150 cm/s, depending on the pathologic condition being evaluated.

Artifacts specific to phase-contrast angiography can occur. Aliasing occurs when the maximum velocity in the vessel is greater than the velocity-encoding setting. In this case, the velocities higher than the velocity encoding are represented in the weighted phase image (combination of phase and magnitude) as decreased signal intensity. This most often occurs in the center of the vessel, where velocity is greatest. With a high-velocity encoding setting, which is most sensitive to the fast flow in the center of the vessel, slow flow along the vessel wall may not be visualized because of its small phase shift. In this case, the vessel lumen size is underestimated. Aliasing in a phase image is manifested as flow in apparently the opposite direction.

Phase-contrast techniques are more sensitive to intravoxel phase cancellations than TOF techniques because of

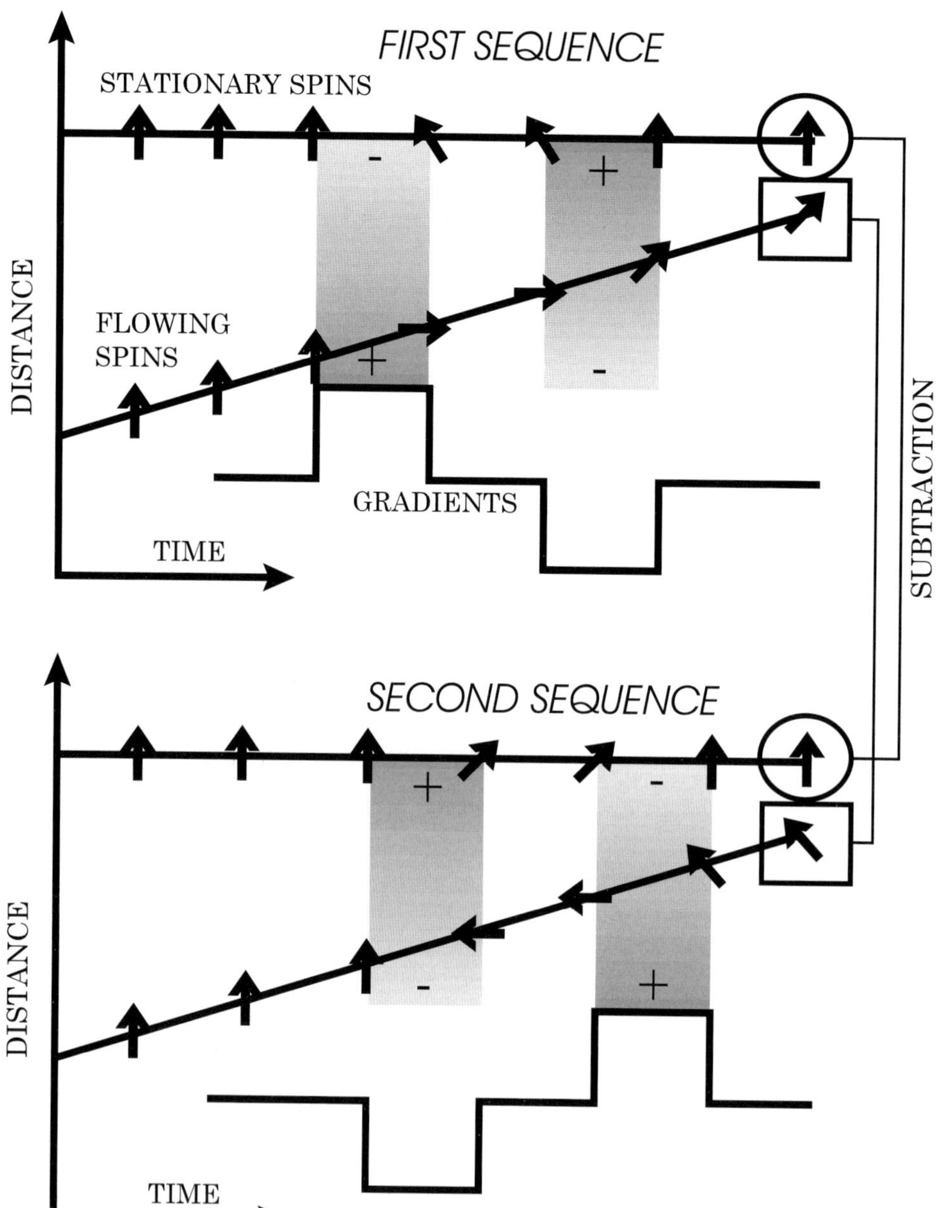


**Fig. 1-8** Phase change of spins with bipolar gradient. Stationary spins have no net phase change after application of the two gradients. Spins that are flowing, however, have a nonzero phase change. A second sequence in which the flow-encoding gradients are reversed produces similar results, with stationary spins having no phase change and moving spins showing a nonzero but different phase change. Subtraction of these two data sets eliminates signal from stationary structures but leaves signal from moving spins. The subtraction might be thought of in this way: For stationary spins with no net phase change, the subtraction would be $5 - 5 = 0$, and for moving spins, the subtraction would be $5 - (-5) = 10$.

the velocity-sensitizing gradients used and the inability to fully flow compensate the sequences. Because the magnetization at each point acquires a phase proportional to its velocity, the spatial averaging of complex flow with many different phases will lead to signal loss (see Case 118). A thick-slab 2D technique is especially prone to this destructive interference of phase shifts because of the large voxel size. Other areas where this phase dispersion is a problem is with tight stenoses with complex or turbulent flow and regions where there are different magnetic susceptibilities (such as the petrous carotid or cavernous carotid resulting from the nearby sinuses). Therefore although thick-slice 2D phase contrast is useful as an evaluation tool for carotid imaging, it is not recommended for detailed examination of carotid bifurcation stenosis. One method to minimize this problem would be to use thinner slices via a 3D or multislice 2D technique. As in TOF imaging, reducing the TE minimizes the dephasing artifacts on phase-contrast MRA

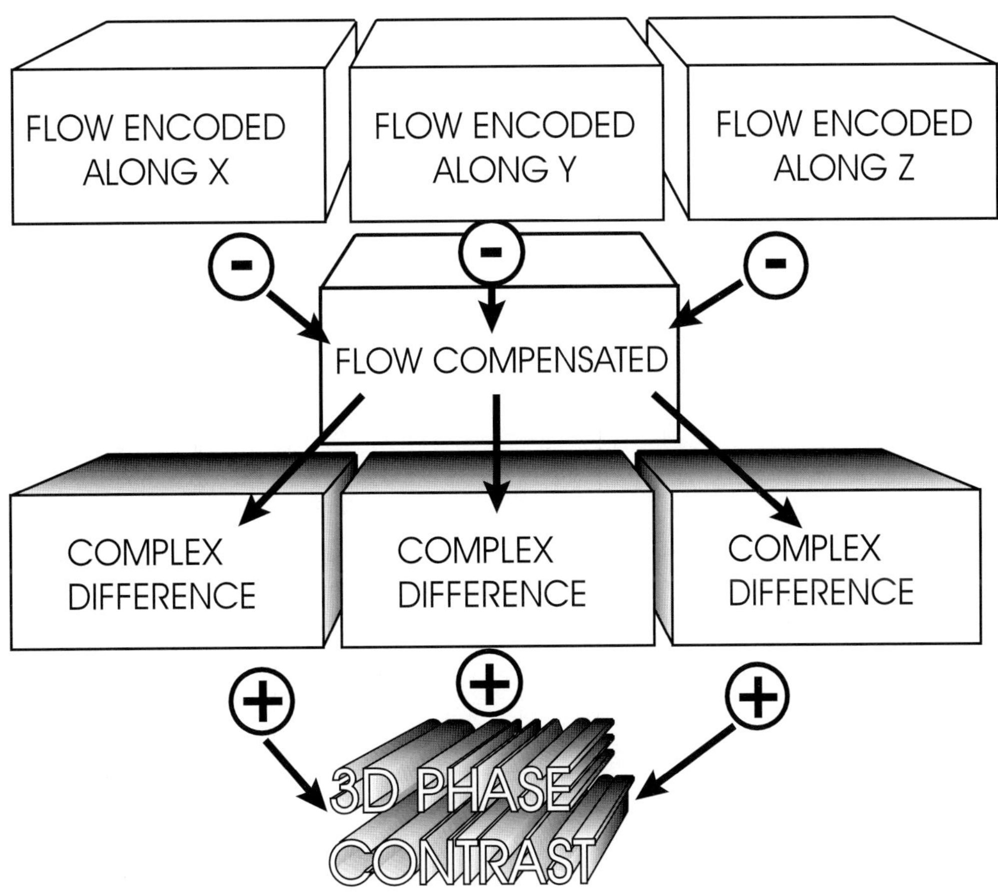


**Fig. 1-9** Schematic of image production for phase-contrast MRA.

without incurring the concomitant increased signal from the background tissue that can occur in TOF imaging. Finally, 3D phase-contrast imaging requires a longer acquisition time than 3D TOF MRA (for equivalent resolutions) because of the necessity to acquire velocity-sensitized sequences in each of the three orthogonal directions.

## REFERENCES

1. Axel A, Shimakawa A, MacFall J: A time-of-flight method of measuring low velocity by magnetic resonance imaging, *Magn Reson Imaging* 4:199-205, 1986.
2. Bradley WG, Waluch V: Blood flow: magnetic resonance imaging, *Radiology* 154:443-450, 1985.
3. Kaufman L, Crooks LE, Sheldon PE et al: Evaluation of NMR Imaging for detection and quantification of obstructions in vessels, *Invest Radiol* 77:554-560, 1982
4. Mills CM, Brant-Zawadzki M, Crooks LE et al: Nuclear magnetic resonance: principles of blood flow imaging, *AJR* 142:165-170, 1984.
5. Bryant DJ, Payne JA, Firmin DN, Longmore DB: Measurements for flow with NMR imaging using a gradient pulse and phase difference technique, *JCAT* 8:588-593, 1984.
6. Young IR, Bydder GM, Payne JA: Flow measurements by the development of phase differences during slice formation in MR imaging, *Magn Reson Med* 3:175-179, 1986.
7. Nishimura DG, Macovski A, Pauly JM: Magnetic resonance angiography, *IEEE Trans Biomed Eng* M15:140-151, 1986.
8. Grant JP, Back C: NMR rheotomography: feasibility and clinical potential, *Med Phys* 9:188-193, 1982.
9. Wedeen VJ, Meuli RA, Edelman RR et al: Projective imaging of pulsatile flow with magnetic resonance imaging, *Science* 230:946-948, 1985.
10. Meuli RA, Weeden VJ, Geller SC et al: MR gated subtraction angiography: evaluation of lower extremities, *Radiology* 159:411-418, 1986.
11. Weeden VJ, Rosen BR, Buxton R, Brady TJ: Projective MRI angiography and quantitative flow-volume densitometry, *Magn Reson Med* 3:226-241, 1986.
12. Moran PR: A flow zeugmatographic interface for NMR imaging in humans, *Magn Reson Imaging* 1:197-203, 1982.
13. Haacke EM, Lenz GM: Improving MR image quality in the presence of motion by using rephasing gradients, *AJR* 148:1251-1258, 1987.
14. Masaryk TJ, Ross JS, Modic MT et al: Magnetic resonance imaging of the carotid bifurcation: work in progress, *Radiology* 166:461-466, 1988.
15. Lenz GW, Haacke EM, Masaryk TJ, Laub G: Pulse sequence design and strategy for in-plane vascular imaging, *Radiology* 166:875-882, 1988.
16. Blackshear WM, Phillips DJ, Chikos PM et al: Carotid artery velocity patterns in normal and stenotic vessels, *Stroke* 11:67-71, 1980.
17. Alfidi RJ, Masaryk TJ, Haacke EM et al: Magnetic resonance angiography of peripheral, carotid and coronary arteries, *AJR* 149:1097-1109, 1987.
18. Masaryk TJ, Ross JS, Modic MT et al: Carotid bifurcation: MR imaging, *Radiology* 166:461-466, 1988.
19. Haacke EM, Lenz GW: *Short echo time, fast gradient-echo imaging.* Presented at 73rd Scientific Assembly and Annual Meeting of RSNA, Chicago, Nov 29 to Dec 4, 1987.

20. Pernicone JR, Siebert JE, Potchen EJ et| al: Three-dimensional phase-contrast MR angiography in the head and neck: preliminary report, *AJNR* 11(3):457-466, 1990.
21. Dumoulin CL, Souza SP, Walker MF, Yoshitome E: Time-resolved magnetic resonance angiography, *Magn Reson Med* 6(3):275-286, 1988.
22. Turski P, Korosec F: Technical features and emerging clinical applications of phase-contrast magnetic resonance angiography, *Neuroimag Clin North Am* 2(4):785-800, 1992.
23. Pernicone JR, Siebert JE, Laird TA et al: Determination of blood flow direction using velocity-phase image display with 3-D phase-contrast MR angiography, *Am J Neuroradiol* 13(5):1435-1438, 1992.
24. Applegate GR, Talagala SL, Applegate LJ: MR angiography of the head and neck: value of two-dimensional phase contrast projection technique, *Am J Roentgen* 159(2):369-374, 1992.
25. Huston J III, Rufenacht DA, Ehman RL, Wiebers DO: Intracranial aneurysms and vascular malformations: comparison of time-of-flight and phase-contrast MR angiography, *Radiology* 181(3):721-730, 1991.
26. McElveen JT Jr, Saunders JE, Meisler WJ et al: Magnetic resonance angiography: technique and skull-base applications, *Am J Otol* 12(5):323-328, 1991.
27. Dumoulin CL, Yucel EK, Vock P et al: Two- and three-dimensional phase contrast MR angiography of the abdomen, *JCAT* 14(5):779-784, 1990.
28. Wagle WA, Dumoulin CL, Souza SP, Cline HE: 3DFT MR angiography of carotid and basilar arteries, *Am J Neuroradiol* 10(5):911-919, 1989.
29. Petereit D, Mehta M, Turski P et al: Treatment of arteriovenous malformations with stereotactic radiosurgery employing both magnetic resonance angiography and standard angiography as a database, *Int J Radiat Oncol Biol Phys* 25(2):309-313, 1993.
30. Ross MR, Pelc NJ, Enzmann DR: Qualitative phase contrast MRA in the normal and abnormal circle of Willis, *Am J Neuroradiol* 14(1):19-25, 1993.
31. Dumoulin CL, Souza SP, Walker MF, Wagle W: Three-dimensional phase contrast angiography, *Magn Reson Med* 9(1):139-149, 1989.
32. Conturo TE, Robinson BH: Analysis of encoding efficiency in MR imaging of velocity magnitude and direction, *Magn Reson Med* 25:233-247, 1992.
33. Pelc NJ, Bernstein MA, Shimakawa A, Glover GH: Encoding strategies for three-dimensional phase-contrast MR imaging of flow, *JMRI* 1:405-413, 1991.

# CHAPTER 2

# Techniques

## CASE 1
## GENERAL THREE-DIMENSIONAL TIME-OF-FLIGHT INTRACRANIAL TECHNIQUE

The basics of three-dimensional time-of-flight intracranial MRA screening technique include an axial volume centered about the circle of Willis and a saturation pulse placed superiorly to eliminate the signal from venous sinus flow. Slice thickness should be around 1 mm or less, with at least 60 slices to provide adequate coverage. Velocity compensation in the frequency- and slice-encoded directions is routine. Evaluation of the posterior circulation requires a more inferior placement of the volume to include the distal vertebral arteries and the origins of the posterior inferior cerebellar arteries.

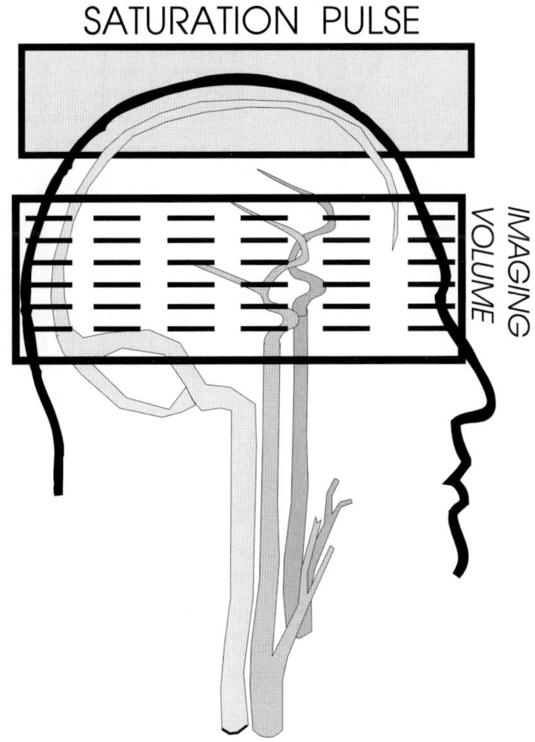


**Setup for three-dimensional intracranial axial volume, anterior circulation.**

**REFERENCES**

Masaryk TJ, Modic MT, Ross JS et al: Intracranial circulation: preliminary clinical results with three-dimensional (volume) MR angiography, *Radiology* 171:793-799, 1989.

Pernicone JR, Thorp KE, Ouimette MV et al: Magnetic resonance angiography in intracranial vascular disease, *Semin Ultrasound CT MR* 13(4):256-273, 1992.

Lewin JS, Laub G: Intracranial MR angiography: a direct comparison of three time of flight techniques, *AJR* 158(2):381-387, 1992.

## CASE 2
## VARIATION OF THE THREE-DIMENSIONAL TIME-OF-FLIGHT TECHNIQUE: MULTIPLE OVERLAPPING SLABS

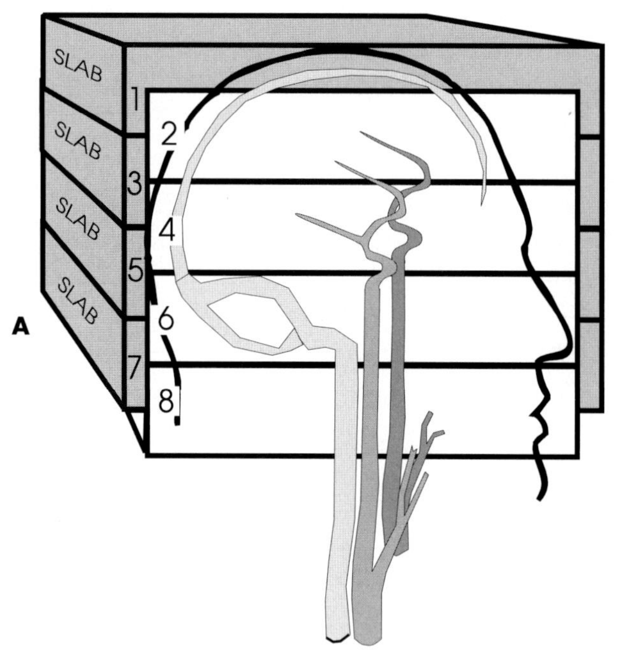


**Diagram of multiple overlapping three-dimensional slabs (drawn with a 50% overlap).**

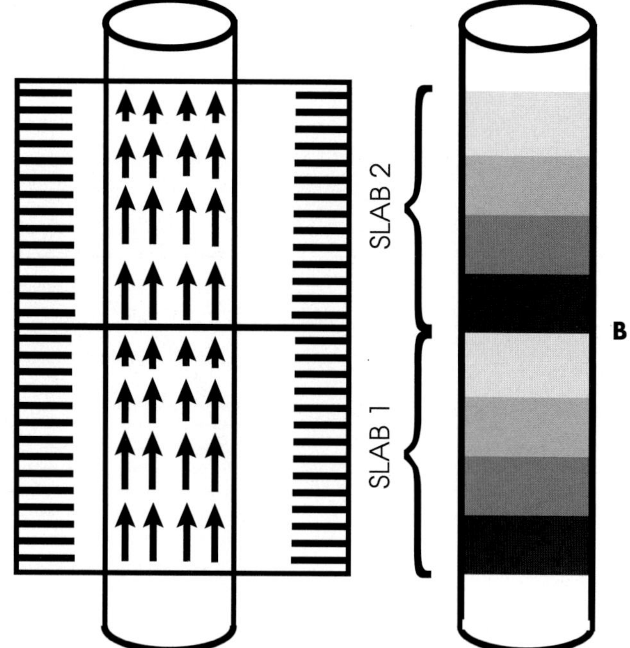


**Diagram of saturation effects with multiple three-dimensional slabs. Flow entering a volume gives more signal than the flow in the distal aspects because of flow saturation. Stacking of multiple volume without correction for this saturation effect gives the venetian blind artifact.**

One limitation of three-dimensional time-of-flight MRA is the presence of flow saturation, which decreases vascular signal within the distal aspects of the imaging volume. This saturation is due to spins experiencing multiple radiofrequency pulses during the imaging acquisition, which does not allow recovery of longitudinal magnetization. One method of limiting this flow-saturation effect for three-dimensional time-of-flight imaging is to use multiple thin slabs that are overlapped, as described by Parker et al, termed *multiple overlapping thin-slab acquisition*. In this technique, the advantages of three-dimensional time-of-flight (i.e., short echo time, motion compensation, good signal-to-noise ratio) are combined with advantages of a two-dimensional type of acquisition (thinner slice with good flow-related enhancement and decreased saturation). Disadvantages of this technique include more complicated postprocessing to combine the various volumes, the presence of venetian blind artifact **(B),** increased imaging time, and the potential for misregistration from patient motion between acquisitions. The venetian blind artifact occurs because there is still some saturation effects within the distal parts of the volumes, even if they are thinner than the standard single-volume time-of-flight techniques. Because of this, the signal within a vessel at the junction of two volumes will not be equal and will have decreased signal at the superior aspect of the lower volume and increased signal at the inferior aspect of the superior volume. The presence of this artifact ties into the other disadvantage of the technique, which is increased imaging time. To limit the venetian blind artifact, several outer slices of the slabs may be excluded from the maximum intensity projection reconstruction, which increases the vessel signal homogeneity. However, discarding these slices necessarily increases the imaging time to cover the same distance. These limitations are in general minor, and this sequence should be considered as a major technique for evaluation of the intracranial and extracranial vasculature. The venetian blind artifact can be almost completely eliminated with appropriate reconstruction of selected aspects of the overlapping volumes **(C** and **D).**

C

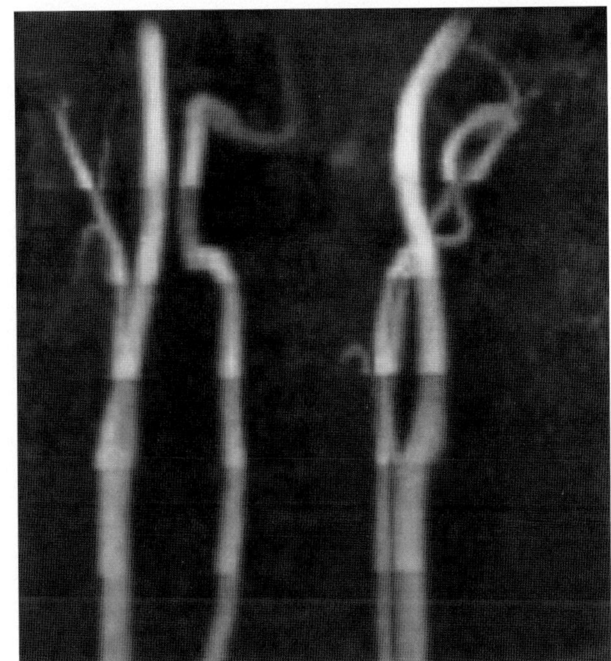

**Venetian blind artifact. Anteroposterior maximum intensity projection view of multiple overlapping slabs (C) shows the venetian blind artifact resulting from the saturation effects within the small three-dimensional volumes as horizontal variations in signal intensity over the imaging area.**

D

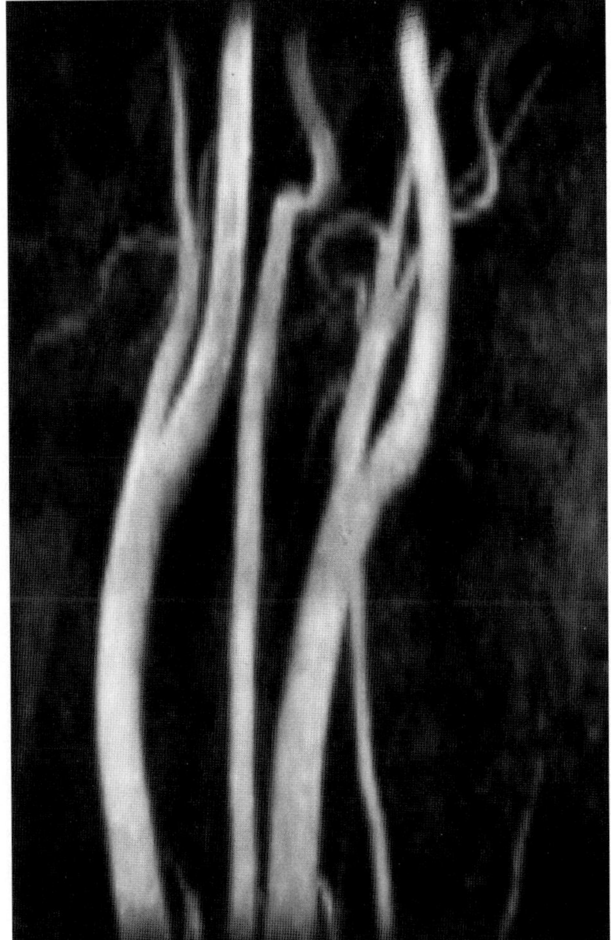

**Overlapping slabs with improved reconstruction. Anteroposterior maximum intensity projection view of three overlapping slabs shows no evidence of the venetian blind artifact. *Technique:* Axial volumes, three overlapping three-dimensional volumes, each 34/10/20, 256 × 128 (½ rectangular field of view), 32 partitions, 42-mm slab, 14.5-cm field of view, total time 9:28.**

Davis et al evaluated three-dimensional time-of-flight single-volume angiography and multiple overlapping thin-slice angiography in 10 volunteers, evaluating each examination for the number of intracranial vessels visualized. Each patient underwent three types of three-dimensional time-of-flight studies (two single volume and one multiple overlapping thin-slab acquisition). (1) Repetition time 45 msec, echo time 4.9 msec, flip angle 15 degrees, field of view 20 cm, 256 × 256 matrix, 12-minute acquisition time. (2) Repetition time 45 msec, echo time 6.8 msec, flip angle 15 degrees, field of view 20 cm, 256 × 256 matrix, 12-minute acquisition time. (3) Multiple overlapping thin-slab acquisition repetition time 45 msec, echo time 6.7 msec, 25-degree flip angle, field of view 20 cm, 256 × 128 matrix, 12-minute acquisition time for 42-ml overall slab thickness. They found improved visualization of vessels with the multiple overlapping thin-slab acquisition technique over the three-dimensional time-of-flight studies (86% of selected vessels on the multiple overlapping thin-slab acquisition vs. 67% with the time-of-flight study). They thought the improvements related primarily to decrease sensitivity to flow saturation with the multiple overlapping thin-slice acquisition.

**REFERENCES**


Davis WL, Warnock SH, Harnsberger HR et al: Intracranial MRA: single volume vs. multiple thin slab three-dimensional time-of-flight acquisition, *JCAT* 17:15-21, 1993.

Blatter DD, Parker DL, Ahn SS et al: Cerebral MR angiography with multiple overlapping thin slab acquisition. II. Early clinical experience, *Radiology* 183:379-389, 1992.

Parker DL, Yuan C, Blatter DD: MR angiography by multiple thin slab 3D acquisition, *Mag Reson Med* 17:434-451, 1991.

Lewin JS, Laub G: *Optimization and evaluation of the multiple-thin volume 3DFT time-of-flight MR angiographic technique.* Paper presented at the Ninth Annual Scientific Meeting of the Society of Magnetic Resonance in Medicine, New York, August 18-24, 1990.

## CASE 3
## VARIATION OF THE THREE-DIMENSIONAL TIME-OF-FLIGHT TECHNIQUE: VARYING THE FLIP ANGLE ACROSS THE VOLUME (TILTED, OPTIMIZED NONSATURATING EXCITATION OR RAMP PULSES)

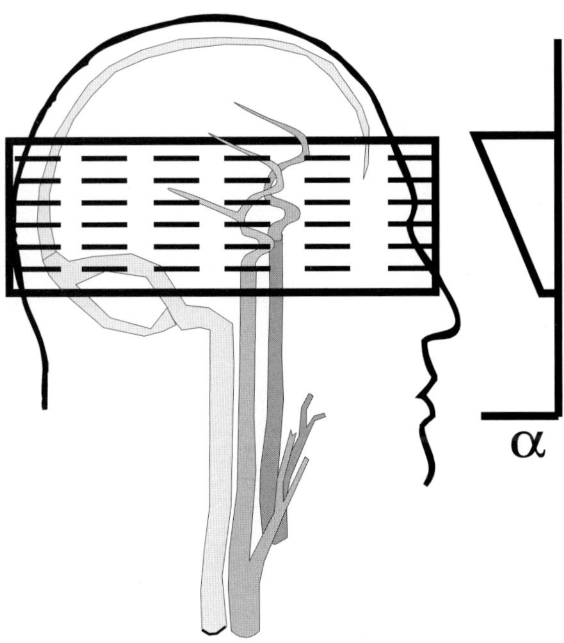


**Schematic of varied flip angle across the volume, with the smaller flip angle at the inferior aspect to minimize saturation effects. (A superior saturation pulse should also be used.)**

The overall saturation of spins as they move into an imaging volume can be decreased by decreasing the flip angle. However, this would also decrease the signal-to-noise ratio of the acquisition. One method to decrease the amount of saturation in time-of-flight MRA is to vary the flip angle across the volume by using a smaller flip angle at the beginning of the volume, which increases as the blood flows through the volume. Thus the blood flowing into the entrance of the imaging volume is receiving less of a radiofrequency pulse, which decreases flow saturation. This technique, called *tilted, optimized nonsaturating excitation* or *ramp pulse* allows use of relatively thick three-dimensional slabs while maintaining good flow-related enhancement and evens out the overall vascular signal across the volume. The optimum flip angle for the central aspect of the volume is around 20 degrees. The ratio of the entrance to exit flip angles can be varied to optimally change the signal distribution across the volume (i.e., 1:2 or 1:3).

#### REFERENCE

Laub G, Purdy DE: *Variable tip angle slab selection for improved three dimensional MR angiography.* In Society of Magnetic Resonance in Medicine: *Book of abstracts 1992,* Berkeley, Calif, 1992, Society of Magnetic Resonance in Medicine.

## CASE 4
## VARIATION OF THE THREE-DIMENSIONAL TIME-OF-FLIGHT TECHNIQUE: MAGNETIZATION TRANSFER BACKGROUND SUPPRESSION

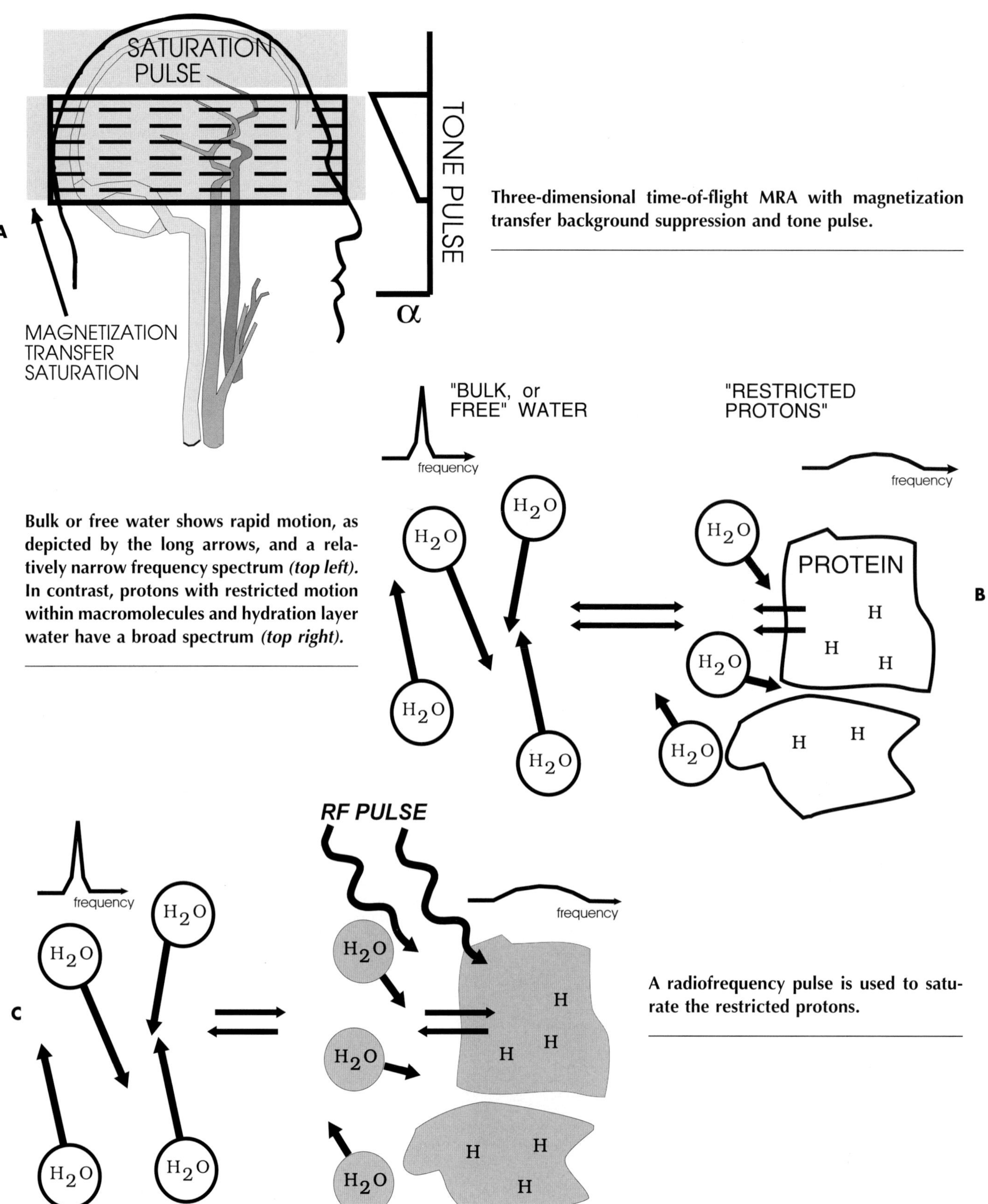


**Three-dimensional time-of-flight MRA with magnetization transfer background suppression and tone pulse.**

**Bulk or free water shows rapid motion, as depicted by the long arrows, and a relatively narrow frequency spectrum *(top left).* In contrast, protons with restricted motion within macromolecules and hydration layer water have a broad spectrum *(top right).***

**A radiofrequency pulse is used to saturate the restricted protons.**

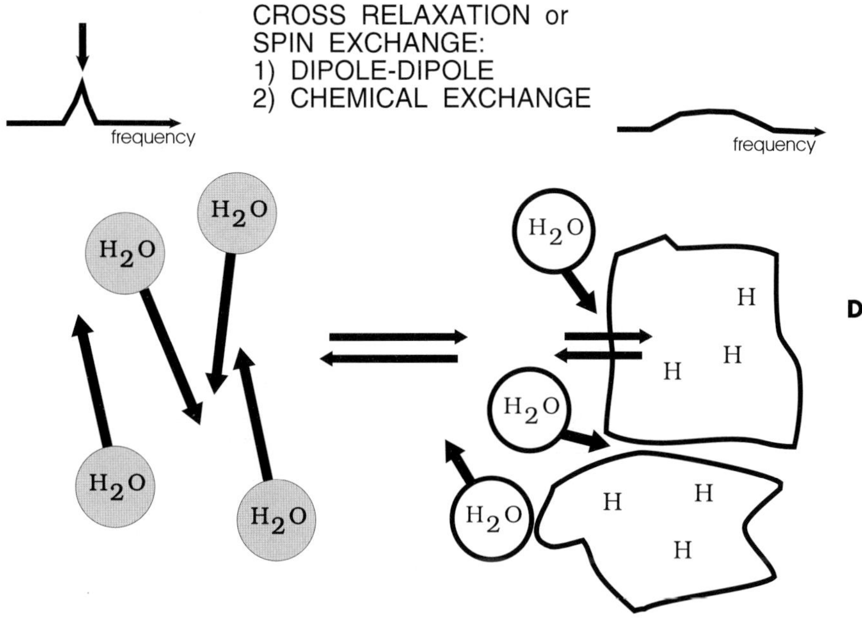


**The saturation is then exchanged with the more mobile free-water protons, which decreases signal intensity on the MR image. (Note the decreased size of the spectral peak of $H_20$ at the top left.)**

Hydrogen in biologic tissues can be considered in two forms, those that are a part of *bulk water*, which can be considered "free," with relatively unrestricted motion, and those that are components of macromolecules and *hydration-layer water*, with relatively restricted motion **(B).** These restricted protons have a broad frequency spectrum *(top right)* compared with the narrow spectrum of free water *(top left)*. Radiofrequency energy (polynomial, Gaussian, or hard pulses) may be applied to saturate these restricted components **(C).** After this saturation pulse is applied, there is exchange of this saturation energy to the freely moving water protons by dipole-dipole interactions or chemical exchange of hydrogen. This transfer of energy then causes saturation of the free-water protons without saturating the signal from blood or cerebrospinal fluid **(D).** This magnetization transfer background suppression reduces the signal of white and gray matter by approximately 50%. When this type of pulse is added to the conventional time-of-flight MRA sequences, markedly improved background suppression is achieved while the high signal from moving blood, which gives better quality maximum intensity projection views with better small vessel conspicuousness, is maintained. Other techniques, such as the tilted, optimized nonsaturating excitation radiofrequency pulse, can be applied with magnetization transfer contrast, as shown in Case 5.

**REFERENCES**

Henkelman RM, Huang X, Qing-San X et al: Quantitative interpretation of magnetization transfer, *Magn Reson Med* 29:759-766, 1993.

Eng J, Ceckler TL, Balaban RS: Quantitative 1H magnetization transfer imaging in vivo, *Magn Reson Med* 17:304-314, 1991.

Pike GB, Hu BS, Glover GH, Enzmann DR: Magnetization transfer time-of-flight magnetic resonance angiography, *Magn Reson Med* 25:372-379, 1992.

Lin W, Tkach JA, Haacke EM, Masaryk TJ: Intracranial MR angiography: application of magnetization transfer contrast and fat saturation to short gradient echo, velocity compensated sequences, *Radiology* 186(3):753-761, 1993.

Edelman RR, Ahn SS, Chien D et al: Improved time of flight MR angiography of the brain with magnetization transfer contrast, *Radiology* 184(2):395-399, 1992.

## CASE 5
## COMPARISON OF VARIOUS BACKGROUND-SUPPRESSION TECHNIQUES FOR TIME-OF-FLIGHT MRA

Base projections of three similar three-dimensional time-of-flight sequences.

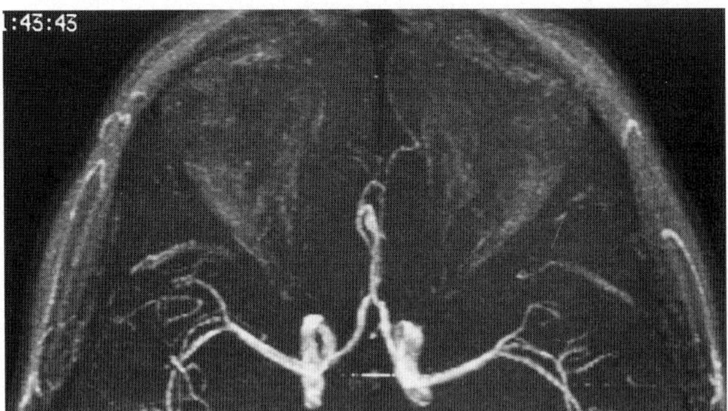


**Conventional three-dimensional time-of-flight sequence with echo time 7 and no special background suppression.**

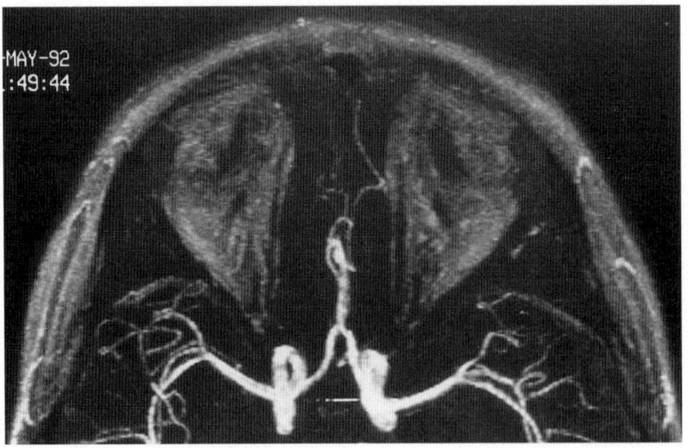


**Same sequence as above except that magnetization transfer background suppression shows decreased signal from the intracranial background but increased conspicuousness of the orbital and subcutaneous fat. The fat is not actually increased in signal by the magnetization transfer pulse but shows up as relatively high signal, since the brain parenchyma is markedly decreased in signal.**

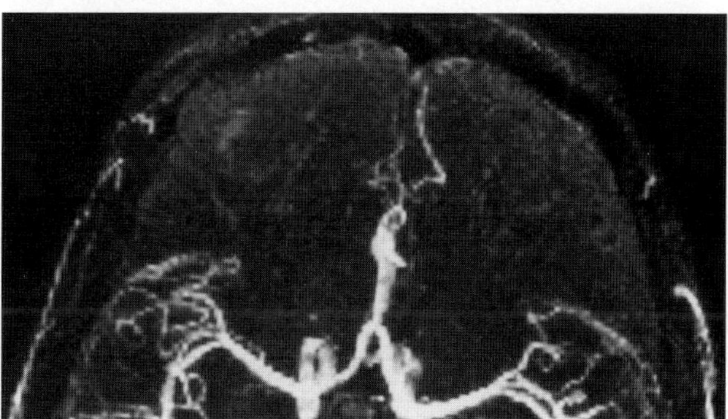

**Same sequence, but now magnetization transfer background suppression and frequency-selective fat suppression eliminate all areas of high signal except from flowing blood (other causes of T1 shortening such as methemoglobin would still be bright even on this three-dimensional time-of-flight sequence).**

## CASE 6
## VARIATION OF THREE-DIMENSIONAL TIME-OF-FLIGHT TECHNIQUE: HIGH RESOLUTION WITH MAGNETIZATION TRANSFER BACKGROUND SUPPRESSION AND TILTED, OPTIMIZED NONSATURATING EXCITATION RADIOFREQUENCY PULSE

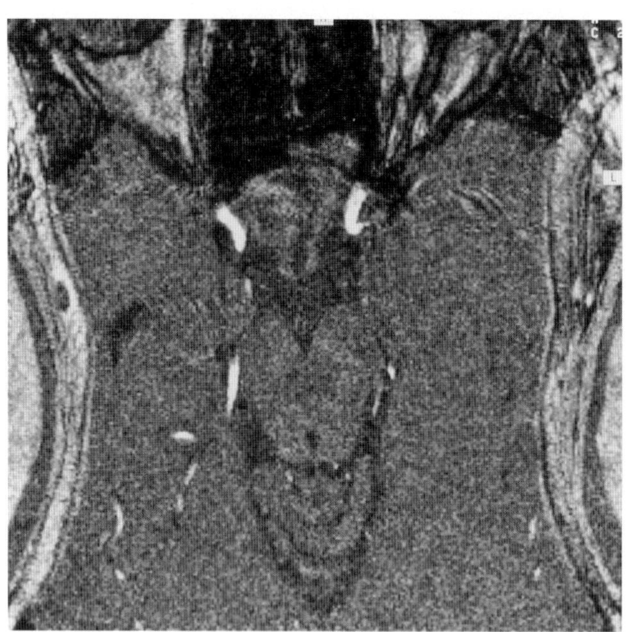

**Base view of high-resolution technique with magnetization transfer background suppression; tilted, optimized nonsaturating excitation pulse; and a 12-cm field of view. Note the small amount of aliasing present with overlap of the pinnae into the area of interest.**

---

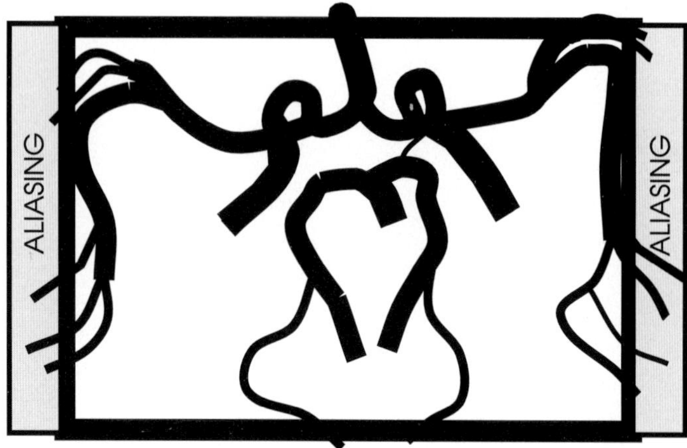


**Schematic of aliasing with a small field of view (12 cm). In general, if the circle of Willis is the area of interest, a 14-cm field of view will provide a good compromise between increased resolution and minimized aliasing. If the middle cerebral branches are of interest, the field of view must be increased to 18 to 20 cm.**

---

In this example, the field of view is reduced to decrease the in-plane voxel dimensions. However, this has positive and negative aspects that must be balanced. Although decreasing the voxel size increases resolution and decreases intravoxel dephasing, it may also be detrimental, since it can introduce the problem of aliasing, also called *wraparound* or *overfolding*. For intracranial imaging, scalp fat and the pinnae may fold over and obscure the distal branches of the middle cerebral arteries. The same problem is encountered if the field of view is held constant and the number of phase-encoding steps is reduced to produce a rectangular field of view. This problem of aliasing may occur along the phase- and frequency-encoding axes in two-dimensional Fourier transform imaging. Any spins that are excited by the radiofrequency pulses in the imaging sequence and that can be detected by the surface coil (as would be used for imaging the cervical carotids) is assigned a spatial location along the imaging gradients. When the body coil is used as a transmitter (surface coils), a considerable amount of tissue may be excited along the imaging plane but outside of the chosen field of view and beyond the physical limits of the receive-only surface coil. Tissues within the field of view are naturally assigned positions in the image based on their individual phases and frequencies. The excited tissue outside the field of view may also be detected by the coil and are assigned phases or frequencies identical to the tissues in the field of view, so these peripheral tissues also appear in the image. Ideally, a surface coil with a well-defined sensitive volume does not detect signal from the peripheral tissue. However, the coils are not constructed that precisely. One strategy to remedy this problem is simply to increase the field of view to a point where the aliasing is eliminated. Alternatively, a commonly used strategy is to oversample the data or acquire additional data at either end of the imaging gradient and then ignore this extra data at the time of image reconstruction. If aliasing still occurs, the redundant data are likely in those segments of data "trimmed off" before reconstruction and do not affect the final image. The acquisition of more data points along the frequency-encoding direction is effectively free because it does not demand additional acquisition time. Some manufacturers automatically incorporate oversampling in all pulse sequences. Although oversampling is also possible in the phase-encoding direction, the examination time increases proportionally. A corresponding reduction in the number of excitations compensates for the increase in examination time without affecting the signal-to-noise ratio. For example, increasing the phase-encoding steps from 128 to 256 and reducing the number of excitations from two to one eliminate the overfolding, maintain the same signal-to-noise ratio, and hold examination time constant. However, if there is physiologic motion in the region to be studied, the motion artifact in the image may be worse, since the signal averaging that occurs with multiple excitations is reduced or eliminated.

## REFERENCE

Ross JS, Ruggieri PM, Tkach JA et al: *High resolution MTS variable flip angle TOF MRA of the intracranial vasculature.* Paper presented at the 78th Annual Meeting of the RSNA, Chicago, Nov 1992.

## CASE 7
## TWO-DIMENSIONAL TIME-OF-FLIGHT TECHNIQUE OF THE CAROTIDS

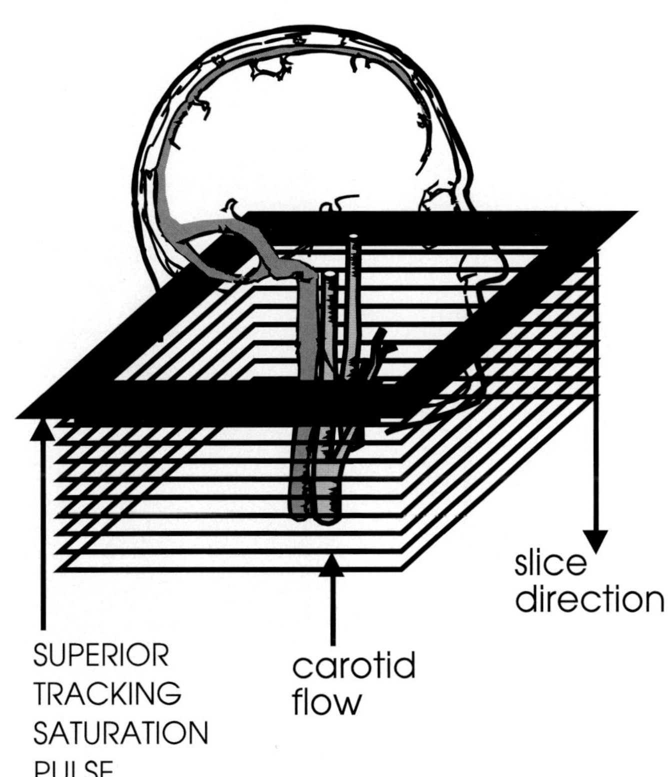


**Schematic of two-dimensional time-of-flight with superior tracking saturation pulse.**

The basic technique of two-dimensional time-of-flight MRA is the acquisition of sequential two-dimensional slices, which are generally obtained in a countercurrent fashion to the blood flow of interest to maximize flow-related enhancement. For arterial flow, this would be acquired from the superior to inferior regions. A saturation pulse is necessary to eliminate venous signal. The saturation pulse can be placed as a fixed pulse superior to the superiormost image slice position, or better, the saturation pulse can be designed to maintain a constant relationship with the moving imaging slice as they are acquired (i.e., a tracking or traveling saturation pulse). The tracking saturation pulse has the advantages of more complete venous suppression and the ability to produce a moderate degree of background suppression within the imaging slice if appropriately positioned. The major advantage of the two-dimensional time-of-flight technique is its sensitivity to flow-related enhancement, which allows visualization of slow and fast flows. The major disadvantage is a relatively thick slice (compared with three-dimensional imaging), which produces dephasing with tight vascular stenoses (greater than 70%).

### REFERENCES

Huston J, Lewis BD, Wiebers DO et al: Carotid artery: prospective blinded comparison of two dimensional time of flight MR angiography with conventional angiography and duplex US, *Radiology* 186(3):339-344, 1993.

Ross JS, Masaryk TJ, Ruggieri P: Magnetic resonance angiography of the carotid bifurcation, *Top Magn Reson Imaging* 3(3):12-22, 1991.

Keller PJ, Drayer BP, Fram EK et al: MR angiography with 2D acquisition and 3D display, *Radiology* 173:527-532, 1989.

## CASE 8
## VARIATIONS IN THREE-DIMENSIONAL TIME-OF-FLIGHT TECHNIQUE OF THE CAROTIDS

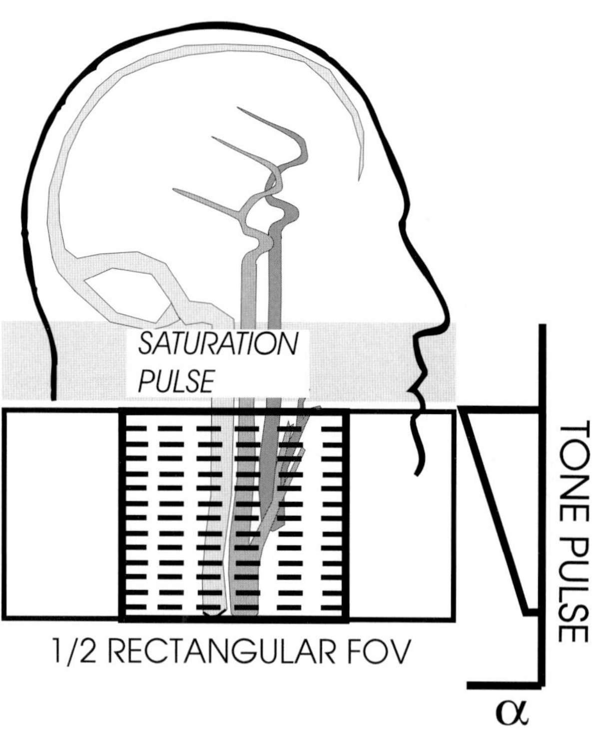


**Schematic of large axial three-dimensional slab with tone radiofrequency pulse and rectangular field of view.**

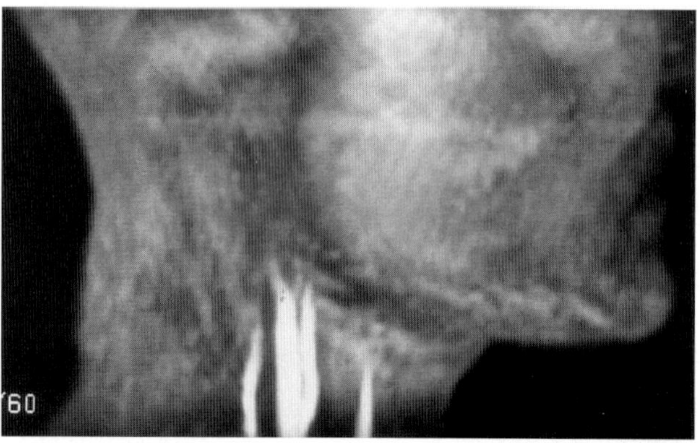

**How *not* to do time-of-flight MRA of the bifurcations. This single lateral maximum intensity projection view displays many aspects of poor technique including (1) large field of view producing poor resolution for the bifurcation; (2) too large of a cephalocaudal volume, which causes marked flow saturation and signal loss of the distal vessels (without the use of additional techniques to minimize saturation effects such as tilted, optimized nonsaturating excitation or multiple thin slabs); (3) short TE of 5 msec (in-phase at 1.5 Tesla), giving bright fat that obscures the vessels on the maximum intensity projection view; (4) no limited-volume maximum intensity projection views (i.e., targeted maximum intensity projection).**

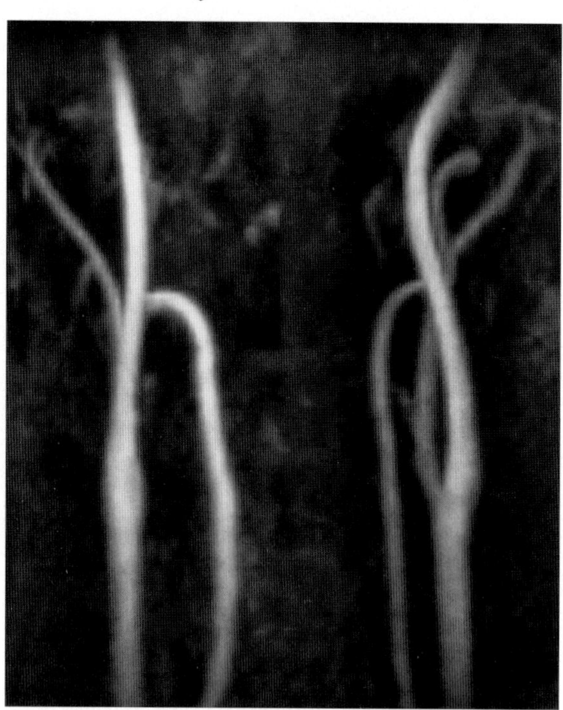

**A 14-cm axial volume length three-dimensional time-of-flight MRA of the carotids. *Technique:* axial volume; three-dimensional time-of-flight; 34/6.4/20 degrees; 128 × 256; 25-cm field of view; ½ rectangular field of view; 128 slices; 140-mm slab; tilted, optimized nonsaturating excitation radiofrequency pulse; 9.3 minutes. Anteroposterior maximum intensity projection view of the carotid bifurcation shows good signal intensity throughout the volume with a good length of coverage.**

**Sagittal slab:** The problem of length of coverage can be addressed by orienting the volume in the sagittal plane. Two 32-slice volumes may be centered about the carotid bifurcations to produce quality MRAs. The disadvantages of this technique are relatively limited flow-related enhancement and in-plane saturation effects. The flow-related enhancement can be maximized by increasing the repitition time to 50 to 80 msec.

A variation on the dual sagittal slab protocol was implemented by Li et al. They angled the slabs obliquely off the sagittal plane so that their inferior margins were more lateral and the superior margins were overlapping medially. With this angulation, the imaging volumes did not saturate the blood flow coming from the aortic arch, which was medial to the inferior margins of the slabs. The sagittal orientation allows for increased length of vessel visualization compared with that for standard single-volume axial sequences and takes less time compared with multislab axial techniques. The disadvantage of this technique and the regular sagittal slab technique compared with the axial orientation is the increased in-plane saturation effects.

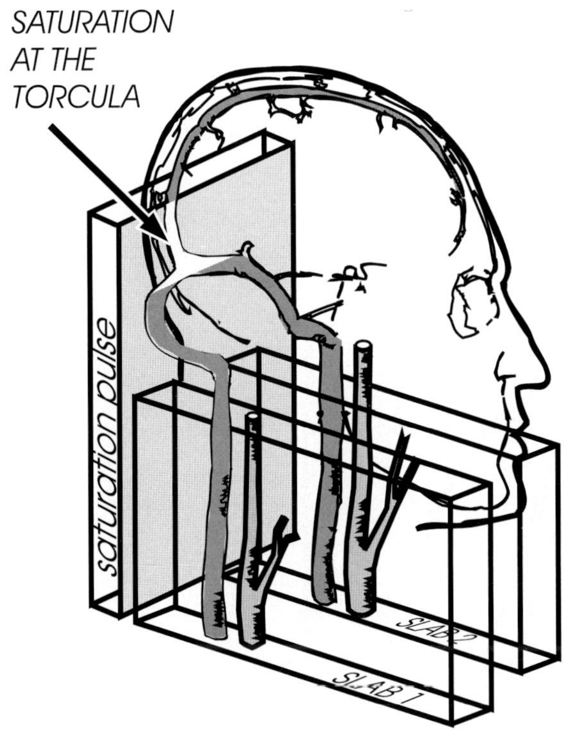


**Dual sagittal slab schematic.**

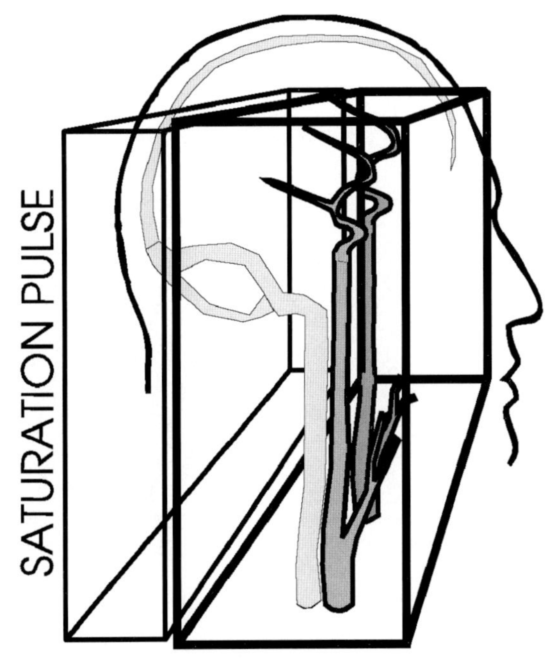


**Coronal slab schematic.**

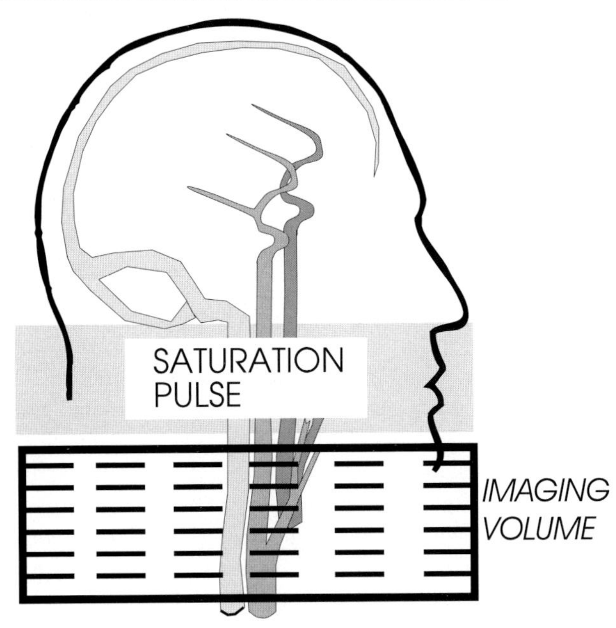


**Axial three-dimensional volume schematic.**

**Coronal slab:** Another method to increase the coverage possible with a three-dimensional time-of-flight technique is to orient the volume in the coronal plane and place a saturation pulse posteriorly to eliminate venous signal at the torcular. Advantages of this technique include a large area of coverage and visualization of the cervical carotids and vertebrals. The major disadvantages are a propensity for in-plane saturation and a larger voxel size because of the increased field of view.

**Axial volume:** Placement of the volume in an axial orientation maximizes flow-related enhancement. The disadvantage of this orientation is the limited length of carotid that can be covered in a reasonable examination time. One solution is to use a smaller number of phase-encoded steps (128) and a rectangular field of view to maintain resolution. The smaller number of phase-encoding steps allows for use of 128 slices, which can span a 140- to 150-mm length. Saturation effects within the distal volume on three-dimensional time-of-flight sequences can be minimized by a variable flip angle across the volume, such as tilted, optimized nonsaturating excitation. The axial orientation is also successfully used with multiple overlapping three-dimensional time-of-flight slabs.

**REFERENCES**

Anderson CM, Haacke EM: Approaches to diagnostic magnetic resonance carotid angiography, *Semin Ultrasound CT MR* 13(4): 246-255, 1992.

Li W, Kramer J, Kleefield J, Edelman RR: MR angiography of the extracranial carotid arteries using a two slab oblique 3-D acquisition, *AJNR* 13:1423-1428, 1992.

Kido DK et al: Clinical evaluation of stenoses of the carotid bifurcation with magnetic resonance angiographic techniques, *Arch Neurol* 48(5):484-489, 1991.

Anderson CM, Soloner D, Lee RE et al: Assessment of carotid artery stenosis by MR angiography: comparison with x-ray angiography and color coded doppler ultrasound, *AJNR* 13(3):989-1003, 1992.

Masaryk AM, Ross JS, DiCello MC et al: 3DFT MR angiography of the carotid bifurcation: potential and limitations as a screening exam, *Radiology* 179:797-804, 1991.

Huston J III, Lewis BD, Wilber DO et al: Carotid artery: prospective blinded comparison of two-dimensional time-of-flight MR angiography with conventional angiography and duplex ultrasound, *Radiology* 186(2):339-344, 1993.

## CASE 9
## TWO-DIMENSIONAL TIME-OF-FLIGHT TECHIQUE FOR VENOUS DISEASE

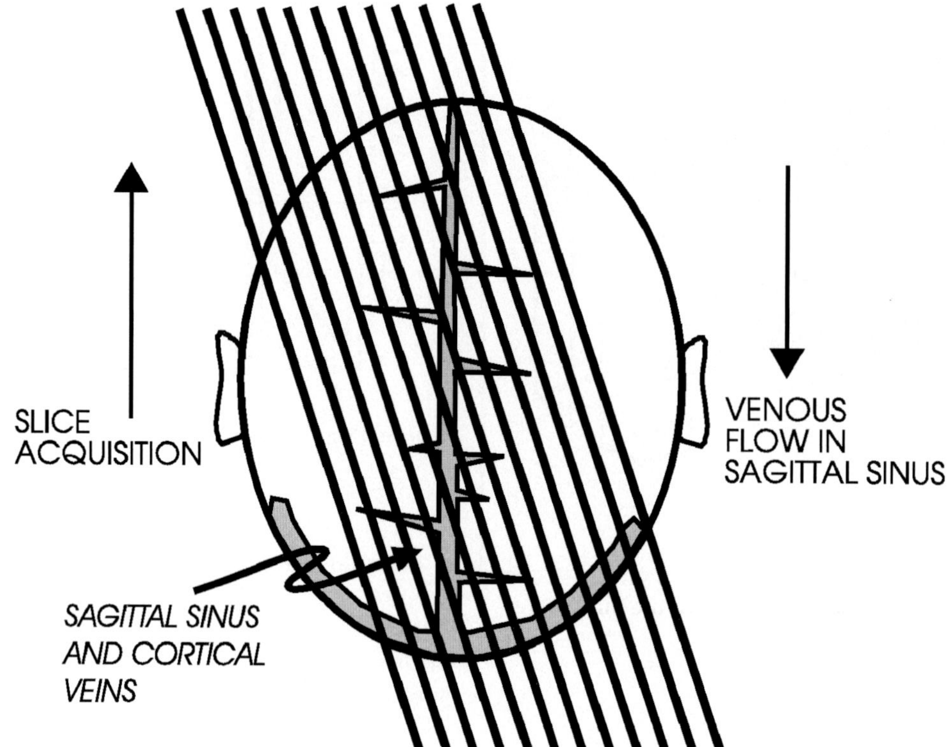


**Schematic of two-dimensional time-of-flight technique for venous sinuses.**

For time-of-flight imaging of the venous system, a two-dimensional technique is used to take maximum advantage of flow-related enhancement and to minimize saturation effects. No single orientation can maximally visualize all the venous sinuses because of the different directions of flow. A sagittal orientation is not recommended because of the increased amount of in-plane dephasing that would be present in the superior sagittal sinus. Coronal imaging provides excellent flow-related enhancement of the superior sagittal sinus and deep veins but can be time consuming to cover the whole head from back to front. However, this complete head coverage is not needed most of the time, since the anterior third of the superior sagittal sinus is variably present or small and of little clinical importance. Imaging of the posterior two thirds of the head encompasses nearly all clinically important venous sinuses. One method around this distance limitation is to obliquely angle the slices as shown in the diagram. Such a position gives good flow-related enhancement while maximizing the overall front-to-back coverage of the head. However, if insufficient slices are acquired, the lateral aspect of the transverse sinuses may not be included in the the images (Fig. 1 [right]).

#### REFERENCE

Lewin JS, Laub G: *Evaluation of the intracranial venous system with the thin-slice oblique acquisition sequentional technique.* Paper presented at the Eighth Annual Meeting of the Society for Magnetic Resonance Imaging, Washington, DC, Feb 18-24, 1990.

## CASE 10
## TWO-DIMENSIONAL PHASE-CONTRAST TECHNIQUE FOR VENOUS DISEASE

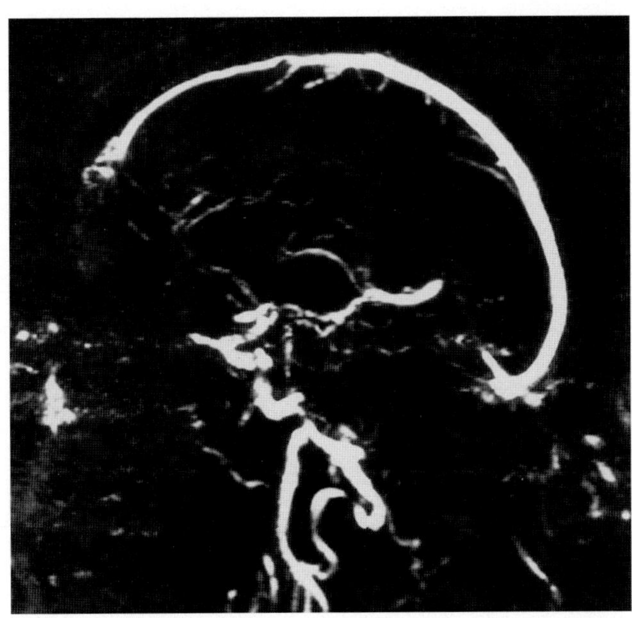

**Sagittal two-dimensional phase contrast of the midline venous sinuses. Technique: two-dimensional phase contrast, 33/8/20, 256 × 192, eight excitations, 60-mm thick section, 10 cm/s velocity encoding for venous disease, 20-cm field of view, 3:25.**

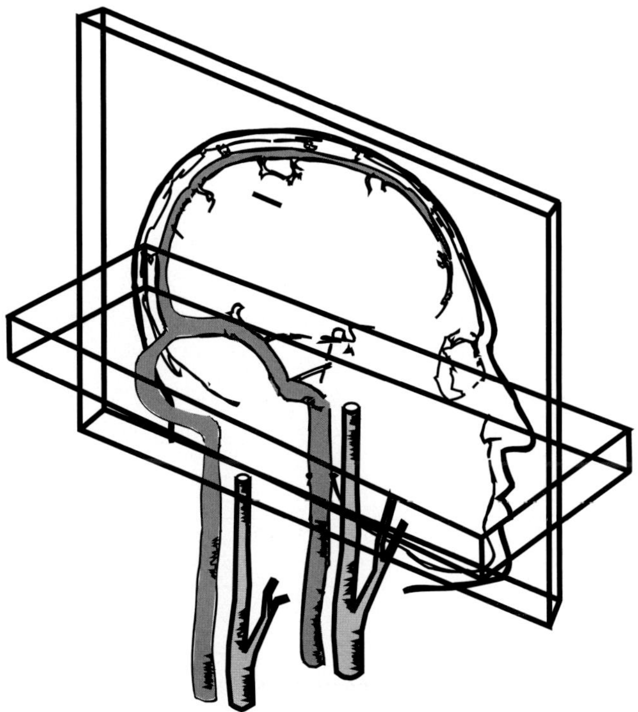

**Schematic of placement of two separate thick single slabs for evaluation of the major sinuses using the phase-contrast technique.**

A quick method for evaluating the venous system is to use single thick-slice two-dimensional phase contrast in the sagittal and axial planes. The sagittal slice is placed in the midline to evaluate the sagittal sinus, and the axial slice evaluates the torcula and transverse sinuses. Each slice takes about 3 to 4 minutes, thus providing a quick and effect method for venous evaluation.

### REFERENCES


Turski PA, Partington C, Kousec Mistretta C et al: *Variable velocity two-dimensional phase contrast MR angiography for the identification of intracranial from states.* Paper presented at the 9th Annual Meeting of the SMRM, New York, 1990.

Dumoulin CL: Phase contrast magnetic resonance angiography. *Neuroimag Clin North Am* 2(4):657-676, 1992.

Applegate GR, Talagala SL, Applegate LJ: MR angiography of the head and neck: value of two-dimensional phase contrast projection technique, *AJR* 159(369-374), 1992.

## CASE 11
## PITFALL: ALIASING ON PHASE-CONTRAST IMAGES

**Technique:** axial two-dimensional phase contrast, 88/8.6/20, 192 × 256, 30-mm single slice, velocity encoding of 30 and 60 cm/s, flow encode right to left, eight excitations, 20-cm field of view, 2:17.

Flow-encode velocity of 60 cm/s **(A)** shows good signal from the middle cerebral arteries with appropriate directional information (i.e., white is flow to the patient's left, and black is flow to the patient's right). With the slower velocity encoding **(B),** there is now low signal within the left middle cerebral artery *(arrow)* resulting from aliasing that could be confused as flow going from the patient's left to right.

If the flow velocity in the vessel exceeds the velocity-encoding setting and the phase shift produced by the flow is greater than 180 degrees, aliasing will occur with apparent flow in the opposite direction. For example, a phase shift of 225 degrees is indistinguishable from a phase shift of −135 degrees (in which the minus is flow in the opposite direction) **(C).**

A

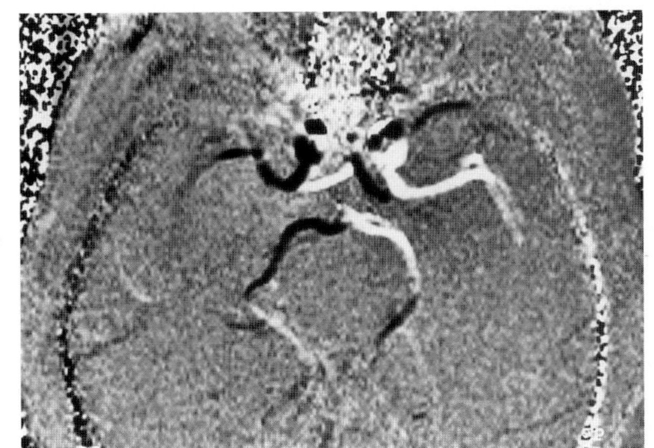

B

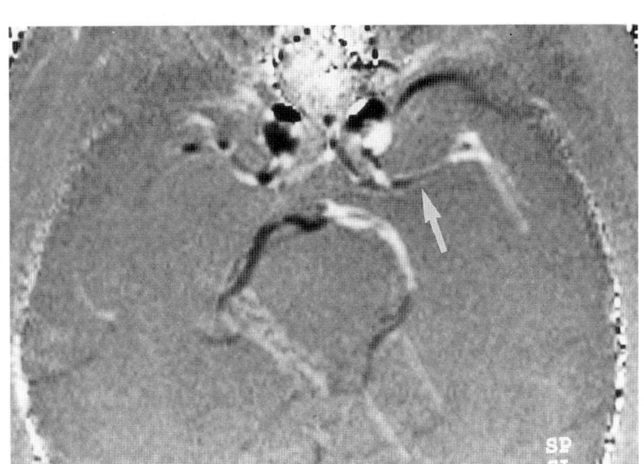

225 degrees

-135 degrees

C

**Schematic of aliasing in which phase shifts of 225 degrees and −135 degrees give the same result.**

## CASE 12
## THREE-DIMENSIONAL PHASE-CONTRAST TECHNIQUE FOR THE BRAIN

Anteroposterior, lateral heads with 10, 30, 60, and 100 cm/s velocity encoding show how the degree of venous and arterial visualization critically depend on the velocity encoding.

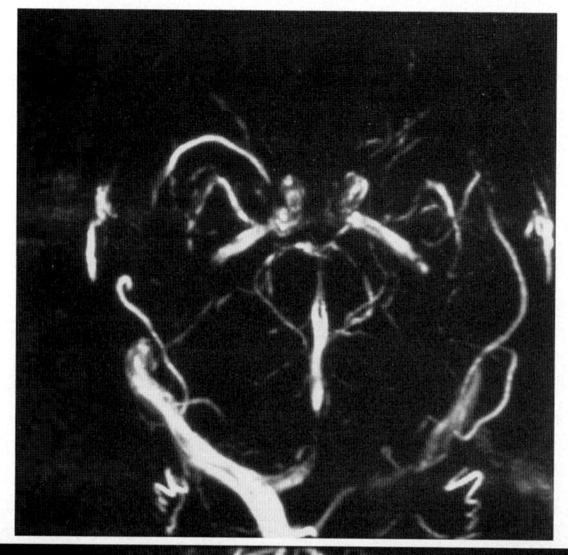
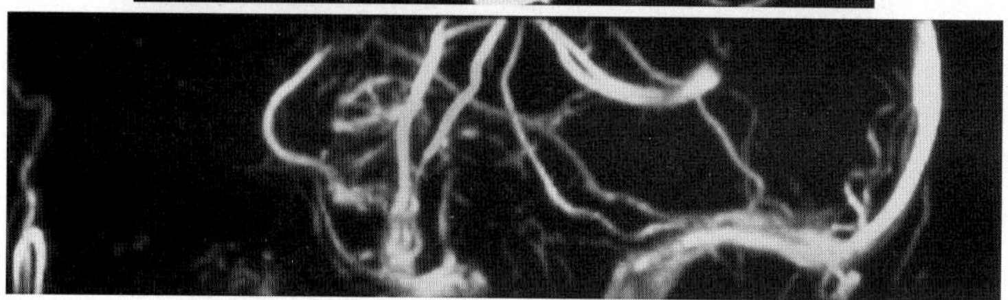

**30 cm/s encoding.**

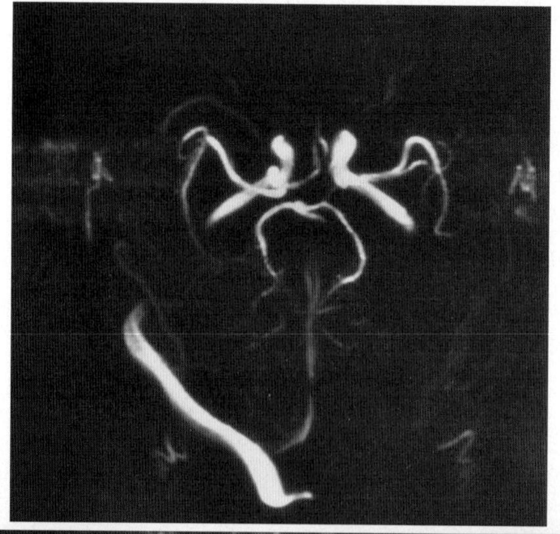
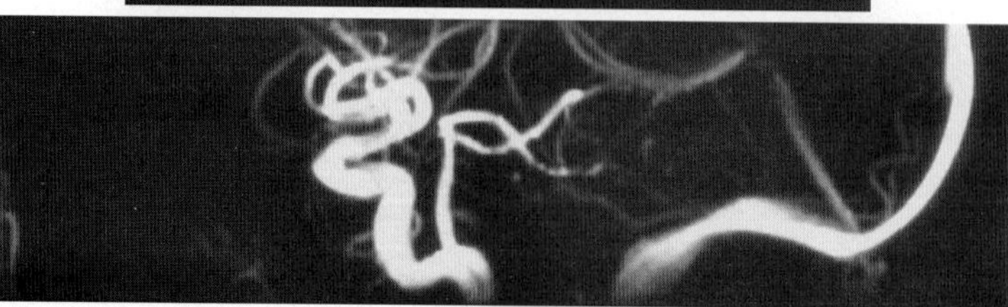

**10 cm/s encoding.**

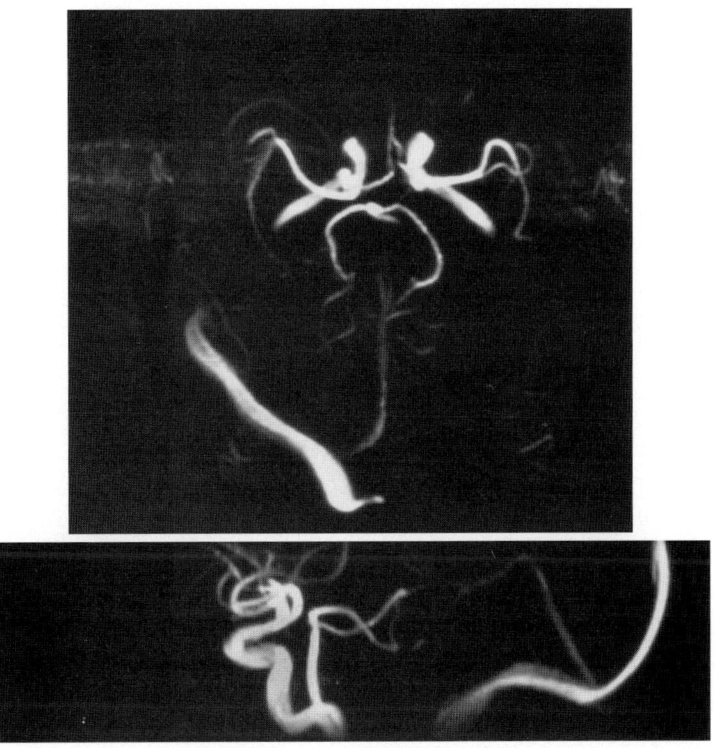

**60 cm/s encoding.**

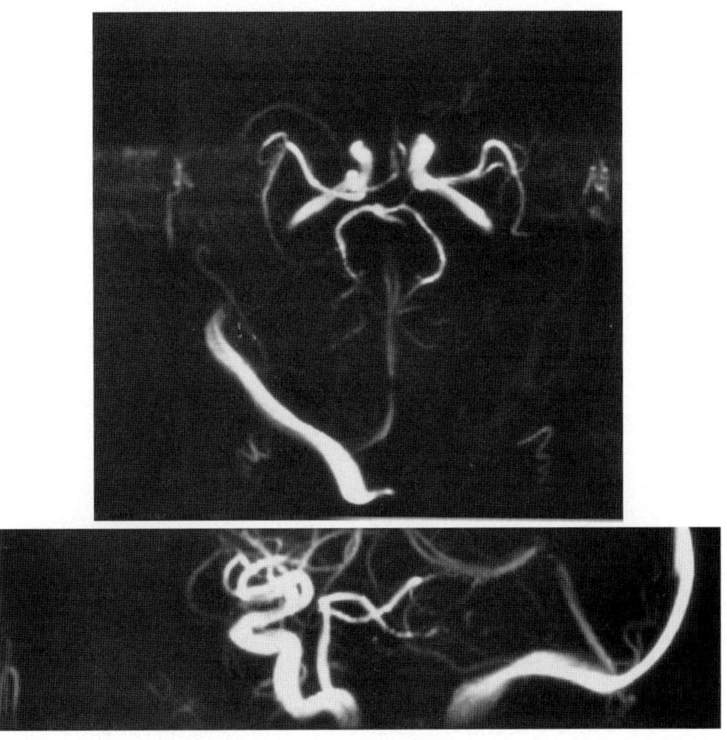

**100 cm/s encoding.**

## CASE 13
## EVALUATION OF DISSECTION USING THE SPIN-ECHO TECHNIQUE

Axial T1-weighted spin-echo images are extremely useful in the evaluation of carotid dissection and should be obtained as a primary diagnostic method, with MRA as an adjunct. The important feature of this sequence is the addition of an inferior saturation pulse to eliminate vascular signal from the carotid, which might be confused with intramural blood. A superior saturation pulse is less necessary for the elimination of venous signal, since the location of signal from the venous side should not be a diagnostic problem relative to arterial dissection. The addition of fat saturation to the T1-weighted spin-echo study facilitates the identification of high-signal-intensity methemoglobin and separating it from perivascular fat. Time-of-flight MRA is useful in the evaluation of dissections, since it allows visualization of the blood flow as well as any surrounding blood products. The downside of this is that the true lumen may be difficult to separate from the blood. Evaluation of the individual partitions usually allows for this distinction.

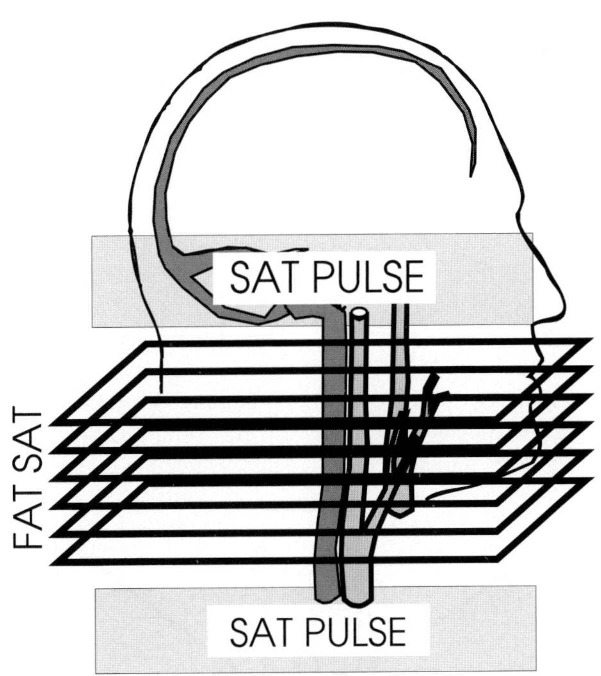


### REFERENCES

Goldberg HI, Grossman RI, Gomori JM et al: Cervical internal carotid artery dissection hemorrhage: diagnosis using MRI, *Radiology* 158(1):157-161, 1986.

Nguyen-Bui L, Brant-Zawadzki M, Veghese P, Gillan G: Magnetic resonance angiography of cervicocranial dissection. *Stroke* 24(1):126-131, 1993.

Ruggieri PR, Modic M, Ross J, Masaryk T: *Neuroradiologic evaluation of carotid dissection.* Paper presented at the 29th Annual Meeting of the American Society of Neuroradiology, Washington, DC, Nov 1991.

Pacini R, Simon J, Ketonen L et al: Chemical-shift imaging of a spontaneous internal carotid artery dissection: case report, *AJNR* 12:360-62, 1991.

## CASE 14
## MAXIMUM INTENSITY PROJECTION

In a maximum intensity projection, parallel rays traverse the entire tomographic volume **(A).** An axis of rotation and angle of projection are chosen to project the parallel rays. The signal intensity is measured in each three-dimensional voxel of each section (partition) encountered by the projected rays. The intensity profile is analyzed along each individual ray. Only the maximum value of each intensity profile is written onto the projected image plane. In these data sets, the maximum intensity value is related to either a vessel or background tissue when the rays do not intersect any vessels. The background intensity can be removed by means of a local threshold algorithm that accepts only pixel intensities above the chosen threshold. Generally, the background is not entirely removed, since it can be used to identify anatomic locations of the reconstructed vessels. Consequently, the maximum intensity projection image shows a two-dimensional projection view of all the vessels within the tomographic volume. Different views are calculated by choosing different angles of projection. These reconstructed projections are displayed on a standard console or in a cine mode.

Because of the thresholding used, the relative signal intensities of vessel blood flow and the background signal are critically important in determining the quality and accuracy of the MRA. The ray tracing algorithm looks for the highest signal as the ray traverses the volume. If the highest signal intensity in the volume relates to blood flow, the MRA will be of good quality and reflect the anatomic structures. However, if by chance the highest signal does not relate to blood flow, the maximum intensity projection will be degraded by underestimation of vessel diameter or failure to visualize vessels entirely. This problem of statistical variation in background signal intensity also explains why it is important to limit the volume of interest in the maximum intensity projection views (i.e., "target" the maximum intensity projection) and to use background suppression techniques for time-of-flight MRA. The less volume involved in the maximum intensity projection, the less statistical chance that the background signal will be higher than the signal from flowing blood. Magnetization transfer background suppression effectively decreases the signal from the brain parenchyma, improving the quality of the maximum intensity projection.

The opposite can also occur; in this case, vital low-signal-intensity structures are obscured by the high-signal-intensity vasculature. This occurs particularly in carotid dissections in which the intimal flap is not visualized or in intraluminal thrombus. This problem is schematically shown in **B,** where a variety of three-dimensional objects with internal signal can give the same projection appearance.

**A**

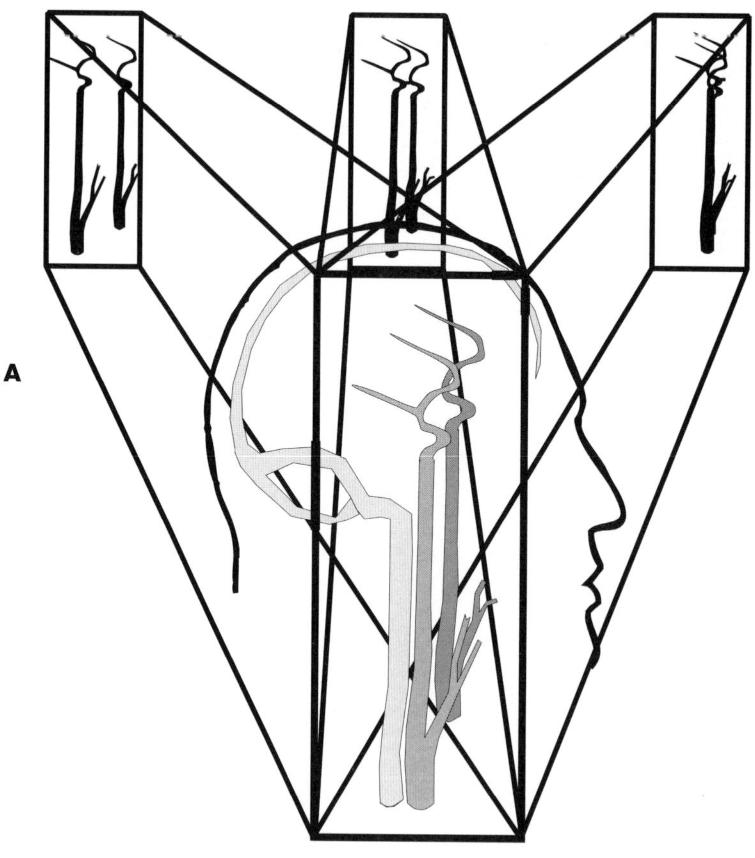

B

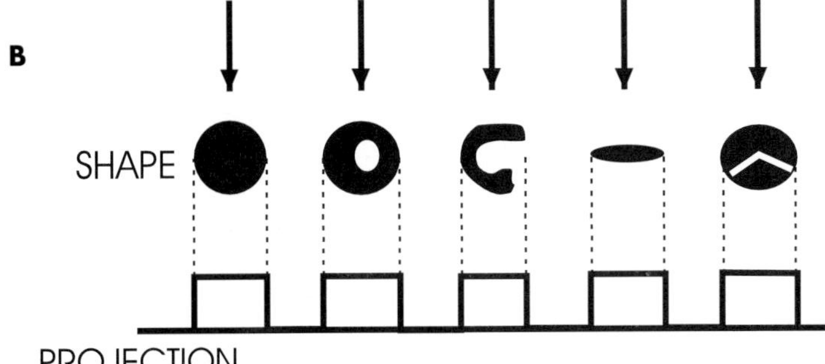


Schematic of outcome of projection for various luminal shapes. Multiple shapes give the same projection outline, making evaluation of the individual MRA partitions necessary.

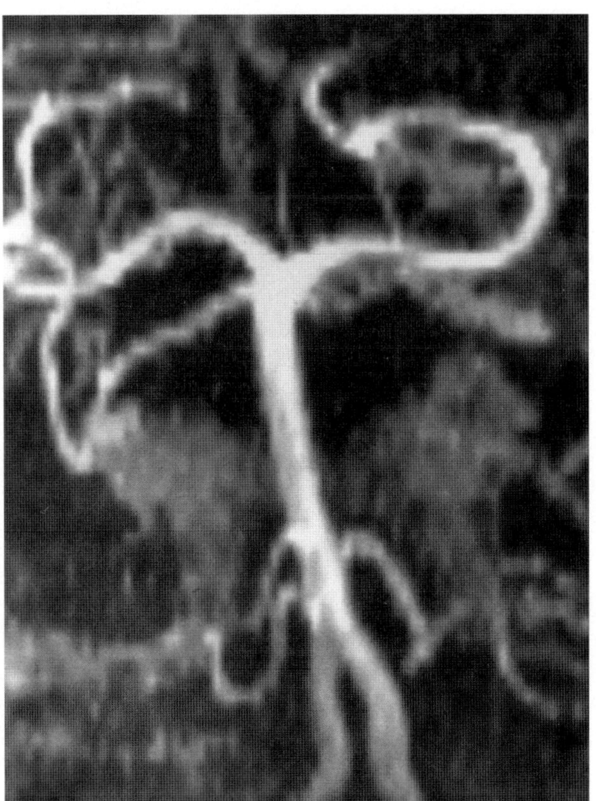

D

C

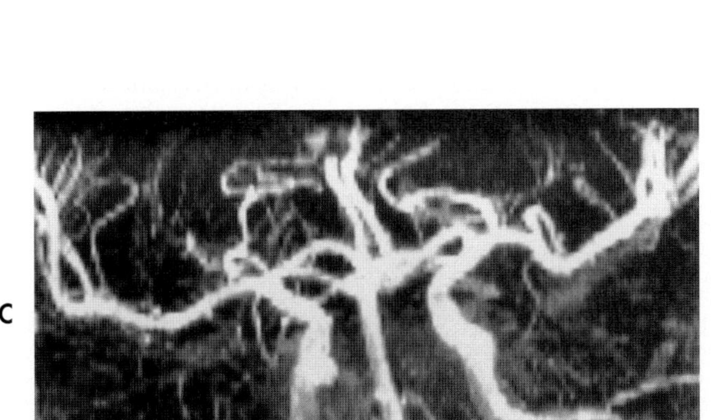

**Improved vessel detection with targeted maximum intensity projection reconstruction. Anteroposterior whole head maximum intensity projection of the intracranial circulation after contrast (C) shows good visualization of the arteries and overlapping of the arterial structures by high signal intensity from venous structures and the nasal mucosa. Targeted anteroposterior maximum intensity projection view (D) of the basilar artery shows improved visualization of the anterior inferior cerebellar artery and posterior inferior cerebellar artery origins compared with maximum intensity projection of the whole head.**

## REFERENCES

Tsuruda J, Saloner D, Norman D: Artifacts associated with MR neuroangiography, *AJNR* 13:1411-1422, 1992.

Cline HE, Dumoulin CL, Lorensen WE et al: Volume rendering and connectivity algorithms for MR angiography, *Magn Reson Med* 18:384-394, 1991.

**TABLE 2-1 Advantages and Disadvantages of Major Techniques**

| Technique | Advantages | Disadvantages | Area of use |
|---|---|---|---|
| Two-dimensional time of flight | Sensitive to slow flow<br>Short scan time<br>Minimized saturation effects | Longer echo time<br>Thicker slices than with three-dimensional techniques<br>Signal loss that is more severe with tight stenosis<br>Motion artifacts<br>Short T1 lesions that simulate flow | Carotid bifurcation<br>Venous disease |
| Three-dimensional time of flight | Short echo time<br>Thin slices<br>Limited signal loss with severe stenosis<br>Short scan time | Insensitivity to slow flow<br>Saturation effects<br>Motion artifacts<br>Short T1 lesions that simulate flow | Carotid bifurcation<br>Intracranial disease |
| Three-dimensional time of flight multislab | Short echo time<br>Thin slices<br>Limited signal loss with severe stenosis<br>Minimized saturation effects | Insensitivity to slow flow<br>Motion artifacts<br>Venetian blind artifact<br>Short T1 lesions that simulate flow | Carotid bifurcation<br>Intracranial disease |
| Two-dimensional phase contrast | Short scan time<br>Slow- or fast-flow view<br>Good background suppression | Large voxel size<br>Long echo time<br>Sensitivity to phase dispersion | Scout for carotid bifurcation<br>Flow direction (crossfilling or subclavian steal)<br>Venous disease |
| Three-dimensional phase contrast | Slow- or fast-flow view<br>Good background suppression<br>Minimized saturation effects<br>Quantitative flow information | Long scan times<br>Longer echo time<br>Sensitivity to phase dispersion | Intracranial disease<br>Venous disease |

# CHAPTER 3

# Normal Anatomy, Variants, and Congenital Anomalies

The intracranial circulation is ideally suited to phase-contrast and time-of-flight techniques because of the absence of gross patient and physiologic motion. Three-dimensional sequences provide the needed spatial resolution to visualize small vessel dimensions and the reconstruction capabilities necessary to display the complex intracranial vessel geometry.

MRA is capable of defining a wide variety of "normal" arterial signals related to age and technique, which must be taken into account to provide maximal diagnostic accuracy. The spatial resolution and contrast-to-noise ratio of MRA makes identification of many congenital vascular anomalies possible; in fact, diagnosis via MRA may even be preferable. To diagnose complex congenital vascular anatomy, the clinician must make use of the maximum intensity projections and, just as important, the individual slices. For instance, the entry site of the persistent hypoglossal artery is characteristic and is easily made only by looking at the individual slices and comparing vascular signal to the surrounding brain parenchyma and skull base anatomy.

## CASE 15
## NORMAL TIME-OF-FLIGHT AND PHASE-CONTRAST MRA IN A NEWBORN

**Technique #1:** axial volume, three-dimensional time-of-flight, 56/6.9/20, 256 × 192, 60 slices, 60-mm slab, magnetization transfer background suppression, ramp radiofrequency pulse, 18-cm field of view, 10:45.

**Technique #2:** axial three-dimensional phase-contrast, 33/8.5/20, 128 × 256, 28 slices, 42-mm slab, velocity encoding of 15 cm/s, flow encoding in all three directions, one excitation, 18-cm field of view, 9:40.

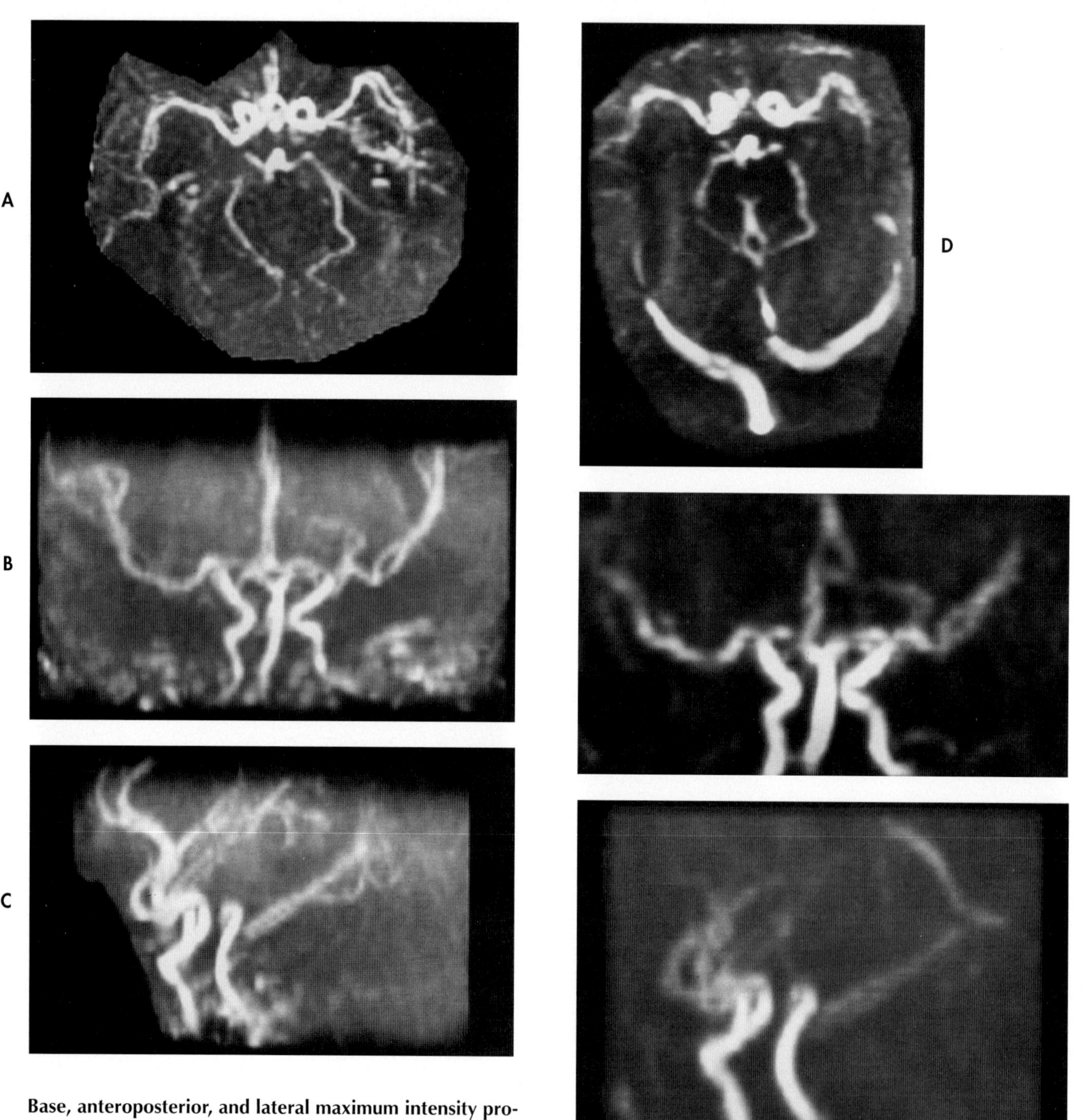


**Base, anteroposterior, and lateral maximum intensity projection views in a 9-day-old infant imaged in a knee coil show good signal intensity in the anterior and posterior circulations on the three-dimensional time-of-flight (A through C) and phase-contrast studies (D through F).**

Cerebral blood flow must be maintained at high levels to sustain adequate substrates for the metabolic activity of the brain. In children younger than 3 years, there is decreased cerebral blood flow; the flow is 30 to 60 ml/100 mg of brain/minute, whereas adult flow is 50 ml/100 mg of brain/minute. Cerebral blood flow increases in 3- to 10-year-old children—up to 100 ml/100 mg of brain/minute. Middle cerebral artery velocity appears to be low at birth—approximately 24 cm/s—but rises in the first few days of life. Velocity appears to peak at around 100 cm/s between the ages of 3 and 6 years. Several factors, such as autoregulation in the mature brain, neuronal activity, perfusion pressure, intracranial pressure, and vascular resistance, control the rate of cerebral blood flow. In the infant, cerebral blood flow may be solely a function of arterial perfusion pressure and intracranial pressure.

These changes in cerebral blood flow may be roughly correlated with the MRA images that can be produced in the various age ranges. Term infants provide a challenge in obtaining quality MRA images, principally because of their small size and the limited spatial resolution of the technique. The relatively decreased cerebral blood flow in the neonatal period does not appear to be a major obstacle to obtaining MRAs by phase-contrast or time-of-flight methods. By 6 months of age, adequate flow and sufficient resolution allow for excellent MRA time-of-flight images because of the fast flow and good flow-related enhancement.

**REFERENCES**

Kirsch JR, Traystman RJ, Rogers MC: Cerebral blood flow measurement techniques in infants and children, *Pediatrics* 75:887-895, 1985.

Volpe JJ, Perlman JM, Hill A et al: Cerebral blood flow velocity in the human newborn: the value of its determination, *Pediatrics* 70:147-152, 1982.

Adams RJ, Nichols FT, Hess DC: *Normal values and physiologic variables.* In Newell DW, Aaslid R: *Transcranial doppler,* New York, 1992, Raven.

Bode H, Wais U: Age dependence of flow velocities in basal cerebral arteries, *Arch Dis Child* 63:606-611, 1988.

## CASE 16
## NORMAL TIME-OF-FLIGHT MRA IN A 13-MONTH-OLD INFANT

**Technique:** axial volume; three-dimensional time-of-flight; 45/7/20; 256 × 256; 64 slices; 60-mm slab; magnetization transfer background suppression; tilted, optimized nonsaturating excitation radiofrequency pulse; 12-cm field of view; 12:20.

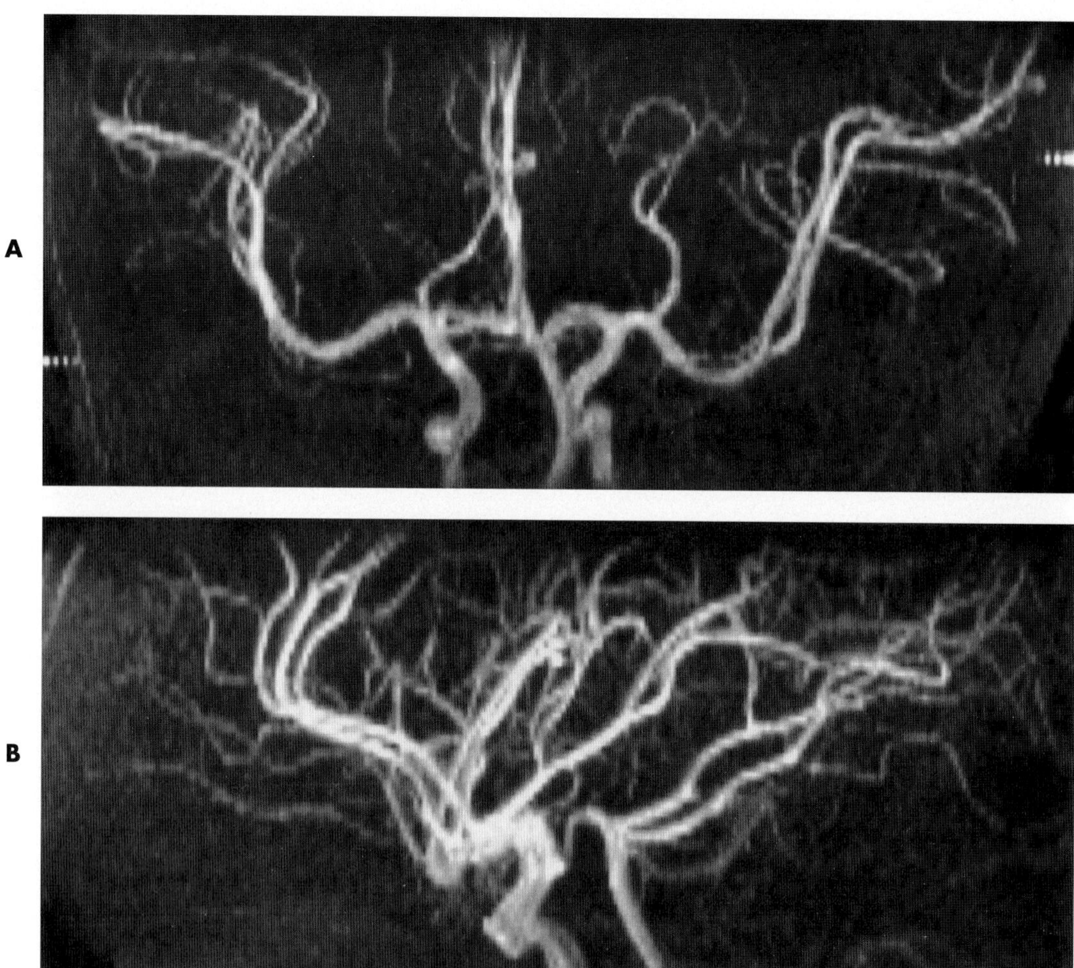


**Anteroposterior (A) and lateral (B) maximum intensity projection views in a 13-month-old child show good signal intensity in the anterior and posterior circulations.**

## CASE 17
## NORMAL PHASE-CONTRAST MRA IN A 2-YEAR-OLD CHILD

**Technique:** axial three-dimensional phase-contrast, 25/8.5/20, 128 × 256, 60 slices, 60-mm slab, velocity encoding of 30 cm/s, flow encoding in all three directions, one excitation, 18-cm field of view, 13:40.

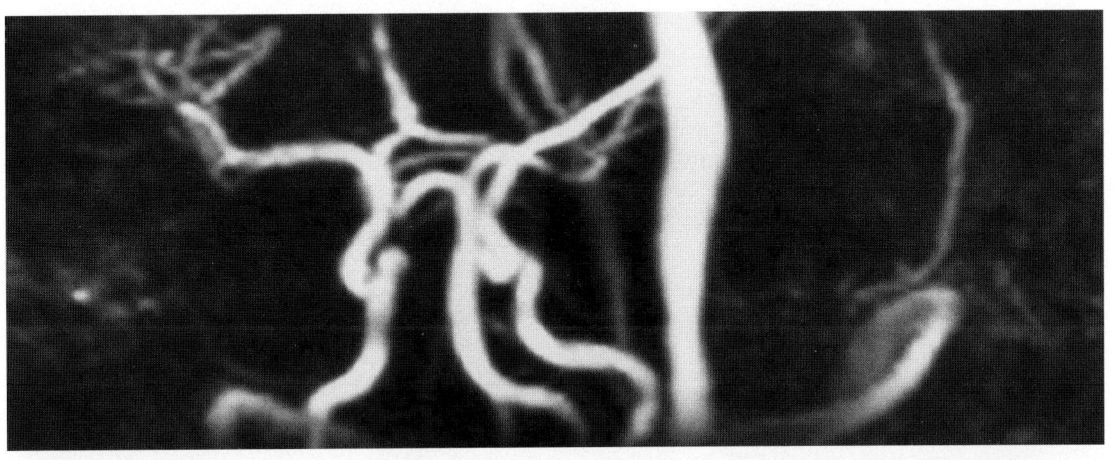

A

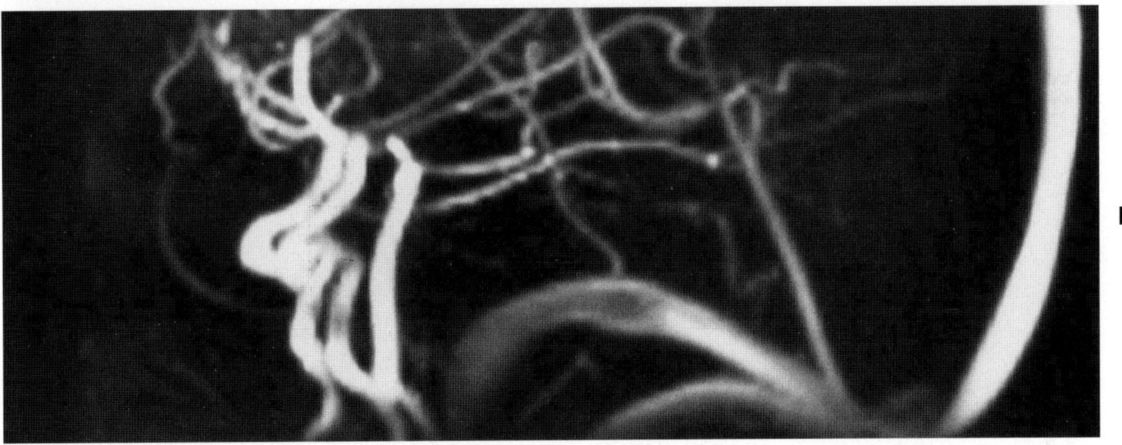

B

**Oblique (A) and lateral (B) maximum intensity projection views show good signal intensity from the anterior and posterior circulations and from the straight, superior sagittal, and transverse sinuses.**

## CASE 18
## NORMAL TIME-OF-FLIGHT MRA IN A 4-YEAR-OLD CHILD

**Technique:** axial volume, three-dimensional time-of-flight, 45/7/20, 256 × 256, 64 slices, 60-mm slab, 12-cm field of view, 12:20.

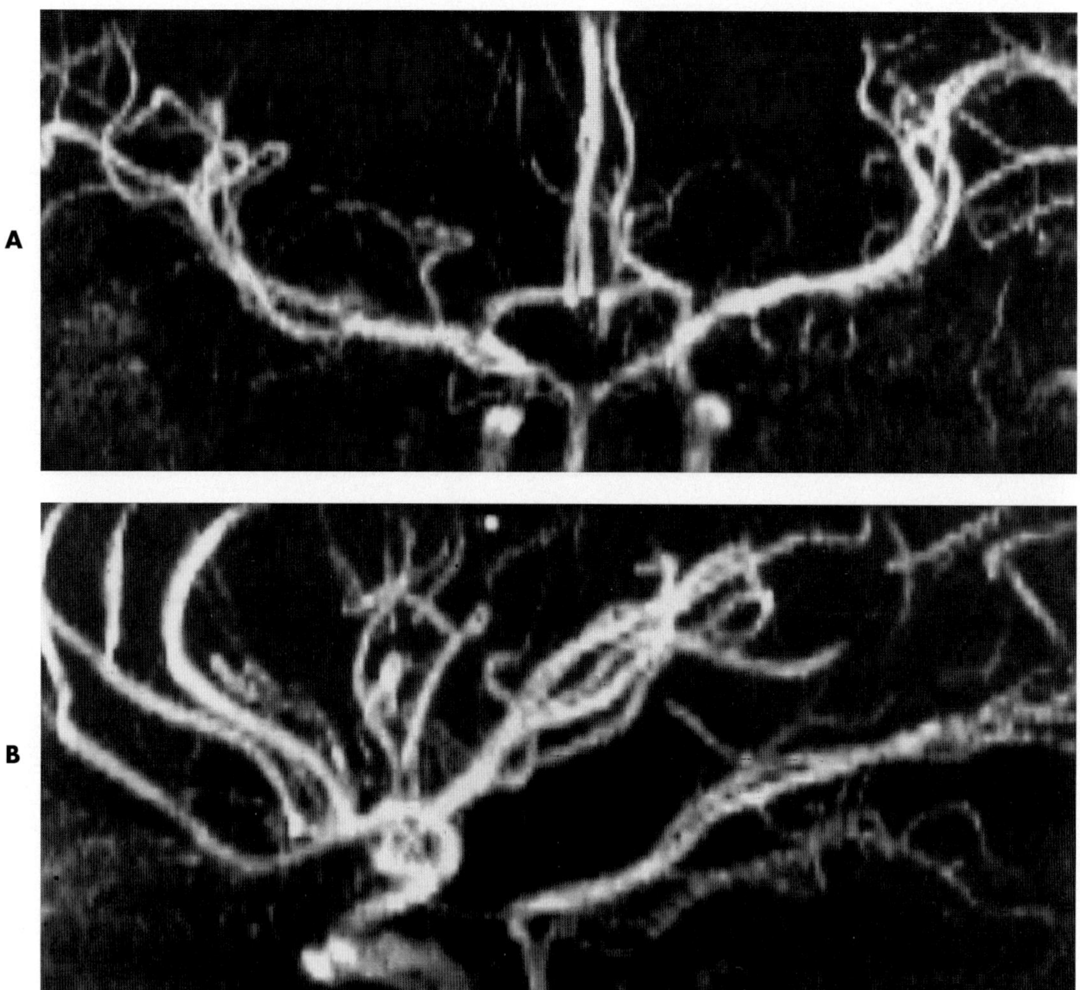

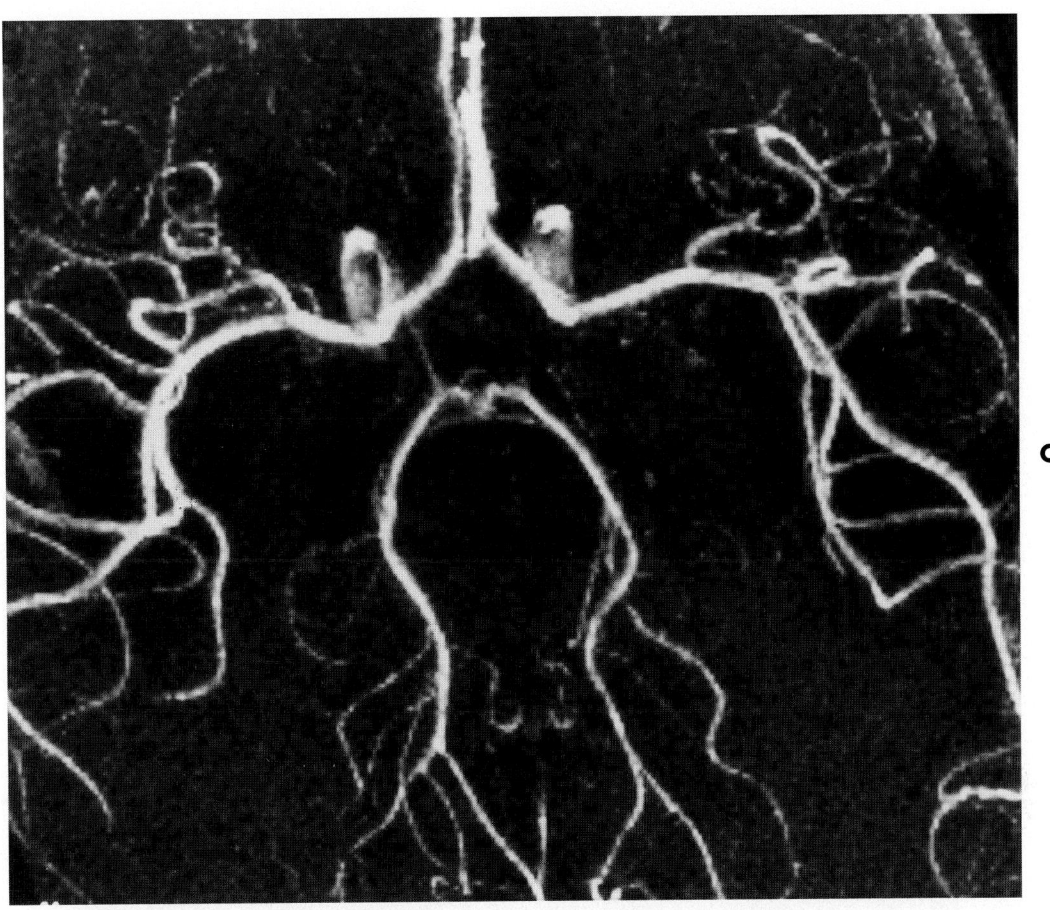

C

**Anteroposterior (A), lateral (B), and base (C) maximum intensity projection views show good signal intensity from all the major intracranial vessels.**

## CASE 19
## NORMAL TIME-OF-FLIGHT STUDY IN AN ADULT

**Technique:** multiple axial volumes; three-dimensional time-of-flight; 43/10/20; 256 × 256; three slabs; 40-mm slabs; 37% overlap; 20-cm field of view; magnetization transfer background suppression; tilted, optimized non-saturating excitation radiofrequency pulse; 9:20.

**A**

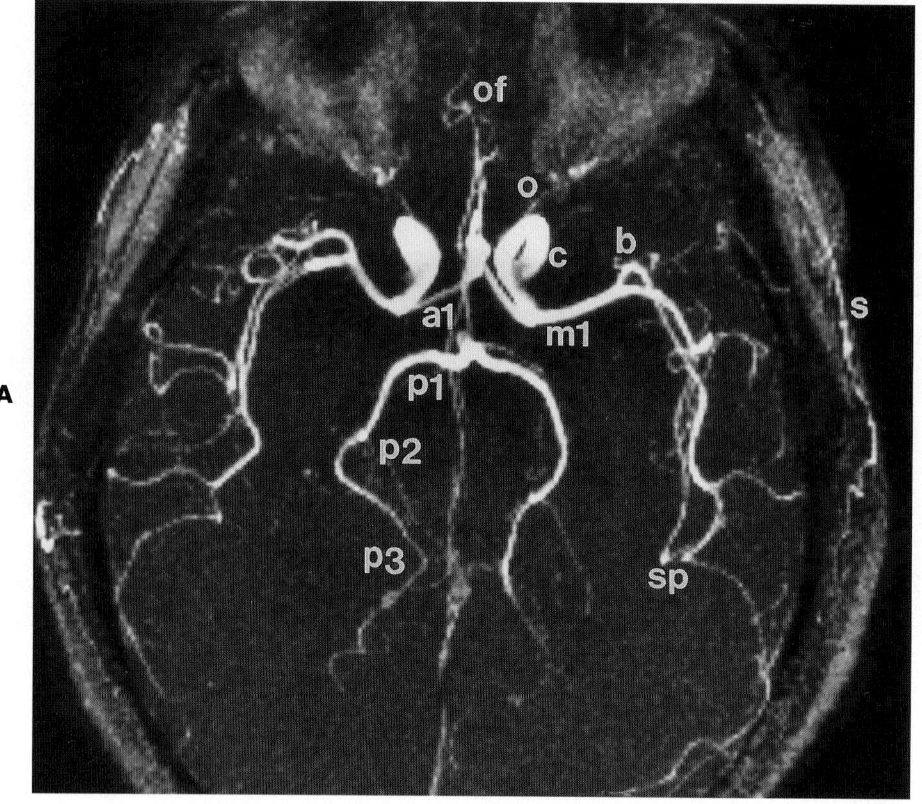

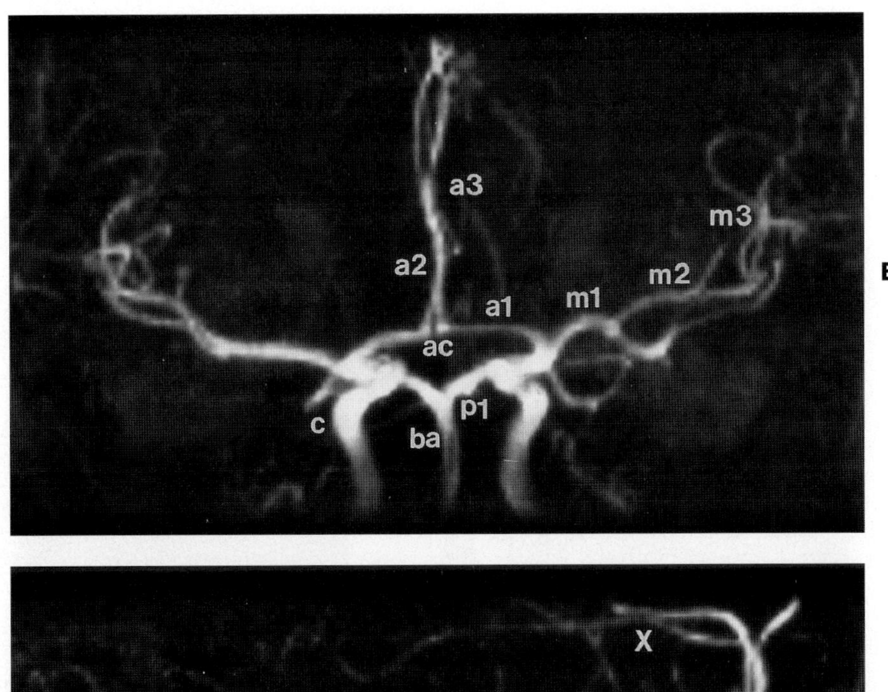


B

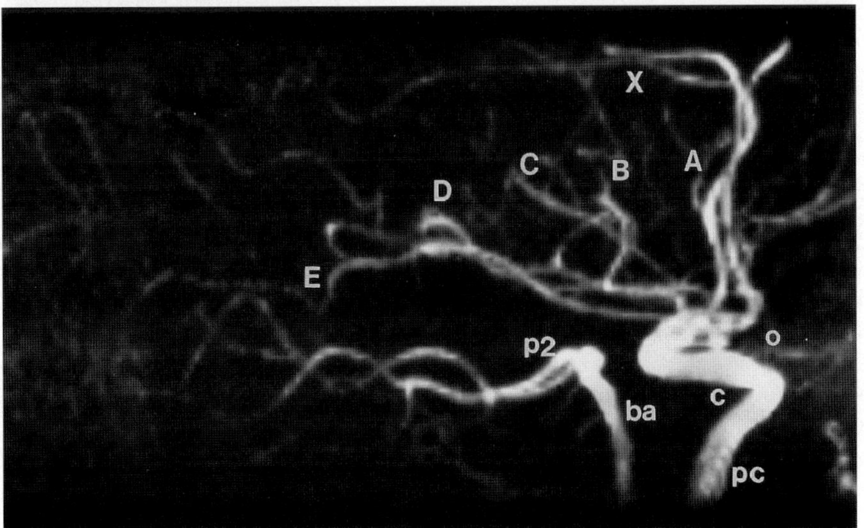


C

Base (A), anteroposterior (B), and lateral (C) maximum intensity projection views depict normal anatomy. *a1,* Horizontal anterior cerebral artery; *a2,* vertical portion of the anterior cerebral artery; *a3,* anterior cerebral at the genu of the corpus callosum; *ac,* region of the anterior communicating artery; *m1,* horizontal middle cerebral artery; *m2,* insular middle cerebral branches; *m3,* opercular middle cerebral branches; *A,* prefrontal branch of the middle cerebral artery; *B,* prerolandic branch of the middle cerebral artery; *C,* rolandic branch of the middle cerebral artery; *D,* parietal branch of the middle cerebral artery; *E,* angular branch of the middle cerebral artery; *p1,* proximal posterior cerebral artery (between basilar tip and posterior communicating artery); *p2,* circummesencephalic or ambient segment; *p3,* segment posterior to the midbrain in quadrageminal cistern; *b,* middle cerebral bifurcation; *ba,* basilar artery; *c,* carotid siphon; *o,* ophthalmic artery; *of,* orbitofrontal branches of the anterior cerebral artery; *pc,* petrous carotid artery; *s,* superficial temporal branch of the external carotid artery; *sp,* sylvian point.

# CASE 20
# NORMAL VENOUS ANATOMY

**Technique:** oblique sagittal, two-dimensional time-of-flight, 32/10/30, 256 × 192, 23-cm field of view, 5:58.

A

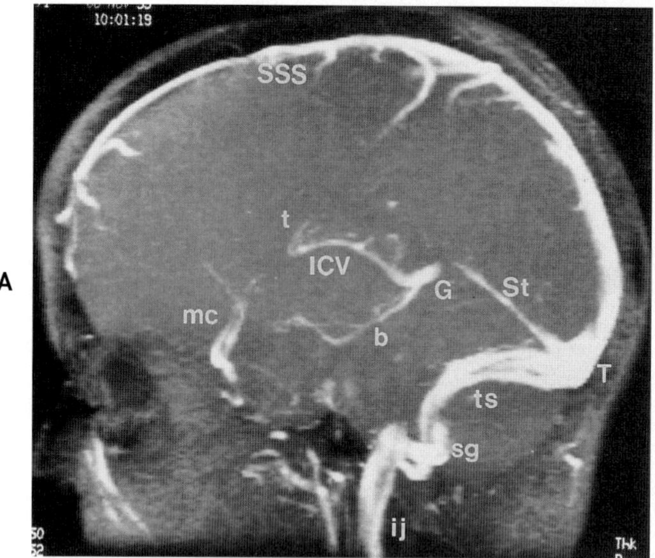


B

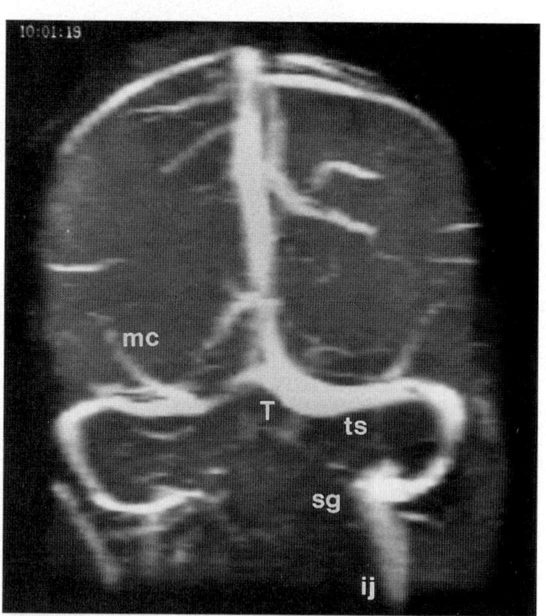


**Lateral (A) and vertex (B) maximum intensity projection views of the two-dimensional time-of-flight MR venogram show the normal-appearing sinuses and cortical veins. Signal loss at the junction of the vein of Galen and straight sinus relates to turbulence and in-plane dephasing on the sagittal-oriented slices. *b,* Basal vein of Rosenthal; *G,* vein of Galen; *ICV,* internal cerebral veins; *ij,* internal jugular vein; *mc,* middle cerebral vein; *SSS,* superior sagittal sinus; *St,* straight sinus; *sg,* sigmoid sinus; *T,* torcular; *t,* thalamostriate vein; *ts,* transverse sinus.**

## CASE 21
## LONG COMMON TRUNK ("AZYGOS") ANTERIOR CEREBRAL ARTERY

**Technique:** axial volume, three-dimensional time-of-flight, 45/7/20, 256 × 256, 64 slices, 60-mm slab, 12-cm field of view, 12:20.

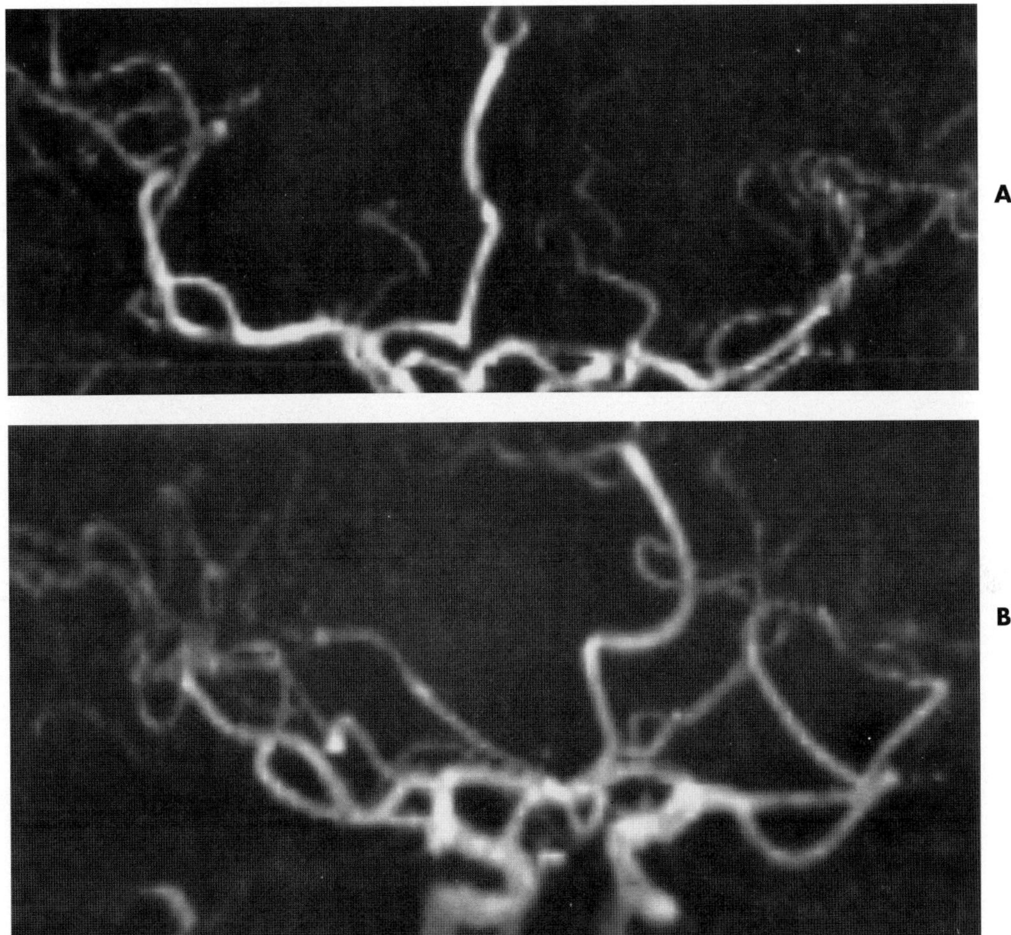


**Anteroposterior and oblique maximum intensity projection views (A and B) show a single anterior cerebral artery fed by the right A1 segment. The anterior cerebral artery then branches beyond the region of the genu of the corpus callosum.**

Many anatomic variations of the anterior cerebral arteries exist. Baptista describes three types of anterior cerebral arteries—unpaired, bihemispheric, and triplicated—in which a single vessel supplies both hemispheres. A single anterior cerebral artery trunk that supplies both hemispheres throughout its course is an uncommon variant, perhaps occurring as rarely as 0.3% of the time (azygos anterior cerebral artery). This vessel should be differentiated from the more common variation, a common trunk of the anterior cerebral artery (either short or long), which occurs in 35% to 5% of cases and is seen in this example.

### REFERENCES

Lasjaunias P, Berenstein A: *Surgical neuroangiography*, vol 3, New York, 1990, Springer-Verlag.

Baptista AG: Studies on the arteries of the brain, *Neurology* 13:825-835, 1963.

Cinnamon J, Zito J, Chilif DJ et al: Aneurysm of the azygos pericallosal artery: diagnosis by MR imaging and MR angiography, *AJNR* 13(1):280-282, 1992.

## CASE 22
## POSTERIOR CEREBRAL ARTERY OF FETAL ORIGIN

**Technique:** axial volume, three-dimensional time-of-flight, 40/7/15, 256 × 256, 64 slices, 60-mm slab, 23-cm field of view, 10:57.

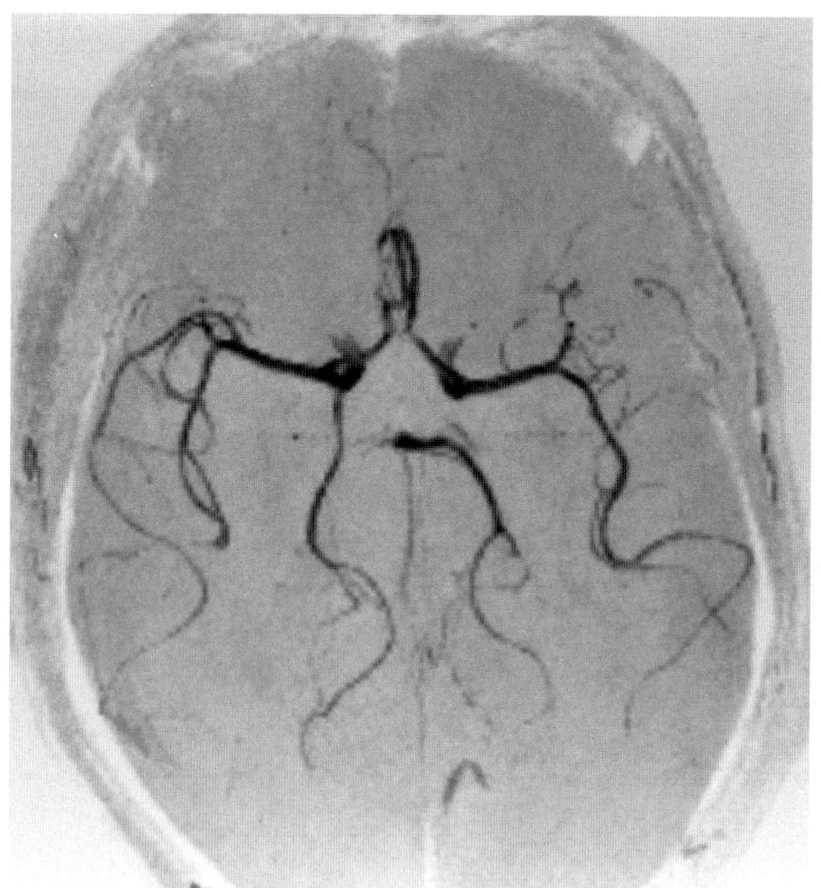

**Maximum intensity projection base view shows the fetal origin of the right posterior cerebral artery from the distal internal carotid artery and the absence of the right P1 segment.**

The embryonic pattern of the posterior cerebral artery arising off the distal internal carotid artery is found on the right in 10.4% of cases, on the left in 9.5% of cases, and bilaterally in 7.7% of cases, according to Wollschlaeger et al.

### REFERENCES

Newton TH, Potts DG: *Radiology of the skull and brain,* vol 2, book 2, St Louis, 1974, Mosby.

Wollschlaeger G, Wollschlaeger PB, Lucas FV, Lopez VF: Experience and result with postmortem cerebral angiography performed as routine procedure of the autopsy, *AJR* 101:68-87, 1967.

## CASE 23
## DUPLICATE SUPERIOR CEREBELLAR ARTERIES

**Technique:** axial volume; three-dimensional time-of-flight; 45/7/20; 256 × 256; 64 slices; 60-mm slab; 12-cm field of view; magnetization transfer background suppression; tilted, optimized nonsaturating excitation radiofrequency pulse; 12:20.

A

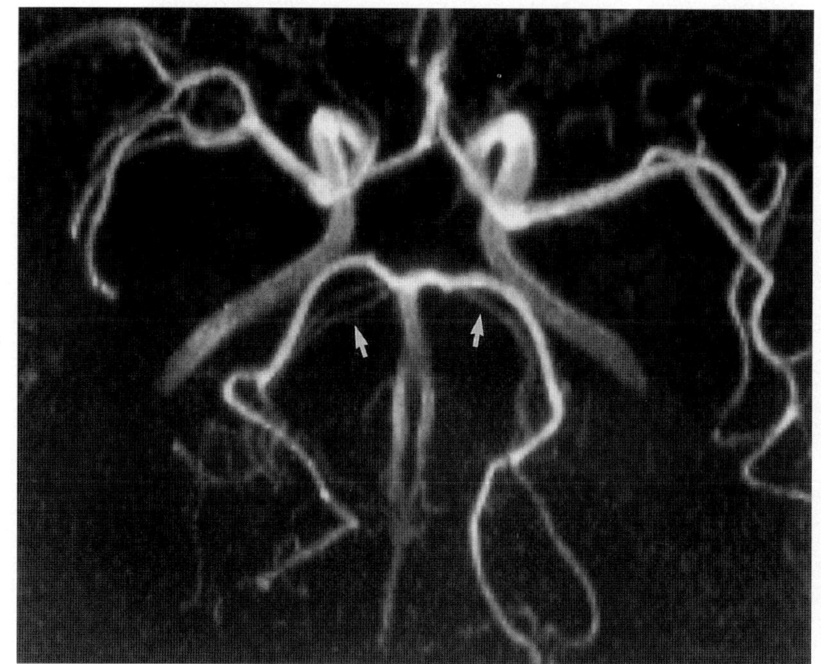

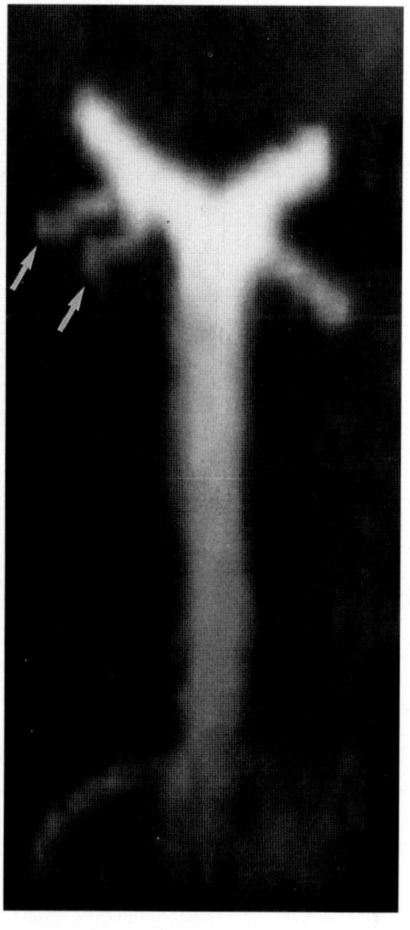

B

**Base maximum intensity projection view shows a normal circle of Willis (A). There are two vessels arising off the distal basilar artery proximal to the posterior cerebral origins on the right *(arrow),* with one superior cerebellar artery on the left *(arrow).* Targeted anteroposterior maximum intensity projection view (B) shows the amputated origins of the posterior cerebral arteries (related to the volume of reconstruction), the left superior cerebellar artery origin, and the duplicated superior cerebellar arteries on the right *(arrows).***

Duplication of the superior cerebellar artery can occur in approximately 28% of the population, with bilateral duplication occurring in approximately 8%. Typically, the upper trunk (medial or superior) supplies the vermian branch, and the lower trunk (lateral or inferior) is the marginal branch.

### REFERENCES

Mani RL, Newton TH: The superior cerebellar artery: arteriographic changes in the diagnosis of posterior fossa lesions, *Radiology* 92:1281-1287, 1969.

Newton TH, Potts DG: *Radiology of the skull and brain,* vol 2, book 2, St Louis, 1974, Mosby.

## CASE 24
## HYPOPLASTIC P1 SEGMENTS BILATERALLY

**Technique:** axial volume, three-dimensional time-of-flight, 45/7/20, 256 × 256, 64 slices, 60-mm slab, 14-cm field of view, 12:20.

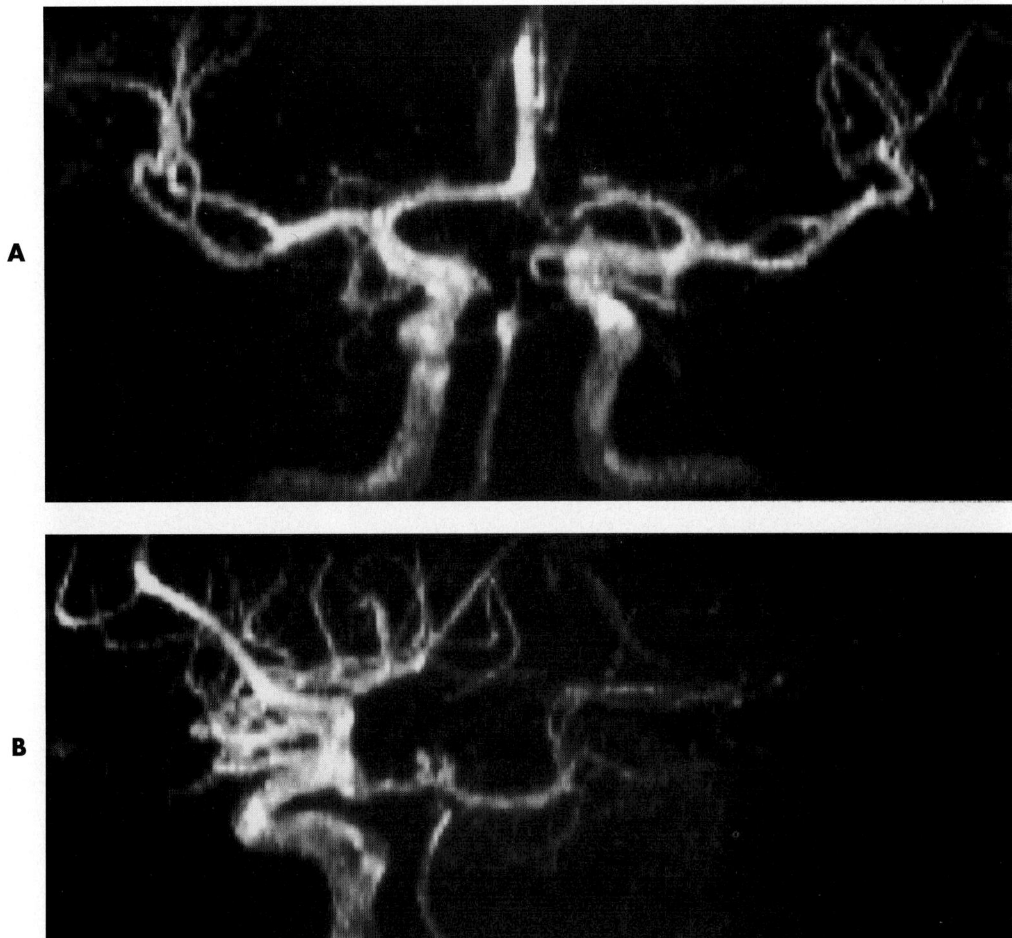

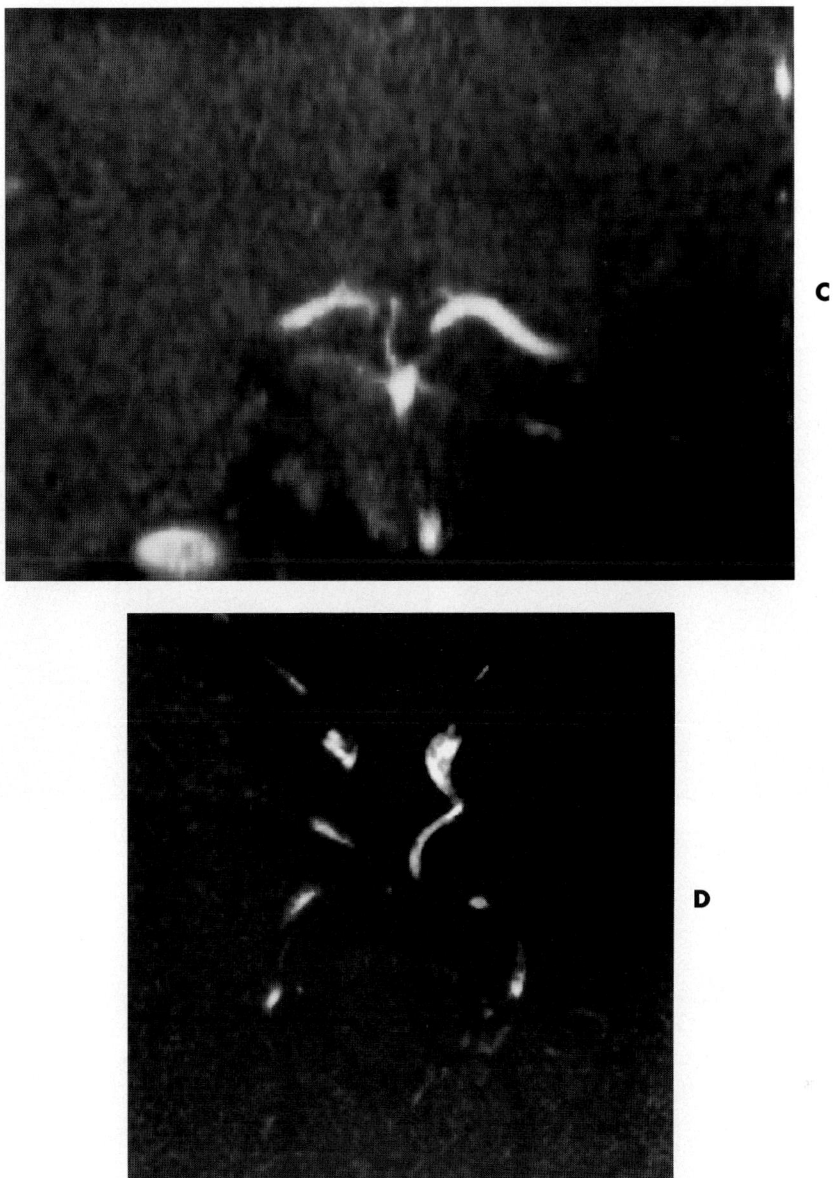


**Anteroposterior and lateral maximum intensity projection views (A and B) show an apparently "short" basilar artery, which does not end in the posterior cerebral arteries. There are fetal origins of the posterior cerebral arteries bilaterally.**

The differential would be a congenital variant vs. occlusion of the distal basilar artery. Coronal reformat of the MRA data **(C)** shows the distal basilar artery with very small P1 segments bilaterally (left smaller than right). The origins of the superior cerebellar arteries are also seen. The large posterior communicating arteries are seen bilaterally. Axial individual slice also shows the fetal origins **(D),** the distal posterior cerebral arteries, and the hypoplastic P1 segments. This variation occurs in about 2% of cases.

#### REFERENCE

Newton TH, Potts DG: *Radiology of the skull and brain,* vol 2, book 2, St Louis, 1974, Mosby.

## CASES 25 AND 26
## PERSISTENT TRIGEMINAL ARTERY
## CASE 25

**History:** 36-year-old with vertigo.

**Technique:** axial volume; three-dimensional time-of-flight; 45/7/20; 256 × 256; 64 slices; 60-mm slab; magnetization transfer background suppression; tilted, optimized nonsaturating excitation radiofrequency pulse; 14-cm field of view; 12:20.

A

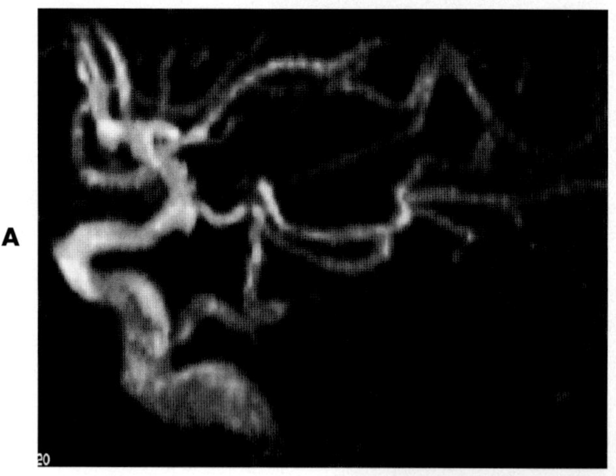

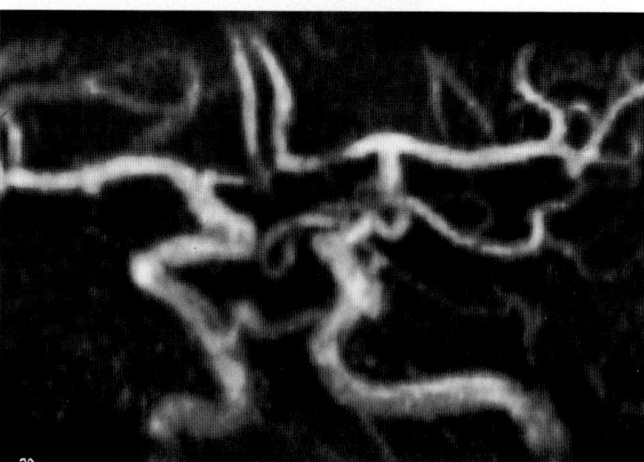

B

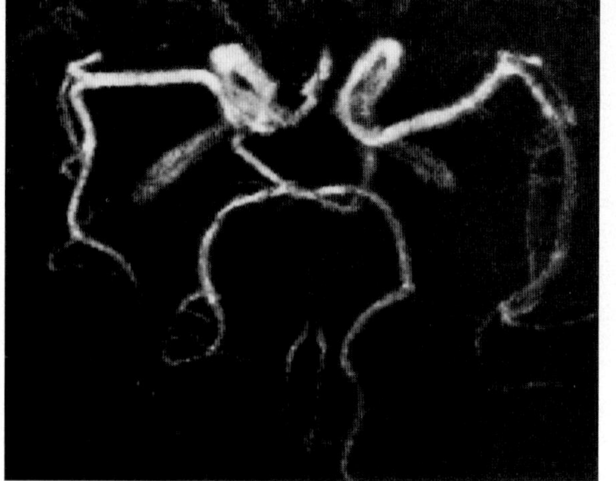

C

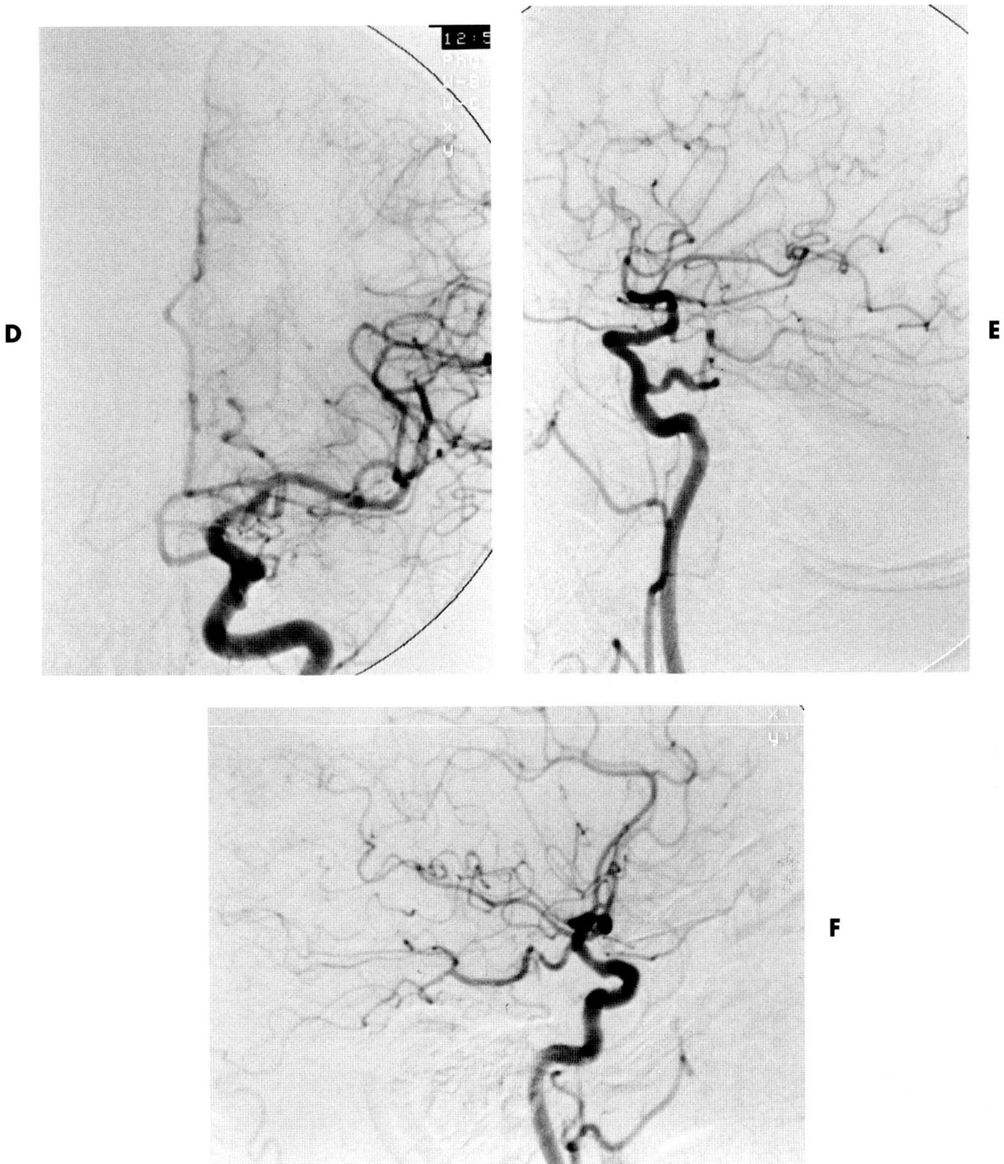


Lateral (A), oblique (B), and base (C) maximum intensity projection views show the typical course for a persistent trigeminal artery arising off the internal carotid artery and supplying the posterior circulation. The three maximum intensity projection views also show a right fetal origin of the posterior cerebral artery. Anteroposterior and lateral conventional angiographic views (D and E) in this patient confirm the anomaly. The right-sided injection confirms the fetal origin of the posterior cerebral artery from the internal carotid artery (F).

## CASE 26

**History:** 55-year-old man with Cushing's disease being evaluated for pituitary adenoma.

**Technique:** axial volume; three-dimensional time-of-flight; 45/7/20; 256 × 256; 64 slices; 60-mm slab; magnetization transfer background suppression; tilted, optimized nonsaturating excitation radiofrequency pulse; 14-cm field of view; 12:20.

A
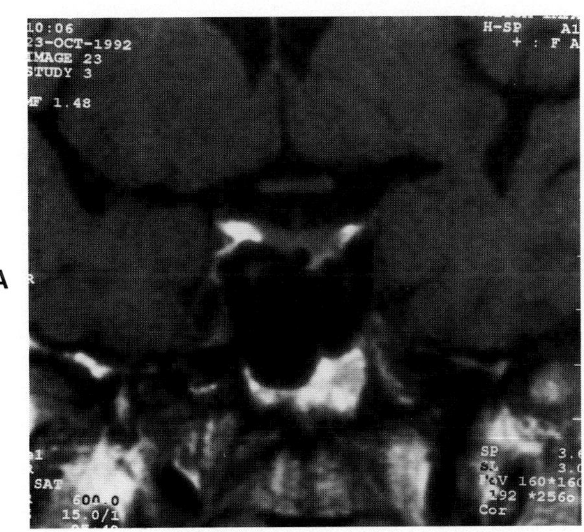


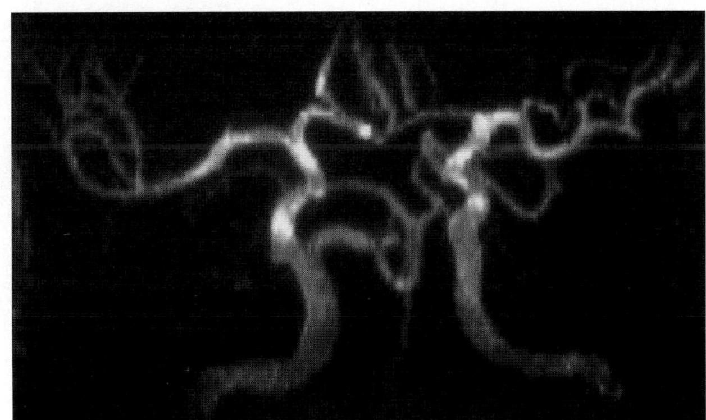
B

**Coronal T1-weighted spin-echo image (A) shows a rounded area of signal void within the base of the pituitary fossa, which appears to be contiguous with the right internal carotid flow void. Anteroposterior maximum intensity projection view (B) shows the persistent trigeminal artery, which takes an intrasellar course.**

The persistent trigeminal artery is the most cephalic and most common of the four types of primitive anastomotic vessels between the carotid and basilar systems. (The four anastomoses between the carotid and vertebral basilar systems in the human embryo are the persistent trigeminal, otic, hypoglossal, and proatlantal arteries.) Angiographic incidence of persistent trigeminal artery is reported at 0.6%. Flow through the persistent trigeminal artery is predominantly from the carotid artery to the basilar artery, although the reverse has been reported. A persistent trigeminal artery is associated with other anomalies of the intracranial vessels, such as asymmetry of the circle of Willis with aplasia or hypoplasia of the posterior communicating artery and hypoplasia of the basilar artery caudal to the anastomosis. Intracranial vascular abnormalities also may exist with the trigeminal artery, the most common being arteriovenous malformations and aneurysms.

The usual course of the persistent trigeminal artery is intracavernous from the posterior lateral wall of the carotid artery to the posterior dural surface of the cavernous sinus, where it exits medial to the sensory root of the trigeminal nerve. However, an occasional trigeminal artery may ascend from the floor of the sella to pierce the dorsum and thus lie intrasellar. Because of this position, the persistent trigeminal artery must be closely inspected, since it would pose a considerable risk for intrasellar or parasellar surgery, as demonstrated in Case 26.

### REFERENCES

Fortner AA, Smoker WRK: Persistent primitive trigeminal artery aneurysm evaluated by MR imaging, *JCAT* 12(5):847-850, 1988.

Fields WS: The significance of persistent trigeminal artery: carotid basilar anastomosis, *Radiology* 91:1096-1101, 1968.

Wollschlaeger G, Wollschlaeger P: The primitive trigeminal artery as seen angiographically at post-mortem examination, *Am J Roentgen Radium Ther Nuclear Med* 92;761-762, 1964.

Schuierer G, Laub G, Huk WJ: MR angiography of the primitive trigeminal artery: report on two cases, *AJNR* 11(6):1131-1132, 1990.

# CASE 27
# PERSISTENT HYPOGLOSSAL ARTERY

**History:** 36-year-old being screened for intracranial aneurysm.

**Technique:** axial volume; three-dimensional time-of-flight; 45/7/20; 256 × 256; 64 slices; 60-mm slab; magnetization transfer background suppression; tilted, optimized nonsaturating excitation radiofrequency pulse; 14-cm field of view; 12:20.

**A**

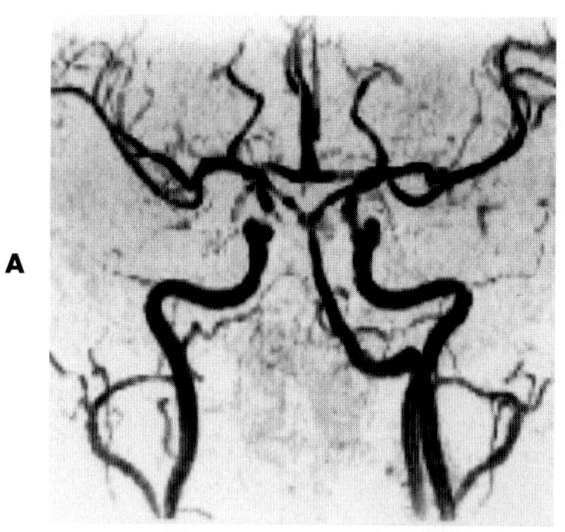

**B**

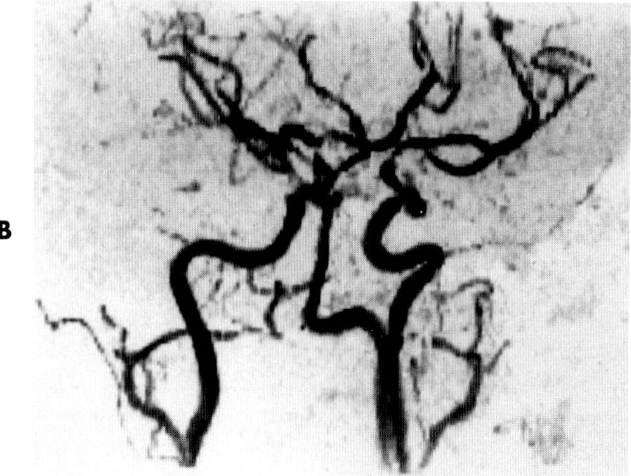

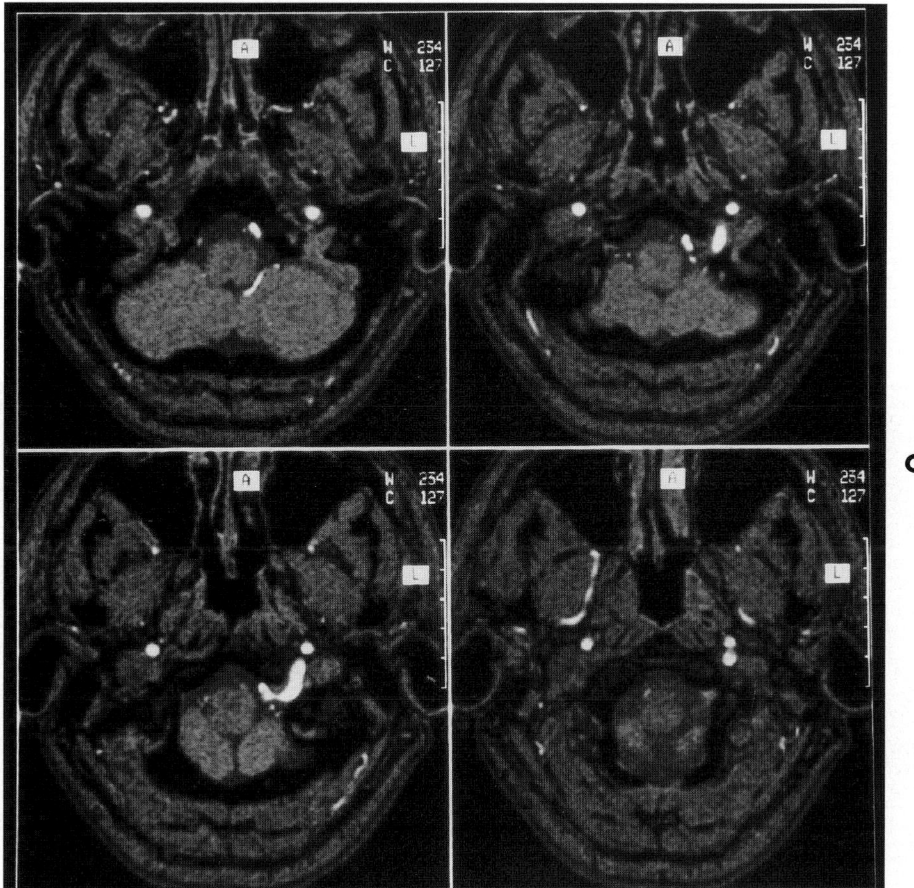


**Anteroposterior (A) and oblique (B) maximum intensity projection views show a large vessel connecting to the basilar artery on the left. The vessel is more lateral and anterior than usual for the vertebral artery. The right vertebral artery is not seen. Four individual slices from the MRA data (C) show the entrance of the anomalous hypoglossal artery intracranially through the hypoglossal canal to join with the basilar artery.**

The frequency of the persistent hypoglossal artery is estimated at around 0.25%. The hypoglossal artery arises from the cervical internal carotid artery at the C1 to C3 level. It then enters into the cranium via the hypoglossal canal (anterior condyloid foramen) with the hypoglossal nerve, where the artery joins the basilar artery to supply the posterior fossa. The vertebral arteries are usually absent or hypoplastic, and the ipsilateral posterior communicating artery cannot be angiographically demonstrated. Concomitant intracranial aneurysms and arteriovenous malformations have been reported.

#### REFERENCES


Mercado RG, Cavazos E, Urrutia G: Persistent hypoglossal artery in combination with multifocal arteriovenous malformations of the brain: case report, *Neurosurgery* 26:871-876, 1990.

Kanai H, Nagai H, Wakabayashi S, Hashimoto N: A large aneurysm of the persistent primitive hypoglossal artery, *Neurosurgery* 30:794-797, 1992.

Hassen-Khodja R, Declemy S, Batt M et al: Persistent hypoglossal artery, *J Cardiovasc Surg* 33:199-201, 1992.

## CASE 28
## HYPOPLASTIC INTERNAL CAROTID ARTERY

**History:** 47-year-old with transient ischemic attacks.

**Technique #1:** carotid/axial volume, three-dimensional time-of-flight, 35/7/20, 128 × 256, rectangular field of view, 128 slices, 25-cm field of view, 9:36.

**Technique #2:** intracranial/axial volume, three-dimensional time-of-flight, 45/7/20, 160 × 512, 64 slices, 24-cm field of view, 7:43.

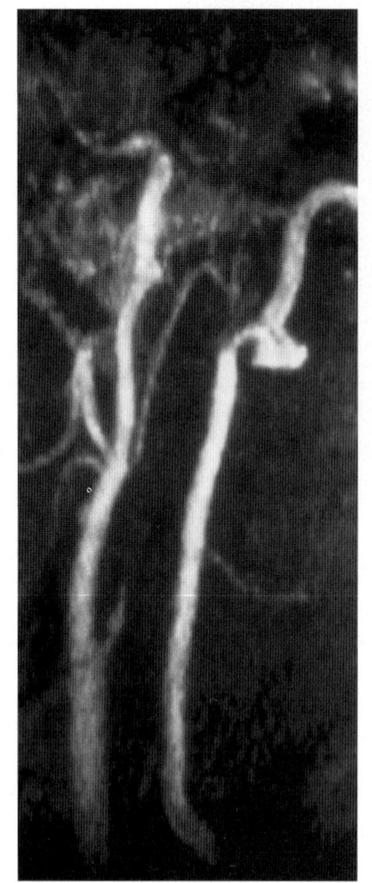


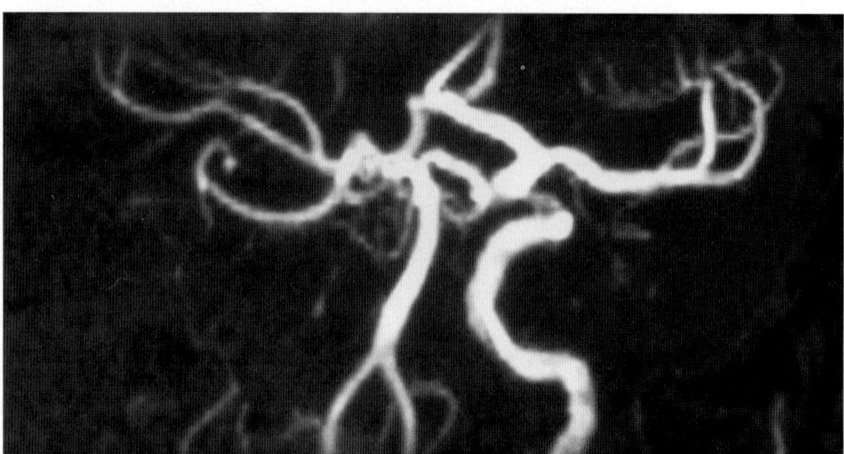


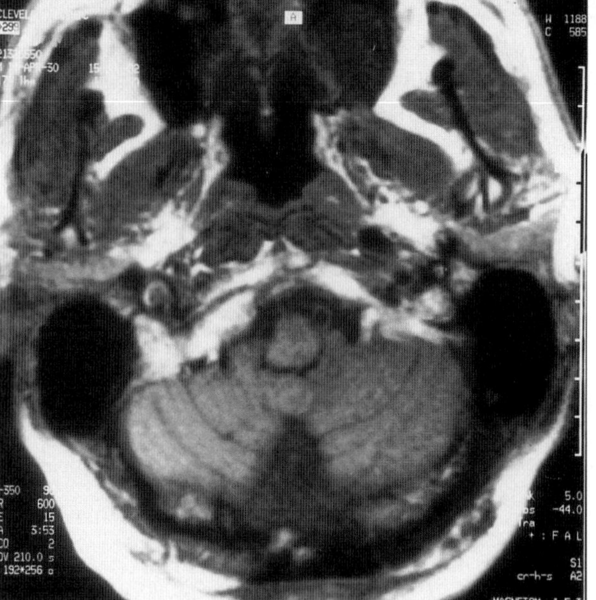


**Lateral maximum intensity projection view of the right carotid bifurcation (A) shows a very small origin of the internal carotid artery without discernible signal in the more distal aspect. The external carotid artery is widely patent. Antero-posterior intracranial maximum intensity projection view (B) shows no signal from the right internal carotid artery. Axial T1-weighted spin-echo image (C) shows no appreciable flow void from the region of the internal carotid artery but just fat signal. There is a normal carotid flow void on the left.**

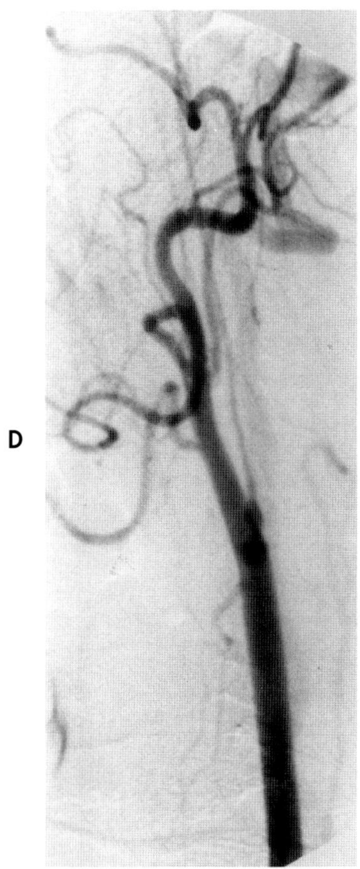

D

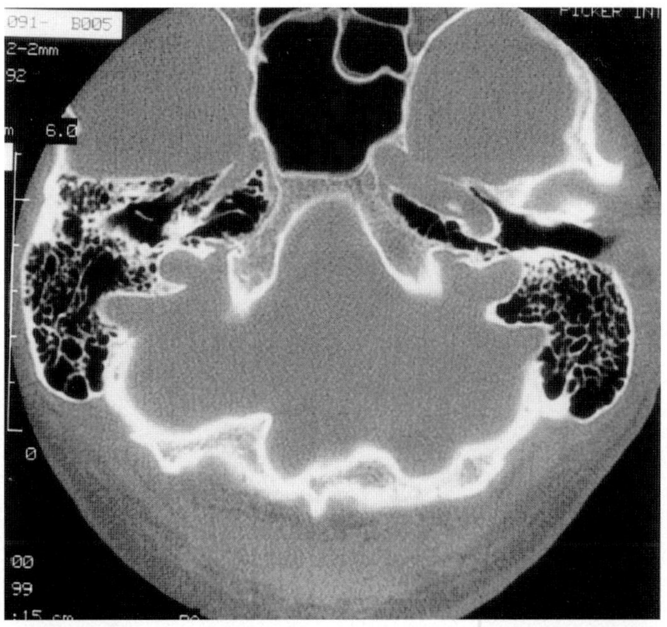

E

**Lateral view of a conventional angiographic right common carotid injection demonstrates a markedly decreased caliber of the internal carotid, which could represent dissection or hypoplasia (D). Axial computed tomographic image of the skull base shows a hypoplastic right carotid canal, confirming the diagnosis of congenital hypoplasia (E).**

Agenesis of the internal carotid artery is total absence of the entire length of the artery, and aplasia occurs when a vestige or portion remains. Aplasia of the internal carotid artery may be unilateral or, rarely, bilateral and is occasionally associated with intracranial aneurysms. According to Cali et al, 62 cases of bilateral internal carotid artery agenesis have been reported since 1913. Aplasia and agenesis of the internal carotid arteries are most often discovered accidentally. Generally, the collateral circulation around the circle of Willis compensates for the congenital anomaly. The main differential of the appearance of the small internal carotid artery on MRA would be severe atherosclerosis at the origin of the internal carotid or carotid dissection. Evaluation of the bony carotid canal by computed tomography allows for distinction of acquired internal carotid pathology, such as dissection from congenital aplasia. With congenital aplasia or agenesis, the canal is small or absent but appears of normal size with the acquired pathology. Quint et al reported on four patients with carotid canal under development that was found on computed tomographic images; two of these patients had circle of Willis aneurysms. Quint et al advocates further evaluation of the intracranial circulation if asymmetry of the bony canals is found. Certainly, MRA would be a useful noninvasive modality in this circumstance.

#### REFERENCES


Lie TA: Congenital anomalies of the carotid arteries. In VanGorcum R, ed: *Excerpta medica,* The Netherlands, 1968.

Breidahl WH, Khangure MS: Case report: MRI diagnosis of congenital absence of the internal carotid artery, *Clin Radiol* 42:354-355, 1990.

Kawai K, Takahashi H, Ikuta F et al: Bilateral hypoplastic internal carotid arteries with multiple cerebral aneurysms, *Clin Neuropathol* 8(6):272-275, 1989.

Cali RL, Berg R, Rama K: Bilateral internal carotid artery agenesis: a case study and review of the literature, *Surgery* 113:227-233, 1993.

Quint DJ, Silbergleit R, Young WC: Absence of the carotid canals at skull base CT, *Radiology* 182:477-481, 1992.

## CASE 29
## ABERRANT INTERNAL CAROTID ARTERY

**History:** 40-year-old with pulsitile tinnitus.

**Technique:** axial volume, three-dimensional time-of-flight, 39/8/15, 512 × 256, 64 slices, 60-mm slab, 22-cm field of view, 10:42.

A

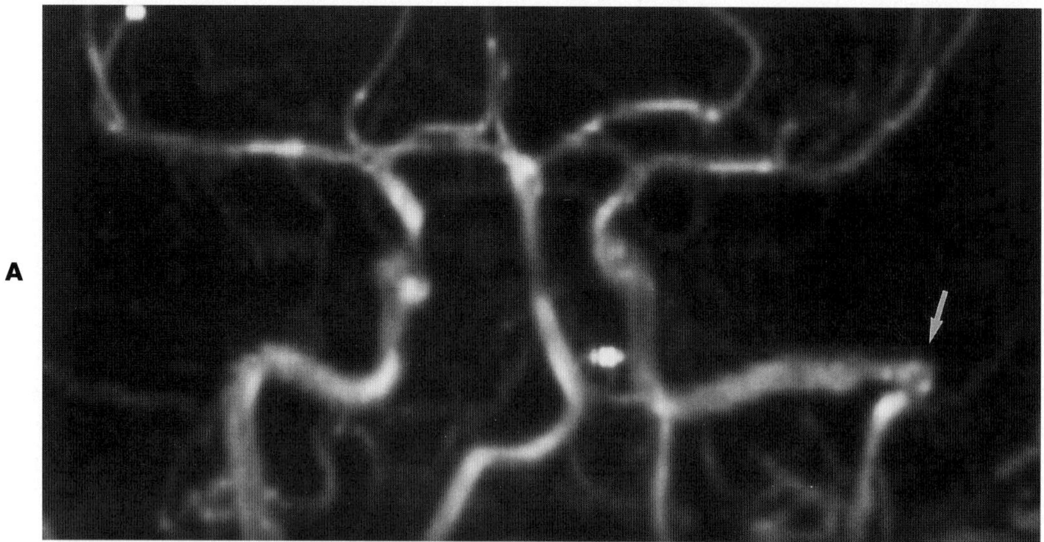

B

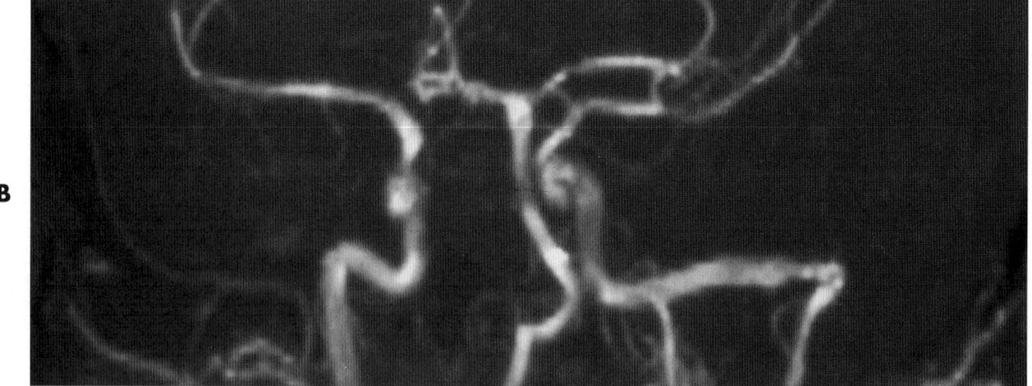

**Anteroposterior (A) and oblique (B) maximum intensity projection views of the MRA data set show an abnormal angulation of the left petrous internal carotid artery, which is more laterally placed than usual *(arrow)* compared with the right internal carotid artery, which is running its normal course. (The dot of high signal in the center of the images is artifact.)**

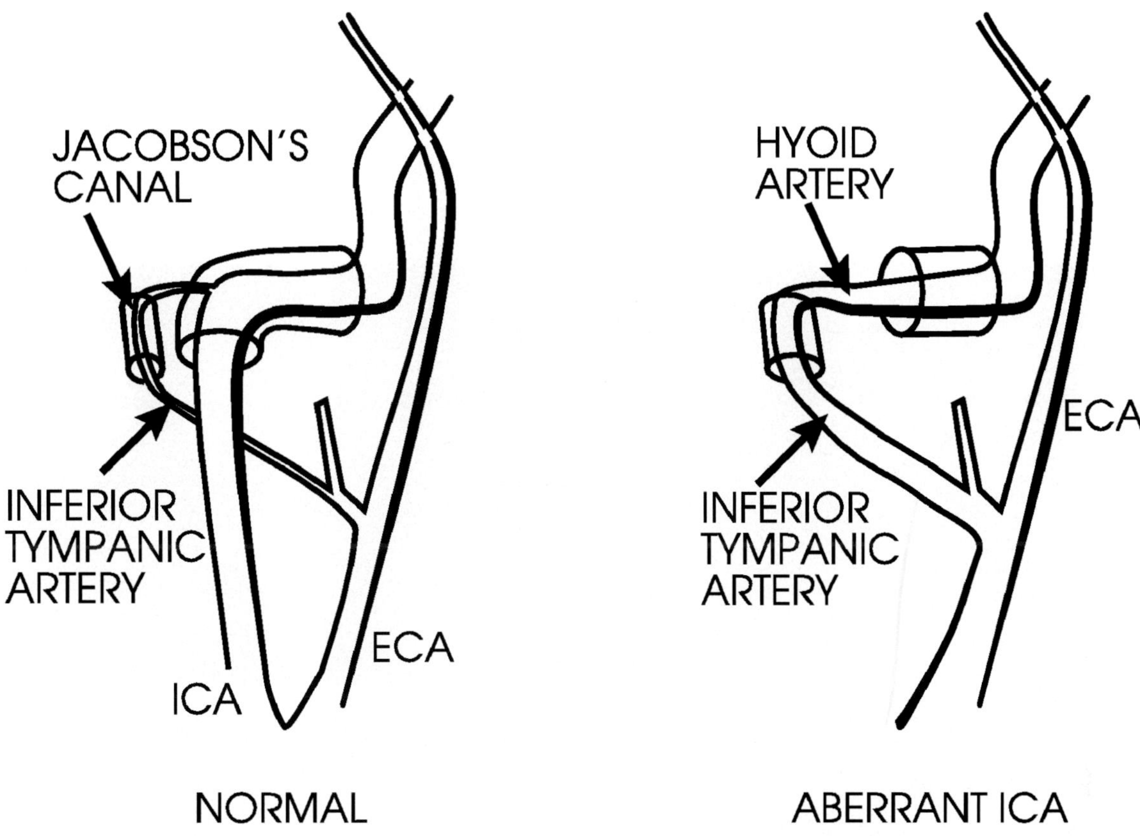


**Schematic of normal and aberrant internal carotid arteries.**

The normally placed internal carotid artery ascends vertically medial and anterior to the middle ear cavity before bending sharply anteriorly and medially below the eustachian tube and cochlea. It passes through the carotid canal into the cranial cavity. Although pinpoint dehiscence of the internal carotid artery may be present in 1% of the population, the incidence of significant congenital bony defects is probably much less than 1%. The abnormality of the internal carotid artery per se is absence of its vertical segment, with the blood supply reaching the horizontal segment via the inferior tympanic and caroticotympanic arteries. This anomalous, narrowed vessel passes into the hypotympanum via the inferior tympanic cannuliculus before joining the horizontal portion. Thus the aberrant internal carotid artery is located anteriorly in the middle ear and presents as a pulsatile mass. Patients may have pulsatile tinnitus, conductive hearing loss, and otalgia.

Computed tomography typically shows absence of the vertical carotid canal, dehiscence of the carotid plate through which the artery enters the horizontal carotid canal, and an enhancing tympanic mass. On coronal computed tomographic images, the key feature is presence or absence of a normal septum between the hypotympanum and carotid canal. Conventional angiography shows the aberrant carotid more laterally and posteriorly placed than normal, so it may lie under the promontory in the middle ear. The vertical segment of the internal carotid artery is not seen, and on anteroposterior view, the conventional angiogram demonstrates an abnormal amount of lateral angulation. MRA should be able to replace conventional angiography as the study of choice for evaluation of vascular mass and pulsatile tinnitus when computed tomography cannot provide definitive information regarding the nature of the mass.

## REFERENCES

Glasscock ME, Dickens JRE, Jackson CG, Wiet RJ: Vascular anomalies of the middle ear, *Laryngoscope* 90:77-88, 1980.

Moret J, Delvert JC, Lasjaunias P: Abnormal vessels in the middle ear, *J Neuroradiol* 9:227-236, 1982.

Phelps PD, Lloyd GAS: Vascular masses in the middle ear, *Clin Radiol* 37:359-364, 1986.

Low WM, Solti-Bohman LG, McElveen JT: Aberrant carotid artery: radiologic diagnosis with emphasis on high resolution computed tomography, *Radiographics* 5:985-993, 1985.

Bold EL, Wanamaker HH, Hughes GB et al: Magnetic resonance angiography (MRA) of vascular anomalies of the middle ear, *Laryngoscope* in press, 1994.

Davis WL, Harnsberger HR: MR angiography of an aberrant internal carotid artery, *AJNR* 12:1225, 1991.

Remley KB, Coit WE, Harnsberger HR et al: Pulsatile tinnitus and the vascular tympanic membrane: CT, MT, and angiographic findings, *Radiology* 174:383-389, 1990.

## CASE 30
## INTERNAL CAROTID DOLICHOECTASIA

**History:** 26-year-old with recurrent right-sided headaches and right optic atrophy.

**Technique:** axial volume, three-dimensional time-of-flight, 41/6/15, 160 × 256, 64 slices, 64-mm slab, 20-cm field of view (3/4 rectangular), 7:02

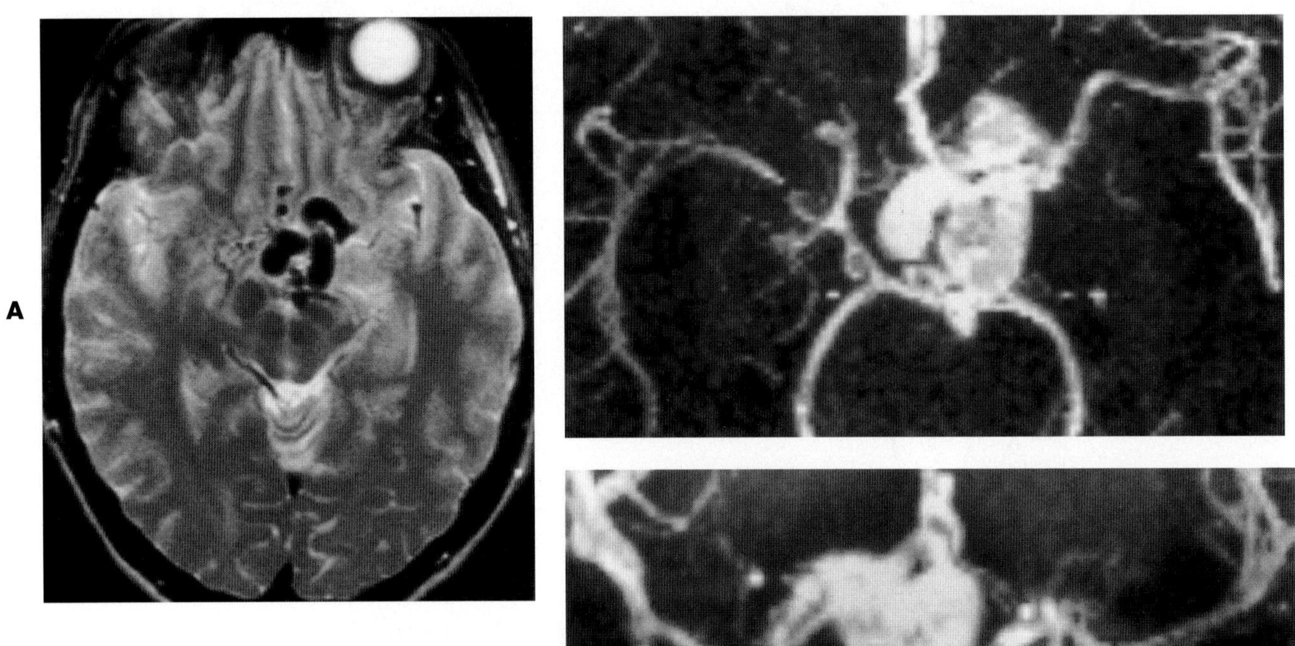

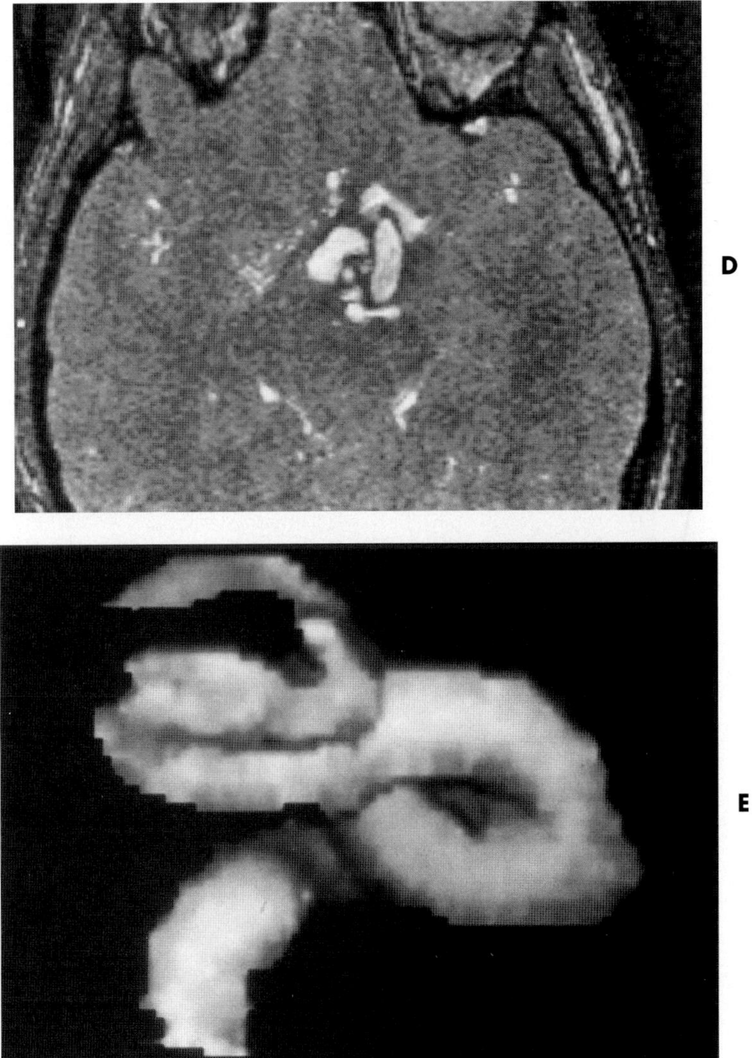


**Axial T2-weighted image shows multiple large areas of flow void centered around the circle of Willis (A). Base and anteroposterior maximum intensity projection views (B and C) and individual slice (D) show a markedly tortuous and fusiformly dilated distal internal carotid artery. This is shown to better advantage on the lateral surface reconstruction of the MRA data set (E). This is presumably congenital in this young woman, with the pressure on the optic apparatus from the massively dilated carotid artery being responsible for the optic atrophy.**

## CASE 31
## FENESTRATION OF THE BASILAR ARTERY

**History:** 44-year-old with chronic headaches.

**Technique:** axial volume, three-dimensional time-of-flight, 40/6/15, 256 × 160 (3/4 rectangular field of view), 64 slices, 60-mm slab, 18-cm field of view, 6:52.

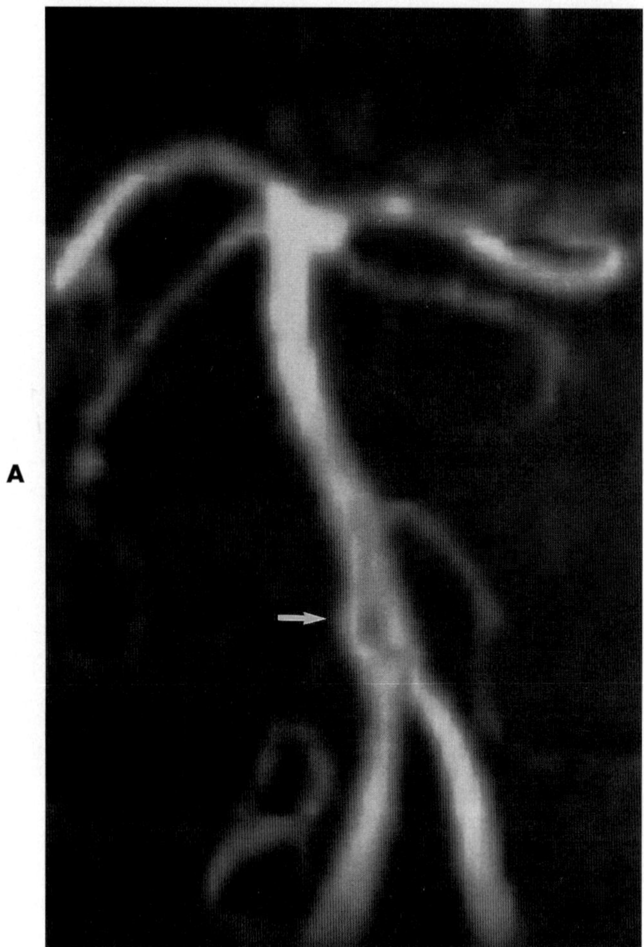

A

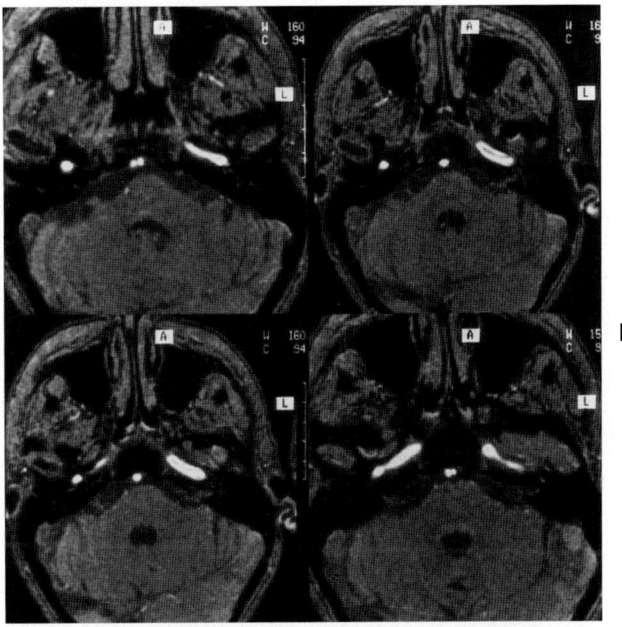

B

**Targeted anteroposterior view (A) shows a focal area of signal loss in the proximal basilar artery, which appears slightly dilated *(arrow)*. The remainder of the study is normal. Individual MRA slices (B) going from inferior *(top left to right)* to superior *(bottom left to right)* show two vertebral arteries joining to form a single basilar artery, which then splits again *(bottom right)*.**

*Fenestration* of the basilar artery refers to a spectrum of congenital anomalies in which there is separation of the vascular lumen into two distinct endothelium-lined channels. The incidence of fenestration is greatest for the vertebral and basilar arteries and more uncommon for the anterior circulation. The angiographic incidence of basilar artery fenestration is reported to be 0.04% to 0.6%. In a review of 5190 angiograms, Sanders et al found an incidence of 0.3%. Case reports have described an association of fenestration of the basilar artery with aneurysms. This has been postulated to occur from a defect in the vessel wall media and altered flow dynamics with turbulence at the proximal end of the fenestration. However, Saunders et al found that the association of a fenestration with an aneurysm at the fenestration site is not different from the typical associations of saccular aneurysms with vessel bifurcations. Fenestrated vessels are very subtle anomalies by current MRA standards of resolution. The identification of fenestration is much more easily made on the individual slices than on the maximum intensity projections.

## REFERENCES

Sanders WP, Sorek PA, Mehta BA: Fenestration of intracranial arteries with special attention to associated aneurysms and other anomalies, *AJNR* 14:675-680, 1993.

Campos J, Fox AJ, Vineula F et al: Saccular aneurysms in basilar artery fenestraion, *AJNR* 8:233-236, 1987.

Teal JS, Rumbaugh CL, Bergeron RT et al: Angiographic demonstration of fenestrations of the intradural intracranial arteries, *Radiology* 106:123-126, 1973.

## CASE 32
## PERINATAL INFARCT WITH DYKE-DAVIDOFF-MASSON SYNDROME

**History:** 16-year-old with severe developmental delay and left hemaparesis.

**Technique:** axial volume; three-dimensional time-of-flight; 45/7/20; 192 × 256; 64 slices; 60-mm slab; magnetization transfer background suppression; tilted, optimized nonsaturating excitation radiofrequency pulse; 14-cm field of view; 9:15.

A

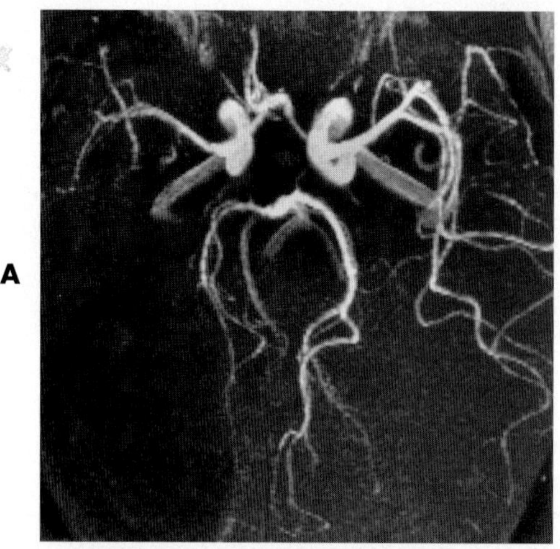

B

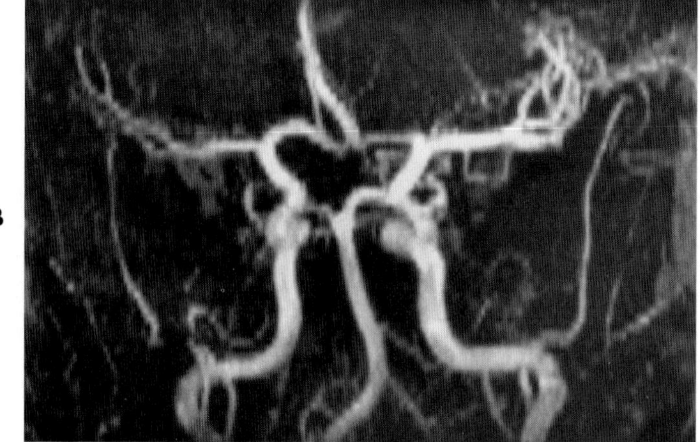

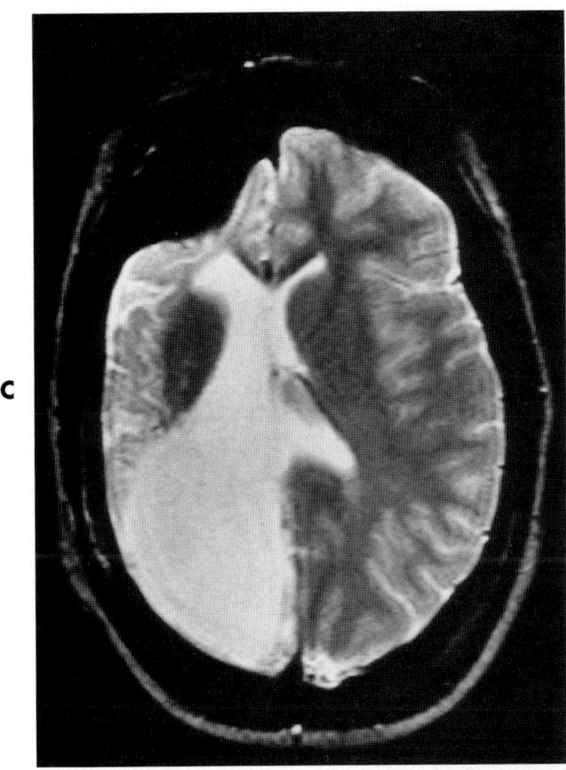

C

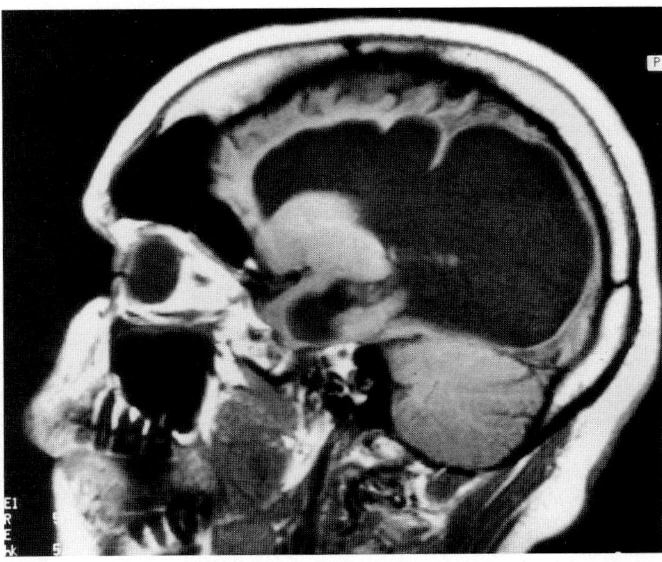

D

**Base (A) and anteroposterior (B) maximum intensity projection MRA views (A and B) show pruning of the distal right middle cerebral and right posterior cerebral branches. Note the small caliber of the right M1 segment compared with that on the normal left side. Axial T2-weighted spin-echo (C) and sagittal T1-weighted spin-echo (D) images show the sequelae of a large right hemispheric infarction with parenchymal volume loss and porencephaly.**

Because of the autopsy of the right hemisphere, there is compensatory dilatation of the right frontal sinus and mastoid aircells (Dyke-Davidoff-Masson syndrome). Thickening of the diploe, which also is part of Dyke-Davidoff-Masson syndrome, is difficult to discern because of the diffuse calvarial thickening related to the anticonvulsant treatment in this case.

**REFERENCES**

Sever RN, Jinkins JR: MR of craniocerebral hemiatrophy, *Clin Imaging* 16(2):93-97, 1992.

Feingold M, Felding J: Dyke-Davidoff-Masson syndrome, *Am J Dis Child* 142(3):304-305, 1988.

## CASE 33
## HYDRANENCEPHALY

**History:** 13-year-old severely disabled child.

**Technique:** axial volume; three-dimensional time-of-flight; 45/7/20; 192 × 256; 64 slices; 80-mm slab; magnetization transfer background suppression; tilted, optimized nonsaturating excitation radiofrequency pulse; 14-cm field of view; 9:15.

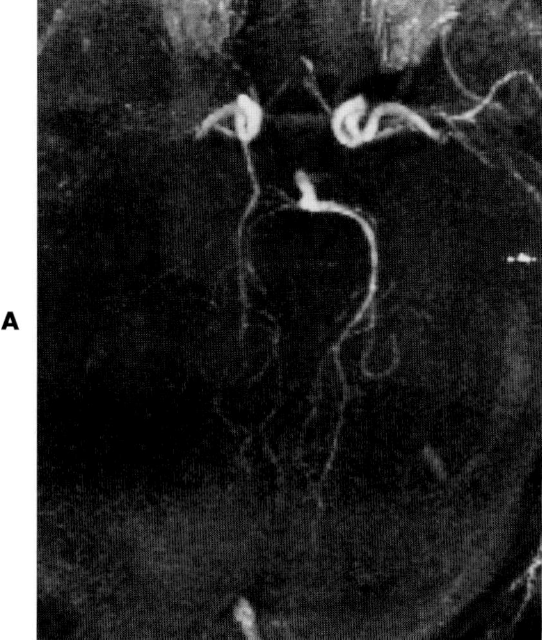

A

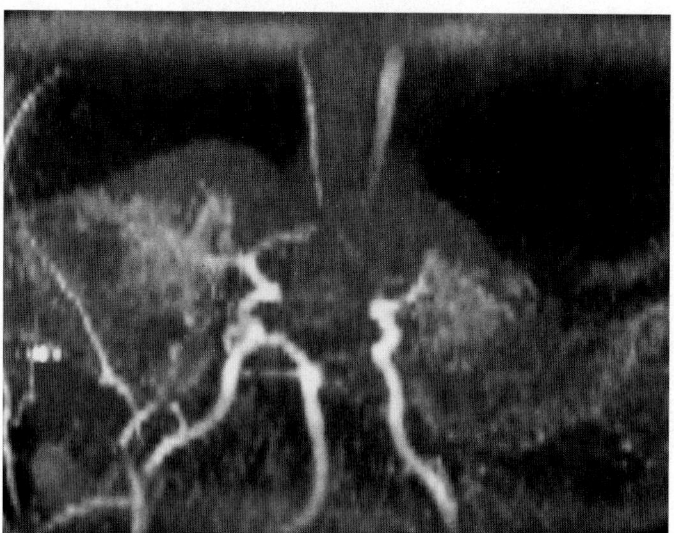

B

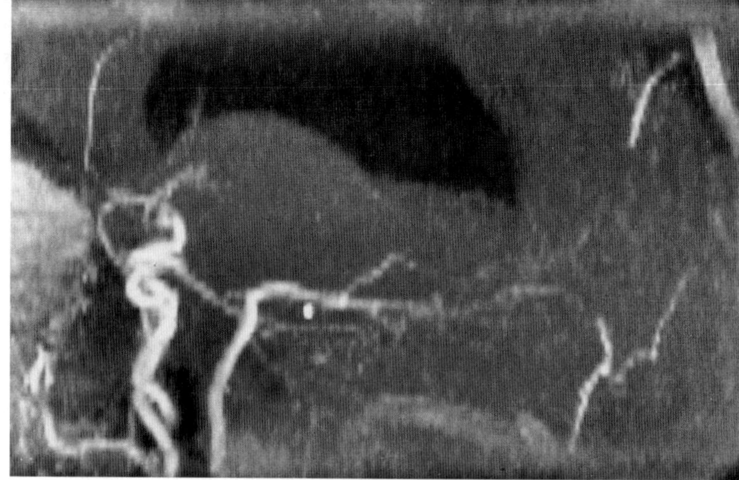

C

D

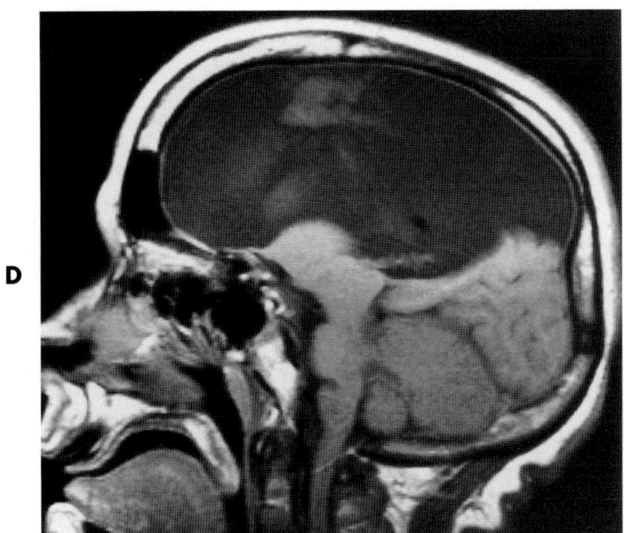

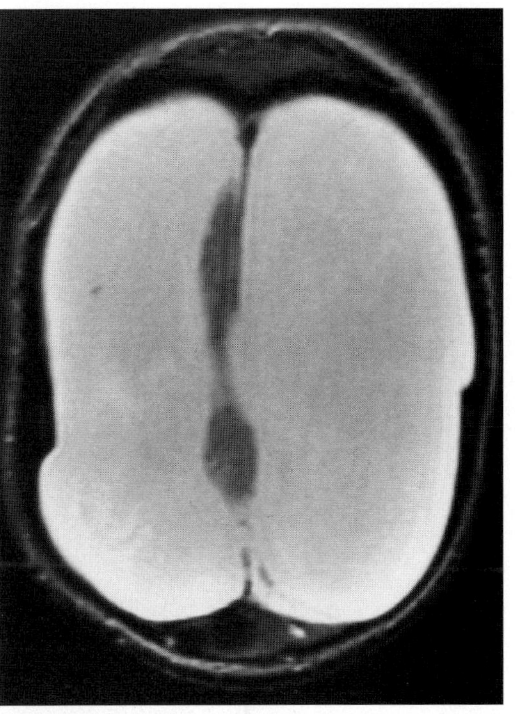

E

**Base (A), anteroposterior (B), and lateral (C) maximum intensity projection views show normal signal from the carotid siphons and basilar arteries. There is almost no visible right middle cerebral or right posterior cerebral vessels and very attenuated left middle cerebral vessels. There is a fetal origin of the right posterior cerebral artery and a relatively normal-appearing left posterior cerebral artery. Sagittal T1-weighted image (D) and axial T2-weighted image (E) show a small amount of brain parenchyma adjacent to a normal falx, with the remainder of the supratentorial space being cerebrospinal fluid.**

The differential diagnosis of this case includes three major entities; hydranencephaly, severe hydrocephalus, and holoprosencephaly. Hydranencephaly is the absence of the majority of the cerebral hemispheres with relatively intact posterior circulation of structures such as the occipital lobes and cerebellum. The remainder of the vault is cerebrospinal fluid that is surrounded by pia arachnoid and that is without glial tissue. These findings most likely represent infarction from occlusion of the supraclinoid internal carotid arteries. This must be distinguished from hydrocephalus, in which neural tissue is present. Holoprosencephaly is excluded in this case by the presence of a normal midline falx. There is a small amount of midline supratentorial brain tissue and some small left middle cerebral branches that might indicate long-standing hydrocephalus. However, the truncated right middle cerebral artery, the normal posterior circulation, and the failure to visualize any brain parenchyma over the convexities strongly indicate hydranencephaly.

**REFERENCE**

Poe LB, Coleman L: MR of hydranencephaly, *AJNR* 10:S61, 1989.

## CASE 34
## STURGE-WEBER SYNDROME

**History:** 14-year-old with seizures and mild left hemaparesis.

**Technique:** two axial volumes, each volume three-dimensional time-of-flight; 45/7/20; 192 × 256; 64 slices; 64-mm slab; magnetization transfer background suppression; tilted, optimized nonsaturating excitation radiofrequency pulse; 18-cm field of view; 9:15.

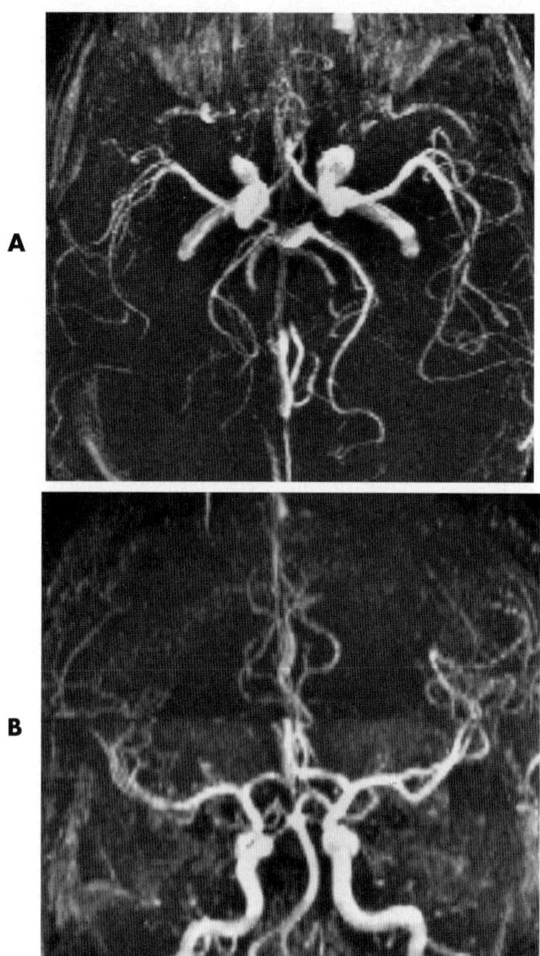

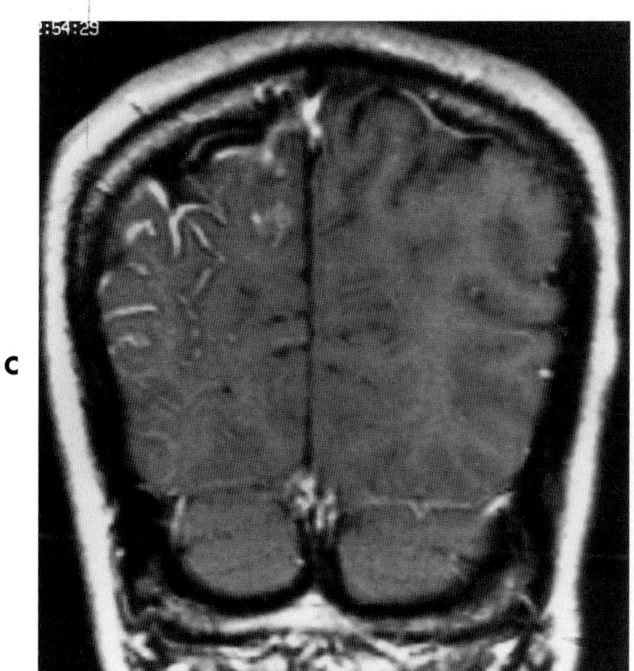


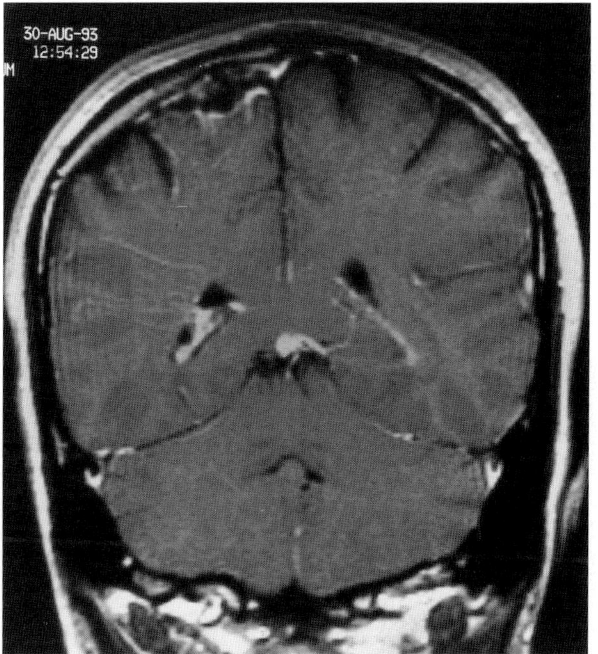


**Base (A) and anteroposterior (B) maximum intensity projection views of an unenhanced three-dimensional time-of-flight MRA show a paucity of distal branches of the right middle cerebral artery. No other abnormality is seen. Coronal T1-weighted spin-echo images after contrast (C) show the gyriform superficial cortical enhancement typical for Sturge-Weber syndrome. Additional coronal T1-weighted image more anterior than C shows abnormally prominent draining medullary veins (D).**

Sturge-Weber syndrome is a phakomatosis classically described by the clinical findings of trigeminal port-wine nevus, seizures, retardation, hemiparesis, and glaucoma. Seizures affect up to 90% of these patients. The imaging features are necessary related to the central nervous system vascular abnormalities seen in Sturge-Weber syndrome: leptomeningeal angiomatosis, abnormal or decreased cortical venous drainage, prominent deep venous drainage, and choroid plexus angiomatous involvement producing enlargement. The typical gyriform calcification may not be visible on MR images, and the diagnosis is established principally by the abnormal enhanced T1-weighted studies. Gyriform enhancement with atrophy, abnormal prominent deep medullary or other draining veins, and enlarged enhancing ipsilateral choroid plexus are typical MR image findings. Time-of-flight MRA for the arterial system may reveal a decreased caliber of the middle cerebral artery branches and pruning of the distal vessels as shown in this case. MR venography with a two-dimensional time-of-flight or phase-contrast technique may show abnormal venous drainage centrally, since there are decreased cortical veins with Sturge-Weber syndrome.

**REFERENCES**

Vogl TJ, Stemmler J, Bergman C et al: MR and MR angiography of Sturge-Weber Syndrome, *AJNR* 14:417-425, 1993.

Benedikt RA, Brown DC, Walker R et al: Sturge-Weber syndrome: cranial MR imaging with Gd-DTPA, *AJNR* 14:409-415, 1993.

Bentson JR, Wilson GH, Newton TH: Cerebral venous drainage pattern of the Sturge-Weber syndrome, *Radiology* 101:111 118, 1971.

## CASE 35
## OCCIPITAL ENCEPHALOCELE

**History:** newborn with occipital mass.

**Technique #1:** oblique coronal, two-dimensional time-of-flight, 30/7.7/30 degrees, 256 × 128, acquired posterior to anterior, 23-cm field of view, 4:20.

**Technique #2:** oblique sagittal, two-dimensional phase-contrast, 38/12.7/30, velocity encoding of 20 cm/sec, 256 × 128, 20-cm field of view, 8:24.

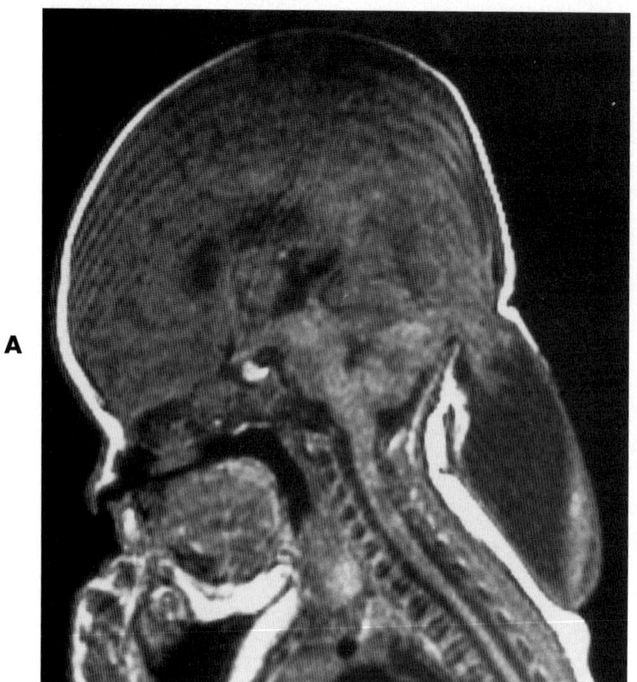

A

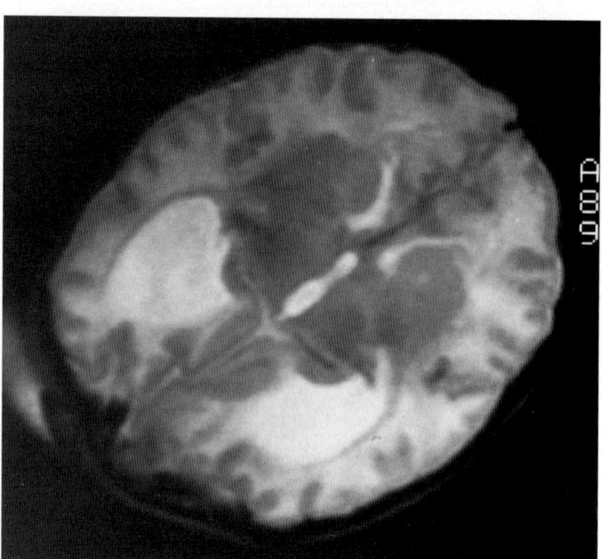

B

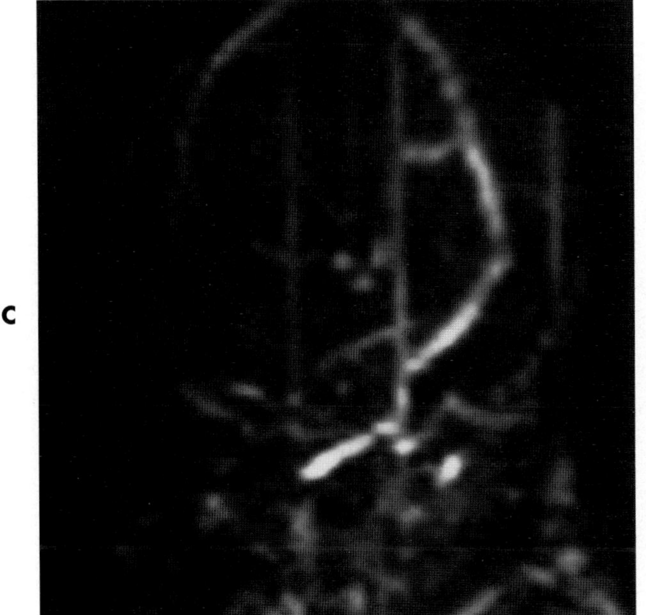

C

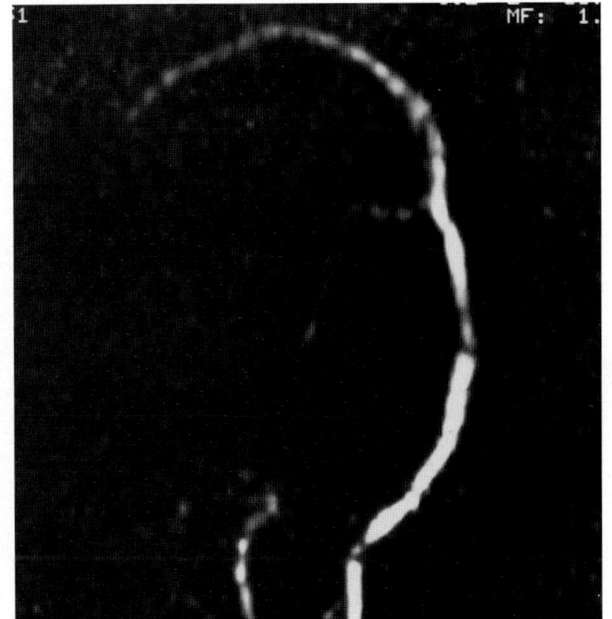


D

Evaluation of this 1-day-old infant with the sagittal T1-weighted image (A) and axial T2-weighted image (B) shows a large occipital encephalocele with a small amount of brain parenchyma herniating into the posterior bony defect. Note the flow void and spatial misregistration of the sagittal sinus to the right of the defect on the T2-weighted study. Lateral maximum intensity projection view of the two-dimensional time-of-flight MR venogram (C) shows a patent superior sagittal sinus that extends not into, but rather around the bony defect of the encephalocele. There is an abnormally high insertion of the straight sinus that is poorly visualized. Overall image quality is degraded by slight patient motion artifact and high signal intensity fat projecting into the maximum intensity projection image. The two-dimensional phase-contrast venogram (D) shows excellent background suppression and better delineation of the venous anatomy compared with the two-dimensional time-of-flight study. Again, note the high insertion of the straight sinus.

# CHAPTER 4

# Aneurysms

Intracranial aneurysm rupture is a disastrous event. Approximately 50% of these people die immediately on rupture, with 50% of the survivors dying within the following 3 days. Half of the remaining patients are left with a permanent neurologic deficit. The proper imaging evaluation of acute subarachnoid hemorrhage is unenhanced computed tomographic scanning followed by conventional intraarterial angiography to define the number and location of aneurysms as well as aneurysm morphology, neck and any associated vasospasm. MRA has a role in the evaluation of symptoms that may be explained by many possibilities, including aneurysm, in the screening of aneurysms in populations at high risk for developing aneurysms, and and in the occasional cases in which the morphology of the aneurysm is unclear even after conventional angiography. The identification of aneurysms on MRA demands meticulous attention to technique, including the evaluation of targeted or limited maximum intensity projections, individual slices, and multiplanar reformats of the original data. A spin-echo study of the brain is also necessary to evaluate for parenchymal sequelae such as infarct, hemorrhage, or edema. The spin-echo study also provides information on portions of large aneurysms, such as the thrombosed area, that may be invisible to the conventional digital subtraction angiography and MRA techniques.

The prevalence of incidental aneurysms in autopsy series is variable and inconsistent, ranging from 1.3% to 7.9%.[1,2] Studies that quote a few autopsy series with high incidences of aneurysms suggest that aneurysms are abundant in the population as a whole and that only a few rupture, making the role of surgical management of incidentally discovered aneurysms unclear. However, a recent report found that the incidence of asymptomatic aneurysms of the anterior circulation was much closer to 1%, making their identification of major clinical significance.[3] That is, the decreased incidence of aneurysms, coupled with the known rate of life-threatening subarachnoid hemorrhage, dramatically increases the risk of having an asymptomatic aneurysm rupture. Although the resolution of MRA does not approach that of conventional arteriography, this does not appear to be a critical shortcoming, since studies suggest that the aneurysms most likely to rupture are of a size that can be easily imaged with MRA. In particular, Locksley[4] and McCormick and Acosta-Rua[5] found no hemorrhages from aneurysms smaller than 3 mm. Current MRA techniques can easily identify aneurysms in that size range, with an in-plane resolution of the gradient-echo technique of less than 0.7 mm. The use of MRA is increased by coupling the technique to that of conventional MR imaging of the brain parenchyma, with less than 15 minutes increase in examination time.

A few retrospective studies have been conducted to test the accuracy of a three-dimensional time-of-flight MRA technique for the detection of intracranial aneurysms compared with intra-arterial digital subtraction angiograms.[6-8] Aneurysms as small as 2 to 4 mm have been detected using a three-dimensional time-of-flight technique. In a series of 21 angiographically confirmed aneurysms in 19 patients, it was demonstrated that there is an incremental increase in sensitivity of 67% when evaluating the MRA images alone compared with a sensitivity of 86% when the MRA images were evaluated using the individual axial slices of the original three-dimensional data set and the spin-echo images. When the maximum intensity projection, individual slices, and spin-echo study are used, the sensitivity would be 95% for the detection of at least one aneurysm; as a result, the study would lead to a traditional angiographic examination.

These studies have shown that there are several limitations and potential pitfalls in the evaluation of the intracranial circulation for aneurysms with MRA using the *three-dimensional Fourier transform time-of-flight* method.

1. The morphology of smaller aneurysms and their relationship to the parent vessel is more accurately reproduced than that of larger aneurysms (those greater than 1 cm). Larger aneurysms or those compressing the parent vessel may reduce the extent of inflow and washout of fresh unsaturated spins within the aneurysm lumen, which gives an apparent reduction of the aneurysm's dimension.[8] This is not a large problem on phase-contrast MRA studies, in which the velocity encoding can be set to enhance the signal from slow flow.
2. The presence of thrombus may provide a variation in the signal intensity within the aneurysm on time-of-

flight MRA images. With an acute or chronic thrombus, the periphery of the aneurysm may not be visible. More typically, subacute thrombus containing hyperintense extracellular methemoglobin is present, causing the periphery of the aneurysm to have a lower signal intensity on the reconstructed MRA images.[9] The residual lumen of the aneurysm is more intensely "opacified" by flow-related enhancement. In giant intracranial aneurysms, thrombus may fill the entire lumen. Such pitfalls are more of a problem with the time-of-flight techniques than with the phase-contrast methods. Nevertheless, larger aneurysms are generally visible on the routine spin-echo images because of the contained blood products, central flow void, and local mass effect.[9] The true aneurysm dimensions can generally be assessed by correlating the individual slices from the MRA data set and/or the multiplanar reconstructions of the original MRA data with the spin-echo images. Similarly, although existing maximum intensity projection software allows the vessels to be viewed from any angle around the three orthogonal axes, some programs do not allow a simultaneous combination of two rotations. Consequently, situations may arise in which the aneurysm neck is not clearly identified in the MRA images, even though the overall relationship to the parent vessel is visible. In most cases, evaluation of the individual slices (partitions) and multiplanar reconstructions of the three-dimensional-data are mandatory for complete evaluation and maximum diagnostic confidence. If vessel overlap presents a problem, it is possible to perform selective MRA studies by using appropriately placed saturation pulses or, more simply, by reconstructing a smaller portion of the overall three-dimensional-volume to eliminate other vascular territories. An additional advantage of this last maneuver is that it reduces the artifacts inherent to the reconstruction with the maximum intensity projection algorithm.

3. Although it is somewhat controversial, conventional MR does not appear to detect acute subarachnoid blood with an adequate degree of sensitivity in this population.[10] In addition, the unstable condition of patients with subarachnoid hemorrhage generally preclude an MR evaluation because of patient motion. If the patient has experienced a sentinel hemorrhage, there may be a component of vascular spasm that could reduce inflow into the aneurysm or even cause thrombosis of the aneurysm lumen. Any substance with a significantly short T1 or high spin density appears bright on the original MRA acquisition and is recognized by the reconstruction program. If the methemoglobin of the subarachnoid hemorrhage surrounds or is superimposed on an aneurysm in a given projection, that aneurysm may not be visualized, or it may be poorly visualized.
4. Identifying the relationship of the aneurysm to the parent vessel may be a problem if the aneurysm arises from an arterial segment that is incompletely seen secondary to motion-induced dephasing. The ability to define carotid siphon pathology is problematic because of significant motion-induced dephasing even on state-of-the-art, quality intracranial MRA. The anterior communicating artery, middle cerebral artery bifurcation, and basilar tip are generally well defined. Signal dropout of varying degrees of severity is a ubiquitous finding within the carotid siphon. Coupled with the anatomic variations of the siphon course, this probably accounts for the majority of missed aneurysms. In particular, if the cephalocaudal height of the siphon is small, the loops tend to merge into one another on the MRA, and the distinction between normal and aneurysmal dilatation may be very difficult.[10,11] A potential solution is the incorporation of shorter echo times and smaller voxels, which should significantly reduce the phase dispersion and signal loss in these problematic vascular segments, which are related to higher-order motion terms and local field inhomogeneities, and to use the information of the individual slices and reformats.[12,13]
5. Volume time-of-flight gradient-echo techniques provide a limited region of interest for intracranial imaging. Imaging the vasculature of the entire head requires at least 128 slices covering 120 to 150 mm. Even with very short TRs, the length of the examination becomes prohibitive at 20 minutes. However, this limited field is generally not a significant problem for the evaluation of aneurysms; in fact, the vast majority of aneurysms are centered about the circle of Willis. Locksley[4] found approximately 10% of single aneurysms involved with subarachnoid hemorrhage in more peripheral branches or within the cerebellar vessels.

## REFERENCES


1. Housepian EM, Pool JL: A systematic analysis of intra-cranial aneurysms from the autopsy file of the Presbyterian Hospital, *J Neuropathol Exp Neurol* 17:409-423, 1958.
2. McCormick WF: *Problems and pathogenesis of intracranial arterial aneurysms.* In Toole JF, Moossy J, Janeway R, eds: *Cerebrovascular disorders,* ed 2, New York, 1971, Grune & Stratton.
3. Atkinson JLD, Sundt TM, Houser OW, Whisnant JP: Angiographic frequency of anterior circulation intracranial aneurysms, *J Neurosurg* 70:551-555, 1989.
4. Locksley HB: *Natural history of subarachnoid hemorrhage, intracranial aneurysms, and arteriovenous malformations: based on 6,368 cases in the Cooperative Study.* In Sahs AL, Perret GE, Locksley HB et al, eds: *Intracranial aneurysms and subarachnoid hemorrhage: a Cooperative Study,* Philadelphia, 1969, Lippincott.
5. McCormick WF, Acosta-Rua GJ: The size of intracranial saccular aneurysms: an autopsy study, *J Neurosurg* 33:422-427, 1970.
6. Masaryk TJ, Modic, MT, Ross JS et al: Intracranial circulation: preliminary clinical results with three-dimensional (volume) MR angiography, *Radiology* 171:793-799, 1989.
7. Ross JS, Masaryk TJ, Modic MT et al: Intracranial aneurysms: evaluation by MR angiography, *AJNR* 11:449-456, 1990.

8. Sevick RJ, Tsuruda JS, Schmalbrock P: Three-dimensional time-of-flight MR angiography in the evaluation of cerebral aneurysms, *JCAT* 14:874-881, 1990.
9. Atlas SW, Grossman RI, Goldberg HI et al: Partially thrombosed giant intracranial aneurysms: correlation of MR and pathologic findings, *Radiology* 162:111-114, 1987.
10. Bradley WG, Schmidt PG: Effect of methemoglobin formation on the MR appearance of subarachnoid hemorrhage, *Radiology* 156:99-104, 1985.
11. Kassell NF, Torner JC, Haley EC et al: The international cooperative study on the timing of aneurysm surgery. I. Overall management results, *J Neurosurg* 73:18-36, 1990.
12. Haacke EM, Masaryk TJ, Wielopolski PA et al: Optimizing blood vessel contrast in fast three-dimensional MRI, *Magn Reson Med* 14:202-221, 1990.
13. Schmalbrock P, Yuan C, Chakeres DW et al: Volume MR angiography: methods to achieve very short echo times, *Radiology* 175:861-865, 1990.

## CASE 36
## PITFALL: TORTUOUS SIPHON

**History:** 55-year-old evaluated for possible vertebrobasilar insufficiency.

**Technique:** axial volume, three-dimensional time-of-flight, 40/7/15, 256 × 160, 64 slices, 60-mm slab, 20-cm field of view, 6:52.

A

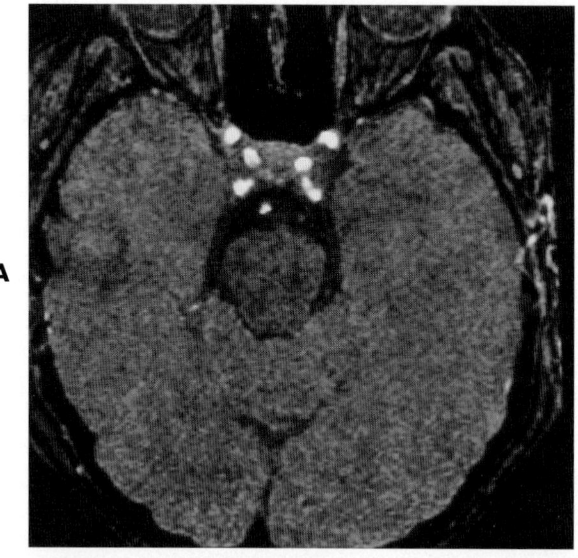

B

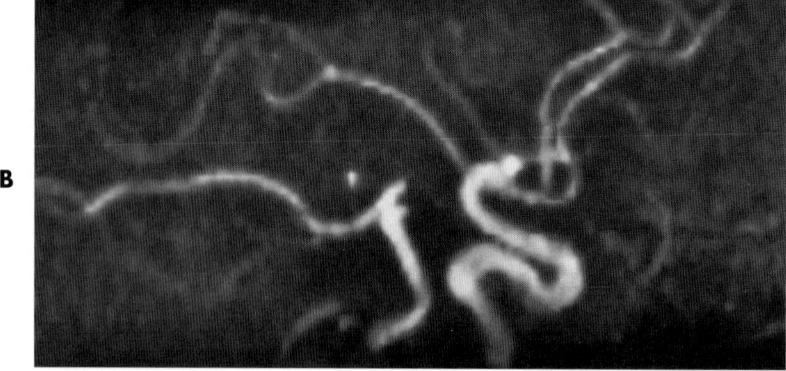

**The individual slice from the MRA data set (A) is confusing, since there are three separate areas of signal intensity from both carotid siphons. The most posterior rounded areas of increased signal could represent posterior communicating aneurysms bilaterally. Evaluation of the targeted maximum intensity projection of the right siphon (B) shows that the cause of the separate signals is from the different loops of a tortuous siphon, as shown schematically in C.**

---

The positioning of the slices with an axially oriented volume through a tortuous siphon can produce multiple separate areas of rounded signal intensity, which must be differentiated from aneurysms. Reformatting of the volume data into the sagittal or coronal planes or targeted maximum intensity projection views will solve this potential area of confusion.

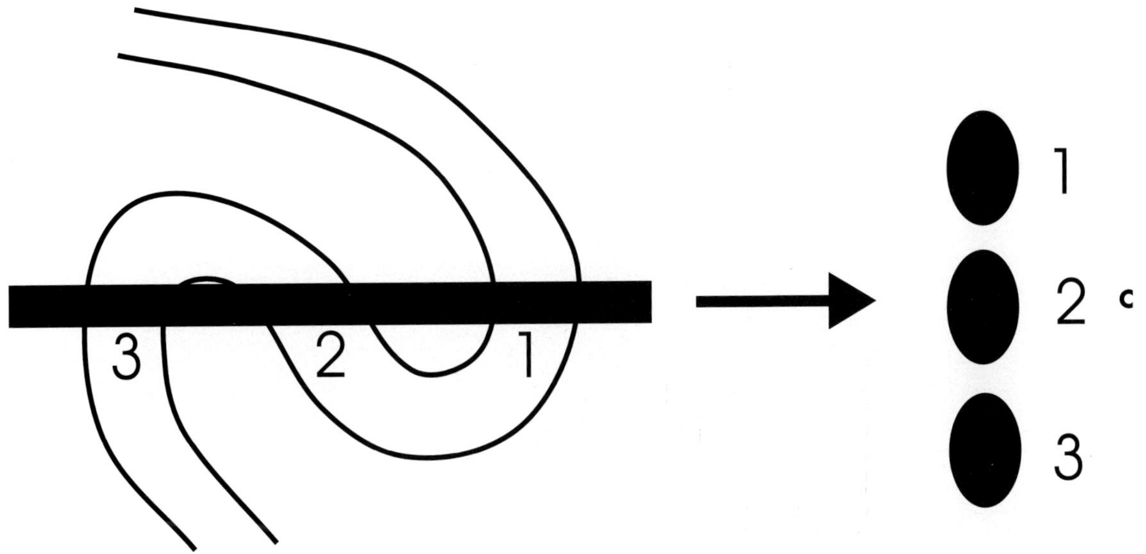


LATERAL VIEW OF SIPHON

MRA INDIVIDUAL SLICE VIEW

**Schematic of tortuous loop causing multiple areas of increased signal on individual axial slices (C). The lateral view of the carotid siphon *(left)*, through which an axial slice is projected *(black line)*, shows multiple areas of increased signal on the axial MRA slices *(right)*.**

## CASE 37
## PITFALL: SUBDURAL HEMATOMA

**History:** 70-year-old with headache and confusion.

**Technique:** axial volume, three-dimensional time-of-flight, 45/7/20, 256 × 128, 60 slices, 60-mm slab, 18-cm field of view, 6:09.

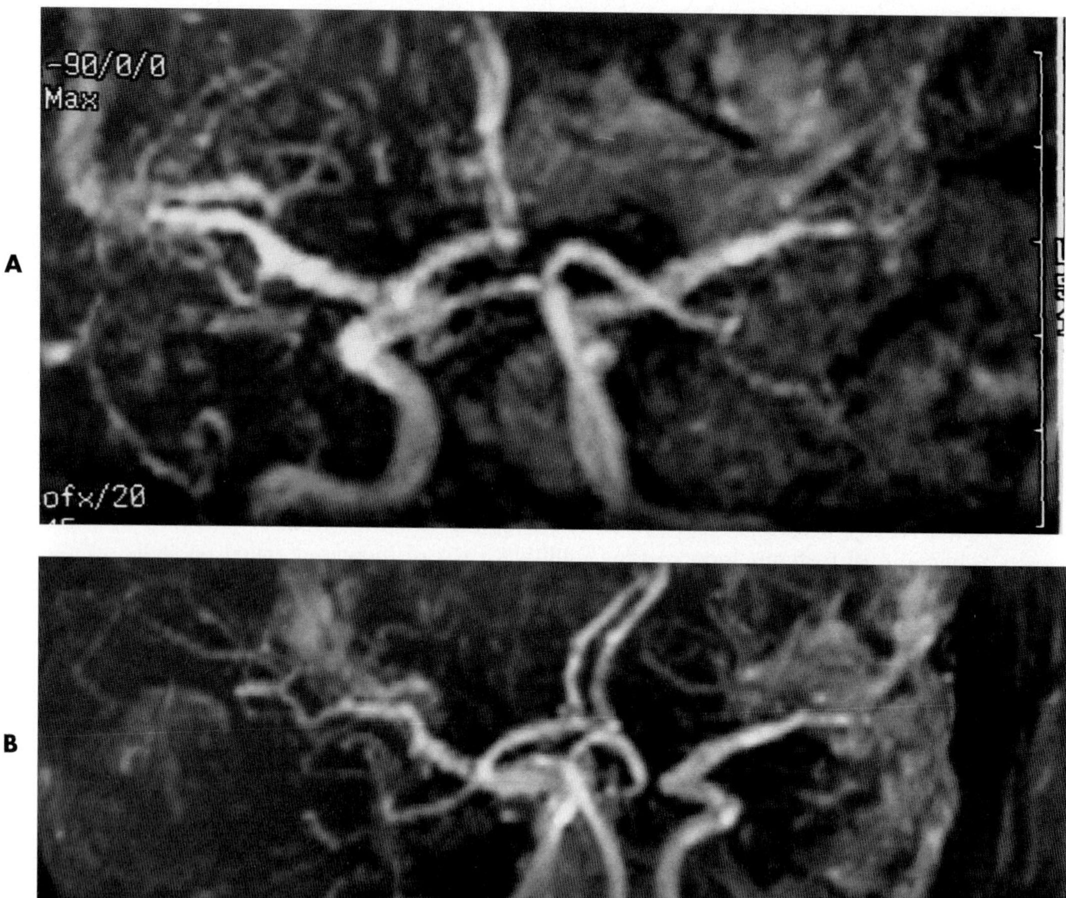


**Anteroposterior (A) and oblique (B) maximum intensity projection views demonstrate a globular increased signal intensity over the left and right intracranial circulations. The left-sided abnormality is much more prominent than the right. T1-weighted axial spin-echo image (C) of the brain shows linear and globular increased signal in the extra axial space over both convexities, representing bilateral subdural hematomas (methemoglobin).**

---

The maximum intensity projection allows for background suppression in time-of-flight MRA and gives a pseudo-N-three-dimensional appearance of the images. However, several inherent limitations of the technique must be recognized. One of the limitations illustrated in this case includes the inability to distinguish various causes of increased signal intensity, such as flow and hemorrhage, on the T1-weighted images. Both flow and hemorrhage have increased signal on the maximum intensity projection views and must be separated by comparing them with other pulse sequences or by performing phase-contrast MRA.

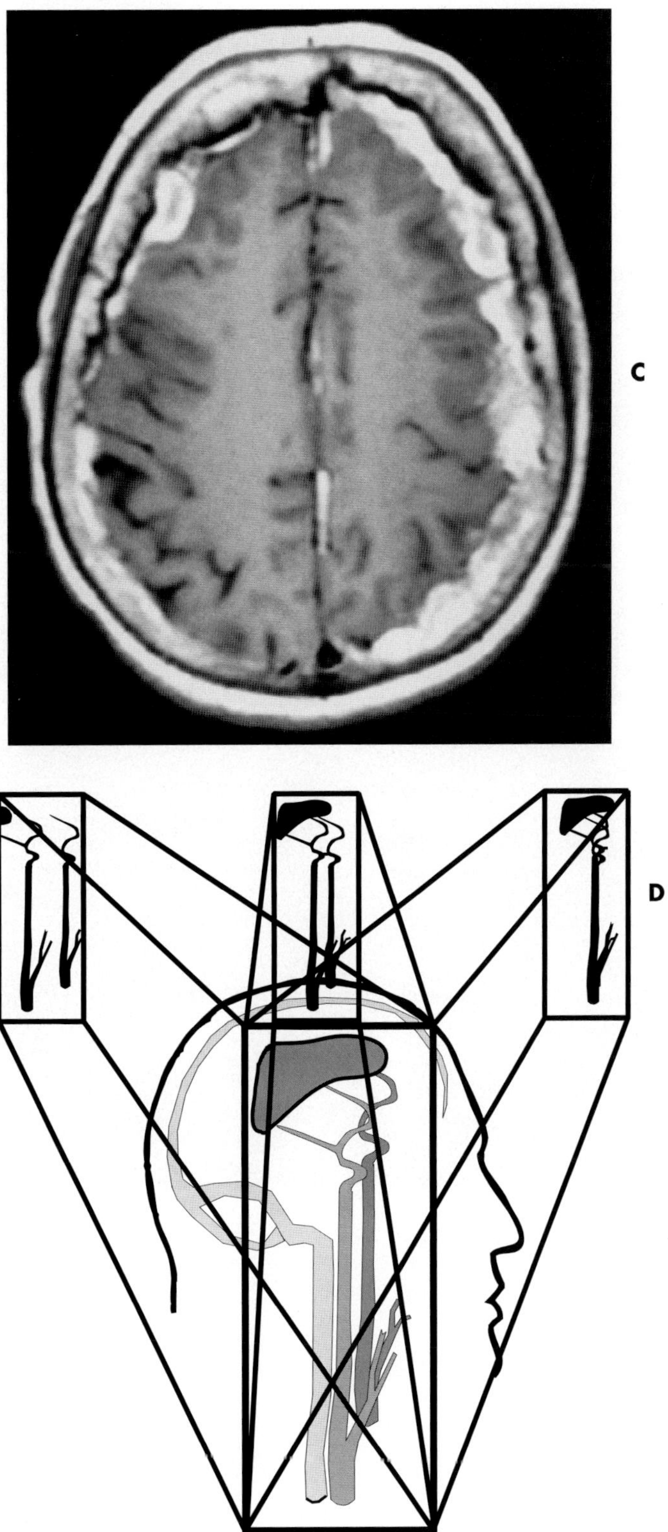


**Three different maximum intensity projections are depicted in this case of a head and neck MRA with a subdural hematoma (D). The high signal intensity methemoglobin appears as increased signal on time-of-flight MRAs related to the sequences' relative T1 weighting.**

## CASE 38
## PITFALL: CONCHA BULLOSA MUCOCELE

**History:** 44-year-old with ataxic gait.

**Technique:** axial volume, three-dimensional time-of-flight, 45/8/20, 256 × 256, 64 slices, 60-mm slab, 15-cm field of view, 12:19.

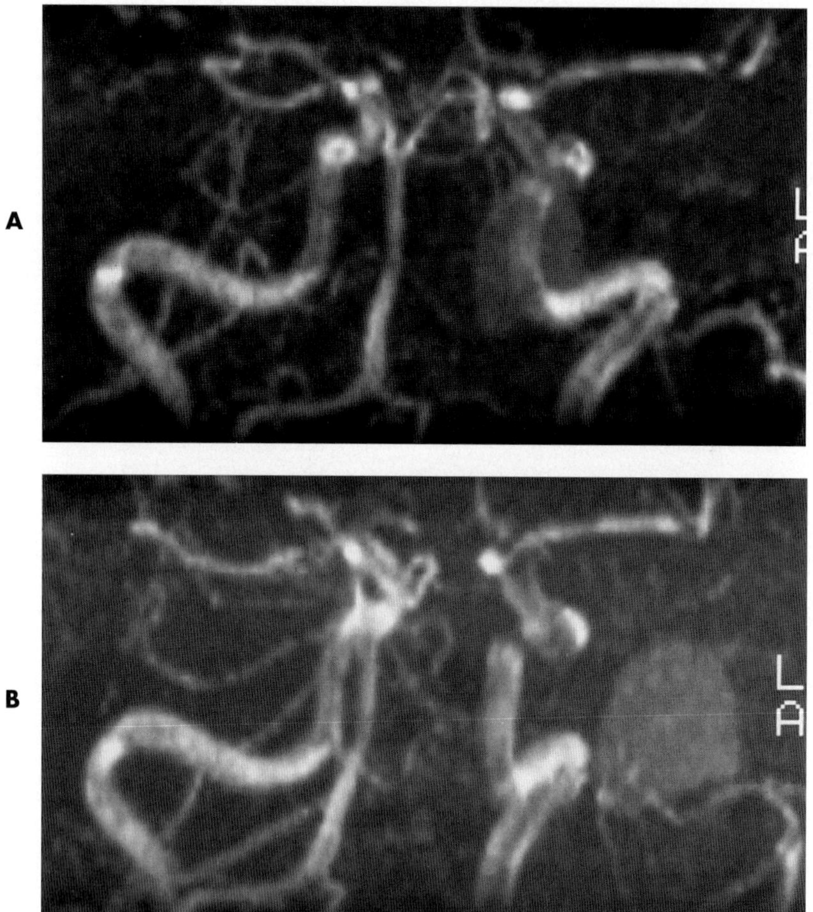

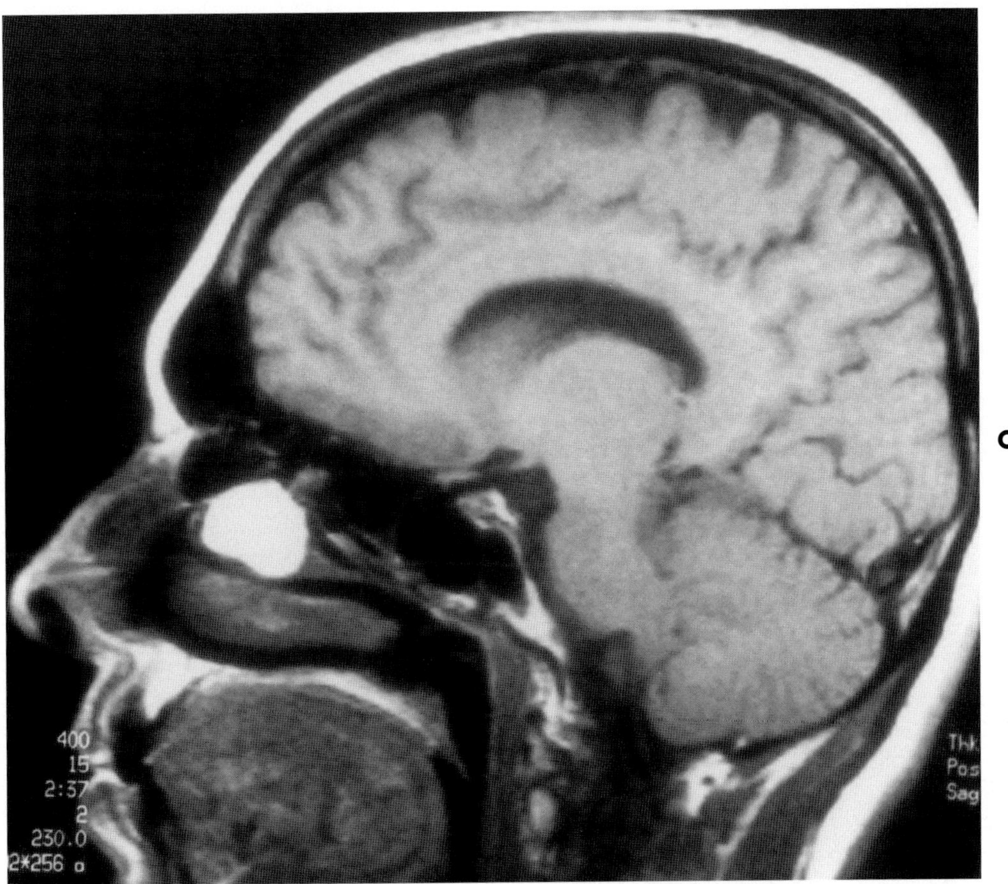


**The anteroposterior view of the maximum intensity projection (A) demonstrates a rounded area of increased signal intensity that projects over the left distal internal carotid artery. On this single view, this could be mistaken for an aneurysm. However, the oblique view (B) demonstrates that this area of increased signal intensity rotates off the carotid and is anterior to the intracranial vasculature. In this instance, the rounded area of increased signal intensity on the maximum intensity projection views relates to the shortened T1 within the chronic secretions of a concha bullosa mucocele, seen on the T1-weighted spin-echo sagittal sequence (C).**

The increased protein content of the secretions within the mucocele contributes to T1 shortening and thus the high signal intensity on T1. The maximum intensity projection postprocessing algorithm does not discriminate between high signal intensity occurring from flow and that occurring from other causes of T1 shortening.

**REFERENCES**

Anderson CM, Saloner D, Tsuruda JS et al: Artifacts in maximum-intensity-projection display of MR angiograms, *AJR* 154:623-629, 1990.

Tsuruda J, Saloner D, Norman D: Artifacts associated with MR neuroangiography, *AJNR* 13:1411-1422, 1992.

Som PM, Dillon W, Fullerton GD et al: Chronically obstructed sinonasal secretions: observations on T1 and T2 shortening, *Radiology* 172:515-520, 1989.

## CASE 39
## PITFALL: FRONTAL SINUS MUCOCELE

**History:** 40-year-old with headaches.

**Technique:** axial volume, three-dimensional time-of-flight, 40/7/15 degrees, 256 × 256, 64 slices, 60-mm slab, 25-cm field of view, 10:57.

A

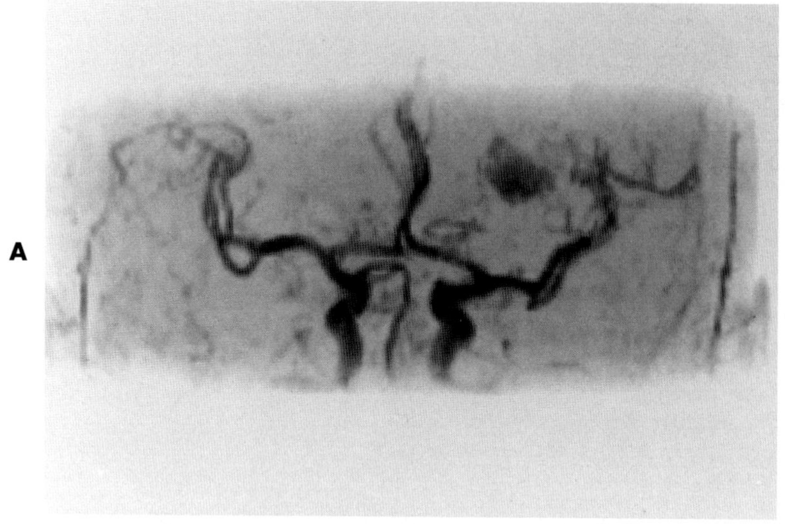

B

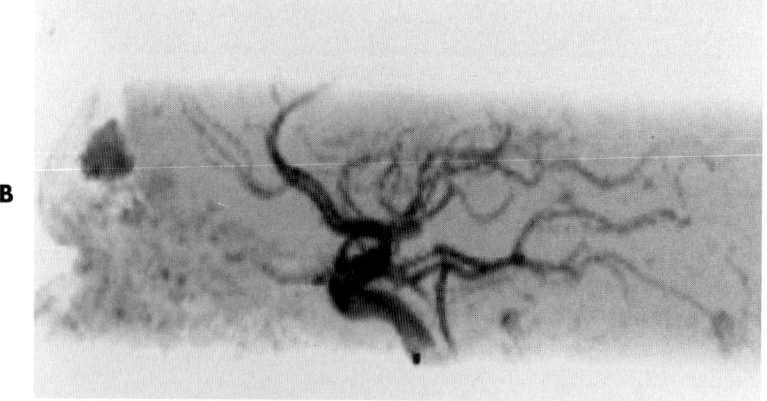

**The anteroposterior (A) and lateral (B) views of the maximum intensity projection demonstrate an ill-defined area of high signal intensity between the distal branches of the left middle and anterior cerebral arteries. Evaluation of the individual slice from the volume three-dimensional time-of-flight angiogram (C) shows that the high signal intensity resides within the left side of the left frontal sinus and represents a small mucocele with inspissated secretions.**

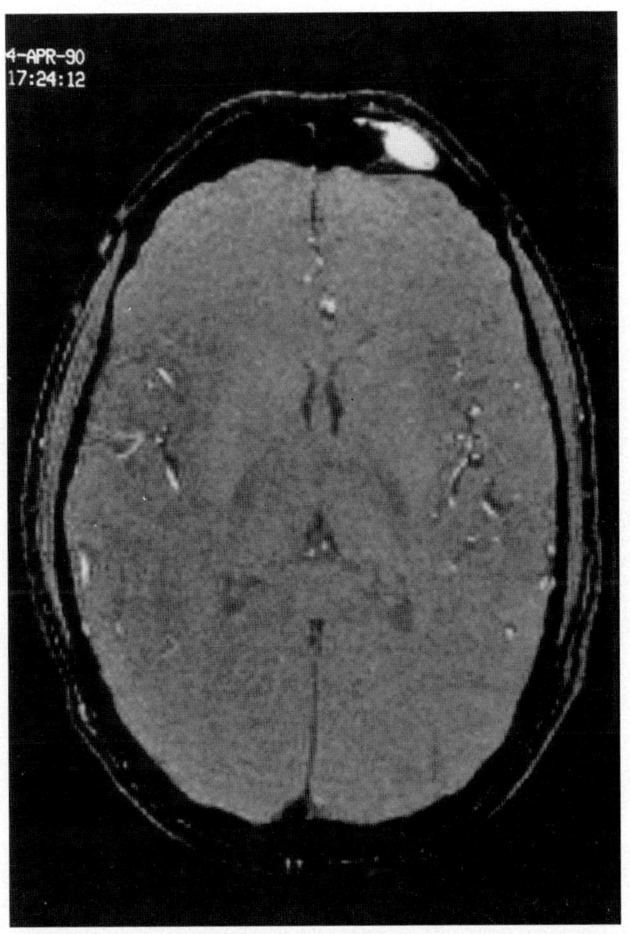


C

This is another example of the failure of maximum intensity projection postprocessing to discriminate between various causes of high signal intensity on T1-weighted images. Thus high signal intensity from flowing blood, hemorrhage (both intracranial and extracranial), protein, and other causes of T1 shortening show up similarly on the maximum intensity projection views.

Som et al have described the signal intensity changes that can occur with chronically obstructed sinonasal secretions on MR images. With obstruction of a sinus, there is an increase in the concentration of macromolecular glycoproteins, an increase in viscosity of the secretions, and a decrease in the free water content of the secretions. With the increase in protein concentration, there is a decrease in the T1 and T2 relaxation times, which accounts for the variable appearance of obstructed sinuses and mucoceles. The decreasing relaxation times are due to the greater contribution to the signal from the bound and structured protons (hydration layer) as the amount of free water decreases. Som et al concluded that an increase in protein concentration from 5% to 25% was sufficient to cause high signal intensity on T1-weighted images. Above a concentration of 25%, the T1 and T2 signal intensities decrease.

**REFERENCES**

Som PM, Dillon W, Fullerton GD et al: Chronically obstructed sinonasal secretions: observations on T1 and T2 shortening, *Radiology* 172:515-520, 1989.

Dillon WP, Som PM, Fullerton GD: Hypointense MR signal in chronically inspissated sinonasal secretions, *Radiology* 174:73-78, 1990.

## CASE 40
## PITFALL: PETROUS APEX CHOLESTEROL GRANULOMA

**History:** 37-year-old with polycystic kidney disease being screened for intracranial aneurysms.

**Technique:** axial volume, three-dimensional time-of-flight, 40/7/15, 256 × 256, 64 slices, 70-mm slab, 25-cm field of view, 10:57.

A

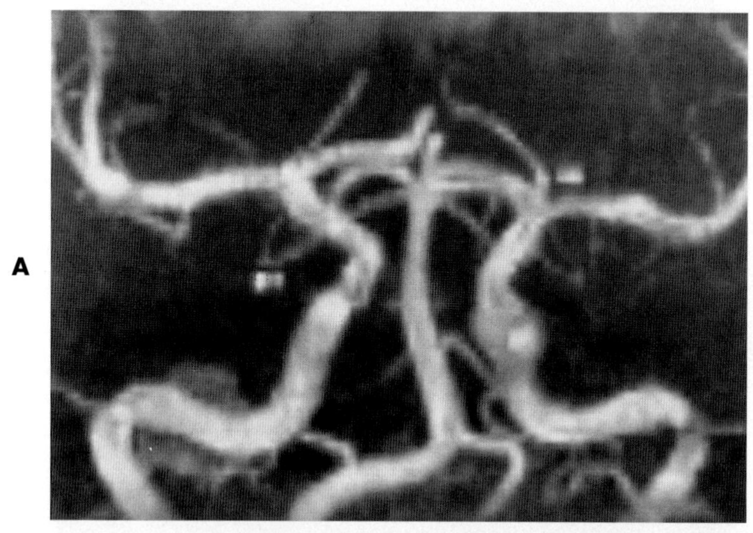

B

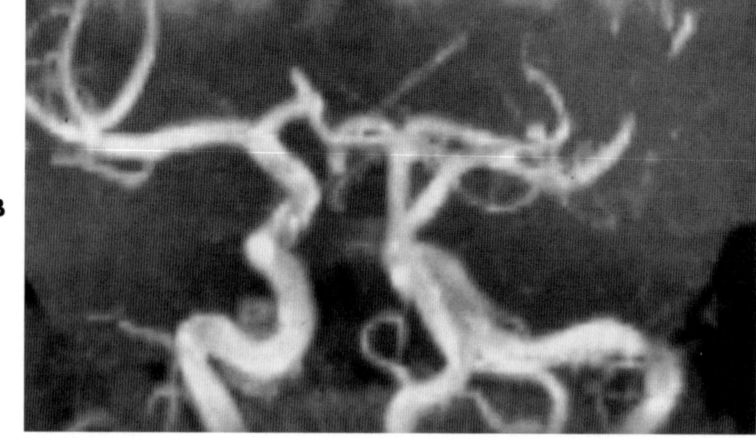

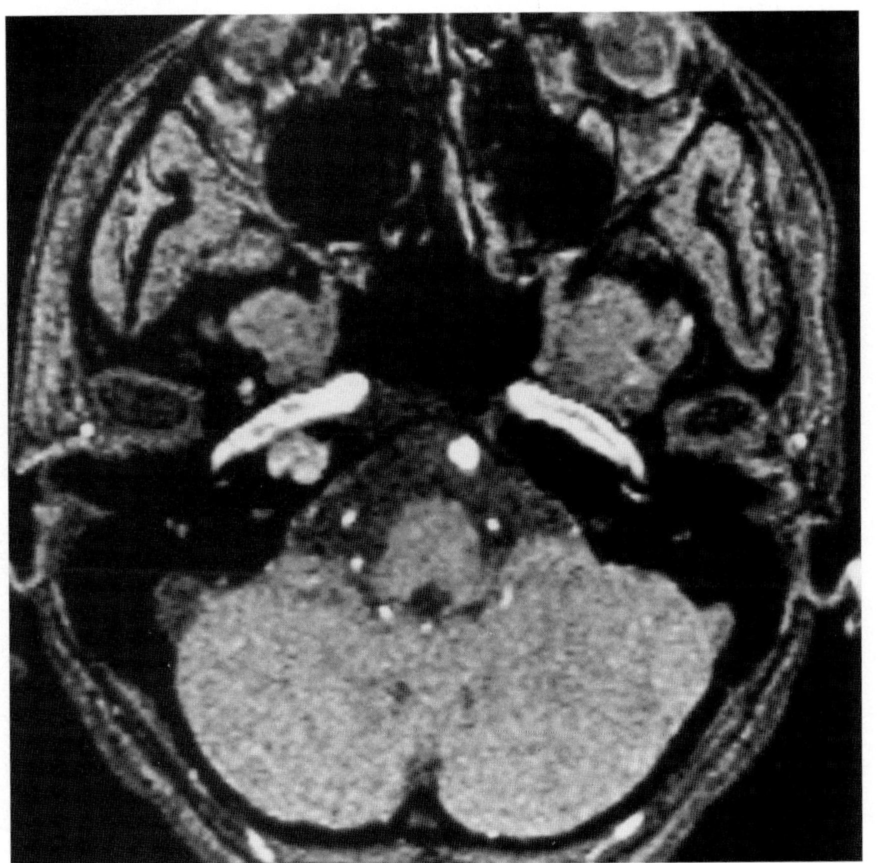


**The anteroposterior (A) and oblique (B) views of the maximum intensity projection demonstrate an ill-defined area of increased signal intensity adjacent to the right petrous carotid artery, which looks suspiciously like a large aneurysm. However, examination of the individual slice from the MRA data (C) shows that the lesion is distinct from the carotid artery and is within the petrous apex, which is typical in signal intensity and position for a petrous apex cholesterol granuloma.**

Petrous apex lesions capable of showing increased signal intensity on T1-weighted images include cholesterol granulomas, cholesteatomas, and mucocele. Cholesterol granulomas are a foreign-body, giant-cell reaction characterized by a fibrous lining; they contain various stages of blood, along with fibrous tissue and cholesterol crystals. They are generally of increased signal on both T1- and T2-weighted images. Other terms used to describe these lesions are *congenital epidermoid cyst* or *giant cholesterol cyst*. The cause of cholesterol cysts is unknown, but one hypothesis is that poor ventilation, interference with drainage, and hemorrhage lead to negative pressure and reabsorption of air, eventually causing a cholesterol cyst. Clinical presentation is by the compression of adjacent structures such as cranial nerves V to VIII, the esutachian tube, and the carotid artery. In their review of 10 cases, Thedinger et al found that headache, diplopia, and dizziness are common presentations. Treatment is generally by drainage and permanent fistulization. Petrous apex cholesteatomas are uncommon but may show increased signal on both T1- and T2-weighted images. Mucoceles of the petrous apex are quite rare. Their signal intensity would presumably be variable, like the signal intensity of mucoceles, because of the variable hydration of the proteinaceous contents.

### REFERENCES


Larson TL, Wong ML: Primary mucocele of the petrous apex: MR appearance, *AJNR* 13:203-204, 1992.

Van Tassel P, Lee Y, Jing B, DePena CA: Mucoceles of the paranasal sinuses: MR imaging with CT correlation, *AJR* 153:407-412, 1989.

Martin N, Sterkers O, Monpoint D et al: Cholesterol granulomas of the middle ear cavities: MR imaging, *Radiology* 172:521-525, 1989.

Thedinger BA, Nadol JB, Montgomery WW et al: Radiographic diagnosis, surgical treatment, and long term follow-up of cholesterol granulomas of the petrous apex, *Laryngoscope* 99:896-907, 1989.

Nagar GT, Vanderveen TS: Cholesterol granulomas involving the temporal bone, *Ann Otol Rhinol Laryngol* 85:204-209, 1976.

Greenberg JJ, Oot RF, Wismer GL et al: Cholesterol granuloma of the petrous apex: MR and CT evaluation, *AJNR* 9:1205-1214, 1988.

# CASE 41
# PITFALL: POSTERIOR PITUITARY

**History:** 15-year-old with minor head trauma.

**Technique:** axial volume, three-dimensional time-of-flight, 45/7/20, 256 × 256, 64 slices, 60-mm slab, 14-cm field of view, 12:20.

A

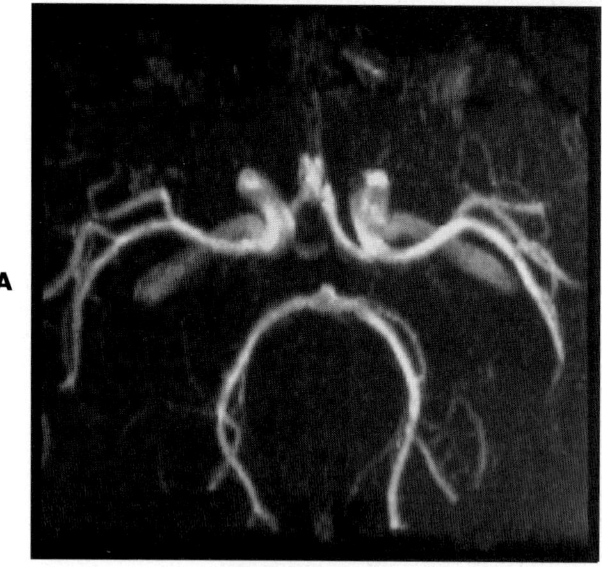

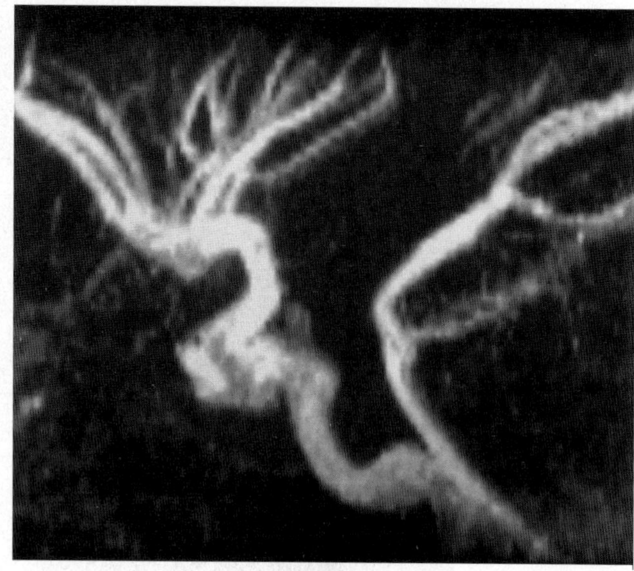

B

C

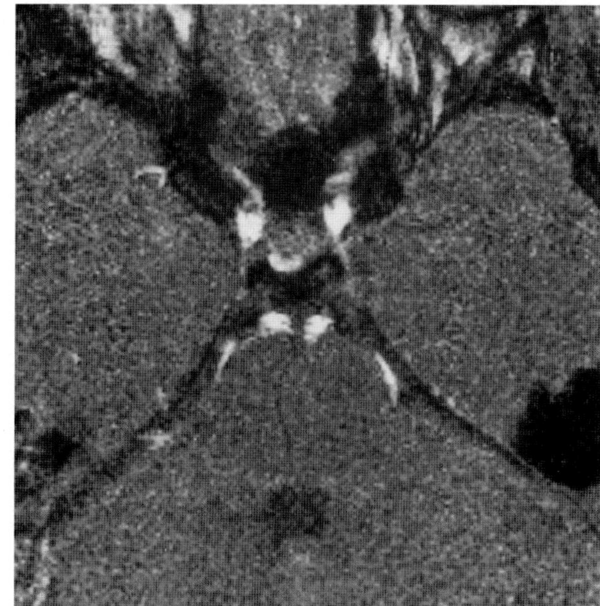

D

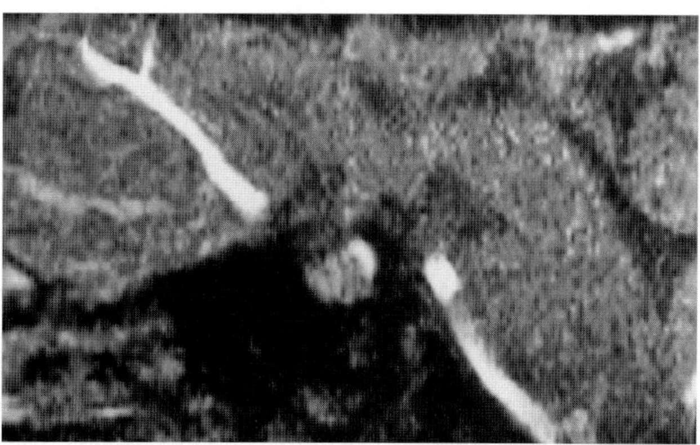

**Base (A) and lateral (B) maximum intensity projection views show a rounded area of increased signal intensity adjacent to the right cavernous carotid, which looks suspiciously like an aneurysm. However, the base angulation shows that the signal is cresent shaped and concave anteriorly, as is the normal posterior pituitary. An individual slice from the MRA data set (C) shows that the high signal intensity from the posterior pituitary between the internal carotid arteries is responsible for the maximum intensity projection signal. Sagittal reformatting of the MRA data (D) also shows the high signal intensity from the posterior pituitary and the high signal from blood flow in the anterior cerebral and basilar arteries.**

The characteristic shape and positioning of the high signal intensity allows for distinction of the normal posterior pituitary bright spot from high signal intensity pathology such as blood or flow.

The source of the signal intensity in the posterior pituitary lobe is a controversial subject. Theories that seek to explain this region of increased signal include phospholipid vesicles in the posterior lobe, lipid in pituicytes of the posterior lobe, neurosecretory granules, and peripituitary fat. Mark et al found that in the vast majority of cases the high signal intensity posterior pituitary did not suppress fat, excluding the signal coming from sellar fat or fat in the dorsum sellae.

**REFERENCES**

Mark LP, Haughton VM, Hendrix LE et al: High-intensity signals within the posterior pituitary fossa: a study with fat-suppression MR techniques, *AJNR* 12:529-532, 1991.

Kucharczyk W, Lenkinski RE, Kucharczyk J, Henkelman RM: The effect of phospholipid vesicles on the NMR relaxation of water: an explanation for the MR appearance of the neurohypophysis? *AJNR* 11:693-700, 1990.

Nishimura K, Fujisawa I, Togashi K et al: Posterior lobe of the pituitary: identification by lack of chemical shift artifact in MR imaging, *JCAT* 10:899-902, 1986.

Kucharczyk J, Kucharczyk W, Berry I et al: Histochemical characterization and functional significance of the posterior pituitary hyperintensity, *AJNR* 9:1079-1083, 1988.

## CASE 42
## PITFALL: INTRACRANIAL HEMORRHAGE OBSCURING AN ANTERIOR COMMUNICATING ARTERY ANEURYSM

**History:** 45-year-old with "worst headache of life."

**Technique:** axial volume, three-dimensional time-of-flight, 40/7/15, 256 × 256, 64 slices, 70-mm slab, 25-cm field of view, 10:57.

A

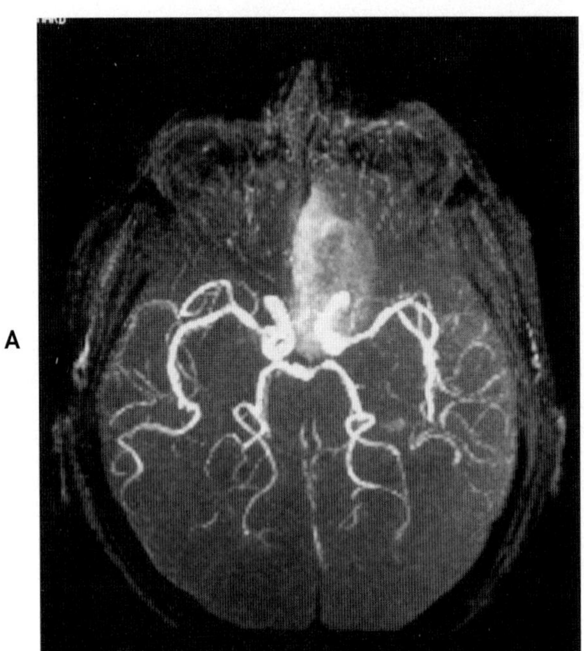

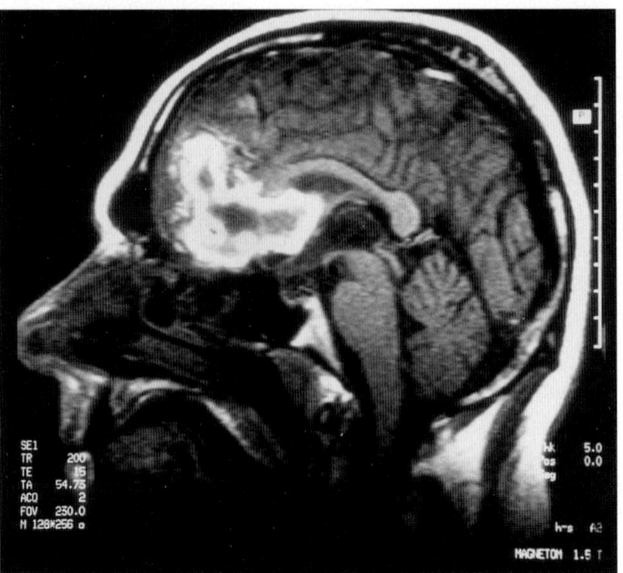


B

C

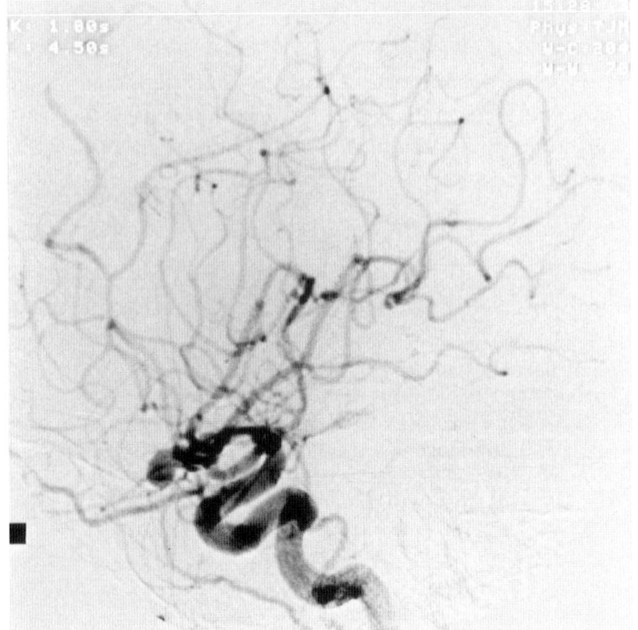

**Base view of the maximum intensity projection (A) shows an irregular area of increased signal intensity involving the interhemispheric fissure. The proximal anterior cerebral arteries are not well visualized. Evaluation of the sagittal T1-weighted spin-echo image (B) shows that there is a large septal and interhemispheric hematoma, demonstrating high signal intensity resulting from the methemoglobin content. Lateral view from a conventional intraarterial angiogram (C) shows a large anterior communicating artery aneurysm that is not visible on the MRA. (From Ruggier P, Masaryk T, Ross JS, Modic M: *Invest Radiol* 27[suppl 2]:*S*33-*S*39, 1992.)**

The maximum intensity projection technique cannot discriminate among various causes of high signal intensity. The septal and interhemispheric hematoma shows up as high signal intensity on the maximum intensity projection views and obscures any high signal intensity that may be arising from the flow within the aneurysm itself. In a similar manner, essentially all of the proximal anterior cerebral artery is obscured, since it is in the region masked by the septal hematoma. For these reasons, time-of-flight MRA is not recommended in the evaluation of patients with acute subarachnoid hemorrhage. In this case, high signal intensity within the subarachoid space might mask the underlying vascular abnormalities. Phase-contrast MRA does not have this problem, since that technique is sensitive only to flow and not the T1 signal intensity. Nevertheless, patients continue to be evaluated for acute subarachnoid hemorrhage with conventional computed tomographic scanning, lumbar puncture, and conventional intraarterial angiography.

Although acute subarachnoid hemorrhage can be detected by MR imaging, its sensitivity (particularly to small amounts of subarachnoid blood) remains unknown. The signal emitted from blood is related to the oxidative state of hemoglobin and its breakdown products. The environment of cerebrospinal fluid is quite different than that of brain parenchyma, which explains the striking contrast between intraaxial and extraaxial hemorrhages. In acute subarachnoid hemorrhage there is very slight T1 shortening of cerebrospinal fluid, which results in slight increases in signal intensity on the short repetition time–echo time images. It takes several days for a significant amount of deoxyhemoglobin to convert to methemoglobin, resulting in obvious increased signal intensity in short repetition time–echo time images. This is probably related to the high oxygen tension in cerebrospinal fluid (versus that of a typical intraparenchymal hematoma). Since there is ongoing resorption of red blood cells from cerebrospinal fluid, MR visualization of small subarachnoid hemorrhages may be impossible. Thus computed tomography remains the diagnostic test of choice for acute subarachnoid hemorrhage. MR imaging can elegantly detect the complications of subarachnoid hemorrhage, specifically ischemia, infarction, and hemosiderosis.

Although MR imaging is not sensitive to small, acute subarachnoid hemorrhages, it more easily demonstrates larger subarachnoid hemorrhages or a small parenchymal hematoma adjacent to an aneurysm. This may be important with multiple cerebral aneurysms when one has ruptured and in which there are no angiographic or computed tomographic findings to suggest the location of the aneurysm rupture. (See Case 52 for further discussion of subarachnoid hemorrhage.)

**REFERENCES**

Bradley WG Jr, Schmidt PG: Effect of methemoglobin formation on the MR appearance of subarachnoid hemorrhage, *Radiology* 156:99-103, 1985.

Hackney DB, Lesnick JE, Zimmerman RA et al: MR identification of bleeding site in subarachnoid hemorrhage with multiple intracranial aneurysms, *JCAT* 10(5):878-880, 1986.

Stone JL, Crowell RM, Gandhi YN, Jafar JJ: Multiple intracranial aneurysms: magnetic resonance imaging for determination of the site of rupture—report of a case, *Neurosurgery* 23(2):97-100, 1988.

## CASE 43
## PITFALL: MISREGISTRATION ARTIFACT IN ANTERIOR LIMB OF CAROTID SIPHONS

**History:** 47-year-old with left-sided numbness.

**Technique:** axial volume, three-dimensional time-of-flight, 45/7/20, 256 × 256, 64 slices, 60-mm slab, 14-cm field of view, 12:20.

A

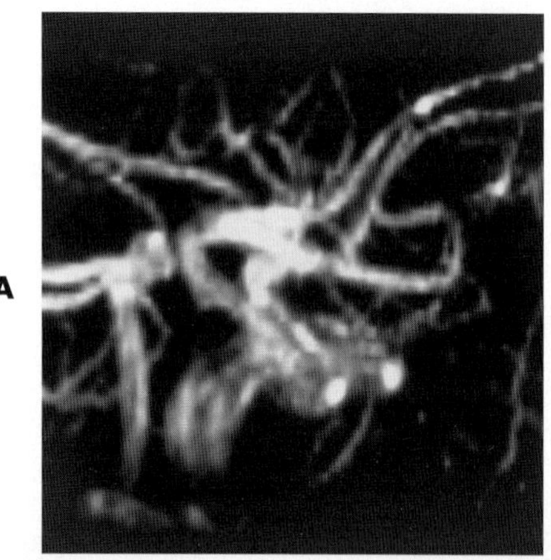

B

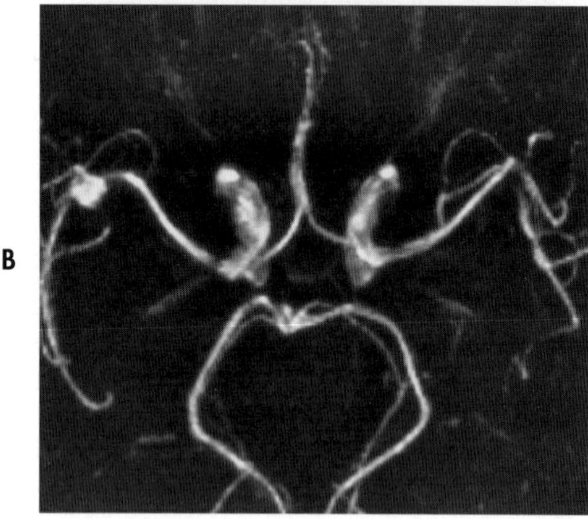

C

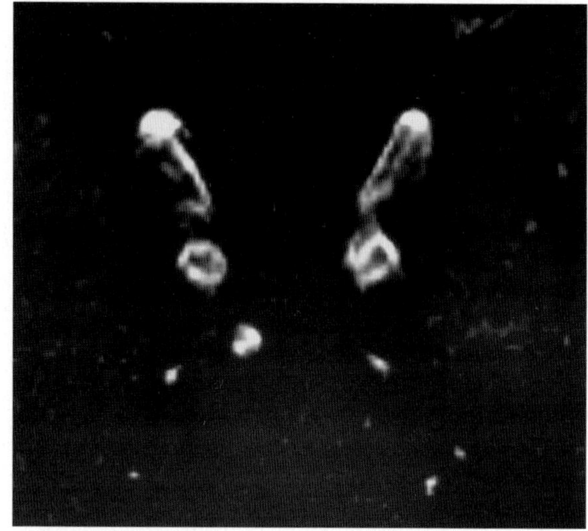

D

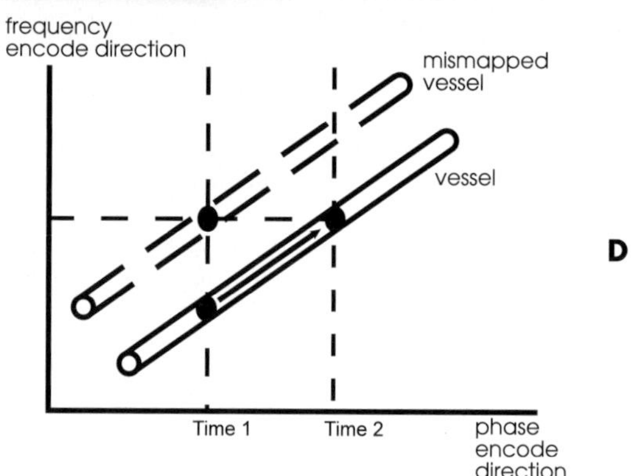


**Oblique and base views of the maximum intensity projection (A and B) show increased signal intensity from the anterior aspect of both siphons. These artifactual globular areas mimicking aneurysms should be differentiated from the globular increased signal from the right middle cerebral bifurcation in this patient, which is an aneurysm. The cause of the carotid siphon bright seen, particulary at the anterior margin of the carotid siphon bend, is artifactual and represents spatial mismapping of flow signal. This increased signal is also shown on the individual slice of the MRA data (C) and with a narrowed window to simulate the appearance on the maximum intensity projection. D shows spatial mismapping. (D redrawn from Larson TC, Kelly WM, Ehman RL, Wekrli FW: *AJNR* 11:1041-1048, 1990.)**

The cause of this mismapping is the interval between the applications of the phase encoding and read gradients during the gradient-echo imaging sequence. Flowing blood is first given a coordinate in space by the phase-encoding gradient. However, when the read gradient is then applied later in the sequence, the flow has moved the position of the spin downstream from its initial starting point **(D).** This mismapping of signal gives a dot (in the case of the carotid siphon, or a line for a length of vessel) that is high in signal intensity because of the summation of signals from adjacent normal parenchyma and the mismapped flow signal. There is also adjacent decreased signal from the opposite side of the vessel, where the signal of the mismapped spins is lost.

### REFERENCE

Larson TC III, Kelly WM, Ehman RL, Wehrli FW: Spatial misregistration of vascular flow during MR imaging of the CNS: cause and clinical significance, *AJNR* 11:1041-1048, 1990.

# CASES 44 AND 45
# PITFALL: ANEURYSM CLIPS
## CASE 44

**History:** 40-year-old tested for follow-up status after aneurysm clipping.

**Technique:** axial volume, three-dimensional time-of-flight, 40/7/15, 256 × 256, 64 slices, 60-mm slab, 25-cm field of view, 10:57.

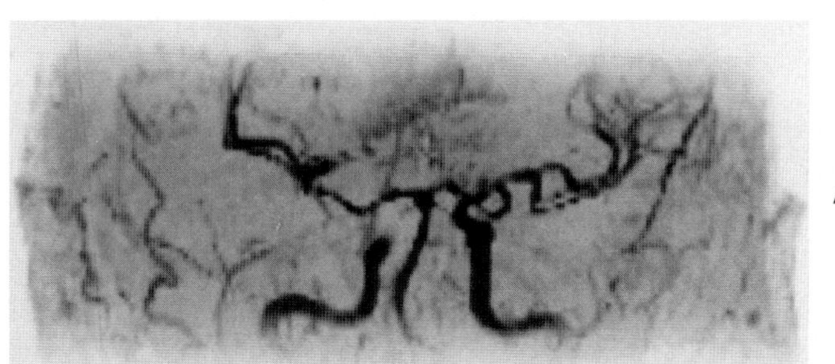

**A**

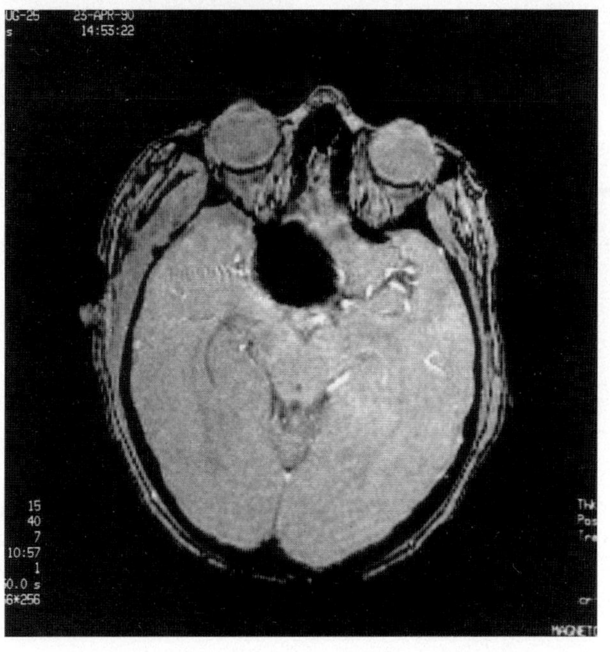


**B**

**AP maximum intensity projection (A) show loss of signal intensity involving the distal right internal carotid artery, as well as lack of signal from the proximal M1 and anterior cerebral circulations. Although internal carotid occlusion with collateral flow could cause a similar pattern, evaluation of the individual slices shows that the loss of signal relates to magnetic susceptibility artifact from a previously placed aneurysm clip (B). Loss of signal intensity within vessels can occur not only in situations such as this (i.e., those with gross susceptibility artifact), but also in more subtle situations such as at junctions of the sinuses with vessels (as around the sphenoid sinus and cavernous carotid artery).**

## CASE 45

**History:** 52-year-old who was tested for status after clipping of an anterior communicating artery aneurysm and who now has a gradual onset of headache.

**Technique:** axial volume; three-dimensional time-of-flight; 45/7/20; 256 × 192; 64 slices; 80-mm slab; 14-cm field of view; magnetization transfer background suppression; tilted, optimized nonsaturating excitation radiofrequency pulse; 9:15.

A

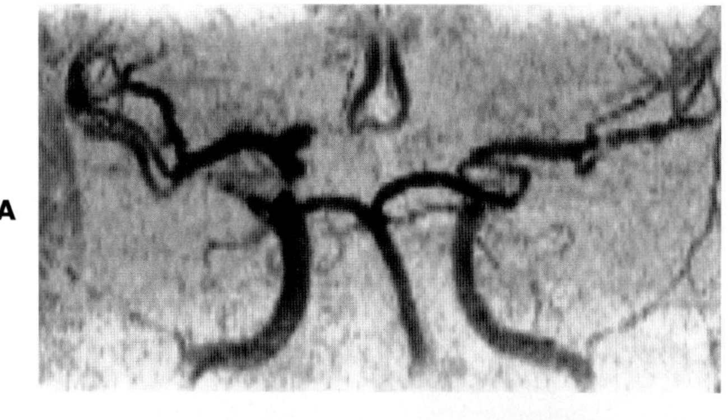

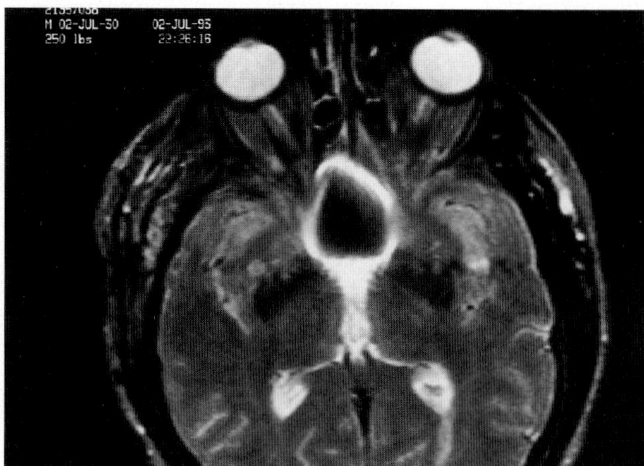


C

B

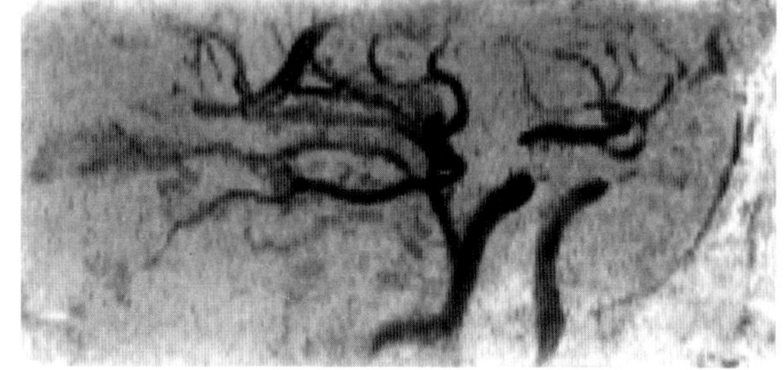

**AP (A) and lateral (B) maximum intensity projection views show complete loss of signal from portions of both carotid siphons, as well as the A1 segments. The proximal A2 segments appear attenuated in size. The axial T2-weighted image (C) shows signal loss with a peripheral high-signal halo typical for metal artifact.**

There are several studies that suggest that postoperative MR imaging of patients with successfully clipped aneurysms is safe and provides more useful information than computed tomography. Regardless of the clips, most computed tomographic images are markedly degraded by beam-hardening artifacts that arise from the aneurysm clip. The artifacts on MR images are caused by paramagnetic properties of the alloys within the surgical clips, resulting in local distortion and inhomogeneities of the magnetic field. With computed tomography and MR imaging, the region immediately adjacent to the clip is markedly degraded and uninterpretable. The amount of artifact created on both imaging modalities relates to not only the clip size, but also to the type of material used in production of the clip.

Nonferromagnetic aneurysm clips that are not deflected in a magnetic field have been available for several years from many manufacturers. The difficulty arises in distinguishing the ferromagnetic from the nonferromagnetic clips after they have been placed in patients. This becomes especially important in imaging patients with remote placement of aneurysm clips. Complete documentation of the brand and the exact metal of the clip should be noted in all cases. This allows patients with nonferromagnetic clips to have access to MR imaging. Several authors have studied and compiled lists of aneurysm clips that have no deflection in magnetic fields and that are therefore safe for MR imaging. The safety of a metallic clip for imaging does not imply that there will be no artifact; rather it implies that there will be no deflection with resulting risks of dislodging of the aneurysm clip.

The importance of adequate documentation of the type of aneurysm clip is strikingly highlighted by a report of a fatal outcome of placement of a patient with a ferromagnetic aneurysm clip into an MR field. The personnel at the site knew that the patient had an aneurysm clip, and the patient's family reported that it was a Yasargil clip (reported to be nonferromagnetic in the literature). It was determined that the aneurysm clip was in reality a Variangle aneurysm clip (which is ferromagnetic) only after a fatal intracranial hemorrhage, which appeared to result from clip motion in the static MR field. Klucznik et al concluded that verbal information should not be relied on and that only the written operative note should be used to prove clip identity.

## REFERENCES

Klucznik RP, Carrier DA, Pyka R, Haid RW: Placement of a ferromagnetic intracerebral aneurysm clip in a magnetic field with a fatal outcome, *Radiology* 187:855-856, 1993.

Kanal E, Shellock FG: MR imaging of patients with intracranial aneurysm clips, *Radiology* 187:612-614, 1993.

Shellock FG, Curtis JS: MR imaging and biomedical implants, materials, and devices: an updated review, *Radiology* 180:541-550, 1991.

Holtas S, Olsson M, Romner B et al: Comparison of MR imaging and CT in patients with intracranial aneurysm clips, *AJNR* 9:891-897, 1988.

Becker RL, Norfray JF, Teitelbaum GP et al: MR imaging in patients with intracranial aneurysm clips, *AJNR* 9:885-889, 1988.

Brothers MF, Fox AJ, Lee DH et al: MR imaging after surgery for vertebrobasilar aneurysm, *AJNR* 11:149-161, 1990.

## CASE 46
## PITFALL: POSTERIOR CEREBRAL LOOP MIMICKING ANEURYSM

**History:** 4-year-old with headaches.

**Technique:** axial volume, three-dimensional time-of-flight, 40/7/15, 256 × 256, 64 slices, 70-mm slab, 25-cm field of view, 10:57.

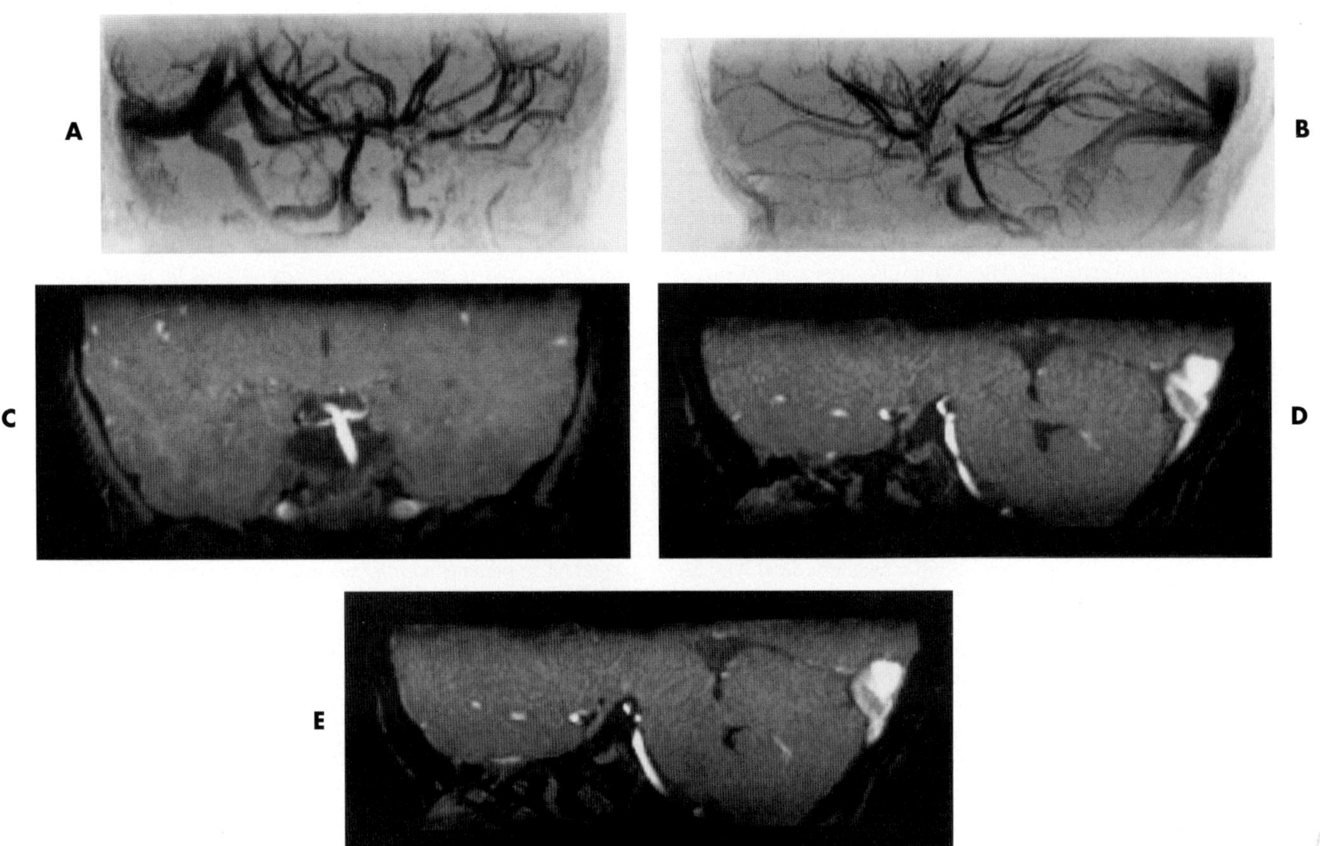


**Right anterior oblique (A) and lateral maximum intensity (B) projections demonstrate an apparent high signal intensity outpouching off the region of the distal basilar artery, which is suspicious for basilar tip aneurysm. However, evaluation of coronal (C) and sagittal (D and E) multiplanar reformats from the original MRA data set show that the apparent aneurysm is, in fact, a cephalic loop of the right P1 segment, a normal anatomic variant.**

Adequate assessment of a MRA data set for aneurysms must rely not only on the maximum intensity projections, but also on routine evaluation of the individual slices, targeted maximum intensity projections, and in questionable areas, multiplanar reformats.

## CASE 47
## PITFALL: FALSE ANEURYSM RESULTING FROM PLACEMENT OF TARGETED MAXIMUM INTENSITY PROJECTION VOLUME

**History:** 30-year-old with headaches.

**Technique:** axial volume, three-dimensional time-of-flight, 40/7/15, 256 × 256, 64 slices, 60-mm volume, 25-cm field of view, 10:57.

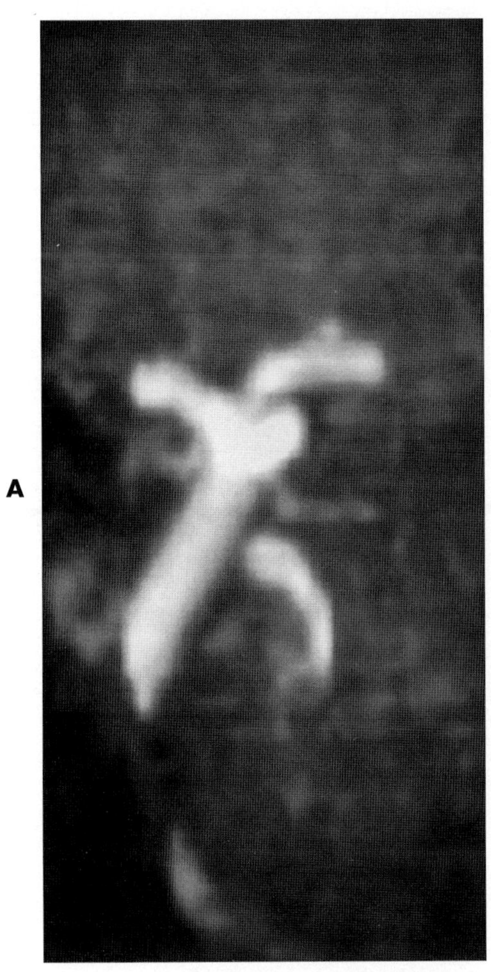
A

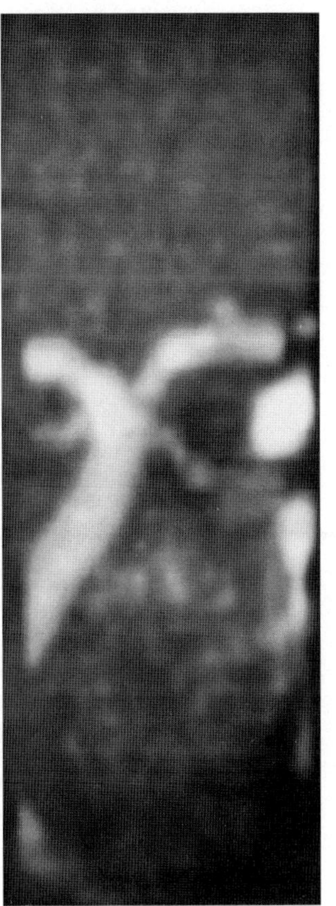
B

**A targeted anteroposterior maximum intensity projection of the posterior circulation (A) demonstrates an apparent aneurysm arising off the distal basilar artery, between the left P1 segment and the origin of the left superior cerebellar artery. However, evaluation of the more lateral projection of the targeted maximum intensity projection (B) shows that this focal high signal intensity represents the posterior aspect of the carotid siphon, which has been inadvertently included in the maximum intensity projection reconstruction.**

Targeted or limited volume maximum intensity projections must be carefully scrutinized to ensure that extraneous portions of the vasculature, which might give false appearances, have not been included.

## CASE 48
## PITFALL: AERATED ANTERIOR CLINOID

**History:** 65-year-old with confusion.

**Technique:** axial volume, three-dimensional time-of-flight, 43/6/20, 512 × 256 matrix, one excitation, 60 slices, 60-mm slab, 18-cm field of view, 11:00.

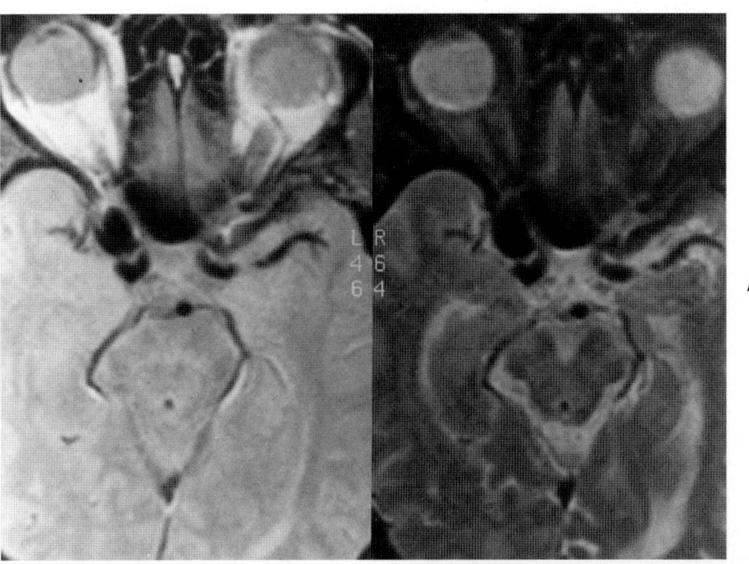

A

B

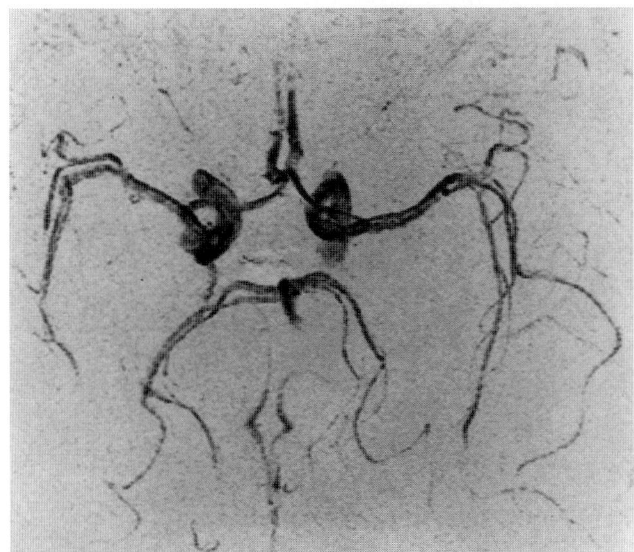

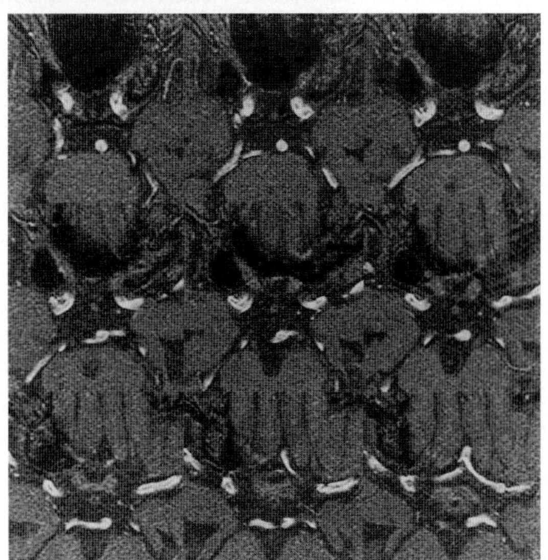

C

**Axial spin density and T2-weighted images (A) demonstrate a rounded area of low signal intensity just anterior to the distal right internal carotid artery and lateral to the optic canal that is suspicious for aneurysm. Base maximum intensity projection view of the MRA (B) demonstrates no abnormality in the region of the distal right internal carotid artery. This is further confirmed on the series of nine individual slices from the study, which demonstrate that the lack of signal intensity relates to an aerated anterior clinoid and not to any vascular abnormality (C). (Courtesy John Huston, Mayo Clinic, Rochester, Minn.)**

Differential diagnosis in this location would be a flow void related to vessel or aneurysm, an aerated anterior clinoid, or a calcified mass. The MRA shows no signal from the lesion, which excluded the possibility of patent aneurysm lumen causing the signal void on the spin echo study.

## CASE 49
## PITFALL: INFUNDIBULAR DILATATION

**History:** 36-year-old with a known left posterior communicating artery aneurysm.

**Technique:** axial volume, three-dimensional time-of-flight, 45/7/20, 256 × 256, 64 slices, 60-mm slab, 15-cm field of view, 12:19.

A

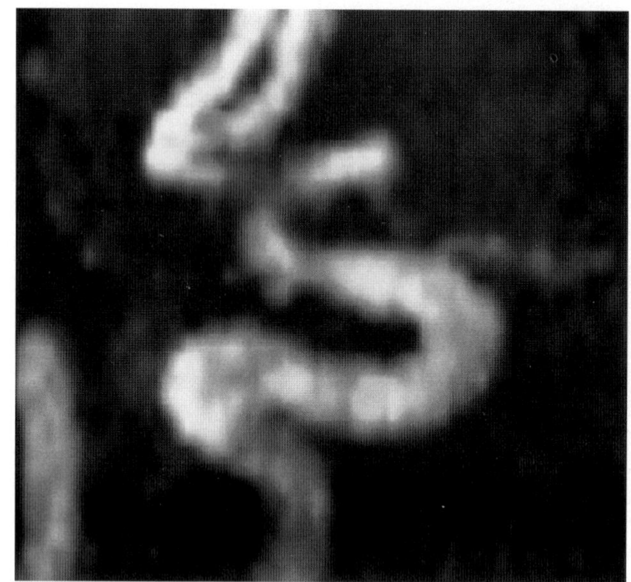

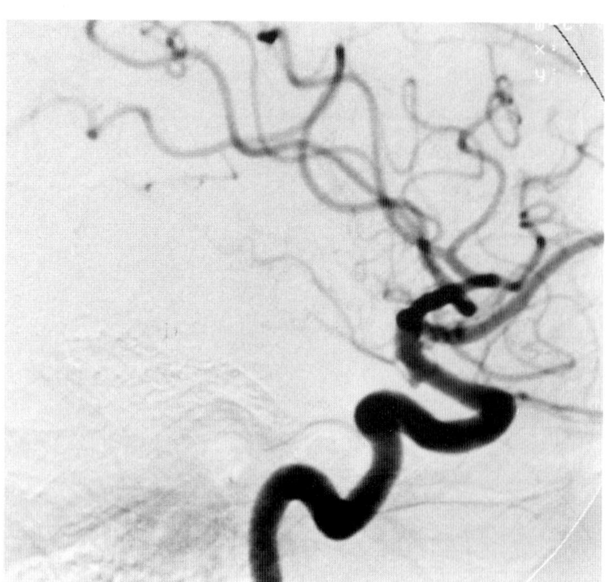

B

**Lateral view targeted maximum intensity projection (A) of the right carotid siphon shows a small focal area of increased signal arising off the posterior aspect of the distal internal carotid artery. The differential at this location would be either a small aneurysm or infundibulum. Lateral view from the conventional angiogram (B) shows this to be an infundibulum, since the base is broader than the apex and the posterior communicating artery is seen arising from its tip.**

The spatial resolution of MRA is becoming such that areas presenting diagnostic problems and controversies on conventional intraarterial angiography are also being manifested by MRA. One such area is the infundibular dilatation of the posterior communicating artery, also called simply an *infundibulum* or *junctional dilatation*. The *infundibulum* refers to the funnel-shaped dilatation of the origin of the posterior communicating artery off of the internal carotid artery. The angiographic diagnosis of an infundibular dilatation is defined by Pool and Potts: (1) maximum diameter of 3 ml or less, (2) a round or conical (but not saccular or irregular) shape, and (3) an infundibulum free of an aneurysm-like neck. Further, the posterior communicating artery should be seen at the tip of the infundibulum. A specific problem on the MRA, as shown in this case, is when an infundibular dilatation occurs when the posterior communicating artery is quite small and not visualized. Thus only the infundibular dilatation is seen, and this mimics a small posterior communicating artery aneurysm.

The incidence of infundibular dilatation is between 10% and 17% of cases studied. Controversy surrounds the issue of whether infundibular dilatation is preaneurysmal. Autopsy studies of patients with infundibular dilatation have noted large medial defects and loss of the internal elastic lamina that resembles the appearance of aneurysm, which could suggest a congenital friability and fragility. Some authors have reported a normal-appearing arterial wall structure. This most likely represents a spectrum ranging from a normal arterial wall structure dilatation to a larger and more round aneurysm-like structure. Ebina et al (1986) suggested that more aggressive follow-up or active treatment should be pursued in patients in whom there is an associated posterior communicating artery aneurysm on the opposite side, in young patients, in patients with hypertension, and in patients with divergent angles of the dilatation with respect to the internal carotid artery. Yearly follow-ups have been suggested, since any infundibular dilatations that converted to aneurysms did so within 5 to 10 years.

## REFERENCES

Ebina K, Suzuki M, Andoh A et al: Recurrent of cerebral aneurysm after initial neck clipping, *Neurosurgery* 11:764-768, 1982.

Epstein F, Ransohoff J, Buzdilovich GN: The clinical significance of junctional dilatation of the posterior communicating artery, *J Neurosurg* 33:529-531, 1970.

Hassler O, Saltzman GF: Angiographic and histologic changes in infundibular widening of the posterior communicating artery, *Acta Radiol* 1:321-327, 1963.

Nukui H, Nagaya T, Miyagi O et al: Development of new aneurysm and enlargement of small aneurysm, *Neurol Med Chir* 22:437-445, 1982.

Patrick D, Appleby A: Infundibular widening of the posterior communicating artery progressing to true aneurysm, *Br J Radiol* 56:59-60, 1983.

Pool JL, Potts DG: *Aneurysms and arteriovenous anomalies of the brain: diagnosis and treatment,* New York, 1965, Harper & Row.

Ebina K, Ohkuma H, Iwabuchi T: An angiographic study of incidence and morphology of infundibular dilatation of the posterior communicating artery, *Neuroradiology* 28:23-29, 1986.

# CASE 50
# PITFALL: INFUNDIBULUM

**History:** 34-year-old with headaches.

**Technique #1:** axial volume, three-dimensional time-of-flight, 43/6/20, 512 × 256 matrix, one excitation, 60 slices, 42-mm slab, 18-cm field of view, 11:00.

**Technique #2:** axial volume, three-dimensional phase-contrast, 26/9/15, 256 × 128 matrix, one excitation, 60 partitions, 42-mm slab, velocity encoding of 30 m/sec, 18-cm field of view, 14 minutes.

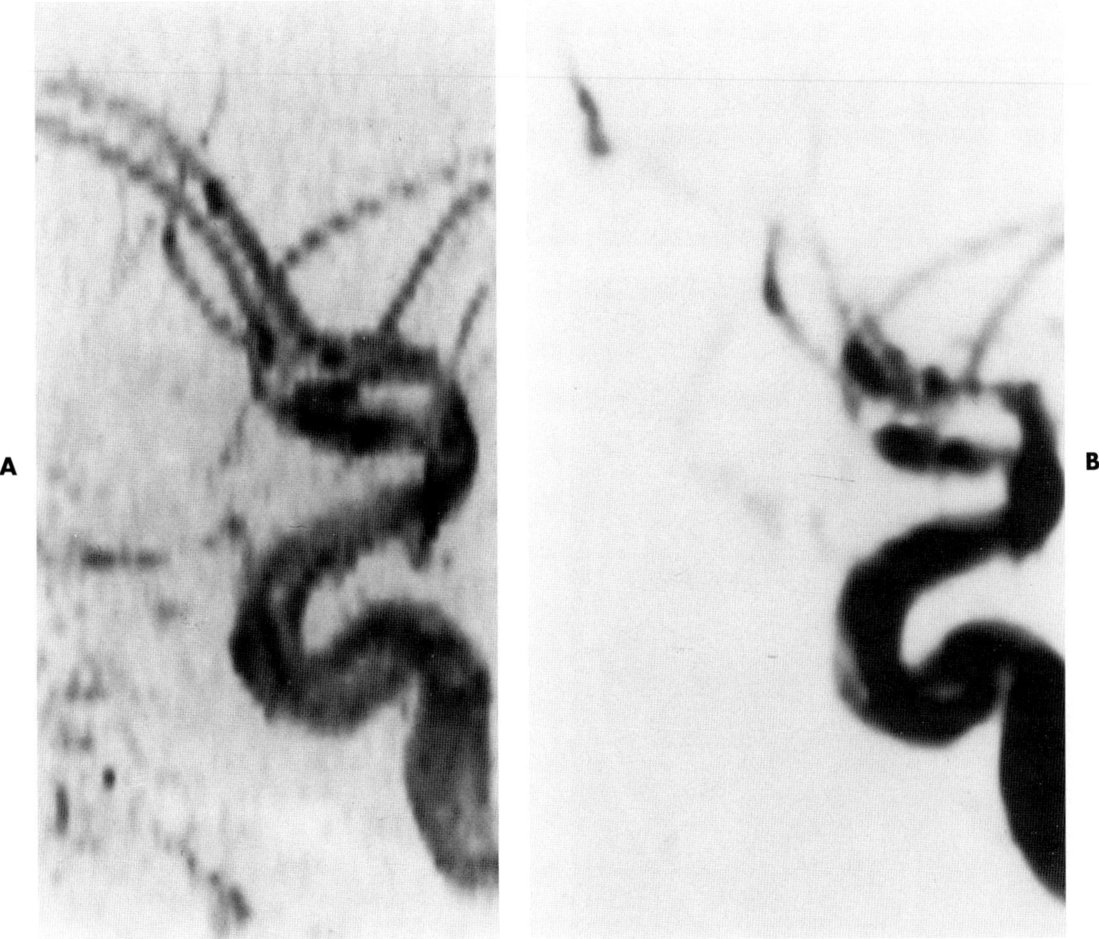


**Lateral view targeted maximum intensity projection time-of-flight angiogram of the carotid siphon (A) shows a triangular projection off the posterior aspect of the distal internal carotid, which represents an infundibulum. The lateral view maximum intensity projection of the phase-contrast study with a 30 m/sec velocity encoding (B) does not show the infundibulum. (Courtesy John Huston, Mayo Clinic, Rochester, Minn.)**

The three-dimensional time-of-flight MRA with superior resolution (512 × 256 matrix) shows smaller vascular structures when compared with a three-dimensional phase-contrast study with worse resolution (256 × 128 matrix). Although the solution may seem to increase the matrix on the phase-contrast study to allow visualization of smaller structures, a 256 × 256 matrix has a prohibitively long examination time for all but the most cooperative patients and forgiving time schedules. See discussion of infundibular dilatations in Case 49.

## CASE 51
## ANTERIOR COMMUNICATING ARTERY ANEURYSM

**History:** 65-year-old with previous subarachnoid hemorrhage and occlusion of the left internal carotid for a parasellar aneurysm now being tested for follow-up.

**Technique:** axial volume, three-dimensional time-of-flight, 40/7/15, 256 × 256, 64 slices, 60-mm slab, 25-cm field of view, 10:57.

A

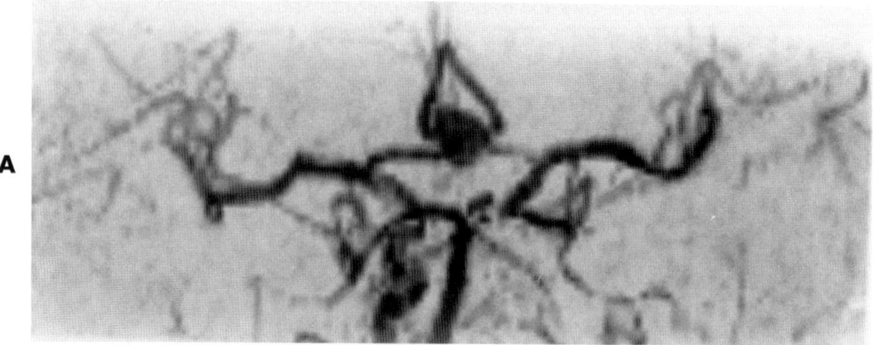

B

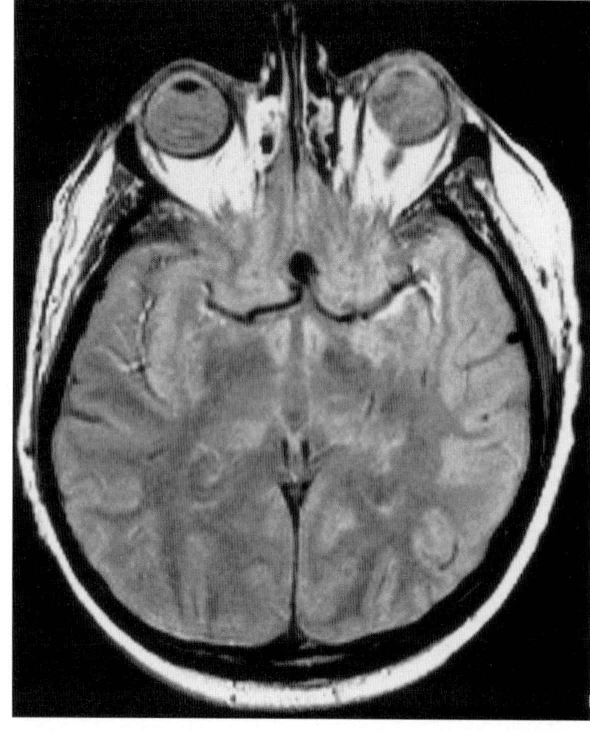

C

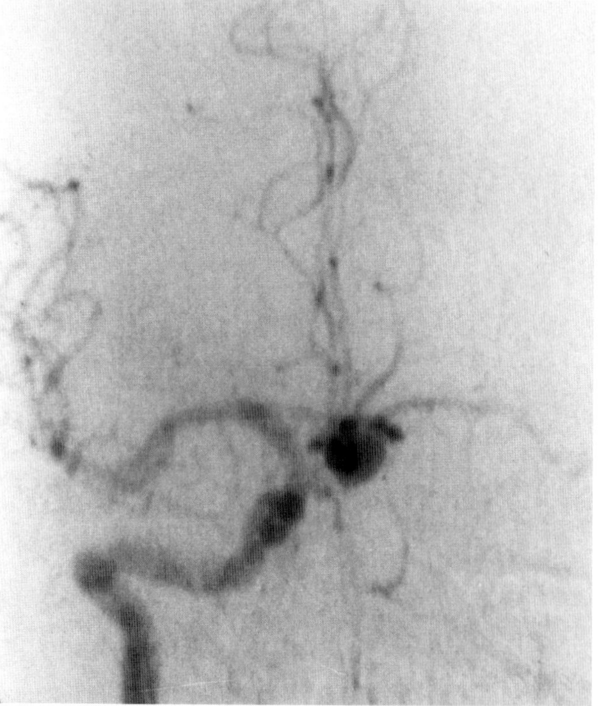

**Anteroposterior maximum intensity projection (A) shows a rounded area of abnormally increased signal intensity involving the anterior communicating artery, which is an anterior communicating artery aneurysm. There is a large right A1 and a small left A1 segment. There is also lack of signal intensity involving the distal left internal carotid artery resulting from the internal carotid artery occlusion. The axial spin-density image of the brain demonstrates the aneurysmal flow void in the midline (B). Anteroposterior view of the right common carotid injection shows the anterior communicating artery aneurysm, with crossfilling to the left side (C).**

There are five types of intracranial aneurysms. These include *berry* (saccular), *mycotic, fusiform* (atherosclerotic), *traumatic,* and *neoplastic.* Rare causes include dissection and syphilis. The prevalence of aneurysms in the North American population is estimated to be 2000 per 100,000. Aneurysms are generally identified in patients between 40 and 60 years of age, with an overall female-to-male ratio of 3:2. However, women have a higher rebleeding rate, more problems with vasospasm, and a higher morbidity and mortality rate after rupture and subarachnoid hemorrhage.

*Berry* aneurysms of the circle of Willis are by far the most common type, as seen in this particular case. *Mycotic* aneurysms are usually peripheral compared with saccular aneurysms, which are around the circle of Willis. The identification of multiple peripheral aneurysms should raise the concern of embolic infectious aneurysms. Valvular heart disease with endocarditis is the main cause, and the overall mortality rate is around 46%. *Atherosclerotic* aneurysm is a fusiform dilatation of a vessel in which the wall has undergone atheromatous degeneration. Atherosclerotic aneurysms may be a fusiform dilatation of main trunk arteries (such as the basilar) or a saccular-appearing aneurysm with sclerosis of the parent vessel. The majority of cases involve the vertebrobasilar system in patients over 40 years of age who are hypertensive. Subarachnoid hemorrhage is uncommon with this type of aneurysm. Clinical findings relate to enlargement and compression of parenchyma and to the underlying atherosclerosis (cranial nerve dysfunction, ischemia). *Traumatic* aneurysms are also referred to as *false aneurysms,* since the majority occur by the recanalization of periarterial hematomas around vessel lacerations related to conditions such as fractures and foreign object penetration. These lesions tend to involve the large basal arteries and middle meningeal artery. When peripheral traumatic aneurysms occur, they involve the middle cerebral artery and anterior cerebral artery distributions.

**REFERENCES**

Kassell NF, Drake CG: Review of the management of saccular aneurysms, *Neurol Clin* 1(1):73-84, 1983.

Bohmfalk GL, Story JL, Wissinger JP et al: Bacterial intracranial aneurysm, *J Neurosurg* 48:369-382, 1978.

Ohara H, Sakamoto T, Suzuki J: *Sclerotic cerebral aneurysms.* In Suzuki J: *Cerebral aneurysms,* Tokoyo, 1979, Neuron.

## CASE 52
## ANTERIOR COMMUNICATING ARTERY ANEURYSM WITH SUBARACHNOID HEMORRHAGE

**History:** 77-year-old with subarachnoid hemorrhage 10 days before.

**Technique:** axial volume, three-dimensional time-of-flight, 40/7/15, 256 × 160, 64 slices, 60-mm slab, 20-cm field of view, 6:52. The matrix size was decreased to shorten the examination time because of patient motion.

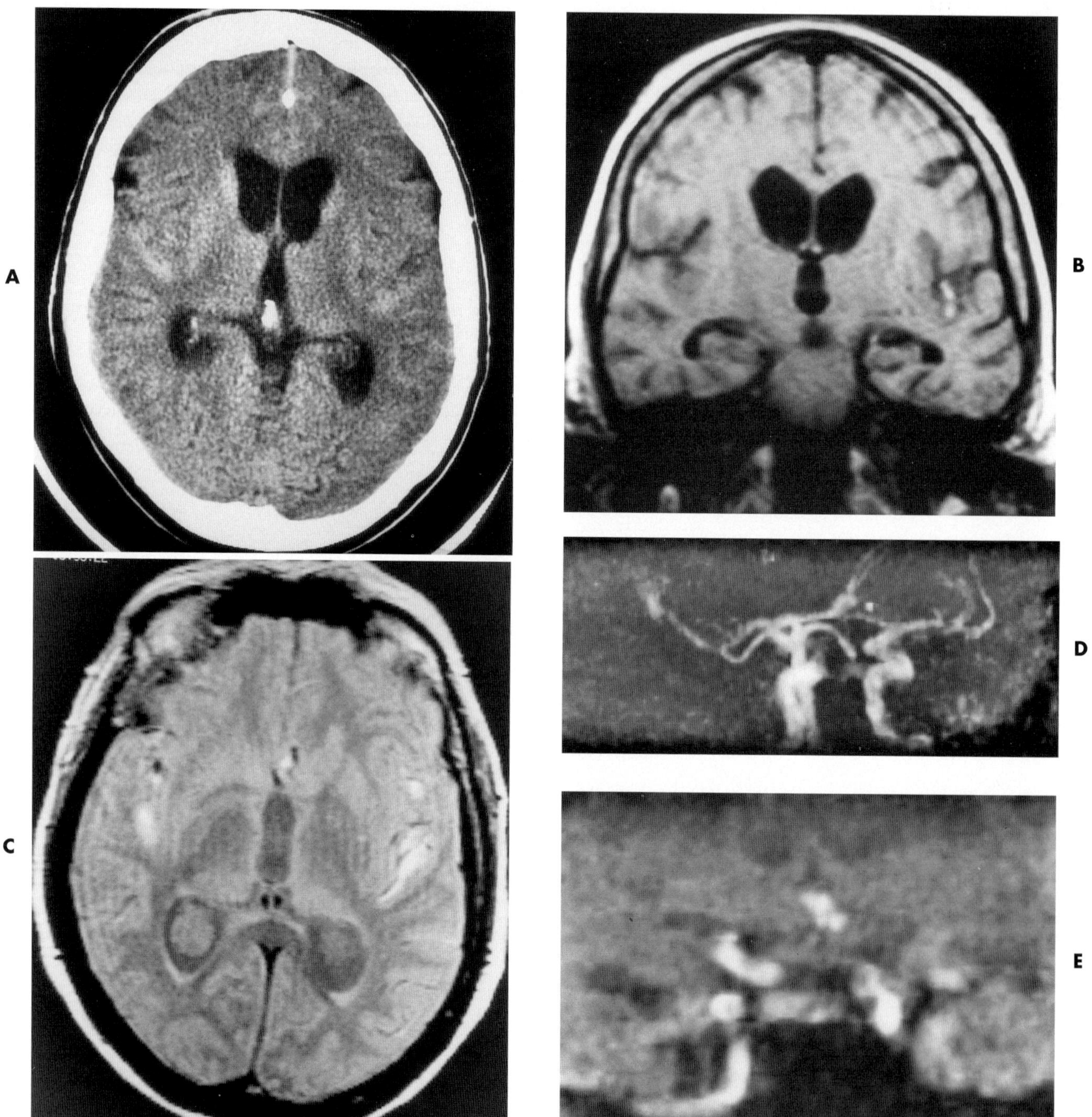

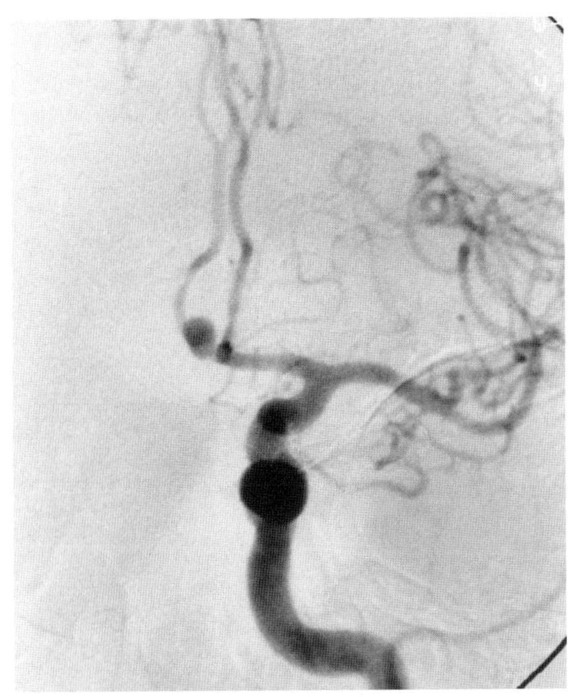

F

**Axial unenhanced computed tomogram (A) shows extensive subarachnoid hemorrhage in the Sylvian fissures and interhemispheric fissure. The coronal T1-weighted spin-echo study (B) shows abnormal increased signal within the left Sylvian fissure. The axial spin density image (C) also shows abnormal increased signal from both Sylvian fissures related to the subarachnoid hemorrhage. Oblique maximum intensity projection view from a time-of-flight MRA (D) demonstrates a globular area of increased signal intensity in the region of the anterior communicating artery and in the Sylvian fissure. Coronal reformat of the MRA data (E) shows the globular area of abnormal increased signal that could represent an aneurysm of the anterior communicating artery or subarachnoid methemoglobin mimicking an aneurysm. Anteroposterior intracranial view of the conventional angiogram left carotid injection (F) shows the anterior communicating artery aneurysm and mild anterior cerebral artery vasospasm.**

The dogma that acute subarachnoid hemorrhage is difficult to detect has been recently challenged by Ogawa et al. The authors evaluated the MR appearance of subarachnoid hemorrhage in 33 patients at O.5Tesla and found almost 100% sensitivity using proton density–weighted images. The appearance of acute subarachnoid hemorrhage causes increased signal intensity within the subarachnoid space on the photon density images, with T1-weighed and T2-weighted images being less sensitive. The cause of the high signal on the photon density images remains unknown. Theories include shorting of the T1 by methemoglobin or water binding of protein associated with the clotting mechanism. The clinical impact and claimed sensitivity of MR to subarachnoid hemorrhage has been challenged. It can be stated that detection of subarachnoid hemorrhage is possible with MR, and subarachnoid hemorrhage must be added to the differential considerations when there is increased signal intensity in the subarachnoid space on photon density–weighted images (such as meningitis). However, computed tomography, not MR, is the imaging modality of choice for the diagnosis of subarachnoid hemorrhage.

**REFERENCES**

Atlas SW: Devil's advocate: MR imaging is highly sensitive for acute subarachnoid hemorrhage . . . Not! *Radiology* 186:319-322, 1993.

Ogawa T, Uemura K: Devil's advocate: reply, *Radiology* 186:323, 1993.

Ogawa T, Inugami A, Shimosegawa E et al: Subarachnoid hemorrhage: evaluation with MR imaging, *Radiology* 186:345-351, 1993.

Jenkins A, Hakley DM, Teasdale GM et al: Magnetic resonance imaging of acute subarachnoid hemorrhage, *J Neurosurg* 68:731-736, 1988.

## CASE 53
## ANTERIOR COMMUNICATING ARTERY ANEURYSM

**History:** 75-year-old being evaluated for vertigo.

**Technique #1:** axial three-dimensional time-of-flight, 43/6/20, 512 × 256 matrix, one excitation, 60 slices, 60-mm slab, 18-cm field of view, 11:00.

**Technique #2:** axial volume, three-dimensional phase-contrast, 26/9/15, 256 × 128 matrix, one excitation, 60 slices, 60-mm slab, velocity encoding of 30 cm/second, 18-cm field of view, 14 minutes.

A
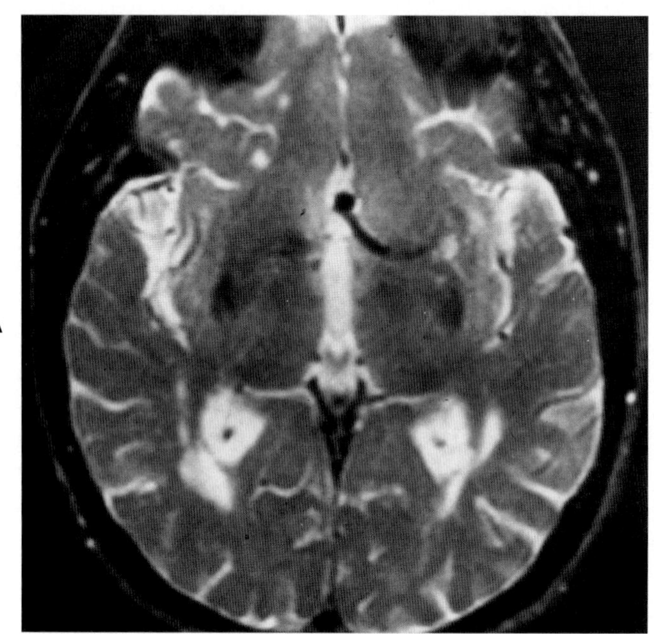

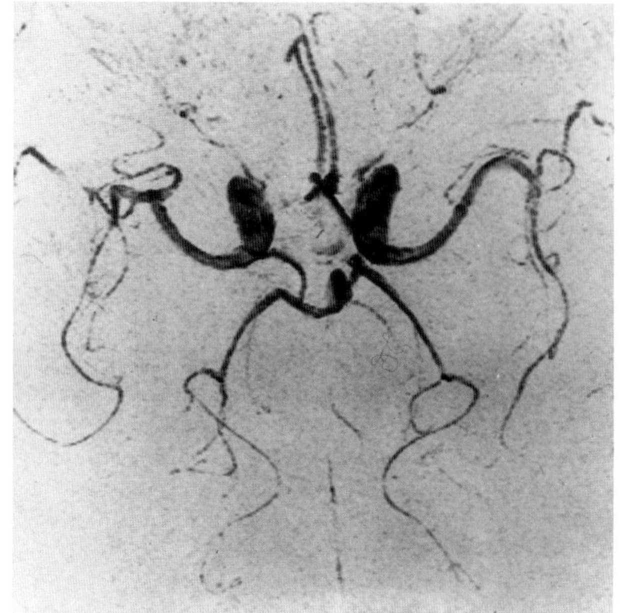
B

C
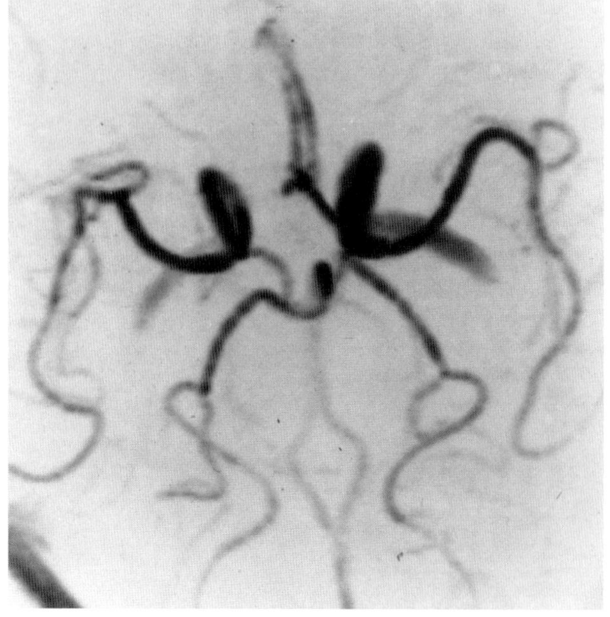

D

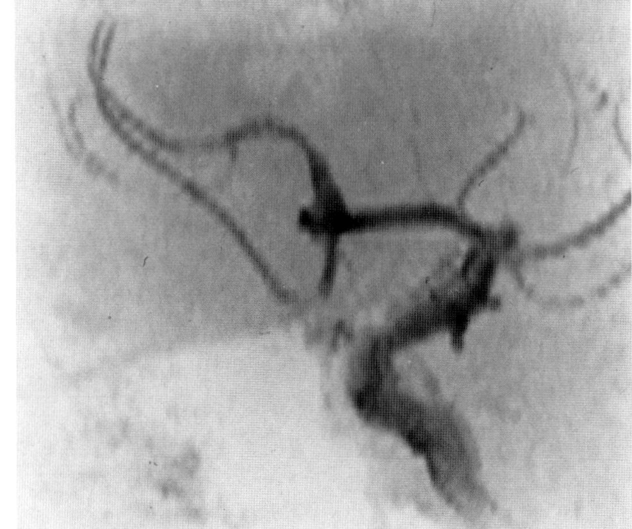

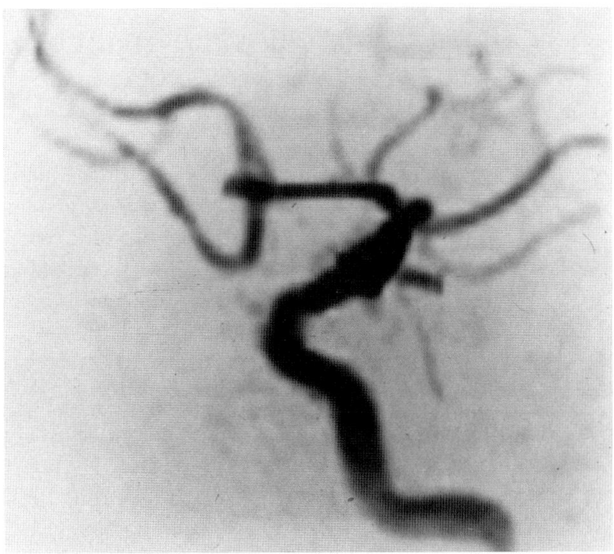

E

There is a suspicious rounded area of decreased signal in the region of the anterior communicating artery on the conventional T2-weighted spin-echo study (A). Base maximum intensity projection views of a three-dimensional time-of-flight (B) and three-dimensional phase-contrast study (C) show no definite abnormality, although there is a slight increase in signal intensity in the region of the anterior communicating artery. However, targeting the maximum intensity projections for both the three-dimensional time-of-flight (D) and the phase-contrast study (E) in the lateral projection demonstrate the small anterior communicating artery aneurysm arising between the two A2 segments bilaterally. Note the hypoplastic right A1 segment. (Courtesy John Huston, Mayo Clinic, Rochester, Minn.)

## CASE 54
## THROMBOSED ANTERIOR COMMUNICATING ARTERY ANEURYSM

**History:** 55-year-old with a history of aneurysm.

**Technique:** axial volume, three-dimensional time-of-flight, 40/7/15, 256 × 256, 64 slices, 60-mm slab, magnetization transfer background suppression, 23-cm field of view, 10:57. The magnetization transfer background suppression is recognizable, since the background signal is so low that the orbital fat signal becomes much more apparent.

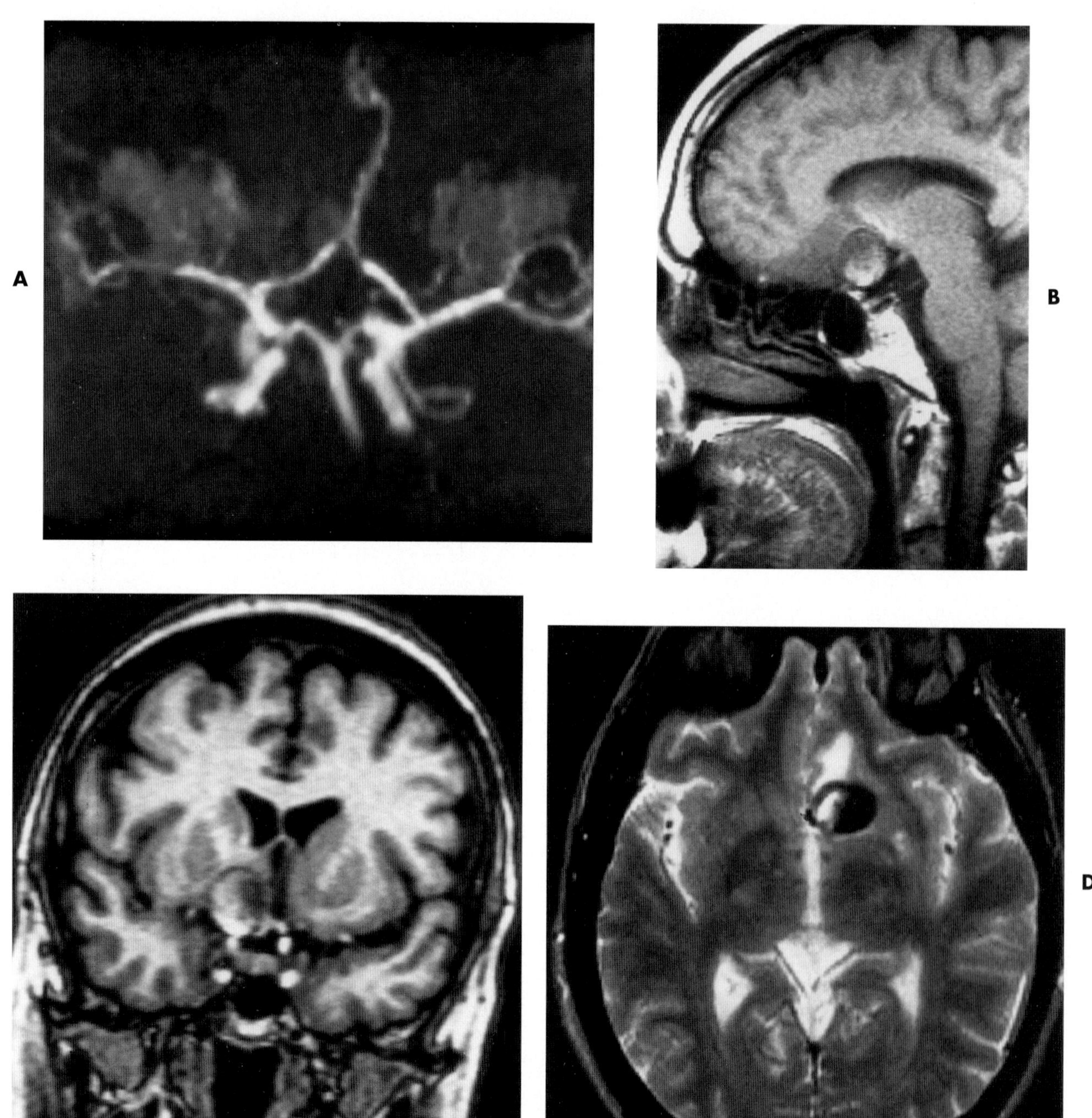

**The Water's type of view of the maximum intensity projection (A) demonstrates only a faint area of increased signal intensity to the right of the junction of the right A1 with the anterior communicating artery, which is not distinguishable from other areas of increased signal overlaying the middle cerebral arteries because of orbital fat. However, the sagittal (B) and coronal (C) T1-weighted images and the axial T2-weighted image (D) demonstrate a rounded mass in the region of the anterior communicating artery, which is consistent with a completely thrombosed anterior communicating artery aneurysm. The small amount of high signal intensity seen on the maximum intensity projection and T1-weighted images relates to the methemoglobin within the thrombosed aneurysm. As with the case of giant intracranial aneurysms with slowed flow, the presence of a thrombosed aneurysm necessitates conventional spin-echo imaging for full evaluation and identification of the vascular lesion.**

The anterior communicating artery is the most common location for intracranial aneurysms. These lesions most often present with subarachnoid hemorrhage, since there are no cranial nerves around this area to provide a clinical presentation as there are for the posterior communicating artery. Anterior communicating artery aneurysms tend to arise toward the side of the larger-feeding A1 segment or in the middle of the anterior communicating artery if the A1 segments are of equal size **(E).** The anterior communicating artery can have may congenital variations and may be multiple or fenestrated.

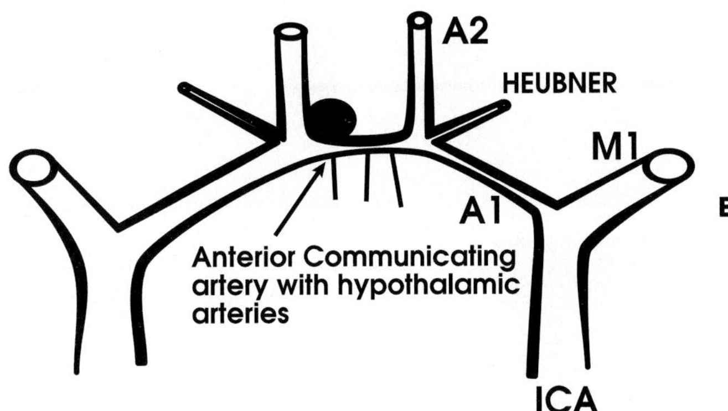


**Typical location and relationships of an anterior communicating artery aneurysm (E).**

**REFERENCE**

Yasargil MG: *Microneurosurgery,* vol 2, New York, 1984, Thieme.

# CASE 55
# MIDDLE CEREBRAL ARTERY ANEURYSM

**History:** 65-year-old with ataxia.

**Technique:** axial volume, three-dimensional time-of-flight, 40/7/15, 256 × 256, 64 slices, 60-mm slab, 25-cm field of view, 10:57.

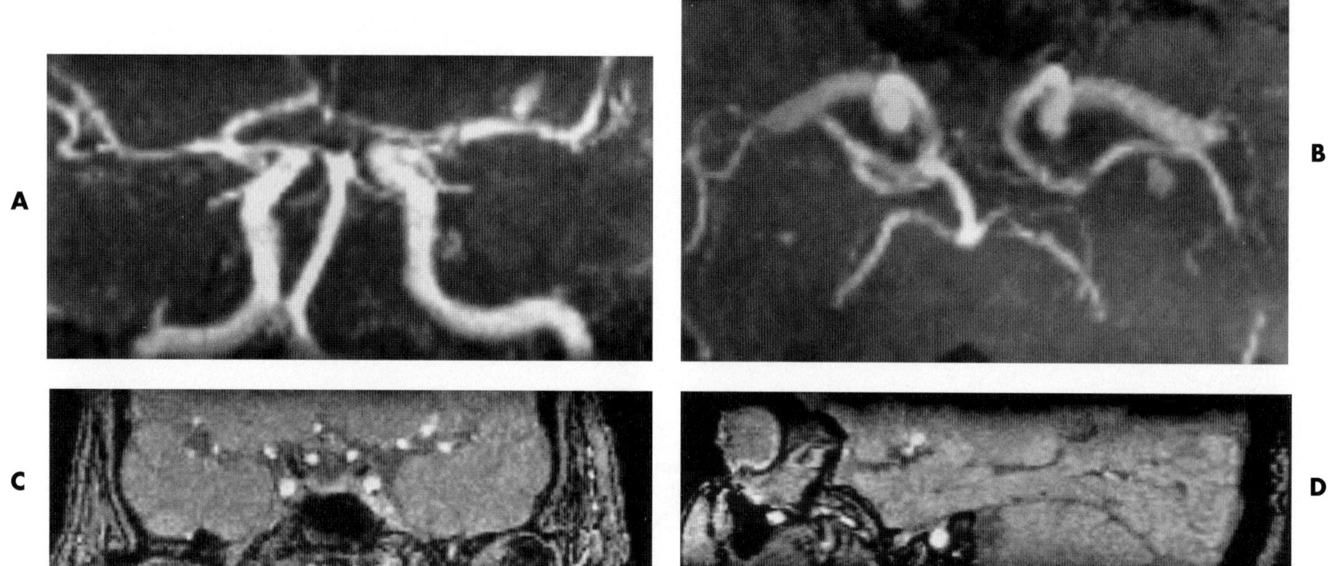


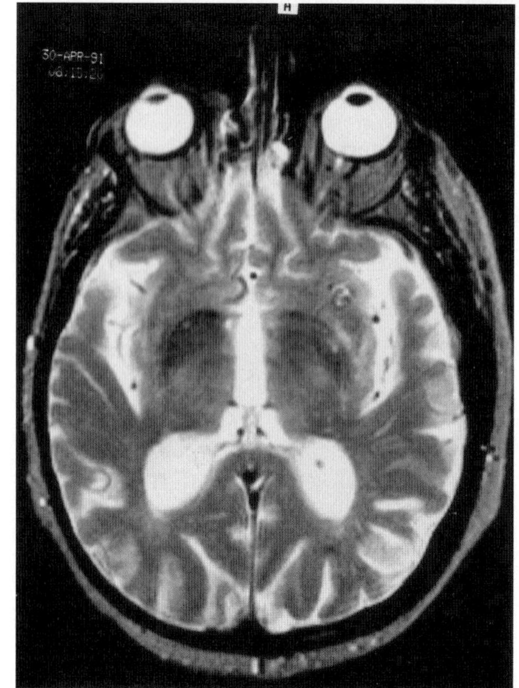


**Anteroposterior (A) and base (B) views of the maximum intensity projection demonstrate an ill-defined, globular area of abnormally increased signal intensity arising off of the region of the distal left M1 segment, which is suspicious for aneurysm. This suspicion is confirmed on the coronal (C) and sagittal (D) reformats of the MRA data, which clearly demonstrate the aneurysm arising superiorly off the distal M1 segment. The axial T2-weighted image of the head (E) demonstrates an ill-defined area of mixed signal intensity in the region of the aneurym resulting from complex flow within the lesion.**

Middle cerebral artery bifurcation aneurysms constitute approximately 18% of aneurysms. These lesions are often multiple and multilobular. The most common locations are at the bifurcation of the M1 segment and the proximal M1 and distal branches. Conditions commonly associated with an increased incidence of intracranial aneurysms include-polycystic kidney disease, coarctation of the aorta, Ehlers-Danlos syndrome, arteriovenous malformations, pseudoxanthoma elasticum, moyamoya disease, and fibromuscular dysplasia; trauma is also associated with an increased incidence. A familial history of aneurysms may also occur.

# CASE 56
# MIDDLE CEREBRAL ARTERY ANEURYSM

**History:** 50-year-old with transient numbness in the left arm.

**Technique #1:** axial volume, three-dimensional phase-contrast, 24/8.1/20, 256 × 128, velocity encoding of 100 cm/sec, 60 slices, 60-mm slab, 16-cm field of view, 13:08.

**Technique #2:** axial volume, three-dimensional time-of-flight, 50/5.0/35, 256 × 192, 60 slices, 60-mm slab, 16-cm field of view, 10:16.

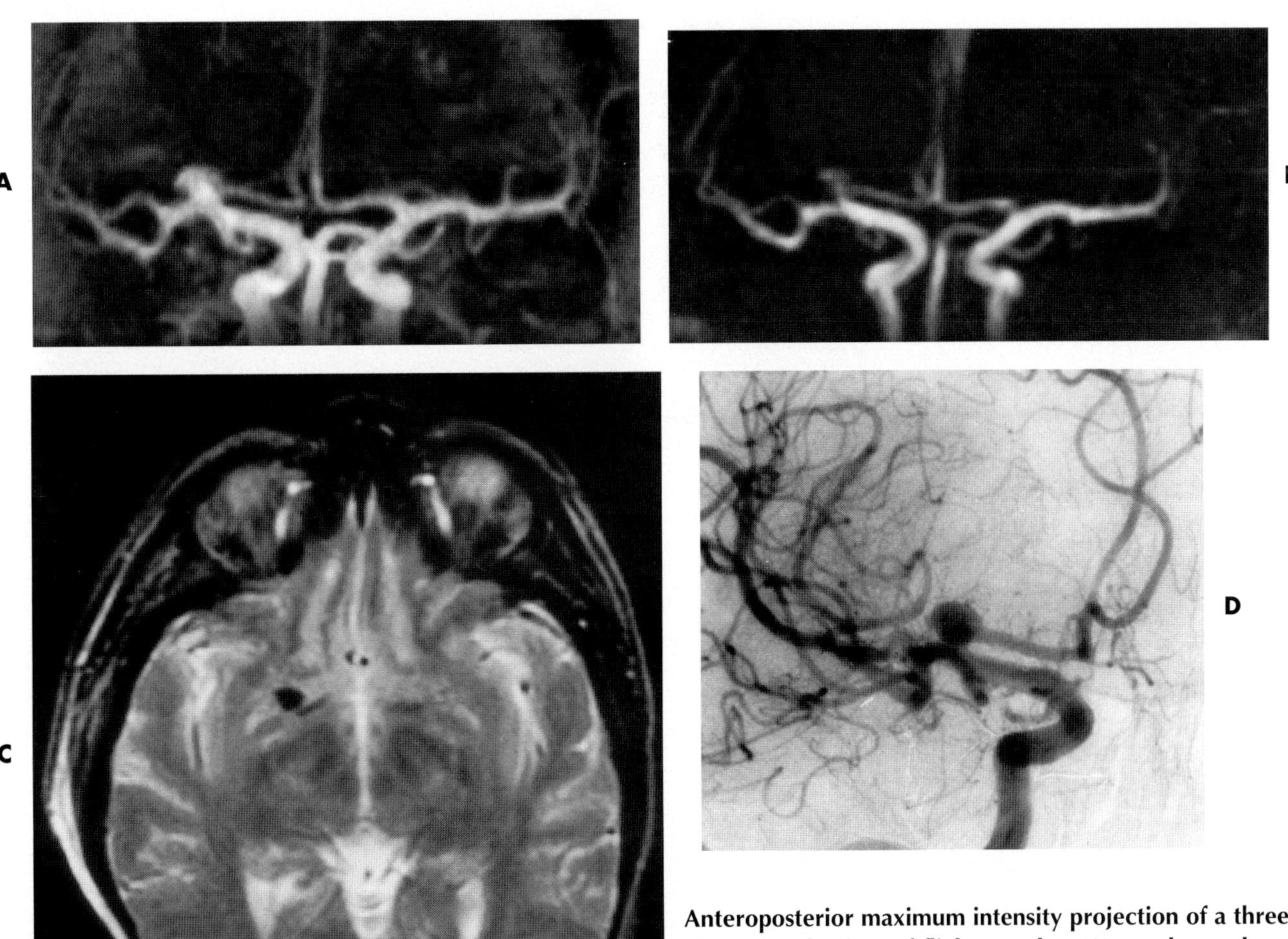


**Anteroposterior maximum intensity projection of a three-dimensional time-of-flight study (A) and a three-dimensional phase-contrast study (B) demonstrate an abnormal outpouching of increased signal intensity arising at the bifurcation of the distal internal carotid artery into the M1 and A1 segments; this represents an aneurysm that is projecting superiorly.**

The aneurysm appears slightly better defined on the three-dimensional time-of-flight study, which may be because of less spin dephasing resulting from the shorter echo time. In addition, the phase-contrast study has a relatively high velocity encoding at 100 cm/sec, which decreases its sensitivity to slower flow. The aneurysm is also identified on the axial T2-weighted study of the head **(C)** as a well-defined area of flow void. An oblique view from an internal carotid artery injection **(D)** demonstrates the aneurysm arising superiorly from the distal internal carotid bifurcation.

## CASE 57
## LEFT MIDDLE CEREBRAL BIFURCATION ANEURYSM

**History:** 49-year-old with headaches.

**Technique #1:** axial three-dimensional time-of-flight, 43/6/20, 512 × 256 matrix, 60 slices, 60-mm slab, 18-cm field of view, 11:00.

**Technique #2:** coronal, two-dimensional phase-contrast, 30/8/20, 512 × 256 matrix, eight excitations, 80-mm single slice, velocity encoding of 30-cm/s, 24-cm field of view, 5 minutes.

A

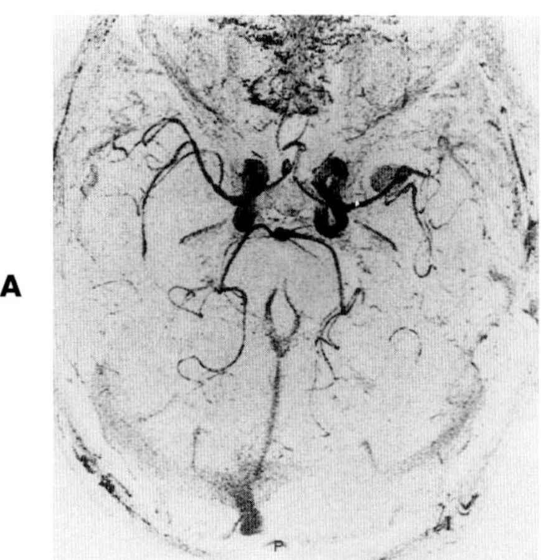

B

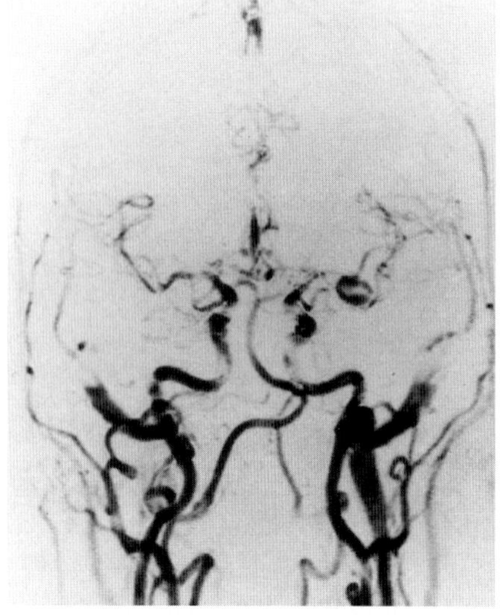

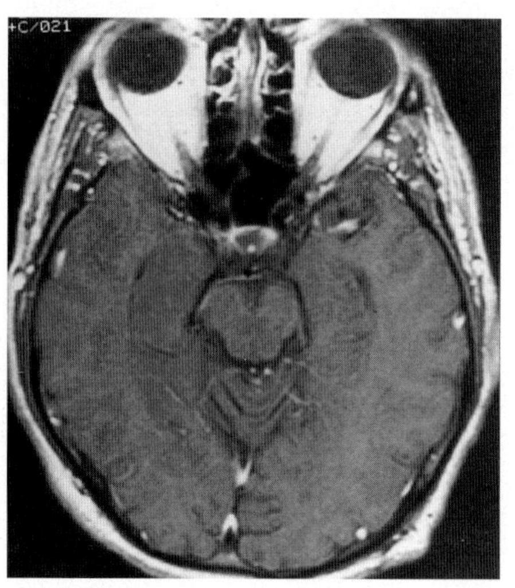


C

**Left middle cerebral bifurcation aneurysm (1.7 cm in size) is well identified in the base projection of the three-dimensional time-of-flight MRA (A) (512 matrix) and the coronal two-dimensional phase-contrast study (B). Both MRA studies were performed after the administration of contrast material. There is overall increased signal intensity from the background on the three-dimensional time-of-flight study because of the enhancement of the nasal mucosa and soft tissues. This is lacking on the two-dimensional phase-contrast study because of the improved background suppression available with this technique. The aneurysm is difficult to detect on the postcontrast axial T1-weighted image (C) because of the T1 shortening of blood that makes the aneurysmal lumen nearly isointense with brain. (Courtesy John Huston, Mayo Clinic, Rochester, Minn.)**

An additional use for phase-contrast MRA, besides identification of flow direction and general aneurysm morphology has been suggested by Meyer et al, who evaluated cine phase-contrast MRA in ruptured and unruptured aneurysms. They demonstrated that ruptured aneurysms increased in volume by up to 50% between systole and diastole, whereas unruptured aneurysms did not increase to such a degree (17.6%). They suggested that cine phase-contrast MRA can detect structural weakness in the aneurysmal wall, which could be of benefit in therapeutic planning.

**REFERENCE**

Meyer FB, Huston John III, Reiderer SS: Pulsatile increases in aneurysm size determined by cine phase-contrast MR angiography, *J Neurosurg* 78:879-883, 1993.

## CASE 58
## GIANT MIDDLE CEREBRAL ARTERY ANEURYSM

**History:** 64-year-old with new onset of seizures.

**Technique:** axial volume, three-dimensional time-of-flight, 40/7/15, 256 × 256, 64 slices, 60-mm slab, 23-cm field of view, 10:57.

A

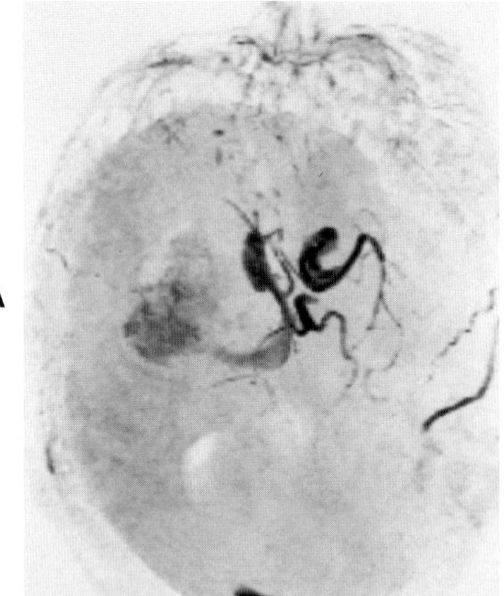

B

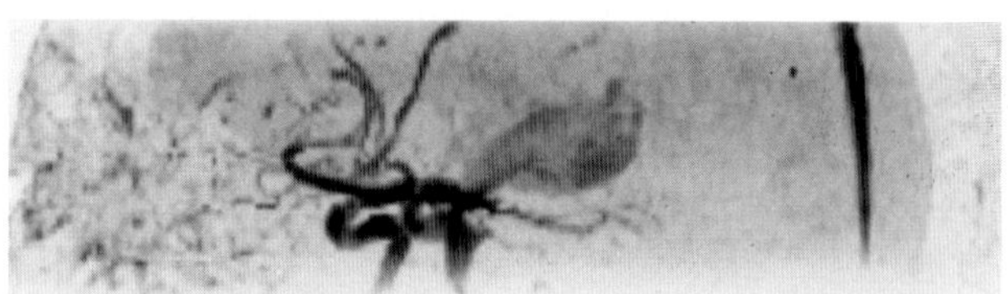

D

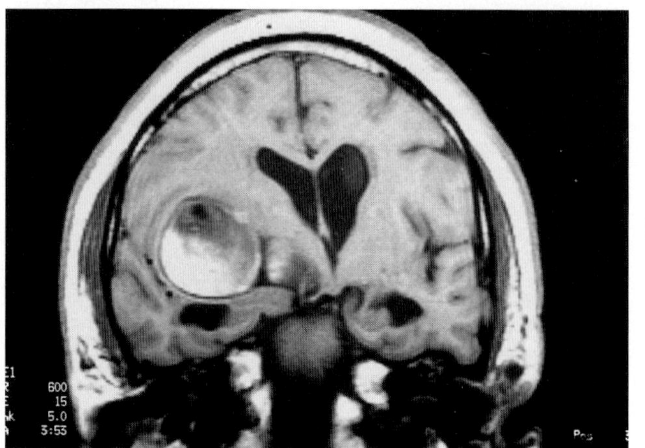

C

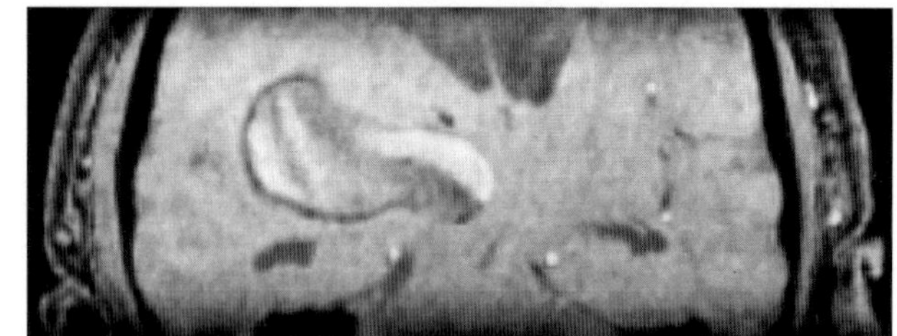

E

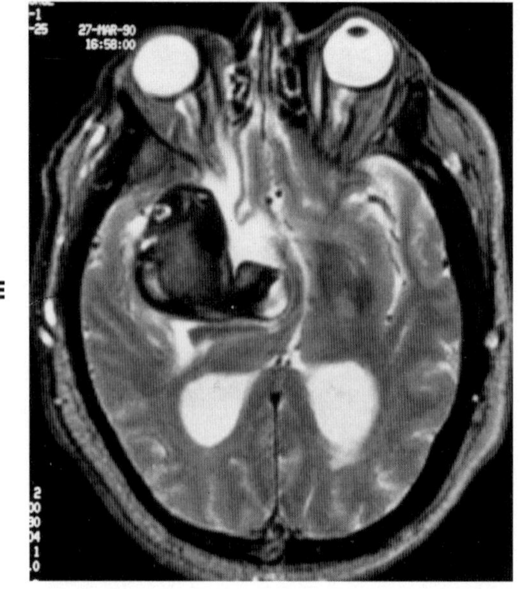

**Oblique (A) and base (B) views of the maximum intensity projection demonstrate a large, ill-defined area of slightly increased signal intensity arising off the region of the distal left internal carotid artery. There is lack of visualization of the left M1 and M2 segments and the distal branches on the MRA. The lesion is better seen on the coronal reformat of the MRA data as a well defined mass of heterogeneous signal intensity (C). T1 coronal (D) and T2-weighted axial (E) views of the head demonstrate a large, lobular, complex mass involving the right middle cerebral distribution, which represents a giant intracranial aneurysm. There is a moderate amount of associated vasogenic edema and midline shift. The lack of visualization of the distal middle cerebral branches relates to slowed and complex flow resulting from the aneurysm. The aneurysm itself is only partially seen, which is also due to a slowed and complex flow, with resultant flow saturation on three-dimensional time-of-flight study.**

Although the aneurysm is not optimally visualized on the time-of-flight study, the conventional T1- and T2-weighted studies confirm the diagnosis of the giant intracranial aneurysm. Typical imaging features of partially thrombosed giant intracranial aneurysms include signal void in the residual patent lumen on spin-echo images, laminated-appearing thrombus, and identification of signal void (spin echo) or increased signal (gradient echo or MRA) from the vessel from which the aneurysm arises. The laminated appearance comes from the histologic appearance of an "onion skin," which is shown on the T2-weighted image and the coronal reformat of the MRA data **(C).** Each layer represents a clot of different age from the neighboring layer. More peripheral layers probably represent more recent clot if growth is occurring because of a new hemorrhage at the periphery of the aneurysm. Layers may also occur inside the lumen of the aneurysm if intraaneurysmal hemodynamics change if or slowed and turbulent flow occurs, thus allowing fresh clot formation.

## REFERENCES

Atlas SW, Grossman RI, Goldberg HI et al: Partially thrombosed giant intracranial aneurysms: correlation of MR and pathologic findings, *Radiology* 162:111-114, 1987.

Schubiger O, Valavanis A, Wichmann W: Growth-mechanism of giant intracranial aneurysms: demonstration by CT and MR imaging, *Neuroradiology* 29:266-271, 1987.

Artman H, Vonofakos D, Muller H et al: Neuroradiologic and neuropathologic findings with growing giant intracranial aneurysm, *Surg Neurol* 21:391-401, 1984.

# CASE 59
## POSTERIOR COMMUNICATING ARTERY ANEURYSM

**History:** 40-year-old with a right-sided third nerve palsy.

**Technique:** axial volume, three-dimensional time-of-flight, 40/8/15, 256 × 128, 64 slices, 60-mm slab, 25-cm field of view, 5:20.

A

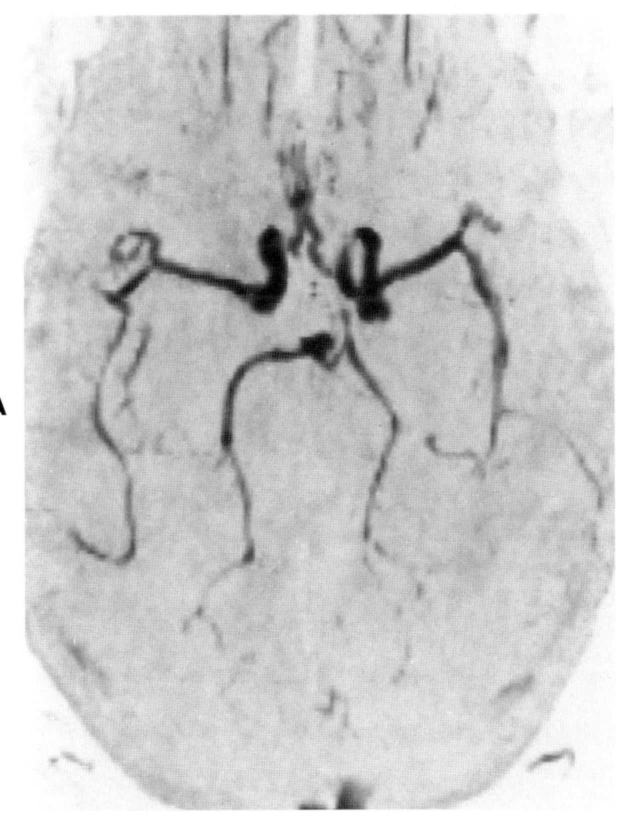

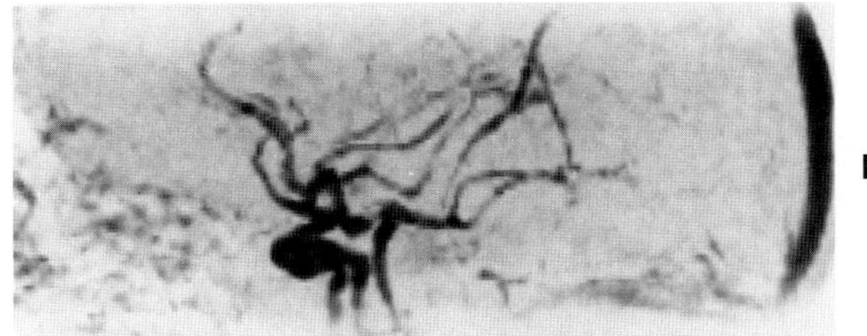

B

**Base (A) and lateral (B) maximum intensity projection views show a rounded outpouching of increased signal intensity arising off the region of the distal left internal carotid artery, which represents a posterior communicating artery aneurysm. Lateral view from the intraarterial angiogram (C) confirms the finding of the posterior communicating artery aneurysm. In this case, there is relatively good definition of the aneurysm neck on the MRA. However, studies with longer echo times may shows a line of signal void separating the distal internal carotid artery and the aneurysm proper, which is caused by dephasing of moving (especially accelerated) spins, particularly at regions of vessel narrowing such as the aneurysm neck. (A from Ross JS, Masaryk T, Modic M et al: *AJNR* 11:449-456, 1990.)**

C

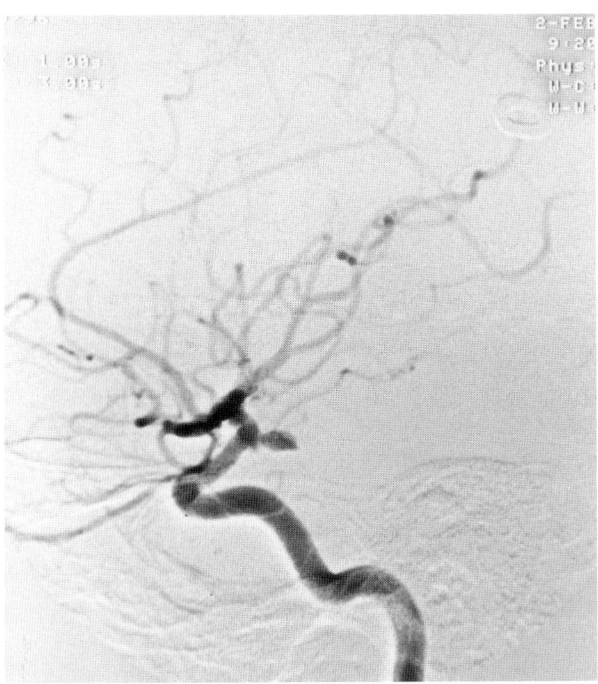

# CASE 60
# POSTERIOR COMMUNICATING ARTERY ANEURYSM

**History:** 43-year-old with bifrontal headaches and a family history of aneurysms.

**Technique #1:** axial volume, three-dimensional time-of-flight, 45/7/20, 256 × 256, 64 slices, 60-mm slab, 15-cm field of view, 12:19.

**Technique #2:** axial volume, three-dimensional time-of-flight, 45/8.5/20, 256 × 256, 64 slices, 60-mm slab, 15-cm field of view, 12:19.

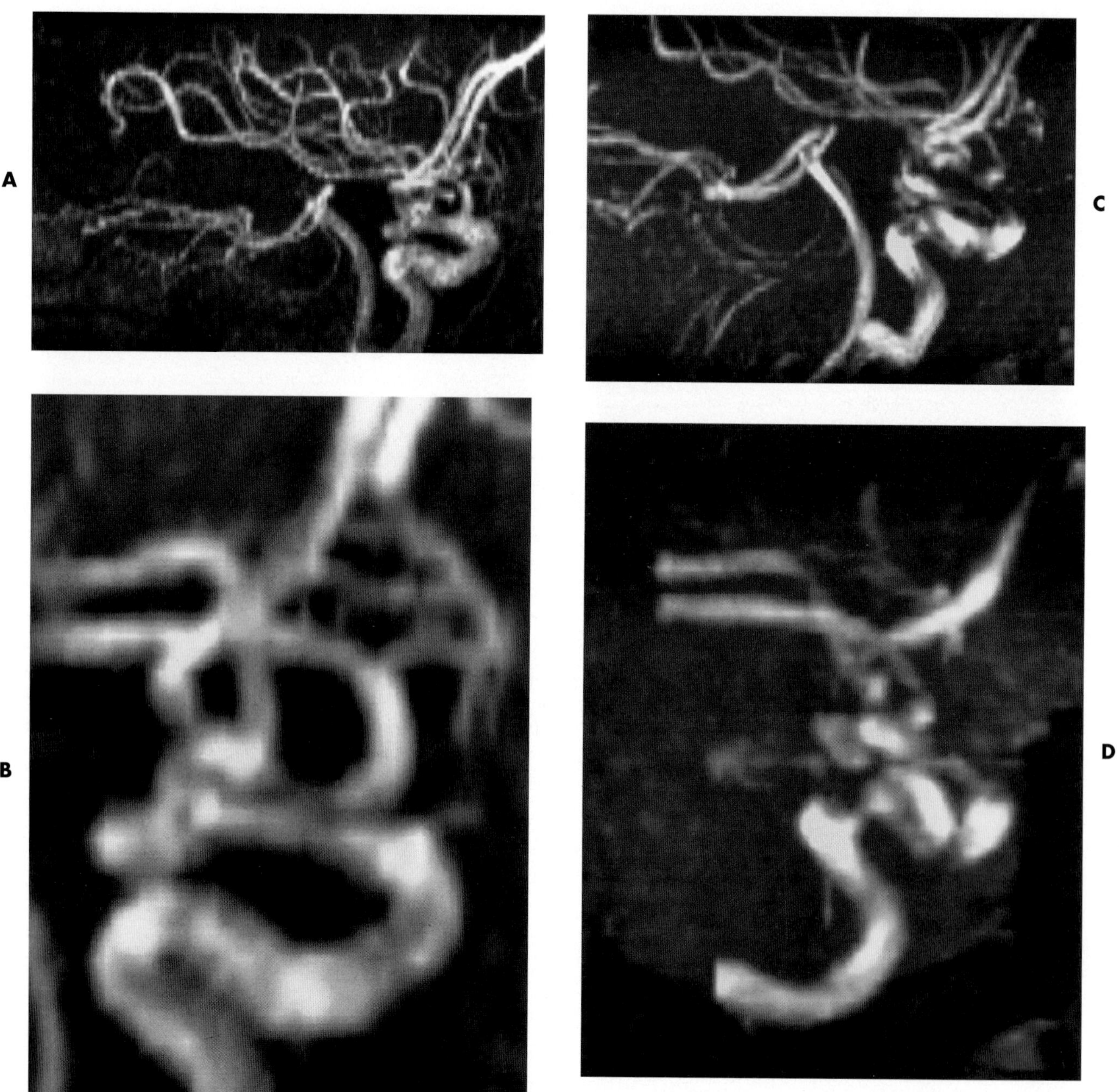

**Lateral maximum intensity projection (A) and targeted carotid siphon maximum intensity projection (B) views with an echo time of 7 show a well-defined posterior communicating artery aneurysm arising off the posterior aspect of the internal carotid artery. The corresponding lateral maximum intensity projection views with an echo time of 8.5 also show the aneurysm (C and D), but it is much less well defined. There is also increased signal loss in the carotid siphon on the longer echo-time study. Lateral targeted maximum intensity projection images with a shorter echo time (B) and a longer echo time (D) show the improvement in image quality that a small change in echo time may produce. (Phase errors increase quadratically with time.) The lateral view of the conventional angiogram (E) shows the posterior communicating artery aneurysm. Both MRA techniques fail to distinguish the origin of the distal internal carotid aneurysm from the adjacent posterior communicating artery infundibulum.**

E

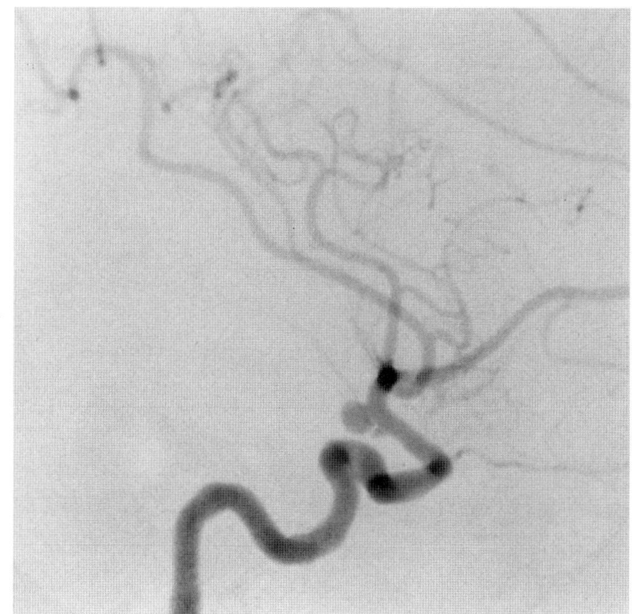

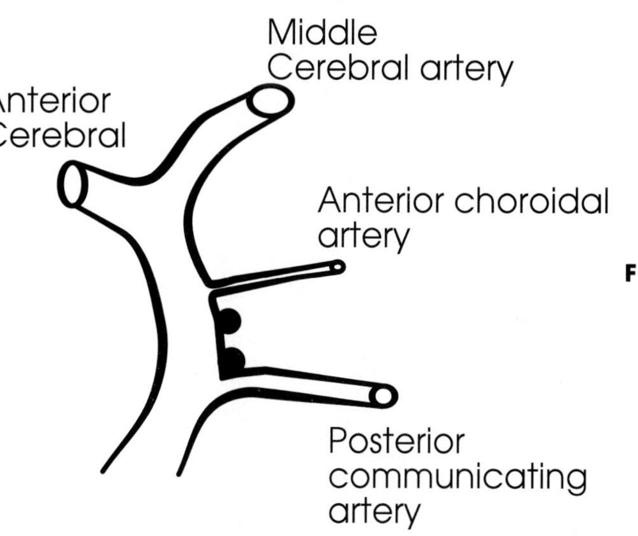


F

**Schematic of posterior communicating artery region aneurysms (F).**

The posterior communicating artery region is the most common site of aneurysm formation on the internal carotid artery, with an incidence of approximately 20%. The anterior choroidal artery just distal to the posterior communicating artery origin (6.6% of internal carotid artery aneurysms in Yasargil's series) may also be involved in aneurysm formation. These lesions commonly compress the third cranial nerve, with up to 40% of patients having third nerve palsy **(F).**

**REFERENCE**

Yasargil MG: *Microneurosurgery,* vol 2, New York, 1984, Thieme.

## CASE 61
## CALCIFIED POSTERIOR COMMUNICATING ARTERY ANEURYSM

**History:** 79-year-old incidentally noted to have intracranial calcification on a tomogram of the temporomandibular joint.

**Technique #1:** axial volume, three-dimensional time-of-flight, 43/6/20, 512 × 256, 60 slices, 60-mm slab, 18-cm field of view, 12:19.

**Technique #2:** axial volume, three-dimensional phase-contrast, 26/9/15, 256 × 128 matrix, one excitation, 60 slices, 60-mm slab, velocity encoding of 30 cm/sec, 18-cm field of view, 14 minutes.

A

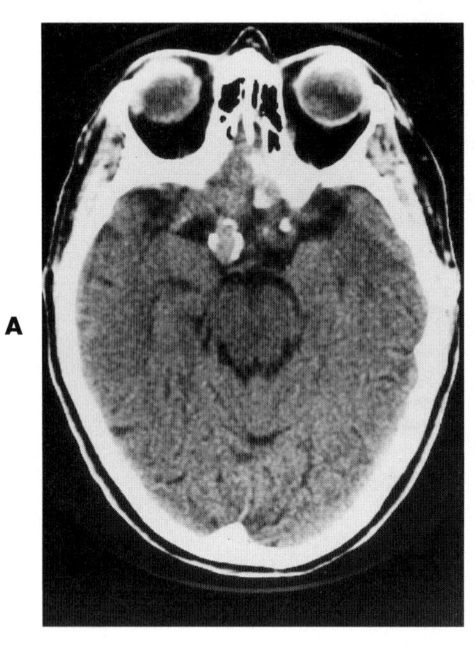

B

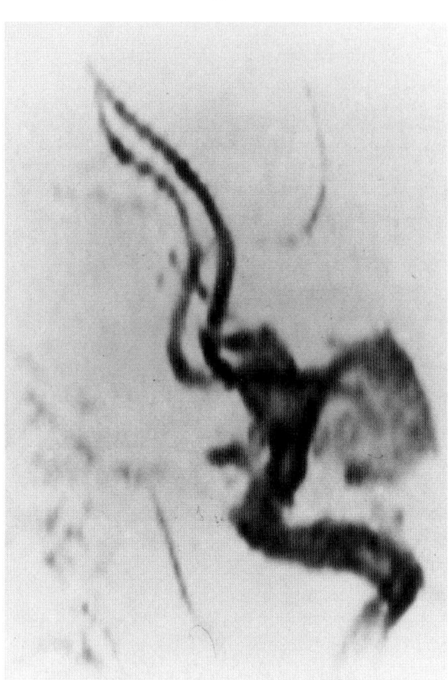

C

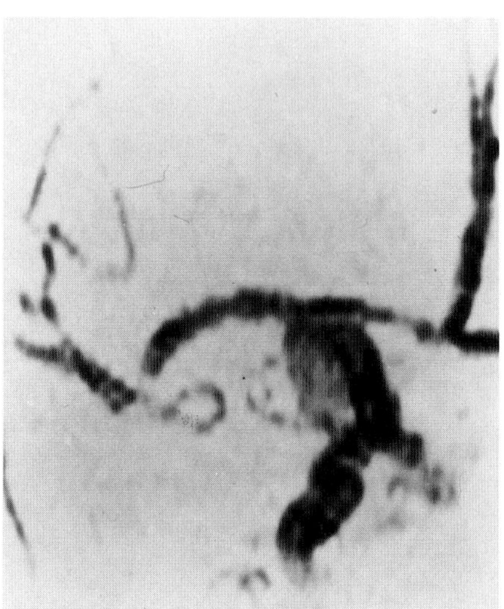

D

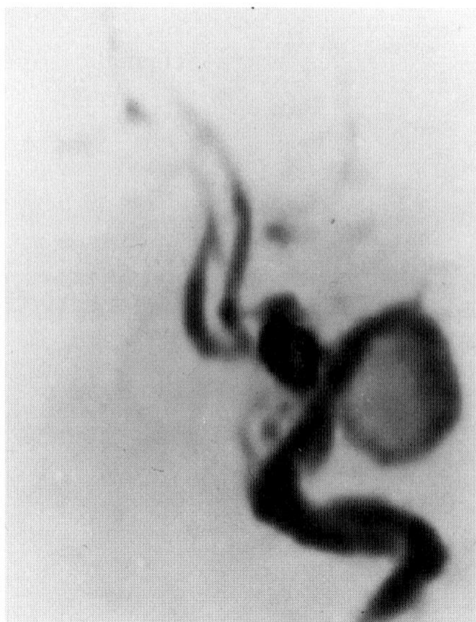

E

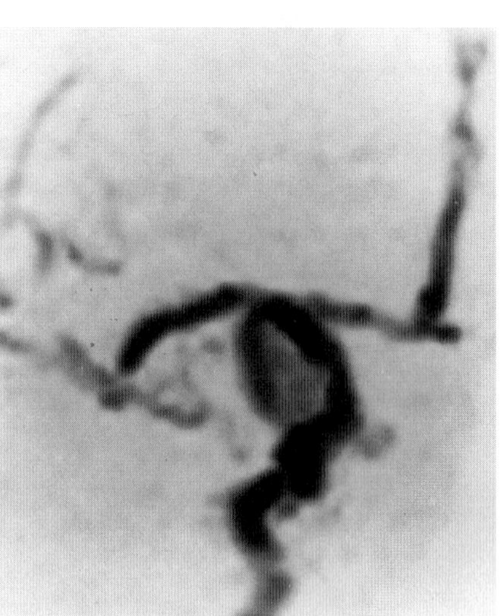

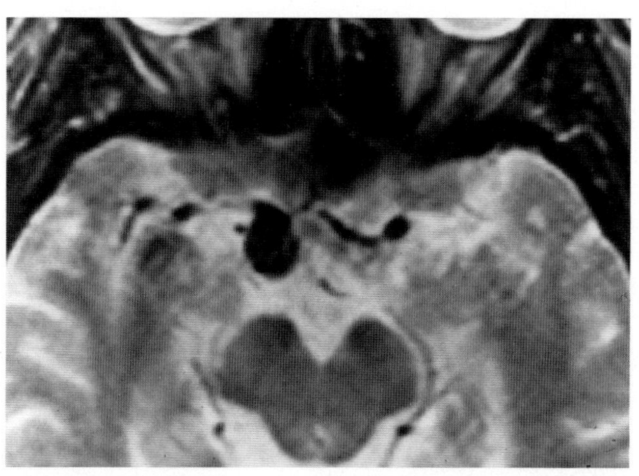


**Axial computed tomographic scan (A) demonstrates a rounded mass in the supersellar cistern on the right, with a peripheral calcification suggesting vascular lesion. Targeted lateral and anteroposterior views from a three-dimensional time-of-flight (B and C) and three-dimensional phase-contrast MRA (30-cm velocity encoding) (D and E) demonstrate the large right posterior communicating artery aneurysm with a superior jet. On the anteroposterior view there is also a small medially projecting distal carotid artery (ophthalmic) aneurysm. This is slightly better identified on the three-dimensional time-of-flight study than on the phase-contrast study, probably because of the shorter echo time of the time-of-flight study. The posterior communicating artery aneurysm is also seen on the axial T2-weighted (F) spin-echo study as an area of flow void. (Courtesy John Huston, Mayo Clinic, Rochester, Minn.)**

## CASE 62
## ANEURYSM OF THE RIGHT INTERNAL CAROTID ARTERY

**History:** 35-year-old with headaches.

**Technique:** axial volume; three-dimensional time-of-flight; 45/7/20; 256 × 256; 64 slices; 60-mm slab; magnetization transfer background suppression; tilted, optimized nonsaturating excitation radiofrequency pulse; 14-cm field of view; 12:20.

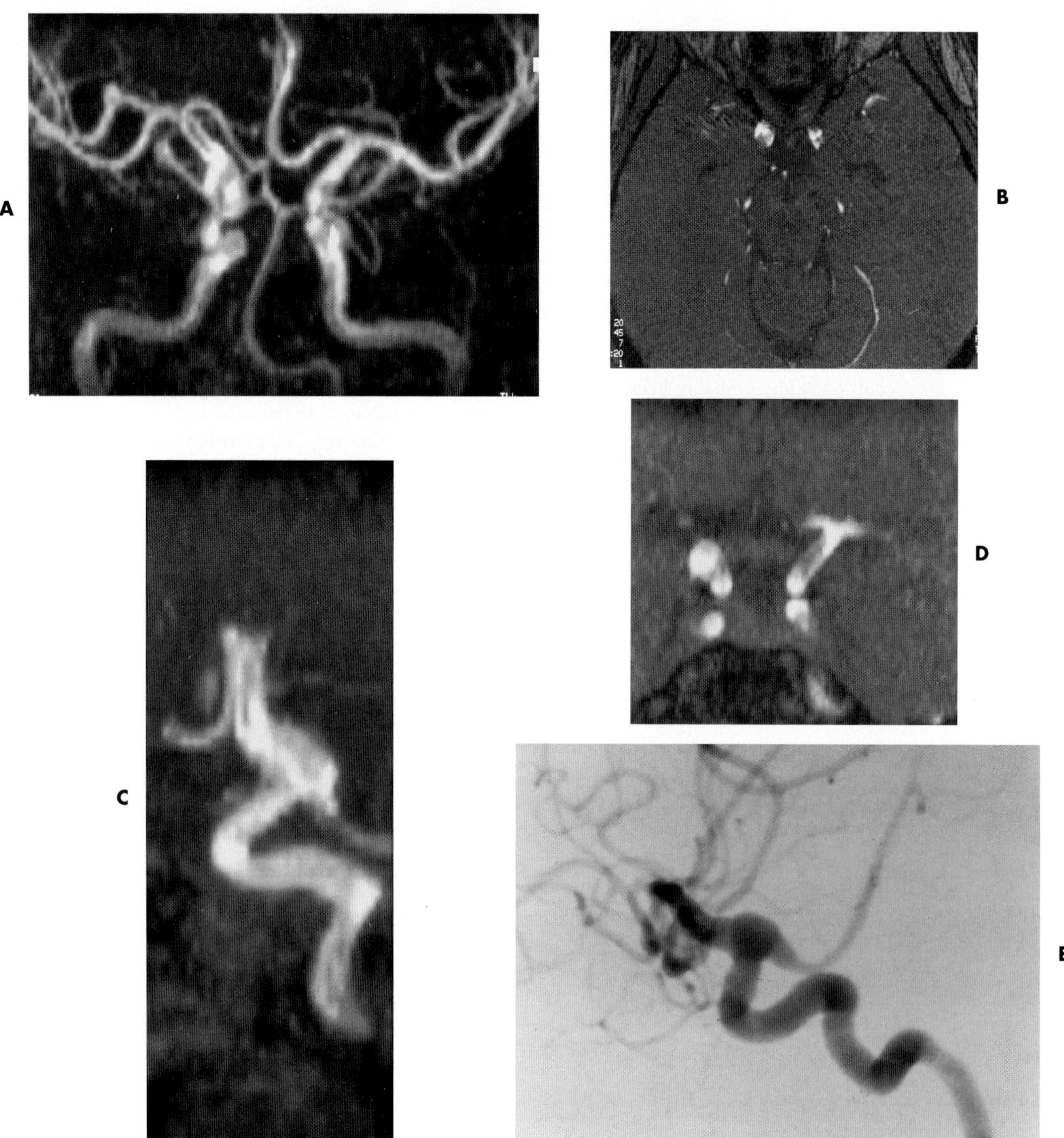

F

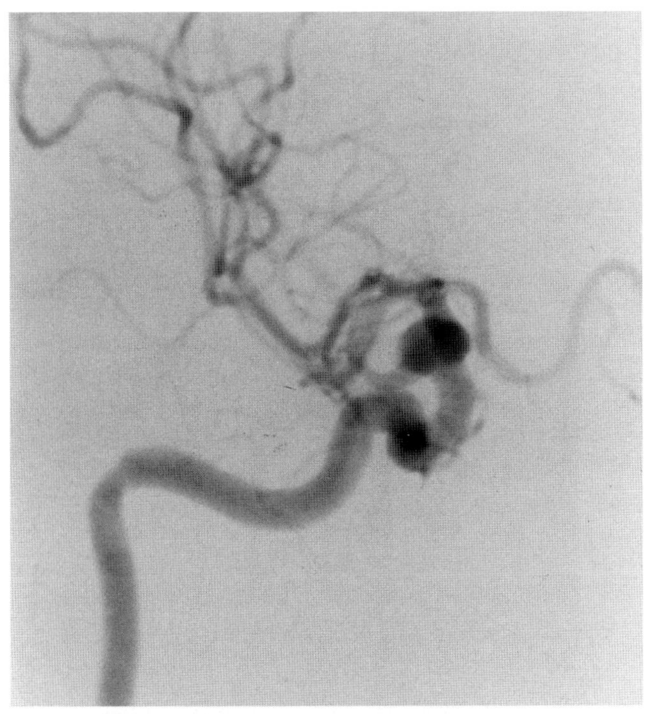

**Anteroposterior maximum intensity projection view of the whole head (A) shows slight bulbous asymmetry in the appearance of the distal right internal carotid signal, which is most apparent on the direct anteroposterior view. Examination of the individual slice (B) more clearly shows the aneurysm of the distal right internal carotid artery as rounded increased signal compared with the normal left side. There is also increased ghosting artifact from the aneurysm along the right-to-left phase-encoding direction, which can indicate an aneurysm. Lateral targeted maximum intensity projection of the distal right internal carotid (C) shows the relationship of the aneurysm to the posterior communicating artery. D, a coronal reformat of the MRA volume, further confirms the pathology and site of origin from the distal internal carotid artery. Lateral and anteroposterior views (E and F) of the right internal carotid injection show the fusiform aneurysmal dilatation of the distal internal carotid artery, including the origin of the posterior communicating artery.**

The annual incidence of subarachnoid hemorrhage from ruptured aneurysm is 12 in 100,000, or approximately 28,000 patients. Approximately 9000 of these patients survive the rupture without major disability or death. The most common locations for intracranial aneurysms are the anterior communicating artery, the distal internal carotid artery at the origin of the posterior communicating artery, and the bifurcation of the middle cerebral artery. The frequency of posterior circulation aneurysms (mainly of basilar tip and posterior internal carotid artery origin) is approximately 10%. The average age at presentation is 46 to 52 years, with a slightly higher incidence in women.

The clinical condition of the patient presenting with a subarachnoid hemorrhage has a major impact on the outcome and clinical management of the patient. The typical grading scale for subarachnoid hemorrhage is:

- Oa Unruptured and without neurologic deficit
- Ob Unruptured and with neurologic deficit (such as third nerve palsy)
- Ia Asymptomatic
- Ib Alert and oriented without meningismus but with focal deficit
- IIa Alert with headache and meningismus
- IIb Alert with headache and meningismus but with deficit
- IIIa Lethargic and disoriented
- IIIb Lethargic and disoriented but with deficit
- IV Semicomatose
- V Comatose

## REFERENCES


Ogawa T, Inugami A, Shimosegawa E et al: Subarachnoid hemorrhage: evaluation with MR imaging, *Radiology* 186:345-351, 1993.

Yasargil MG: *Microneurosurgery,* vol 2, New York, 1984, Thieme.

Locksley HB: *Natural history of subarachnoid hemorrhage, intracranial aneurysms, and arteriovenous malformations: based on 6,368 cases in the Cooperative Study.* In Sahs AL, Perret GE, Locksley HB et al, eds: *Intracranial aneurysms and subarachnoid hemorrhage: a Cooperative Study,* Philadelphia, 1969, Lippincott.

Ross JS, Masaryk TJ, Modic MT et al: Intracranial aneurysms: evaluation by MR angiography, *AJNR* 11:449-456, 1990.

# CASE 63
# PARTIALLY THROMBOSED GIANT INTRACRANIAL ANEURYSM

**History:** 71-year-old with a 3-week history of intense bitemporal headache.

**Technique:** axial volume; three-dimensional time-of-flight; 45/7/20 degrees; 256 × 256; 64 slices; 60-mm slab; magnetization transfer background suppression; tilted, optimized nonsaturating excitation radiofrequency pulse; 14-cm field of view; 12:20.

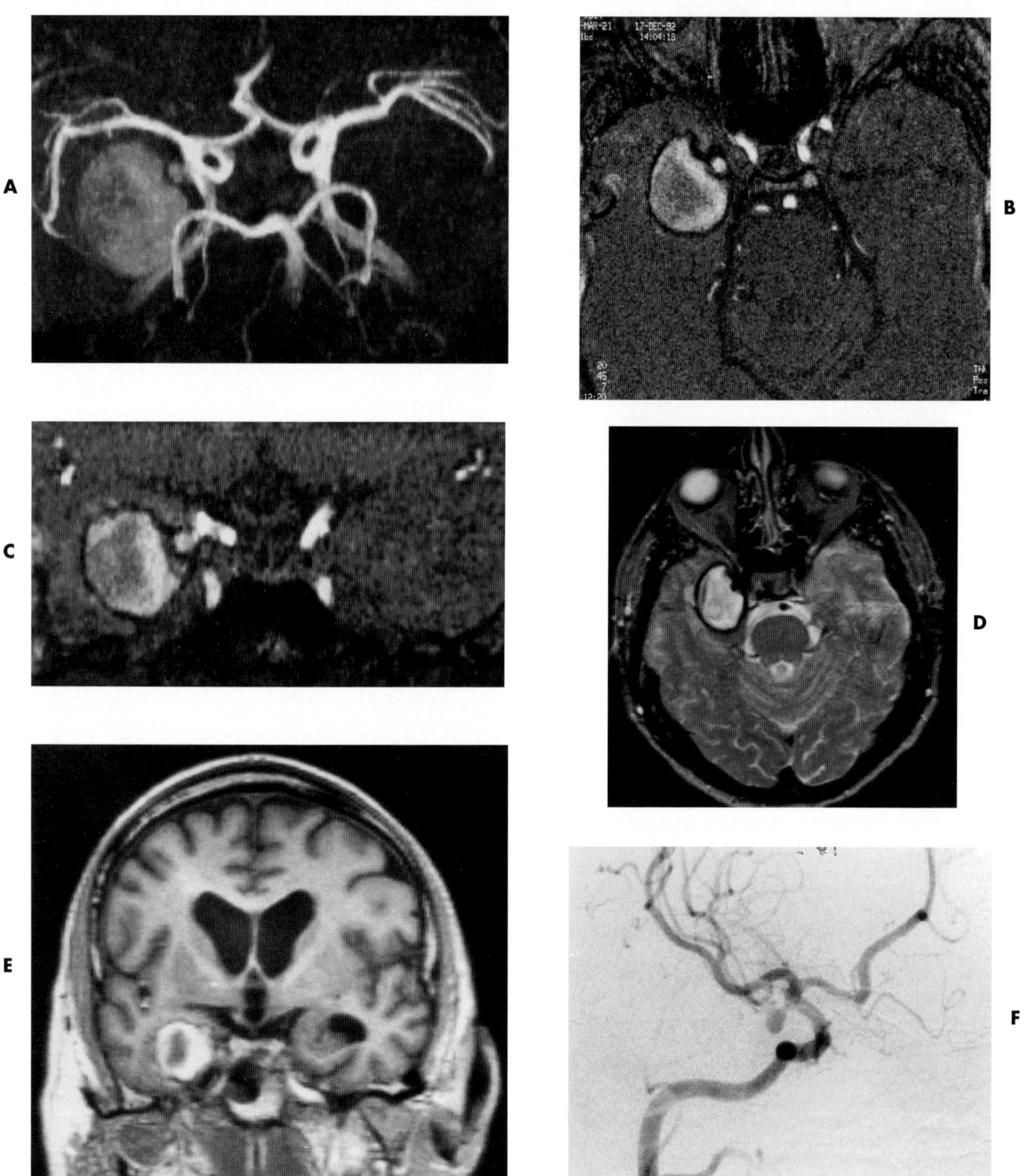

**Base view of the maximum intensity projection (A) demonstrates a large, rounded area of abnormally increased signal intensity adjacent to the distal right internal carotid artery. There is a smaller area of increased signal intensity just lateral and contiguous with the right carotid siphon, which appears separated from the bulk of the lesion by a line of low signal intensity. This is also demonstrated on the individual slices (B), where a more focal area of the residual lumen is separated from the thrombosed portion of the aneurysm. Coronal reformat (C) through the aneurysm demonstrates to a better extent the junction of the internal carotid artery with the true aneurysm lumen and the separation of the true lumen from the thrombosed portion, which has methemoglobin within it. On the axial T2-weighted image (D), the thrombosed portion of the aneurysm shows high signal intensity with a small focal area of signal flow void, which represents the patent lumen. Methemoglobin shows high signal intensity on the predominately T1-weighted volume gradient-echo image (E). Right anterior oblique intracranial view from a common carotid injection (F) demonstrates the small residual patent lumen of the much larger thrombosed aneurysm.**

Giant intracranial aneurysms are defined as larger than 2.5 cm. The incidence of these lesions is approximately 5%, with a 3:1 female-to-male ratio. Giant intracranial aneurysms are one of many aneurysms (not necessarily giant) in 10% to 30% of cases. They tend to present less often with subarachnoid hemorrhage than with saccular aneurysms. Instead, they present with mass effect (hemispheric dysfunction, headache, visual deficit, seizures, and dementia). These lesions vary widely in natural history: (1) Intracavernous and thrombosed aneurysms rarely enlarge or rupture, (2) the aneurysm may remain unchanged in size or even decrease in size, and (3) they may enlarge and rupture. Giant intracranial aneurysms tend to involve the middle cerebral artery (24% of cases), the anterior communicating artery (17%), the internal carotid artery (16%), the basilar artery (12%), the intracavernous carotid artery (11%), and the carotid/ophthalmic region (10%). Giant intracranial aneurysms may grow by recurrent hemorrhage into its wall and behave like a growing encapsulated hematoma.

### REFERENCES


Hosobuchi Y: Direct surgical treatment of giant intracranial aneurysms, *J Neurosurg* 51:743-756, 1979.

Sonntag VKH, Yuan RH, Stein BM: Giant intracranial aneurysms: a review of 13 cases, *Surg Neurol* 8:81-84, 1977.

Creissard P et al: Les anevnismes geants, *Neurochirurgie* 26:309-353, 1980.

Drake CG: Giant intracranial aneurysms: experience with surgical treatment in 174 patients, *Clin Neurosurg* 26:12-95, 1979.

Sundt TM, Piepgras DG: Surgical approach to giant intracranial aneurysms: operative experience with 80 cases, *J Neurosurg* 51:731-742, 1979.

## CASE 64
## BALLOON OCCLUSION OF CAVERNOUS ANEURYSM WITH EXTRACRANIAL-INTRACRANIAL BYPASS

**History:** 48-year-old after balloon occlusion of the left cavernous carotid aneurysm.

**Technique:** axial volume, three-dimensional time-of-flight, 40/6/15, 256 × 160, 64 slices, 60-mm slab, 20-cm field of view (rectangular), 6:52.

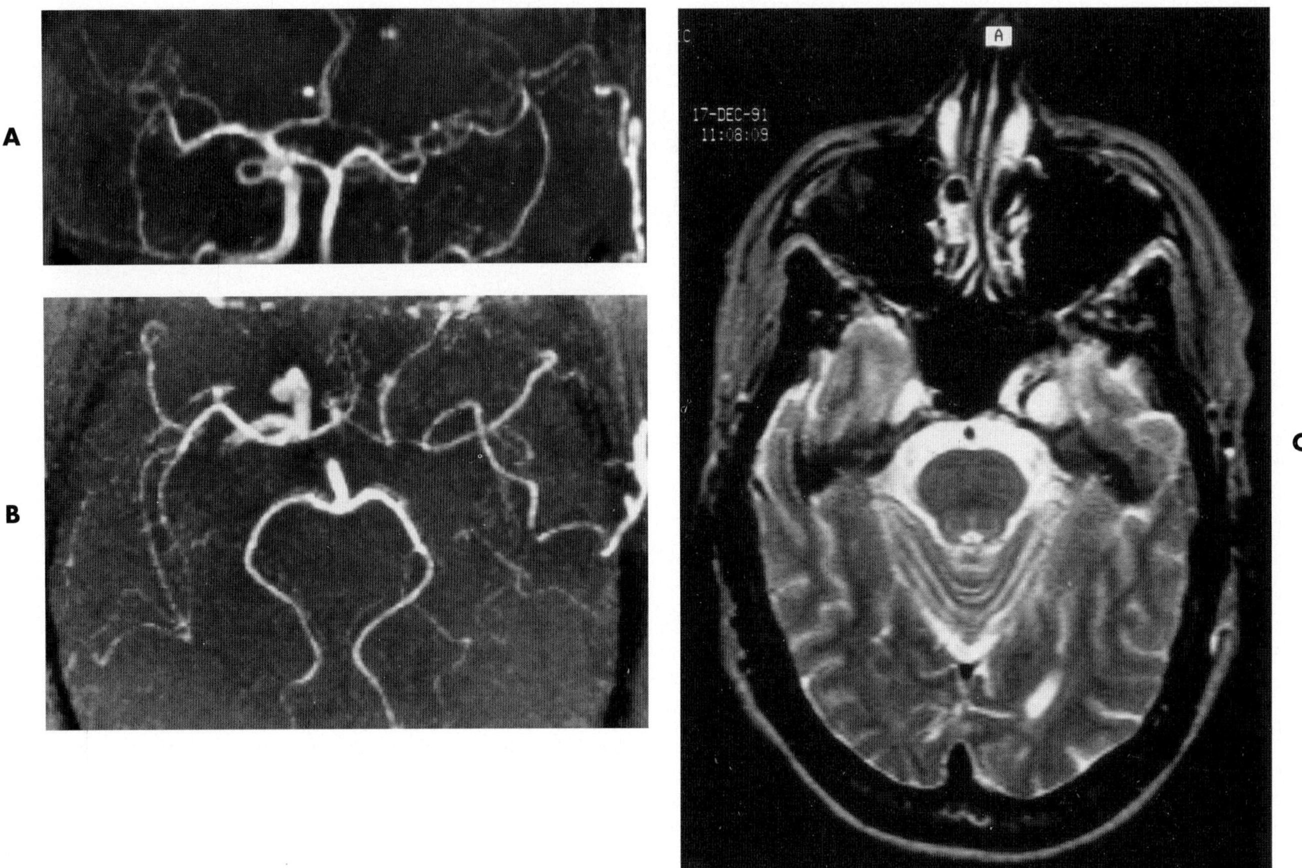


**The anteroposterior (A) and targeted base (B) maximum intensity projections show a lack of flow-related enhancement from the left internal carotid artery. A large external carotid branch is seen coursing sinuously over the left convexity and then connecting with the distal left middle cerebral artery branches, which represents the superficial temporal to middle cerebral artery bypass. The carotid has been therapeutically occluded by balloon placement. T2-weighted axial study of the head (C) demonstrates the thrombosed large distal internal carotid artery aneurysm.**

Extracranial-intracranial bypass surgery is used in the treatment of giant intracranial aneurysms in cases in which direct surgical clipping or ligation is unsuitable. To prevent ischemic complications caused by occlusion of the parent vessel (usually the internal carotid artery or middle cerebral artery), a variety of bypasses have been performed, including superficial temporal to middle cerebral and donor vessels such as middle meningeal artery, occipital artery, and venous interposition grafts. Conventional angiography has been generally used for follow-up of these grafts, but MRA may provide an easy outpatient noninvasive method for determining patency.

In one series, six patients with giant aneurysms thrombosed by balloon embolization were followed with MR imaging. Of the aneurysms that were 100% occluded all demonstrated a decrease in physical size on follow-up MR imaging scans. One patient who had a 90% obliteration of the lumen demonstrated no change in the size of giant aneurysm over a 2-year follow-up period. Thrombus formation in an incompletely thrombosed giant aneurysm is to be differentiated from organizing thrombus in a completely thrombosed aneurysm. The thrombosis after occlusion is due to stasis, a mechanism analogous to venous (red thrombosis) rather than arterial (white thrombosis). This is reflected in the appearance on MR images. Induced thrombosis demonstrates an area of hyperintensity at 5 to 10 days on short repitition–echo time and long repitition time–short echo time images. The long repitition time–echo time images demonstrate hypointensity. At 4 to 6 weeks, induced thrombus was hyperintense on all spin-echo sequences where spontaneous hemorrhage still had areas of hypointensity, but these had increased in signal intensity from the subacute stage (5 to 10 days).

## REFERENCES

Tsuruda JS, Sevick RJ, Halbach VV: Three dimensional time of flight MR angiography in the evaluation of intracranial aneurysms treated by endovascular balloon occlusion, *AJNR* 13:1129, 1992.

Kwan ESK, Wolpert SM, Scott RM, Runge V: MR evaluation of neurovascular lesions after endovascular occlusion with detachable balloons, *AJNR* 9:523-531, 1988.

Strother CM, Eldevik P, Kikuchi Y et al: Thrombus formation and structure and the evolution of mass effect in intracranial aneurysms treated by balloon embolization: emphasis on MR findings, *AJNR* 10:787-796, 1989.

Spetzler RF, Roski RA: The role of EC-IC in the treatment of giant intracranial aneurysms, *Neurolog Res* 2:345-359, 1980.

## CASE 65
## PSEUDOANEURYSM OF THE LEFT CAVERNOUS CAROTID AFTER BALLOON OCCLUSION OF A CAROTID CAVERNOUS FISTULA

**History:** 27-year-old after a motor vehicle accident that produced a left carotid cavernous fistula. The fistula was successfully treated with balloon occlusion.

**Technique:** axial volume, three-dimensional time-of-flight, 45/6.9/15, 256 × 256, 64 slices, 54-mm slab, 15-cm field of view, 12:19.

A

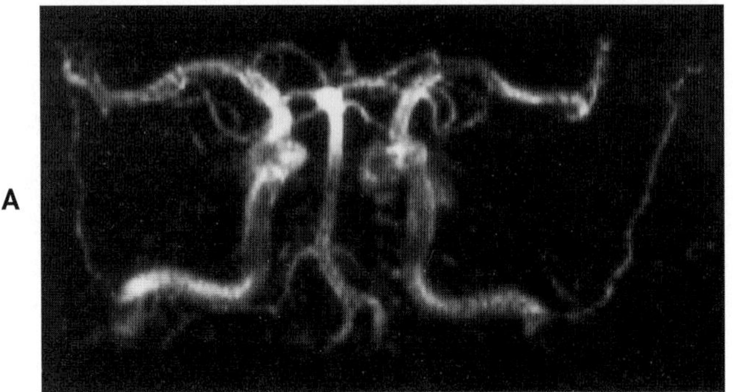

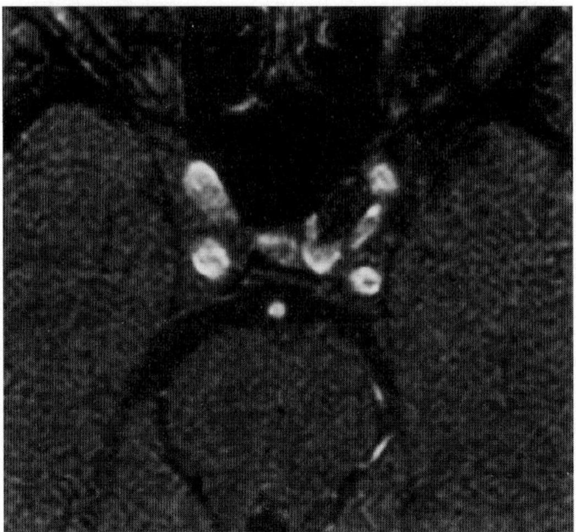

B

C

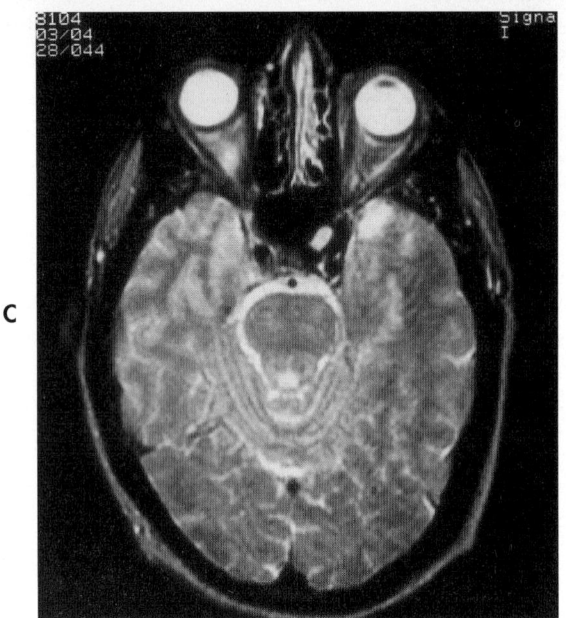


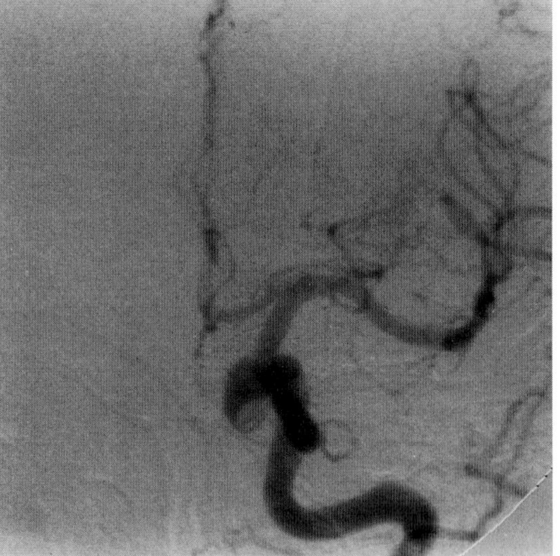

D

**Anteroposterior maximum intensity projection view of the intracranial circulation (A) shows a large, rounded area of increased signal arising off the medial aspect of the left cavernous carotid artery. Evaluation of the individual slices of the MRA data set (B) show the relationship of the low signal intensity balloon with the pseudoaneurysm arising medially, which is increased in signal. T2-weighted image (C) shows the balloon as high signal intensity, whereas the pseudoaneurysm is difficult to detect separate from the normal siphon and the sphenoid sinus. Conventional angiographic anteroposterior intracranial view (D) of a left common carotid injection shows the pseudoaneurysm arising off the carotid, similar to the MRA. In this instance, the MRA is useful to follow the course of the pseudoaneurysm to evaluate enlargement or other complications.**

# CASE 66
# OPHTHALMIC ARTERY ANEURYSM

**History:** 35-year-old with polycystic kidney disease and headaches.

**Technique:** axial volume, three-dimensional time-of-flight, 40/7/15, 256 × 256, 64 slices, 60-mm slab, 23-cm field of view, 10:57.

A
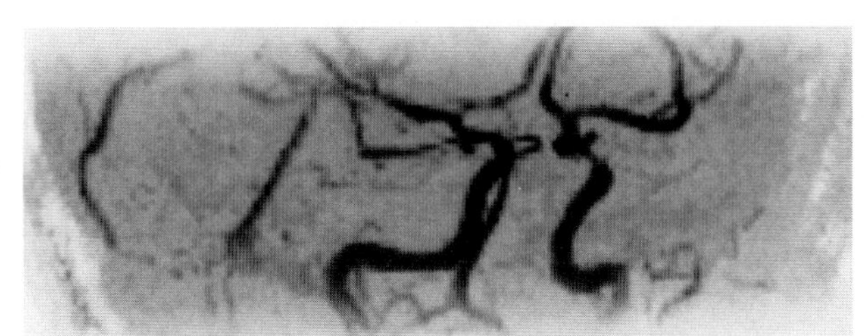

B
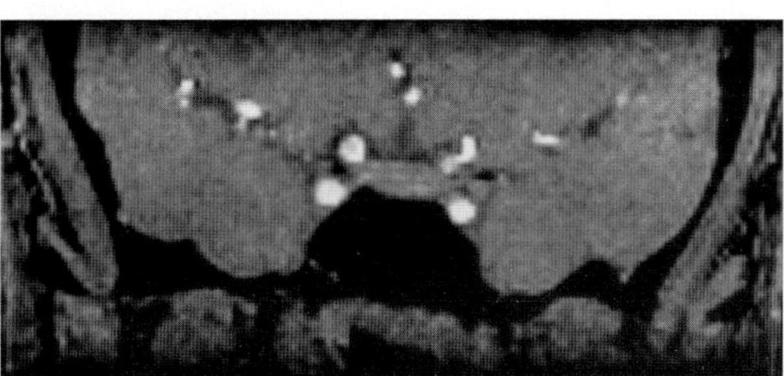

C
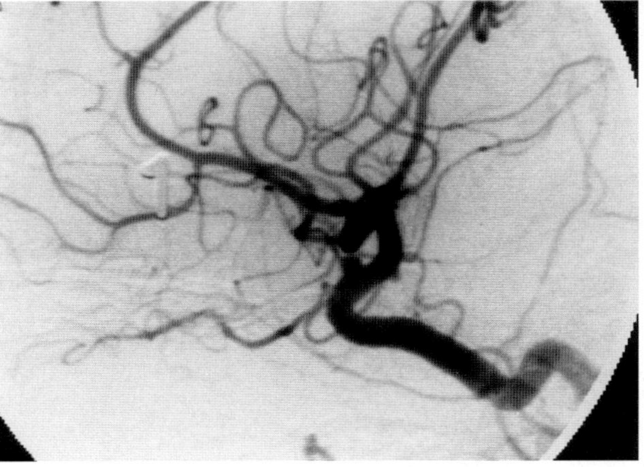

**Right anterior oblique maximum intensity projection view (A) demonstrates a small outpouching of abnormal increased signal intensity arising off the distal left internal carotid artery in the region of the ophthalmic artery origin. This aneurysm is confirmed on the coronal (B) reformat, which definitively shows a small abnormal outpouching of high signal intensity arising off the distal left internal carotid siphon and projecting laterally and superiorly. Lateral view of a conventional angiogram (C) confirms the small ophthalmic artery aneurysm. Small ophthalmic artery aneurysms or siphon aneurysms may be detected only with meticulous attention to the whole head maximum intensity projection, targeted maximum intensity projection, and planar reformats.**

---

Ophthalmic artery aneurysms generally arise off the medial and superomedial wall of the distal internal carotid artery and usually arise just distal to the origin of the ophthalmic artery. These aneurysms constitute 1.3% to 5% of intracranial aneurysms and may be bilaterally symmetrical. Commonly the fundus of the aneurysm is beneath the optic nerve and may elevate and compress it. The ophthalmic artery origin is intradural in 90% of patients, and in approximately 8% of patients, it is extradural.

## REFERENCE

Yasargil MG: *Microneurosurgery,* vol 2, New York, 1984, Thieme.

# CASE 67
# LARGE OPHTHALMIC ARTERY ANEURYSM

**History:** 50-year-old with decreased vision in the left eye.

**Technique:** axial volume, three-dimensional time-of-flight, 30/7/20, 256 × 192, 64 slices, 64-mm slab, 16-cm field of view, 6:11.

A

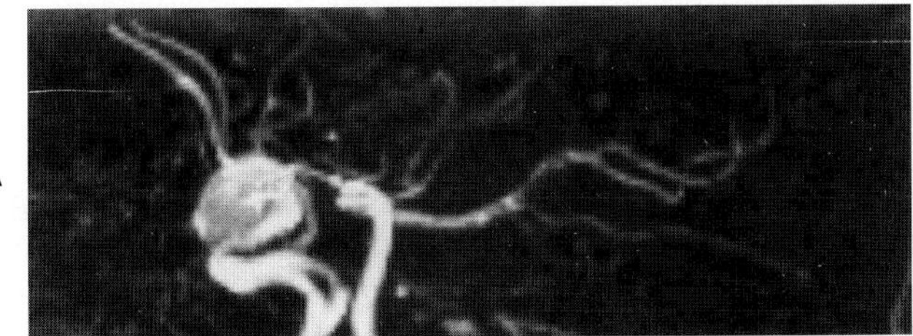

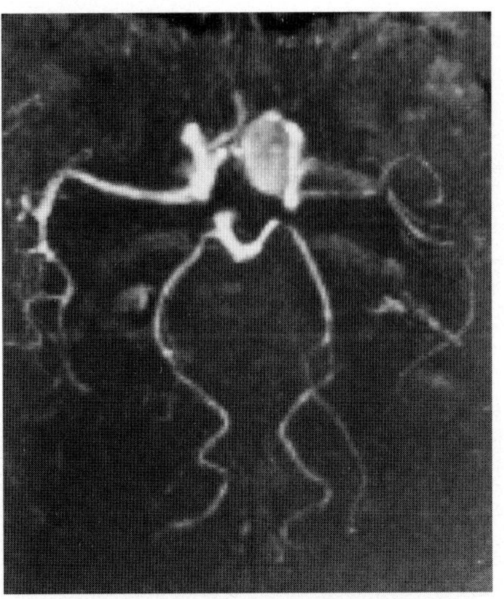

B

C

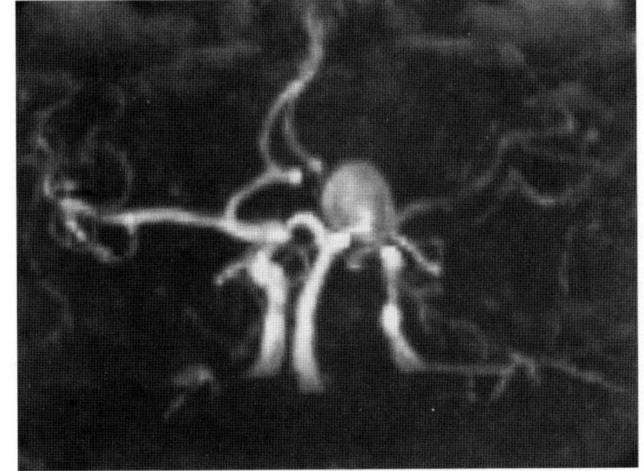

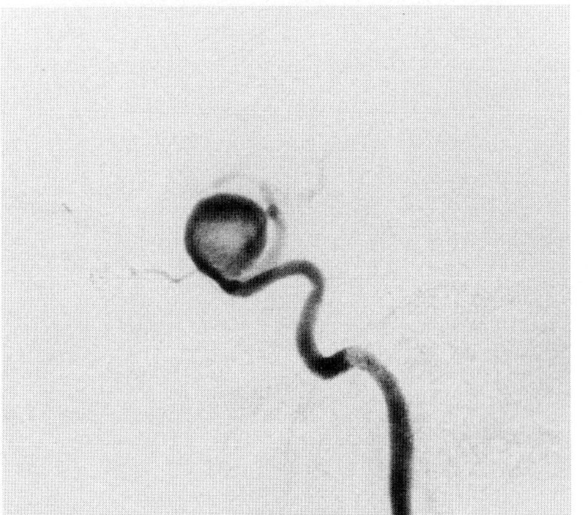

D

**Anteroposterior (A), base (B), and lateral (C) view maximum intensity projections demonstrate a large aneurysm arising off the distal left internal carotid artery and projecting superiorly and anteriorly. Relatively low signal intensity is seen within the central aspect of the aneurysm, which is caused by vortical or slow flow with flow saturation. The periphery of the aneurysm shows relatively higher signal intensity related to faster flow and better flow-related enhancement. This type of pattern is confirmed on the lateral view of the conventional angiographic internal carotid injection (D), which shows the periphery of the jet extending superiorly and circumferentially within the aneurysm and slowed flow within the central portion.**

## CASE 68
## MULITPLE ANEURYSMS

**History:** 40-year-old with a history of polycystic kidney disease.

**Technique:** axial volumes, three-dimensional time-of-flight, 40/6/15, 256 × 160, 64 slices, 60-mm slab, 20-cm field of view (rectangular), 6:52.

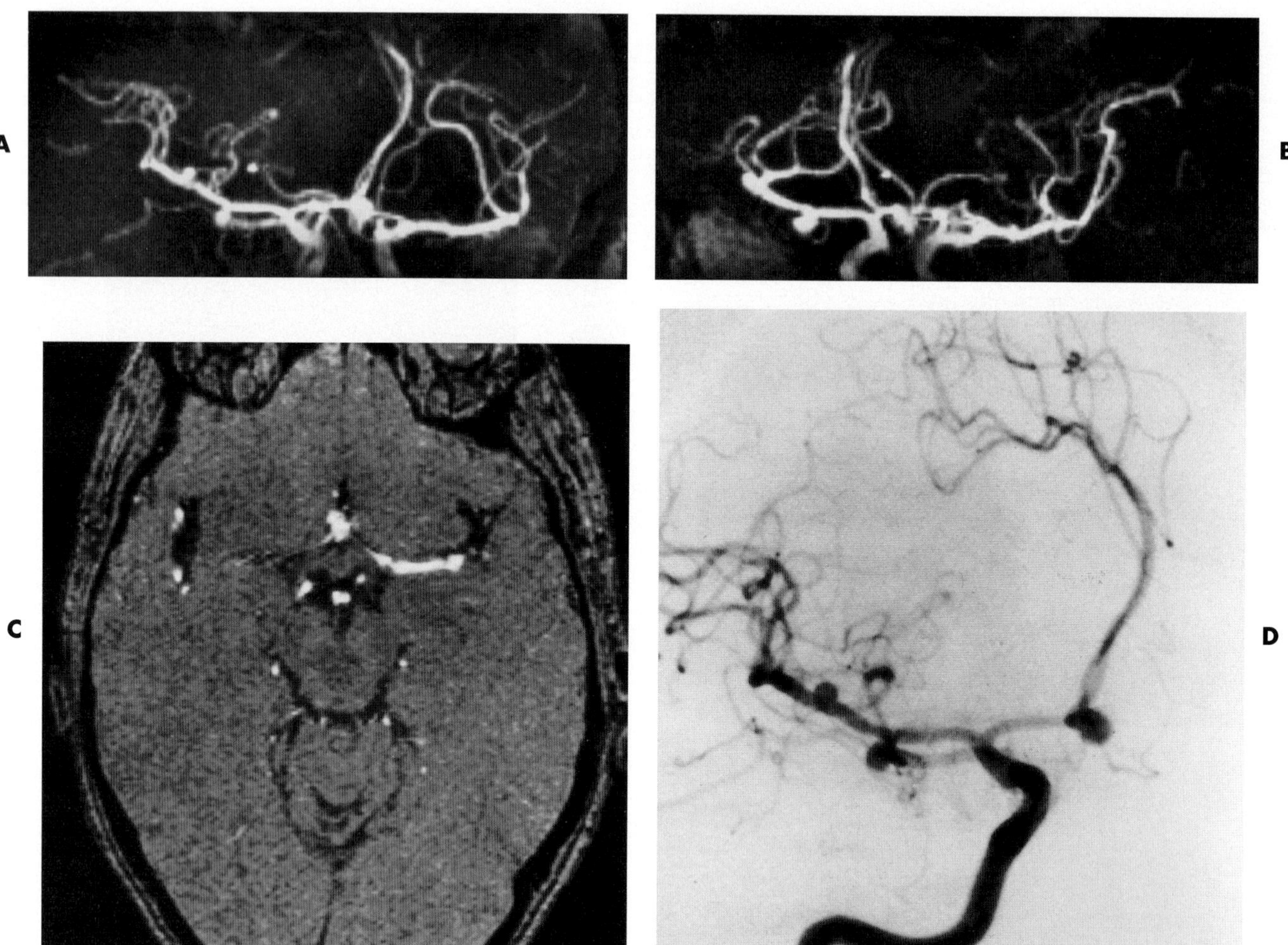


**Right anterior oblique (A) and left anterior oblique (B) maximum intensity projection views of the MRA show three globular areas of increased signal intensity suspicious for aneurysms. These are located in the region of the anterior communicating artery, projecting inferiorly off of the midportion of the left M1 segment, and at the middle cerebral bifurcation. Individual slice of the MRA sequence (C) demonstrates the anterior communicating artery aneurysm. Right anterior oblique view from the conventional angiogram confirms the three aneurysms (D).**

Nehls et al found that multiple aneurysms occur in about a third of patients in whom one aneurysm is found. They also found a female-to-male ratio of 5:1 (11:1 if there are more than 3 aneurysms). The most common locations for multiple aneurysms are the ophthalmic artery, posterior communicating artery, middle cerebral artery, and anterior communicating artery. Previously existing conditions associated with multiple intracranial aneurysms include Ehlers-Danlos syndrome, moyamoya disease, and coarctation of the aorta.

Although patients with adult polycystic kidney disease have been reported to have an increased prevalence of cerebral aneurysms, the estimates have varied, and the methods used to date have had varying degrees of invasiveness, sensitivity, and specificity. This has lead to bias in patient selection and has likely altered the estimates of prevalence. Ruggieri et al evaluated 93 patients with adult polycystic kidney disease by MRA. Pertinent patient demographics, history, and signs and symptoms, including factors suggested to be associated with an increased prevalence of aneurysms, were collected. Each of the participants were studied with conventional spin-echo parenchymal imaging and three dimensional time-of-flight MRA. The MRA images were reconstructed using a targeted maximum intensity projection technique to produce projected angiographic images of the entire anterior circulation, the carotid siphon region, and left and right anterior circulations, and the posterior circulation. Evaluation of the data included a review of the individual slices from each of the two three-dimensional MRA volumes, the postprocessed MRA images described previously, the spin-echo images, multiplanar reconstructions, and/or high-resolution targeted maximum intensity projection images of the MRA data in areas suspicious for an aneurysm. All patients with aneurysms that could require therapy then had cerebral arteriograms. The prevalence values were estimated using the proportions of patients with aneurysms and adjusted for the reported sensitivity and specificity of three-dimensional time-of-flight MRA. A total of 13 aneurysms were identified in 10 patients. Some 11 of the aneurysms were saccular, including 5 intradural anterior circulation, 3 extradural juxtasellar, and 3 petrous internal carotid artery aneurysms. All were 7 mm or smaller. A total of 60% of these patients had a family history of known or suspected aneurysms. Conventional arteriograms were performed in 6 patients, each of which confirmed the findings on MRA. The best estimate of the overall prevalence of cerebral aneurysms is 11.7% in the group with adult polycystic kidney disease, and 25.8% of patients with positive family histories of aneurysm would be predicted to have a saccular intracranial aneurysm. The prevalence of aneurysms in this study of patients, with or without a family history of aneurysm, is greater than that reported for the general population. MR parenchymal imaging with MRA is a useful screening tool for cerebral aneurysms and eliminates the selection bias inherent to an invasive examination.

**REFERENCES**

Ruggieri PM, Poulos N, Lewin JS et al: Screening patients with adult polycystic kidney disease by means of three-dimensional time-of-flight MR angiography, *Abstract Radiol* 185(p):226, 1992.

Ross JS, Masaryk TJ, Modic MT et al: Intracranial aneurysms: evaluation by MR angiography, *AJNR* 11:449-456, 1990.

Sevick RJ, Tsuruda JS, Schmalbrock P: Three-dimensional time-of-flight MR angiography in the evaluation of cerebral aneurysms, *JCAT* 14:874-881, 1990.

Nehls DG, Flom RA, Carter LP, Spetzler RF: Multiple intracranial aneurysms: determining the site of rupture. *J Neurosurg* 63:342-348, 1985.

Levey AS, Pauker SG, Kassirer JP: Occult intracranial aneurysms in polycystic kidney disease: when is cerebral arteriography indicated? *N Engl J Med* 308:986-994, 1983.

## CASE 69
## MULITPLE ANEURYSMS

**History:** 64-year-old with decreased vision in the right eye.

**Technique:** two axial volumes, three-dimensional time-of-flight, 40/7/15, 256 × 256, 32 slices each volume, 30-mm slab, 25-cm field of view, 4:45 per volume.

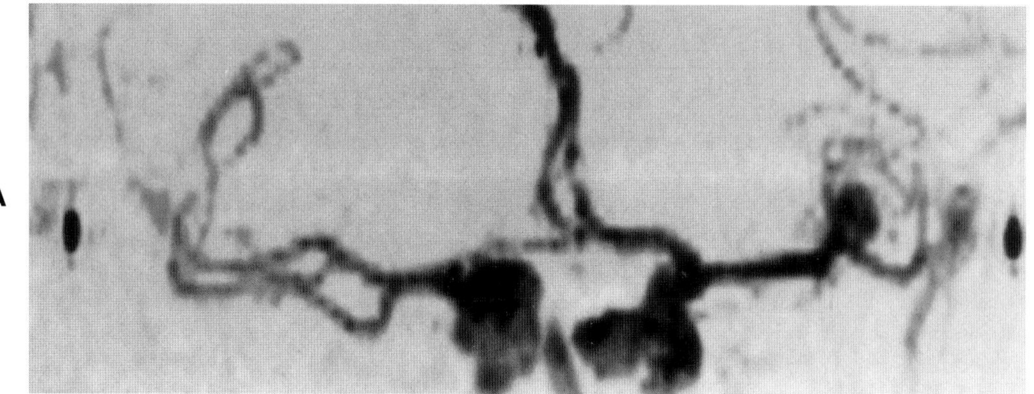


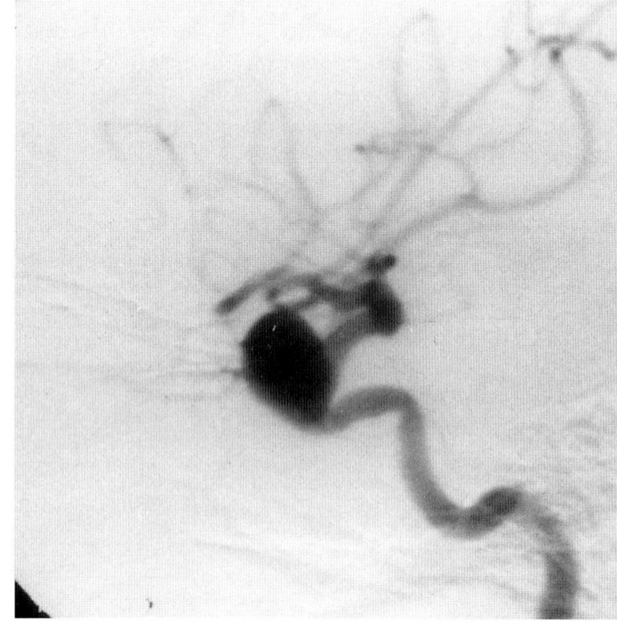


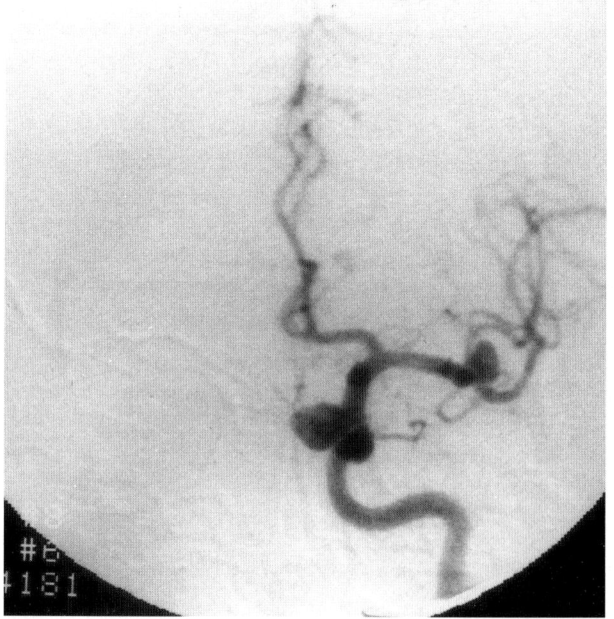


***Study #1:*** **Anteroposterior maximum intensity projection view (A) demonstrates multiple aneurysms seen as abnormal, rounded areas of increased signal intensity involving the right and the left carotid siphons (ophthalmic origins) and the left middle cerebral bifurcation. Conventional angiographic lateral view of the right (B) and anteroposterior view of the left (C) carotid injections confirm the presence and appearance of the three aneurysms.**

D

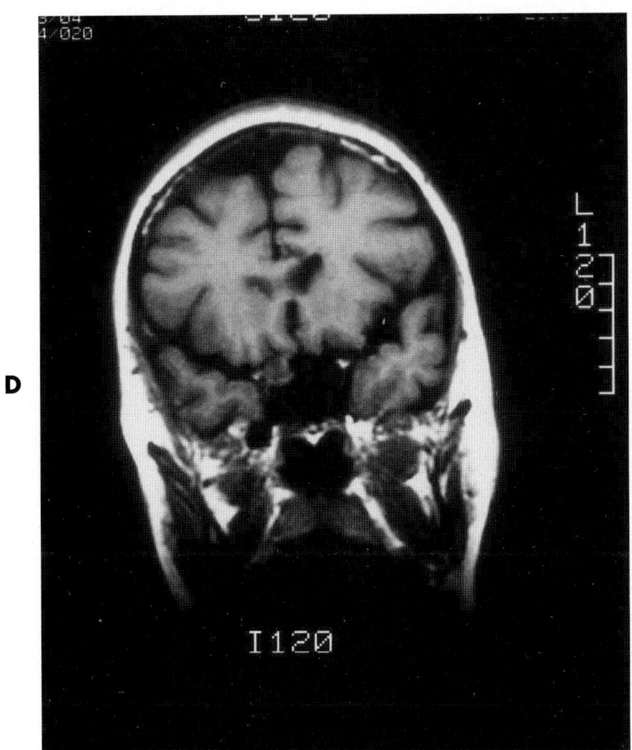


E

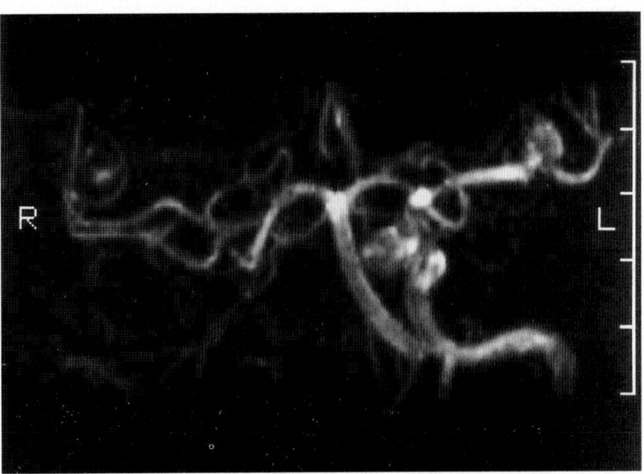


***Study #2:*** **The patient subsequently underwent balloon occlusion of the right internal carotid artery. The occluded right internal carotid aneurysms is seen as intermediate signal thrombus on the coronal T1-weighted spin-echo study (D). Repeat MRA (E) shows the right carotid occlusion, and the large left internal carotid and smaller left middle cerebral bifurcation aneurysms.**

Care must be taken to scrutinize the individual slices of the MRA studies as well as all the projections in patients who may have several aneurysms. In addition, care must be taken in the placement of the axial volumes when an aneurysm is found. In particular, a second volume may be necessary to include the posterior fossa arteries, particularly the origin of the posterior inferior cerebellar artery, which may be excluded in a volume placed for circle of Willis abnormalities.

## CASE 70
## CALCIFIED AND THROMBOSED POSTERIOR CEREBRAL ANEURYSM

**History:** 60-year-old with head trauma after a motor vehicle accident. Computed tomography performed for evaluation of head trauma showed a calcified mass.

**Technique:** axial volume, three-dimensional time-of-flight, 40/7/15, 256 × 256, 64 slices, 60-mm slab, 25-cm field of view, 10:57.

A

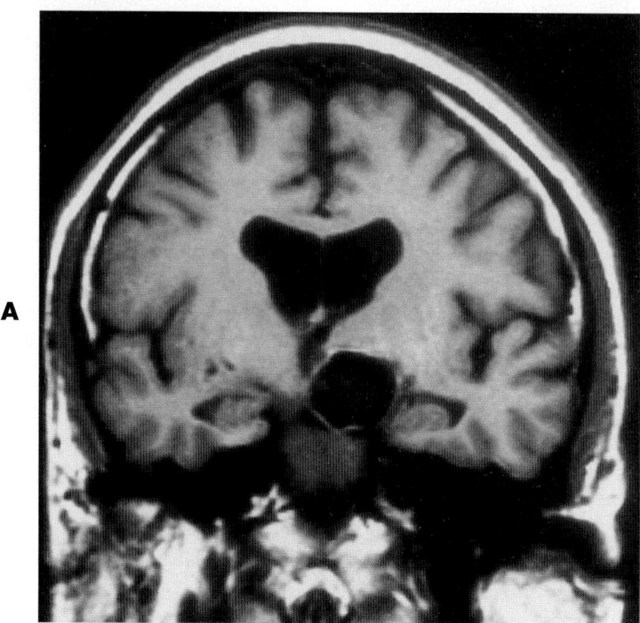

B

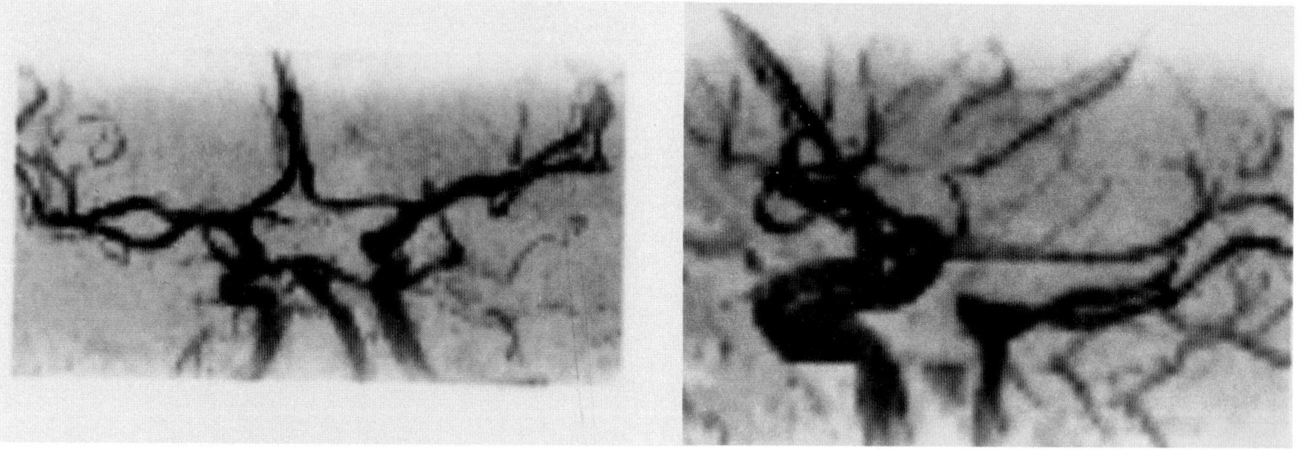

C

D

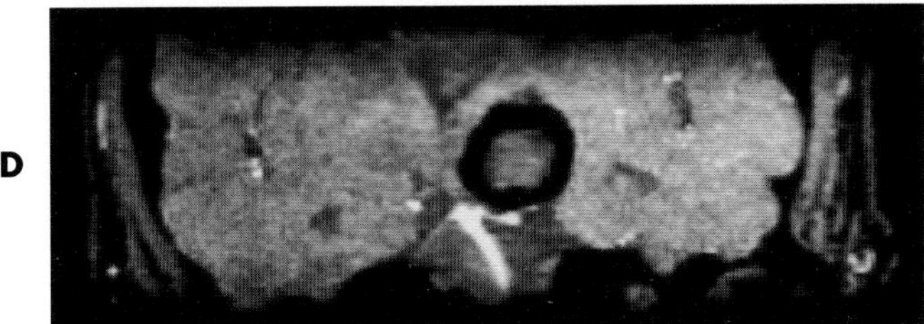

F

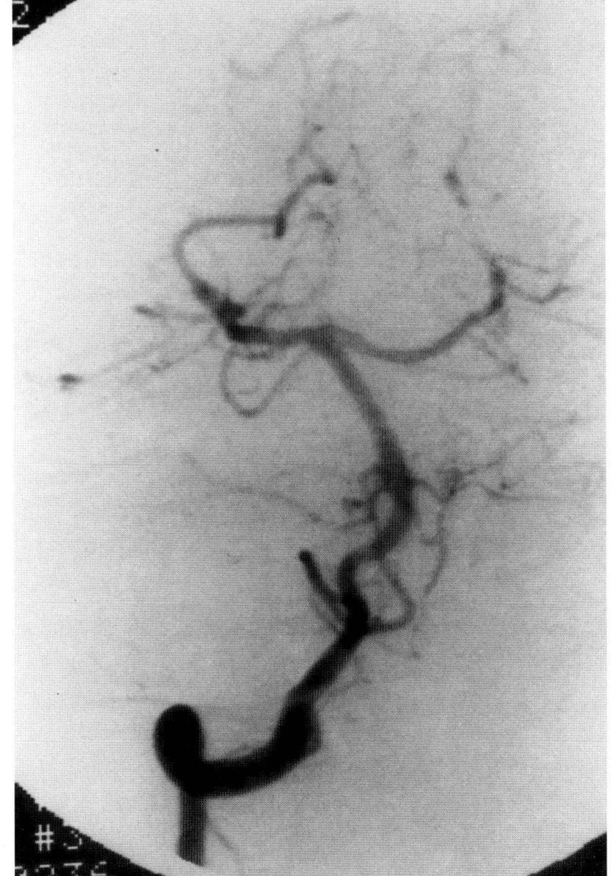

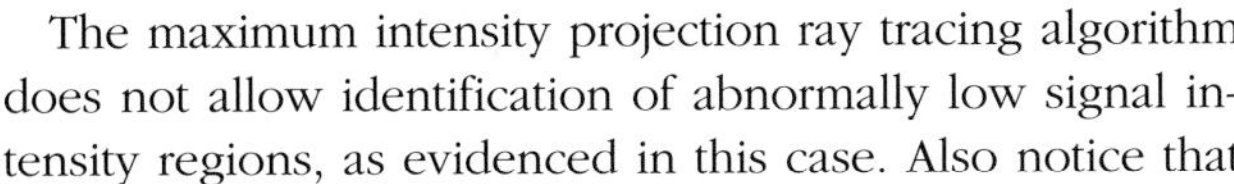

E

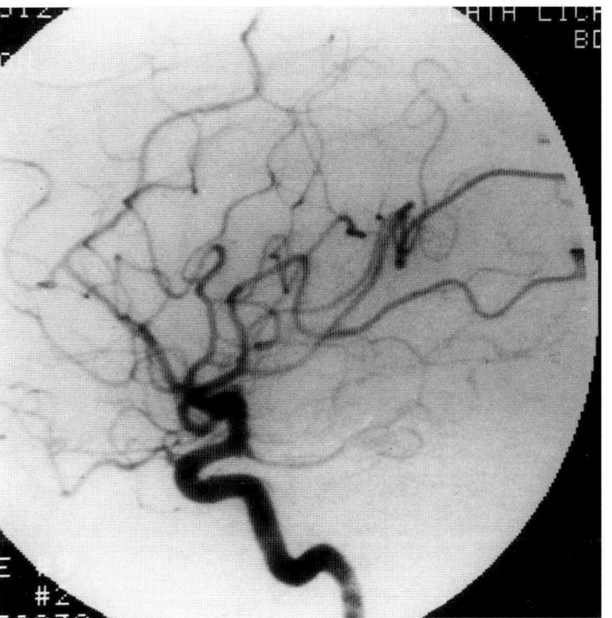

**The T1-weighted coronal image (A) demonstrates a well-defined mass that shows a thick rind of markedly low signal intensity. The anteroposterior (B) and lateral (C) views of the maximum intensity projection demonstrates abnormal inferior displacement of the left P1 segment and slight displacement of the distal basilar artery to the right. This is confirmed on the coronal reformat of the original MRA data (D), which shows a well-defined low signal intensity mass situated above the left P1 segment, causing the displacement. This represents a calcified and completely thrombosed aneurysm. Conventional angiographic lateral internal carotid injection (E) and anteroposterior view of the right vertebral injection (F) show only the mass effect on the proximal posterior cerebral and anterior choroidal arteries.**

The maximum intensity projection ray tracing algorithm does not allow identification of abnormally low signal intensity regions, as evidenced in this case. Also notice that the anterior choroidal artery is not identified on the lateral MRA maximum intensity projection view, in contrast with the conventional angiogram.

# CASE 71
# BASILAR TIP ANEURYSM

**History:** 56-year-old with unsteady gait.

**Technique:** axial volume, three-dimensional time-of-flight, 40/6/15, 256 × 160, 64 slices, 60-mm slab, 20-cm field of view (rectangular), 6:52.

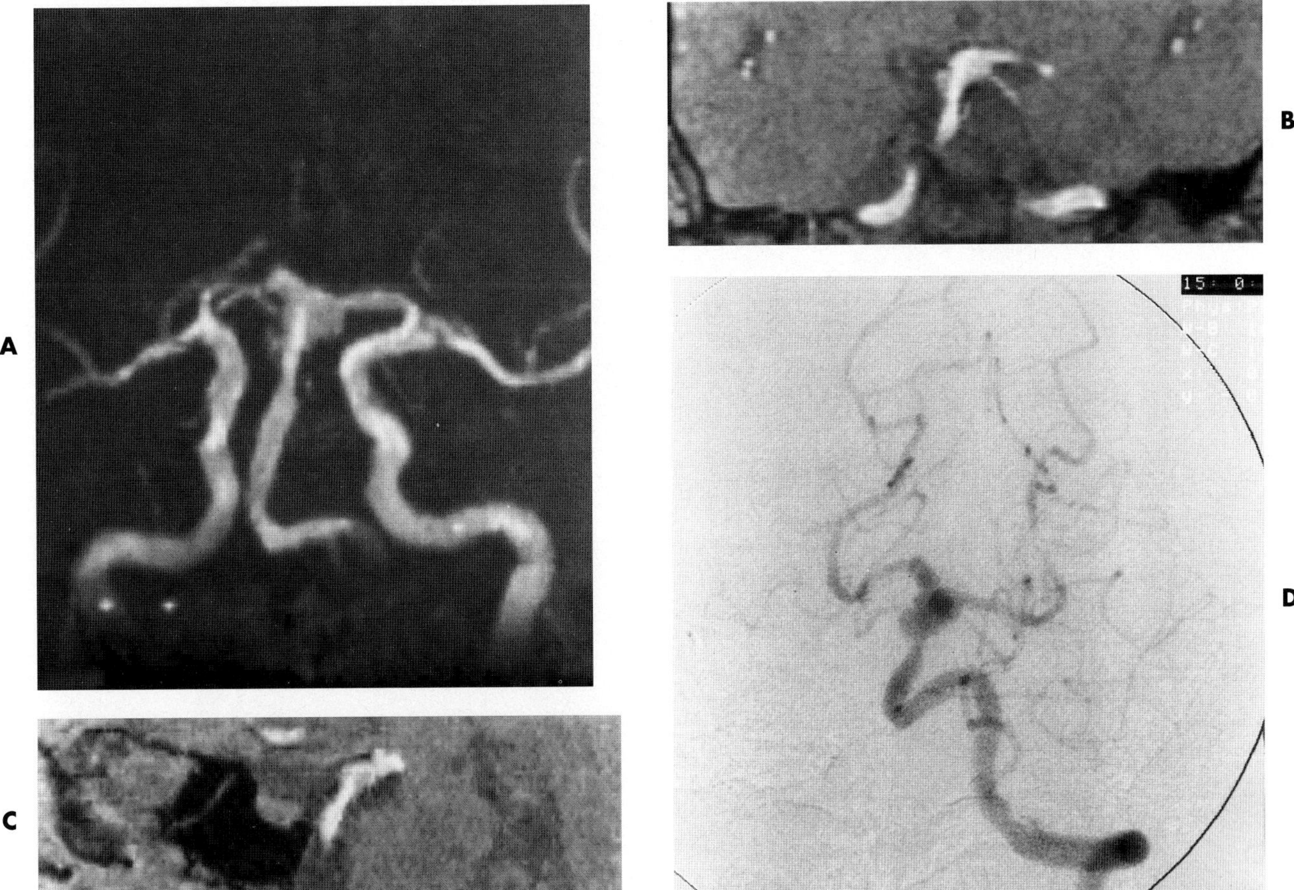


**Water's type of maximum intensity projection (A) shows a lobular, abnormal area of increased signal intensity involving the basilar tip, which is highly suspicious for aneurysm. Coronal (B) and sagittal (C) reformats from the original MRA volume data confirm the presence of a lobular aneurysm involving the basilar tip, with mild mass effect on the inferior third ventricle and hypothalamus. The coronal reformats also show that this broad-based aneurysm involves the origin of the left P1 segment as well as the origin of the left superior cerebellar artery. The shape and size of the basilar tip aneurysm are confirmed on the anteroposterior left vertebral injection of the conventional angiogram (D).**

## CASE 72
## BASILAR TIP ANEURYSM

**History:** 68-year-old with left third nerve palsy.

**Technique:** axial volume, three-dimensional time-of-flight, 40/6/15, 256 × 160, 64 slices, 60-mm slab, 20-cm field of view (rectangular), 6:52.

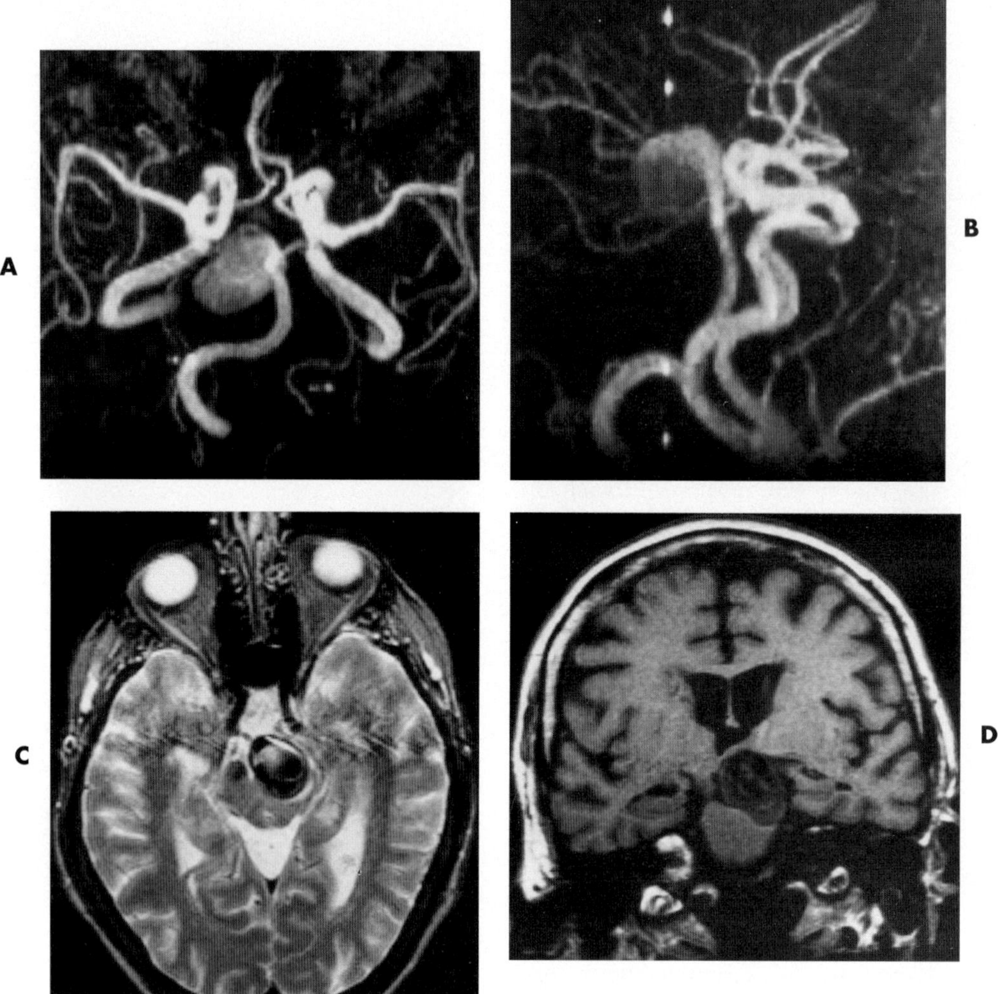


**Base (A) and lateral (B) whole head maximum intensity projection images show a large, rounded outpouching of increased signal intensity arising off the region of the basilar tip. Note the vertically oriented high signal intensity jet involving the dome of the aneurysm. The rest of the aneurysm is of relatively lower signal intensity because of flow saturation related to complex or vortical flow. This pattern is typical of larger aneurysms on three-dimensional time-of-flight MRAs. Axial T2-weighted (C) and coronal T1-weighted (D) spin-echo studies demonstrate an inhomogeneous, large low signal intensity mass that is the aneurysm. There is considerable mass effect on the brainstem (in particular, the left cerebral peduncle). There is characteristic phase-encoding artifact through the level of the aneurysm that extends from right to left. Lateral view of a left vertebral artery injection (E) shows the large aneurysm, as identified on the MRA. Note also the identification of the jet extending superiorly from the neck into the dome of the aneurysm. Delayed view of the conventional angiogram (F) shows continued filling of the aneurysm caused by slow flow, which explains the signal loss caused by slow flow saturation within the bulk of the aneurysm on the MRA.**

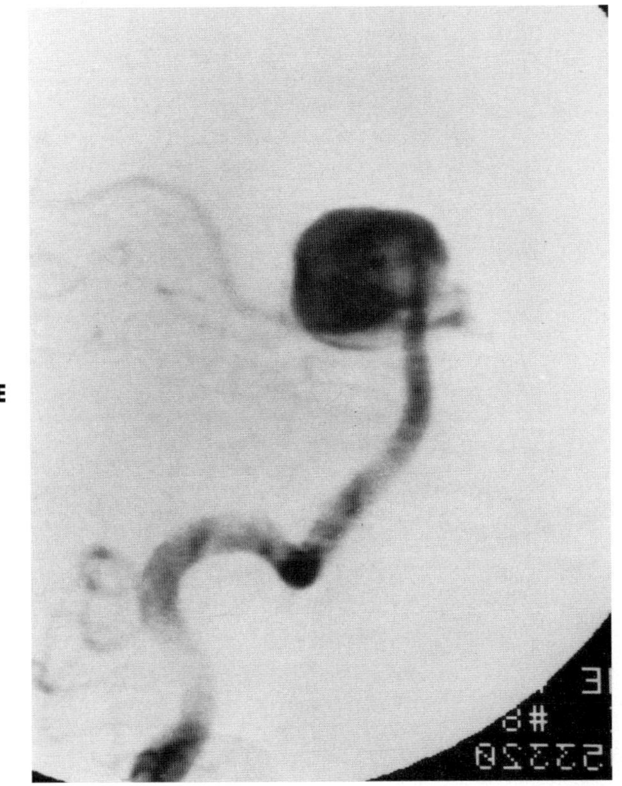


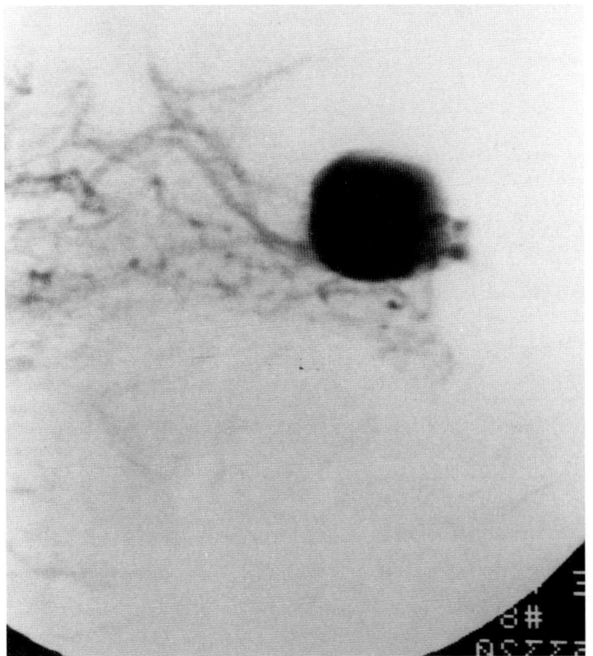


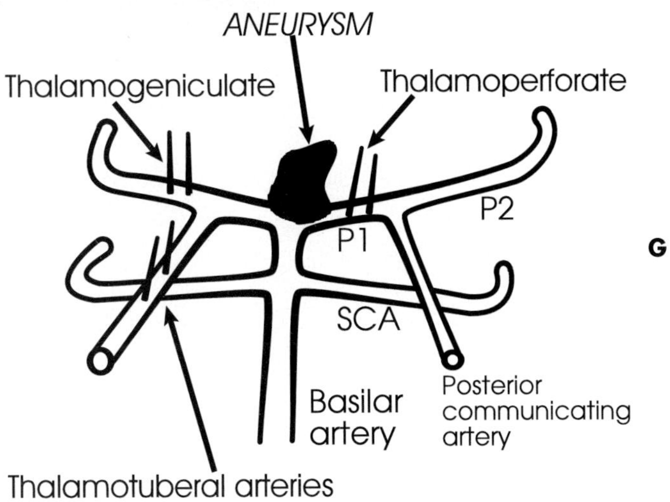


**Basilar tip and perforating vessels.**

Approximately 10% of intracranial aneurysms arise off the posterior circulation, with over half of this coming from the basilar artery bifurcation, as shown in the schematic **(G).** Perforating vessels, which are surgically very important, are not visible with current MRA techniques because of issues relating to spatial resolution and slow flow.

**REFERENCE**

Yasargil MG: *Microneurosurgery,* vol 2, New York, 1984, Thieme.

# CASE 73
# BASILAR TIP ANEURYSM

**History:** 24-year-old with subarachnoid hemorrhage.

**Technique:** axial volume; three-dimensional time-of-flight; 45/7/20; 256 × 256; 64 slices; 60-mm slab; magnetization transfer background suppression; tilted, optimized nonsaturating excitation radiofrequency pulse; 14-cm field of view; 12:20.

A 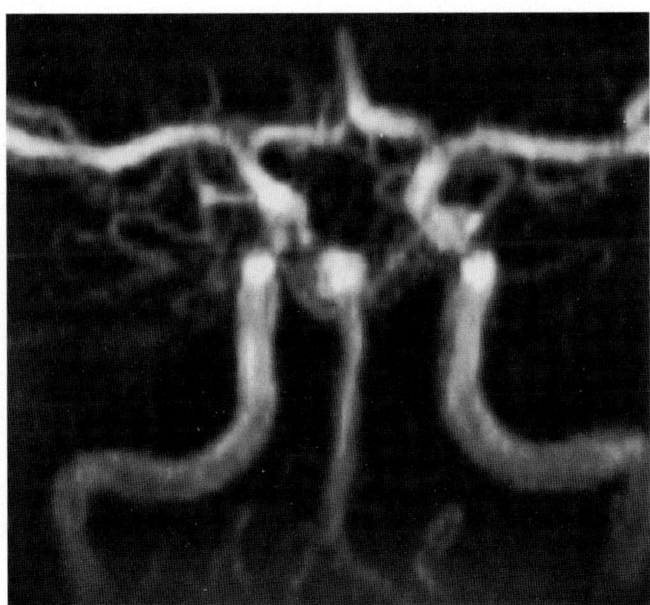

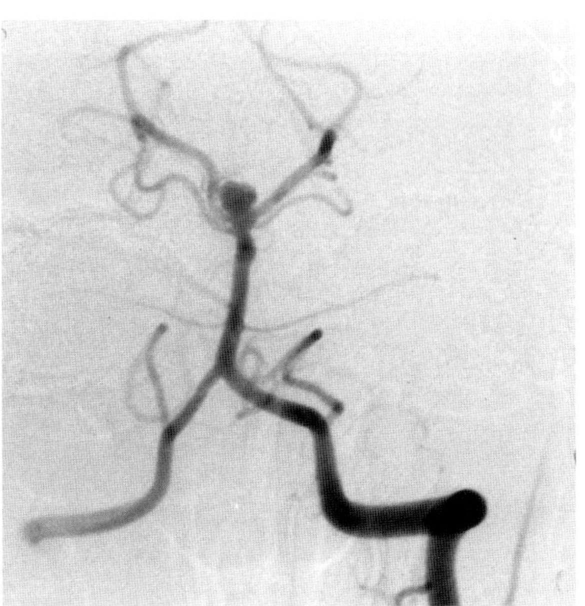 B

**Anteroposterior maximum intensity projection view (A) demonstrates a rounded outpouching of abnormal increased signal intensity arising from the distal aspect of the basilar artery, which represents a basilar tip aneurysm. Anteroposterior projection from a left vertebral injection (B) shows the aneurysm involving the basilar tip.**

Aneurysms ranging in size from 3 to 8 mm generally have fast flow and lend themselves to three-dimensional time-of-flight techniques. Notice the false narrowing of the carotid siphons on the MRA, which is presumably related to complex siphon flow with dephasing and signal loss in this patient with fast flow and good cardiac output.

# CASE 74
# POSTERIOR CEREBRAL ARTERY ANEURYSM

**History:** 38-year-old with dysarthria and memory loss after a motor vehicle accident.

**Technique:** Intracranial/axial volume; three-dimensional time-of-flight; 45/7/20; 256 × 192; 64 slices; 60-mm slab; magnetization transfer background suppression; tilted, optimized nonsaturating excitation radiofrequency pulse; 14-cm field of view; 9:15.

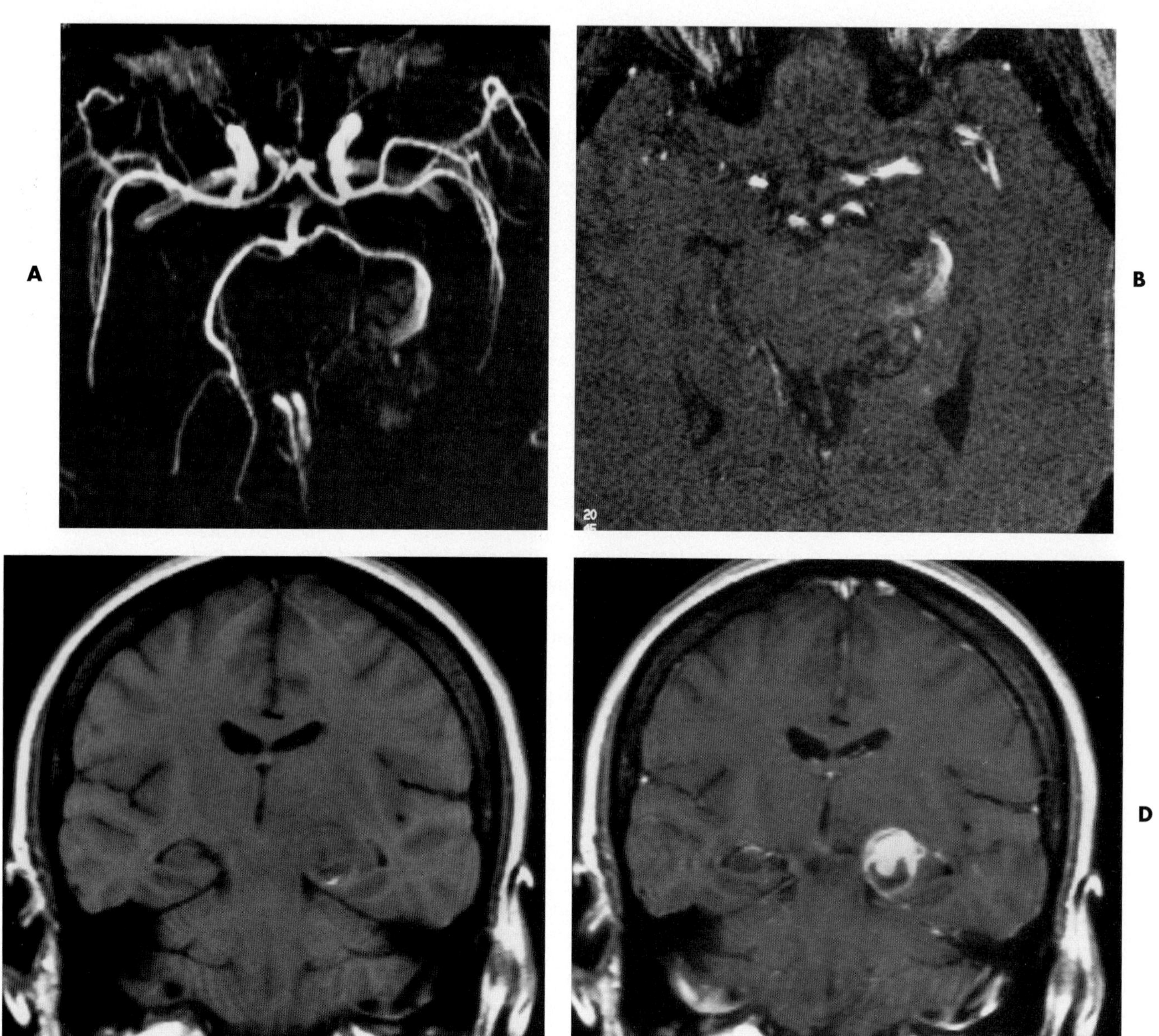

E

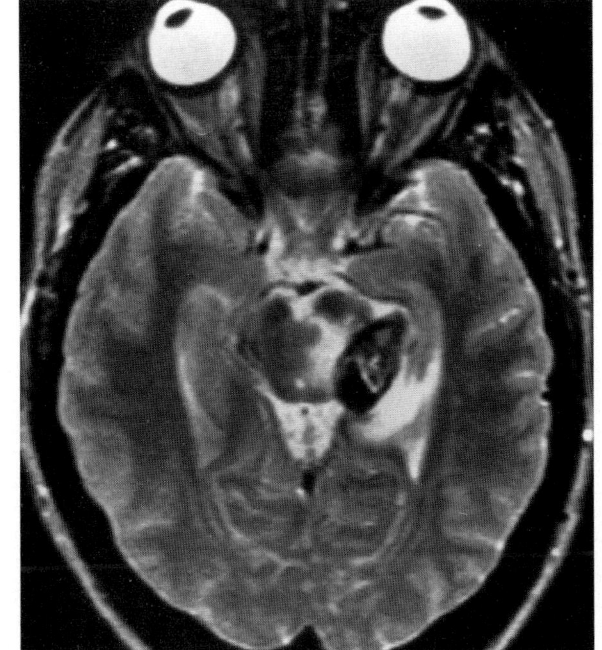

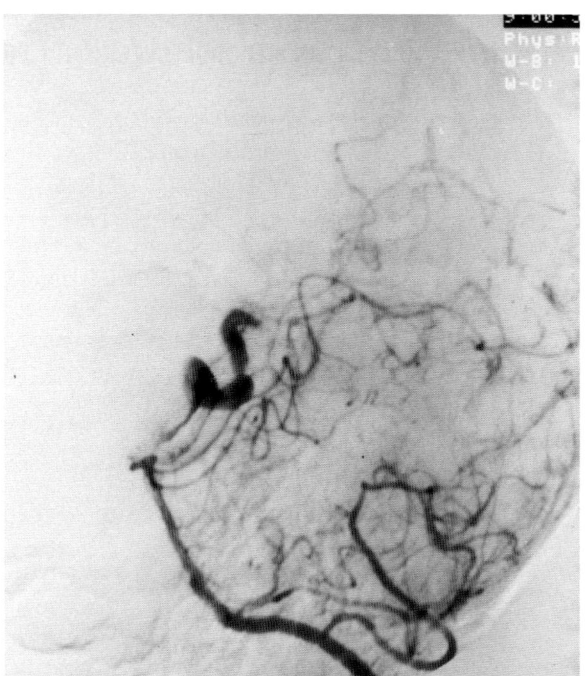

F

**Base maximum intensity projection MRA view (A) shows a fusiformly dilated left posterior cerebral artery, with no visualization of the more distal left posterior cerebral artery as contrasted with the normal-appearing right posterior cerebral artery. Vague increased signal is scattered around the distal aspect of the fusiform aneurysm. Indivdual slice from the MRA data set again shows the fusiform dilatation (B). Coronal T1-weighted spin-echo images before (C) and after (D) contrast show the partially thrombosed lumen as increased signal before contrast and marked enhancement of the lumen and wall. Axial T2-weighted sequence shows a large area of decreased signal intensity in the left circummesencephalic cistern, with associated vasogenic edema of the left midbrain and posterior temporal lobe (E). The decreased signal relates to thrombosis and spin dephasing related to slow flow. Lateral view of the vertebral injection (F) shows the large, slowly filling posterior cerebral fusiform aneurysm.**

## CASE 75
## TOTALLY THROMBOSED POSTERIOR INFERIOR CEREBELLAR ARTERY ANEURYSM WITH NEW HEMORRHAGE

**History:** 57-year-old with previous aortic valve replacement and coronary bypass with new complaints of severe headache, nausea, and vomiting. Computed tomogram is positive for subarachnoid hemorrhage.

**Technique:** axial volume, three-dimensional time-of-flight, 45/8.5/20, 256 × 256, 64 slices, 60-mm slab, 15-cm field of view, 12:19.

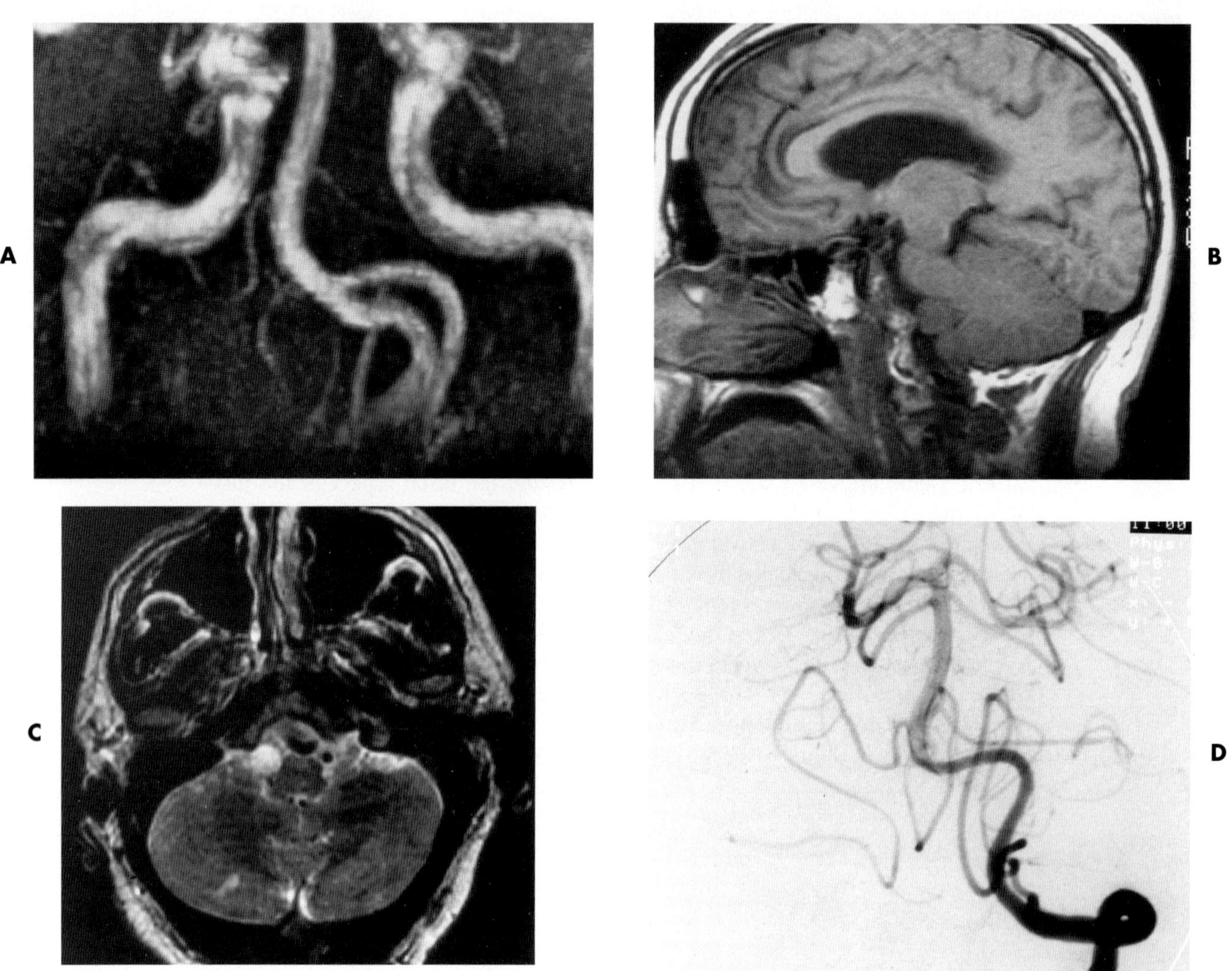


***Study #1:*** **Anteroposterior view from a maximum intensity projection (A) demonstrates a slightly ectatic vertebral basilar junction, but no focal abnormality is identified to suggest aneurysm. However, the T1-weighted sagittal (B) as well as the T2-weighted axial view (C) demonstrate a rounded abnormality involving the right medullary cistern. This demonstrates increased signal intensity on the T2-weighted (and spin density) image (not shown) and is isointense on the T1-weighted sagittal image. Anteroposterior and lateral view from a left vertebral injection (D) demonstrates a combined right and posterior inferior cerebellar artery without evidence of residual patent aneurysmal lumen. The differential at this point is a totally thrombosed aneurysm with unusual thrombus signal intensity or an incidental tumor such as an epidermoid.**

E

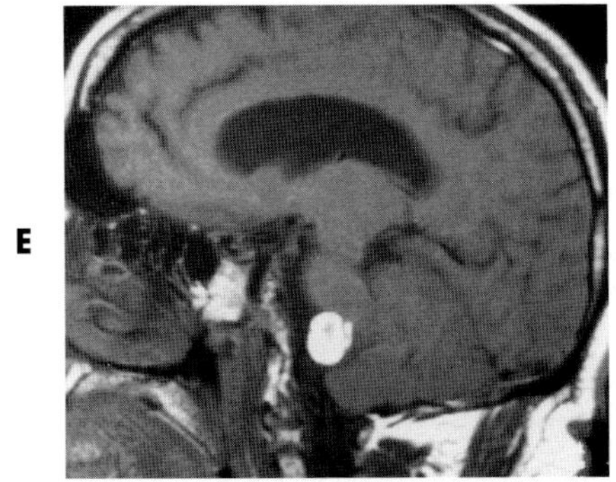

F

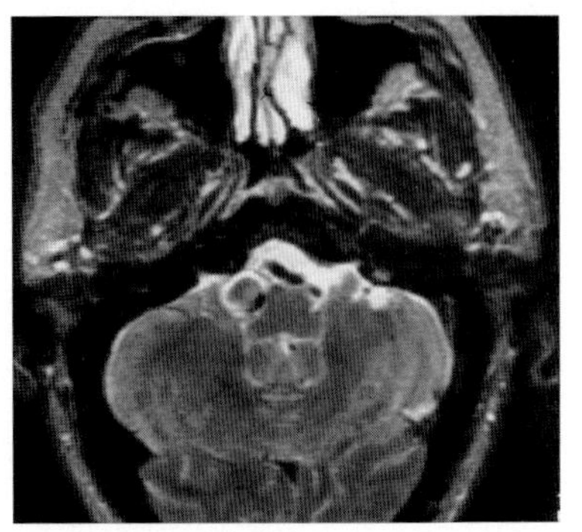

***Study #2:*** **Repeat MR 10 days later shows a striking change in the signal intensity of the mass. The sagittal T1-weighted image (E) shows marked increased signal, whereas the T2-weighted image (F) shows central low signal and peripheral increased signal intensity. This pattern is consistent with fresh hemorrhage (methemoglobin) into the previous chronic aneurysm thrombus.**

G

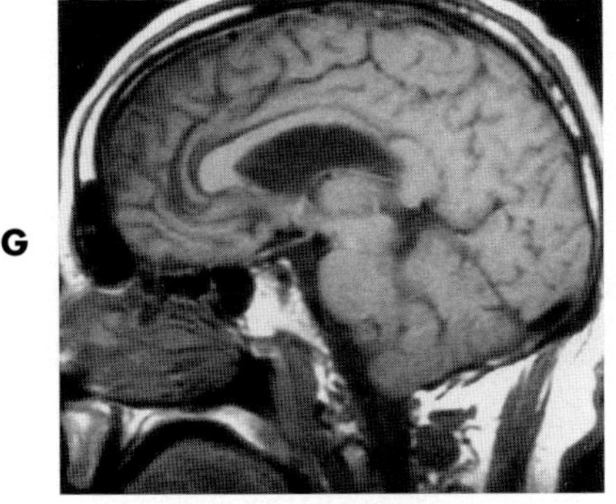

H

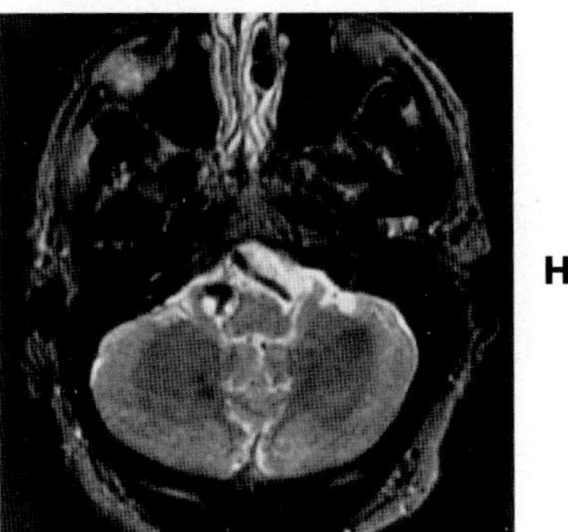

***Study #3:*** **Repeat MR 4 weeks later shows further evolution of the thrombus, with decreasing signal intensity and decreasing aneurysm size on the T1- (G) and T2-weighted (H) images.**

Thrombosed aneurysms may demonstrate a wide variety of signal intensity changes related to the age of the thrombus and presence of rebleeding. These lesions do not show up on MRAs, since there is no patent lumen to provide flow signal. Nonetheless, a well-defined, rounded shape; appropriate location; and low signal intensity on the T2-weighted spin-echo images point to the diagnosis of aneurysm. This aneurysm ultimately rebled as a large posterior fossa subarachnoid hemorrhage that resulted in death. There was pathologic confirmation of the posterior inferior cerebellar artery aneurysm.

Vertebral artery saccular aneurysms often arise at the origin of the posterior inferior cerebellar artery and are in the lateral cerebellomedullary cistern. These lesions often present with subarachnoid hemorrhage, twelfth nerve palsy, ataxia, and nystagmus. Vorkapic et al reviewed a series of 56 patients with gastrointestinal anastomosis, 28 with signs of mass effect and 19 with subarachnoid hemorrhage. A total of 11 cases involved the vertebrobasilar system. The predisposition of giant intracranial aneurysms to subarachnoid hemorrhage is controversial. However, the weight of evidence reveals that subarachnoid hemorrhage is a common manifestation of giant intracranial aneurysms and that mural thrombus does not provide protection from bleeding, as evidenced in this particular case.

**REFERENCES**


Drake CG: Giant intracranial aneurysms: experience with surgical treatment in 174 patients, *Clin Neurosurg* 2:612-695, 1979.

Sonntag VKH, Yuan RH, Stein BM: Giant intracranial aneurysms: a review of 13 cases, *Surg Neurol* 8:81-84, 1977.

Sundt TM, Piepgras DG: Surgical approach to giant intracranial aneurysms: operative experience with 80 cases, *J Neurosurg* 51:731-742, 1979.

Vorkapic P, Czech T, Pendl G et al: Clinico-radiological spectrum of giant intracranial aneurysms, *Neurosurg Rev* 14:271-274, 1991.

## CASE 76
## PARTIALLY THROMBOSED POSTERIOR INFERIOR CEREBELLAR ARTERY ANEURYSM

**History:** 44-year-old with ataxia.

**Technique #1:** Axial three-dimensional phase-contrast, 26/9/15, 256 × 128 matrix, 60 slices, 60-mm slab, velocity encoding of 30 cm/sec, 18-cm field of view, 14 minutes.

**Technique #2:** Axial volume, three-dimensional time-of-flight, 43/6/20, 512 × 256 matrix, one excitation, 60 slices, 60-mm slab, 18-cm field of view, 11:00.

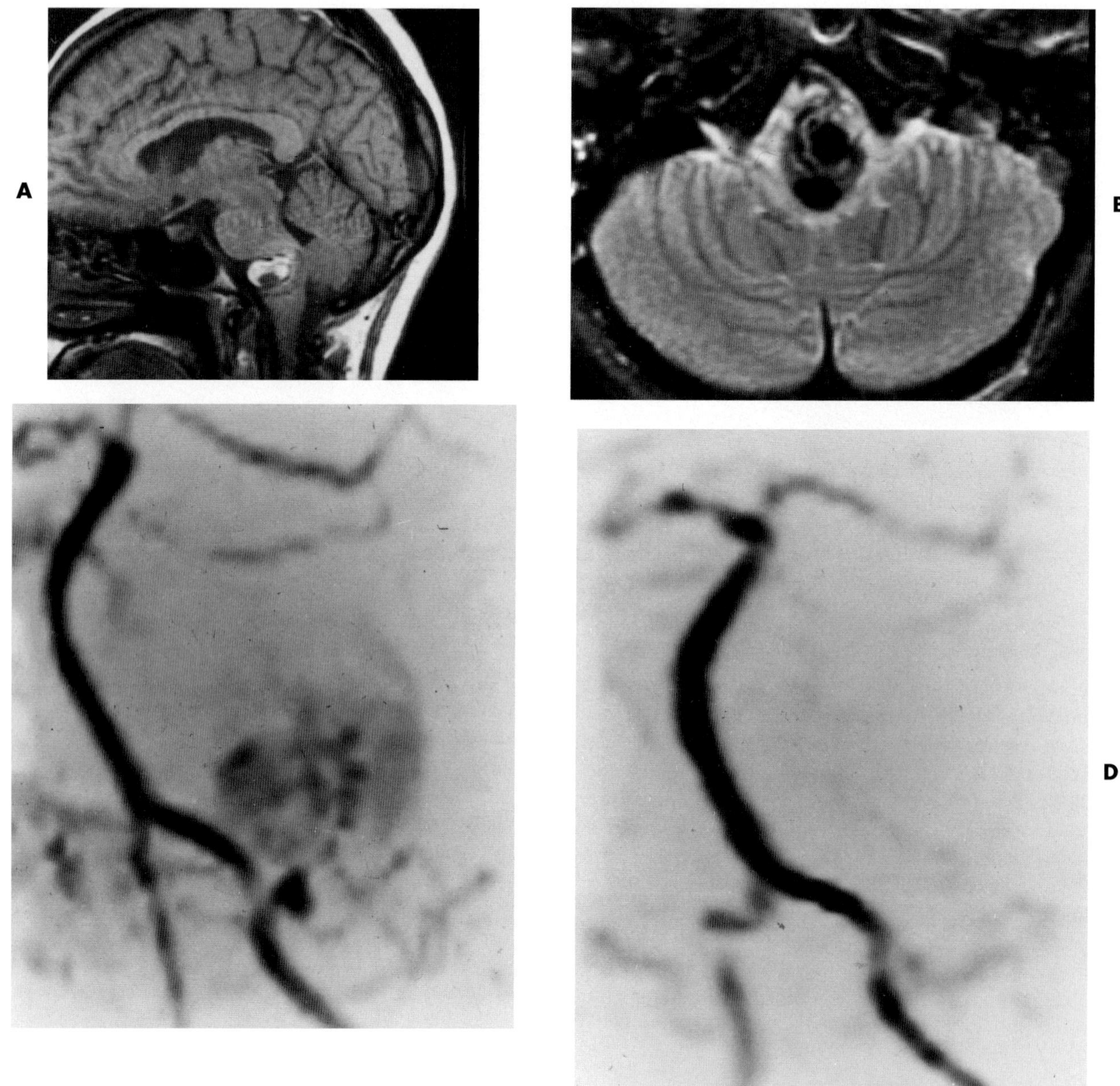

A large, rounded mass of complex signal intensity is present at the pontomedullary junction, with considerable mass effect on the brainstem (A and B). The mass shows increased signal on the T1-weighted spin-echo study (A) and decreased signal on the T2-weighted study (B), consistent with methemoglobin thrombus within an aneurysm. Oblique maximum intensity projection view of the three-dimensional time-of-flight angiogram shows a small rounded area of increased signal intensity arising from the region of the left posterior inferior cerebellar artery origin (C). Notice the considerable "shine through" of the methemoglobin containing thrombus on the time-of-flight maximum intensity projection. Comparable oblique view of the three-dimensional phase-contrast study completely suppresses the potentially confusing signal from the thrombus but shows poor visualization of the true lumen of the small posterior inferior cerebellar artery aneurysm (D). Lateral view of the left vertebral artery injection shows the left posterior inferior cerebellar artery origin aneurysm (E). (Courtesy John Huston, Mayo Clinic, Rochester, Minn.)

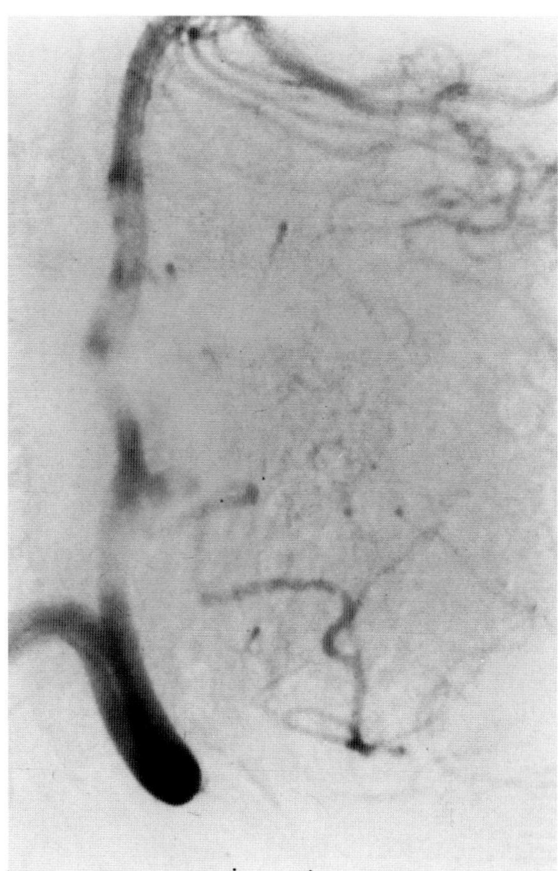
E

## CASE 77
## DOLICHOECTASIA OF THE INTERNAL CAROTID ARTERY

**History:** 44-year-old with right sixth nerve palsy.

**Technique:** axial volume, three-dimensional time-of-flight, 40/7/15, 256 × 256, 64 slices, 60-mm slab, 23-cm field of view, 10:57.

A

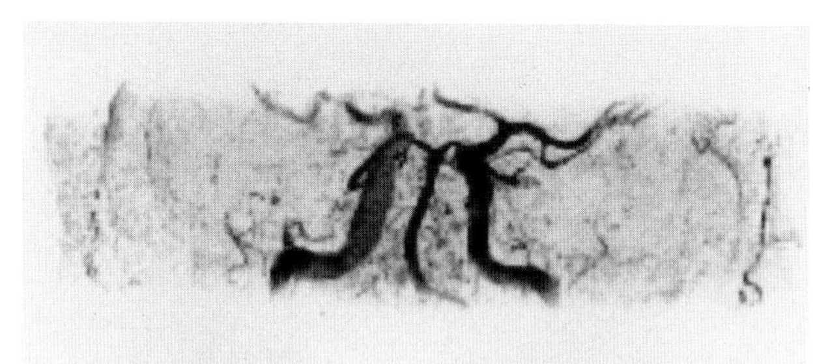

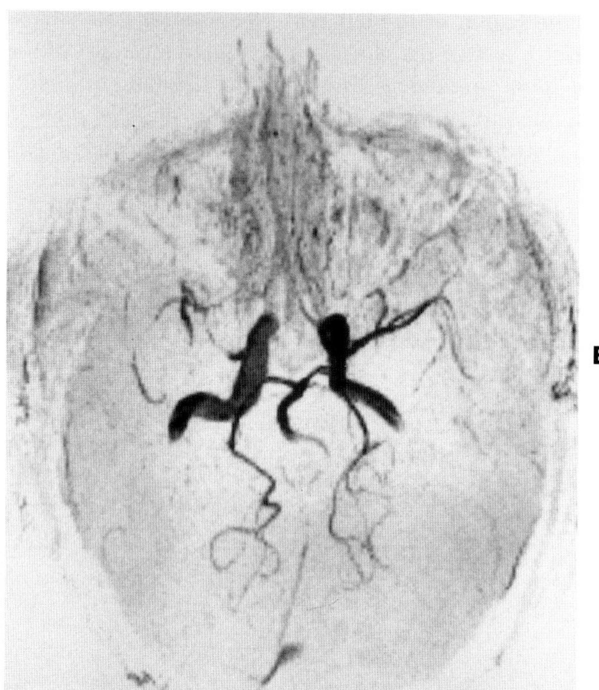

B

C

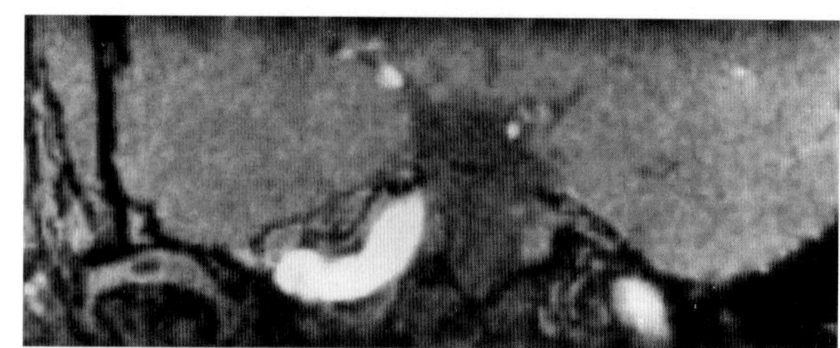

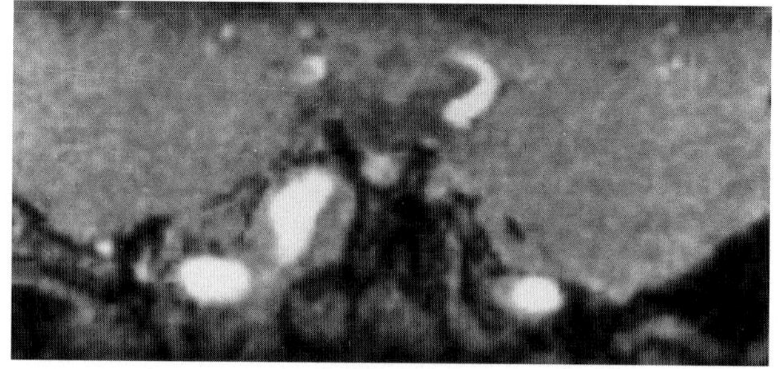

D

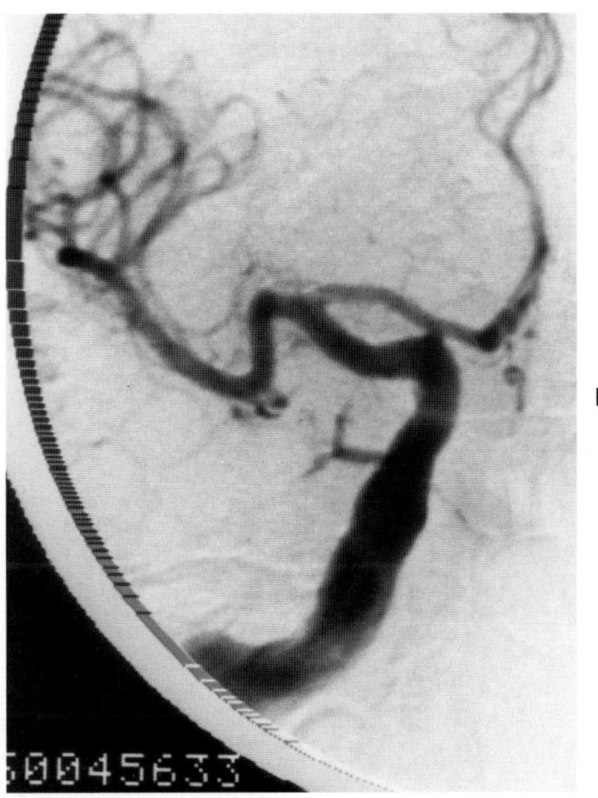

**E**

**AP (A) and base (B) views from the maximum intensity projection demonstrate a diffusely enlarged distal right internal carotid artery up to the level of the supra-clinoid segment. There is slight decreased signal intensity throughout the distal right internal carotid artery related to slowed flow with flow saturation. Coronal reformats through the dolichoectatic internal carotid artery (C and D) demonstrate the relationship of the patent lumen to the thickened, aneurysmal wall. The overall dimension of the aneurysm is considerable larger than that of the patent lumen. This is further confirmed on the anteroposterior projection of the intraarterial digital subtraction angiography (E), which shows the long segment of dolichoectasia but underestimates the size of the aneurysm.**

## CASE 78
## DOLICHOECTASIA OF THE BASILAR ARTERY AND INCIDENTAL MIDDLE FOSSAE MENINGIOMA

**History:** 66-year-old with memory loss.

**Technique:** axial volume, 45/6.9/20 degrees, 256 × 128, 64 slices, 60-mm slab, 18-cm field of view, 6:09.

A

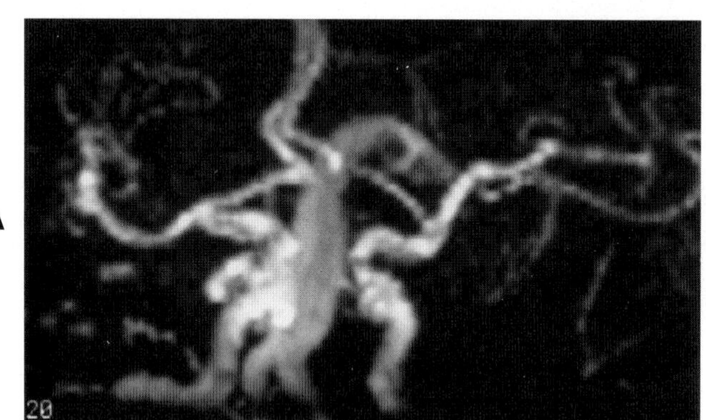


B

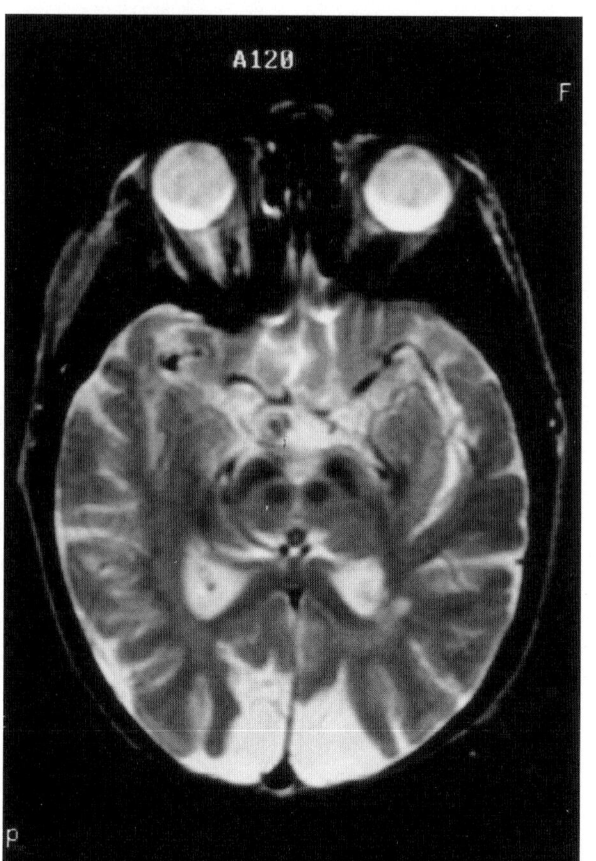


C

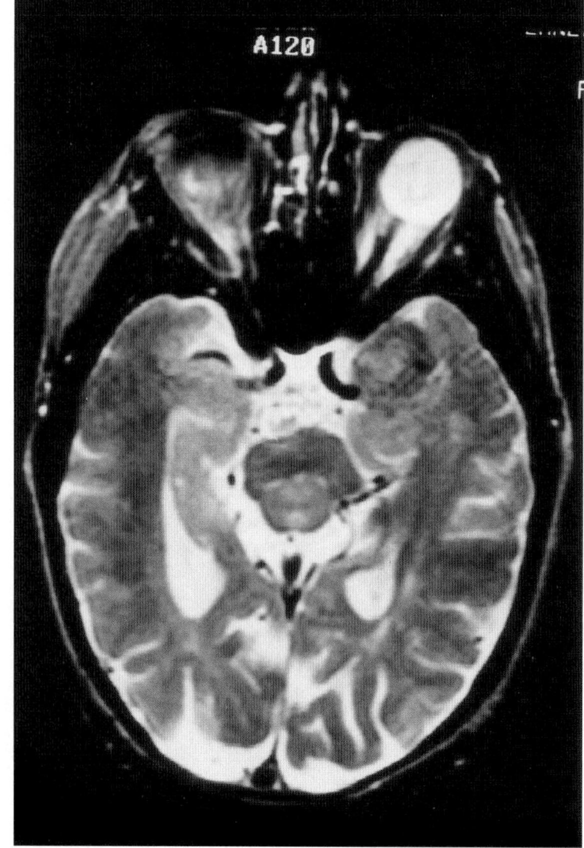


D

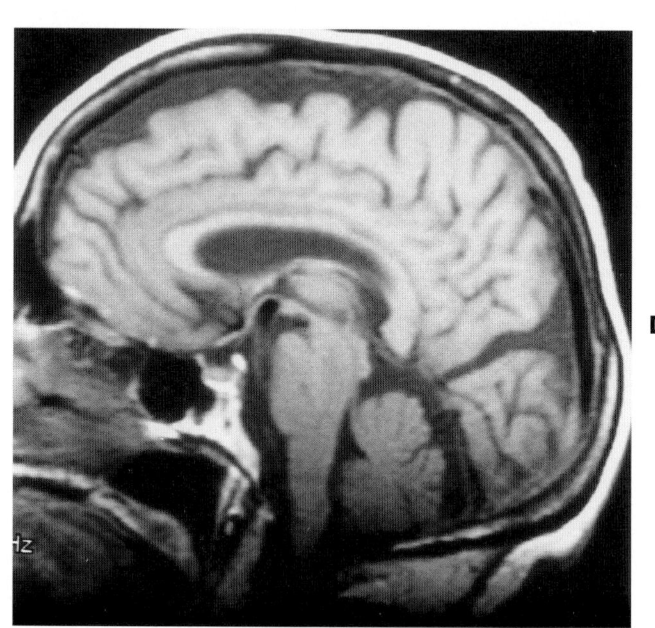

**The right anterior oblique maximum intensity projection (A) demonstrates a fusiformly dilated and ectatic basilar artery, which represents dolichoectasia. The ectasia extends throughout the length of the basilar artery and involves the left posterior cerebral artery. The slightly decreased signal intensity from the dolichoectatic basilar artery in relation to the carotid arteries is caused by flow saturation related to the slowly flowing blood within the fusiform aneurysm. The slow flow is also demonstrated on the T2-weighted axial spin-echo images (B and C), where the dilated basilar artery shows abnormal increased signal intensity instead of the usual flow void, as is present within the carotid arteries. The lengthening of the basilar artery is well seen on the sagittal T1-weighted image by the mass effect on the floor of the third ventricle (D). Incidentally noted is a low signal intensity meningioma involving the left middle cranial fossa (C).**

*Vertebrobasilar dolichoectasia* is a morphologic term, not a pathologic one, and it probably encompasses several different underlying etiologies **(E).** These underlying etiologies would include degenerative atheromatous dilatation and intracranial dissection and/or aneurysm. Mizutani and Aruga described five patients with complex intracranial vertebrobasilar dolichoectasia and identified two types of intracranial vertebrobasilar dissections. The first type is seen as a tight stenosis related to compression of the true lumen by intramural hematoma, and the second has a patent false lumen. Regardless of the underlying cause of the dolichoectasia, this condition has a high morbidity rate because of occlusion of the perforating branches to the brainstem, with resultant ischemia, distal thromboembolism, and rarely subarachnoid hemorrhage. Medical and surgical therapy are not clear-cut responses, since anticoagulation could increase the risk of subarachnoid hemorrhage. Surgical treatment is generally reserved for patients with subarachnoid hemorrhage and may involve wrapping the vessel with muslin or trapping.

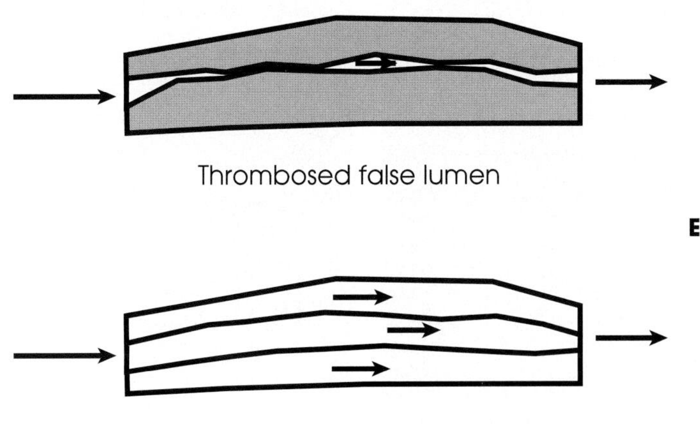


**Dolichoectasia (E) with dilatation and thrombosis *(top)* and dissection *(bottom).***

**REFERENCES**

Iwama T, Andoh T, Sakai N et al: Dissecting and fusiform aneurysms of vertebro-basilar systems. MR imaging, *Neuroradiology* 32:272, 1990.

Mizutani T, Aruga T: "Dolichoectatic" intracranial vertebrobasilar dissecting aneurysm, *Neurosurgery* 31(4):765-773, 1992.

## CASE 79
## MULTIPLE EXTRA AND INTRACRANIAL ANEURYSMS

**History:** 49-year-old with headaches and dizzy spells and a pulsatile mass felt in the left neck.

**Technique #1:** intracranial/axial volume; three-dimensional time-of-flight; 45/7/20; 256 × 192; 64 slices; 60-mm slab; magnetization transfer background suppression; tilted, optimized nonsaturating excitation radiofrequency pulse; 14-cm field of view; 9:15.

**Technique #2:** cervical/axial volume; three-dimensional time-of-flight; 34/6/20; 256 × 128; 128 slices; 140-mm slab; tilted, optimized nonsaturating excitation radiofrequency pulse; 25-cm field of view; 9:19.

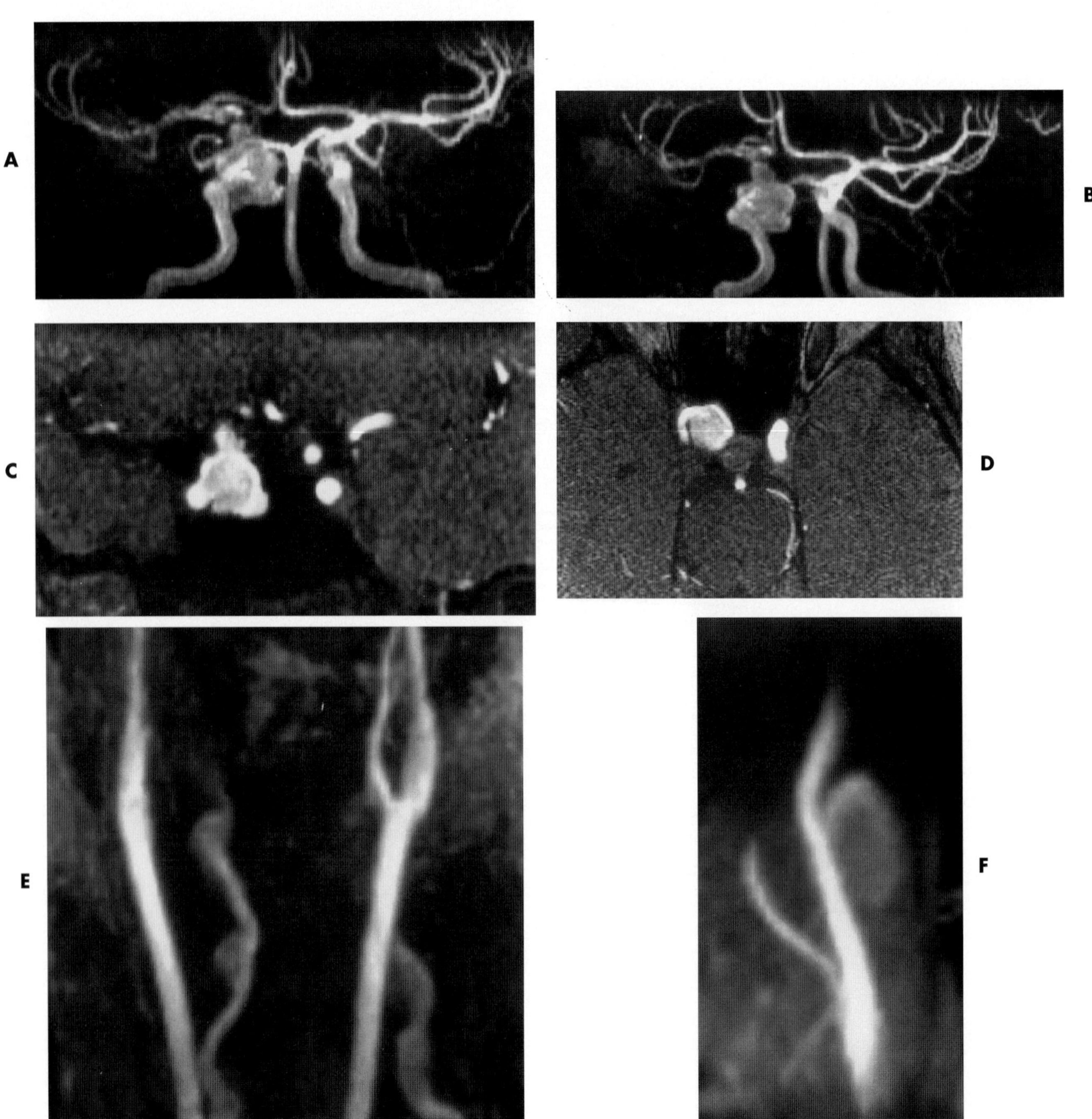

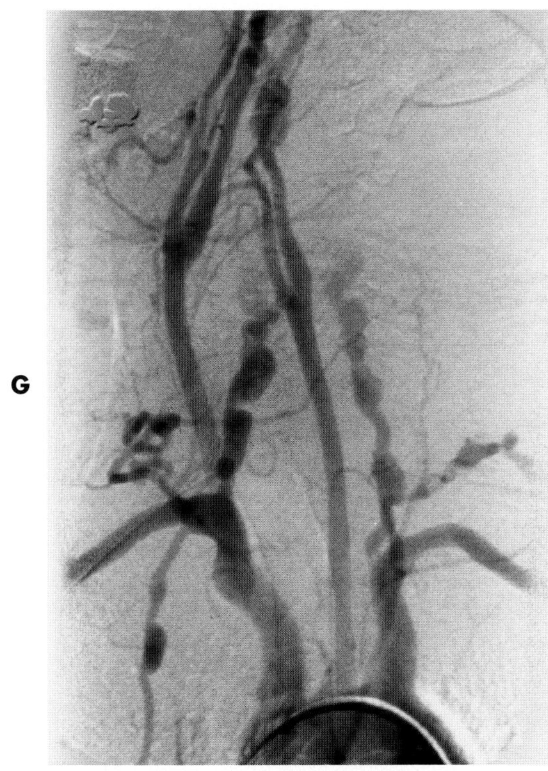

G

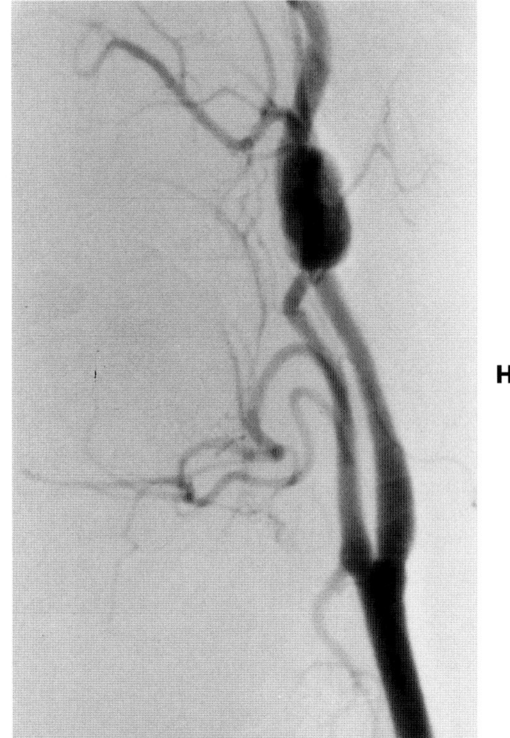

H

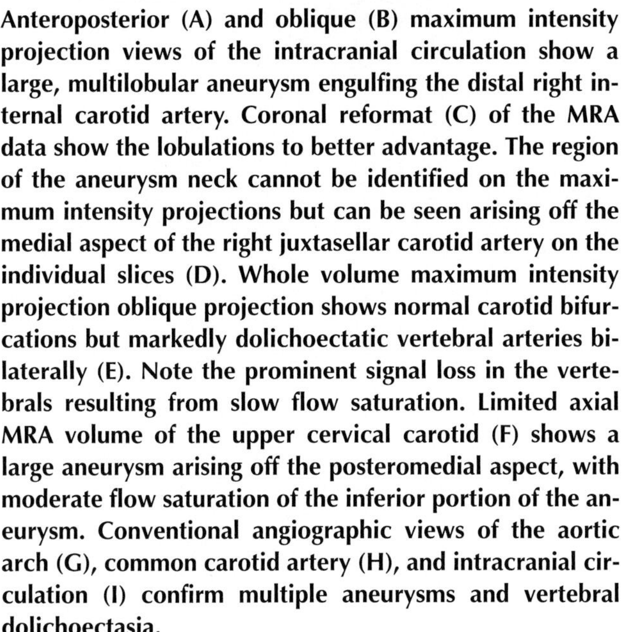

**Anteroposterior (A) and oblique (B) maximum intensity projection views of the intracranial circulation show a large, multilobular aneurysm engulfing the distal right internal carotid artery. Coronal reformat (C) of the MRA data show the lobulations to better advantage. The region of the aneurysm neck cannot be identified on the maximum intensity projections but can be seen arising off the medial aspect of the right juxtasellar carotid artery on the individual slices (D). Whole volume maximum intensity projection oblique projection shows normal carotid bifurcations but markedly dolichoectatic vertebral arteries bilaterally (E). Note the prominent signal loss in the vertebrals resulting from slow flow saturation. Limited axial MRA volume of the upper cervical carotid (F) shows a large aneurysm arising off the posteromedial aspect, with moderate flow saturation of the inferior portion of the aneurysm. Conventional angiographic views of the aortic arch (G), common carotid artery (H), and intracranial circulation (I) confirm multiple aneurysms and vertebral dolichoectasia.**

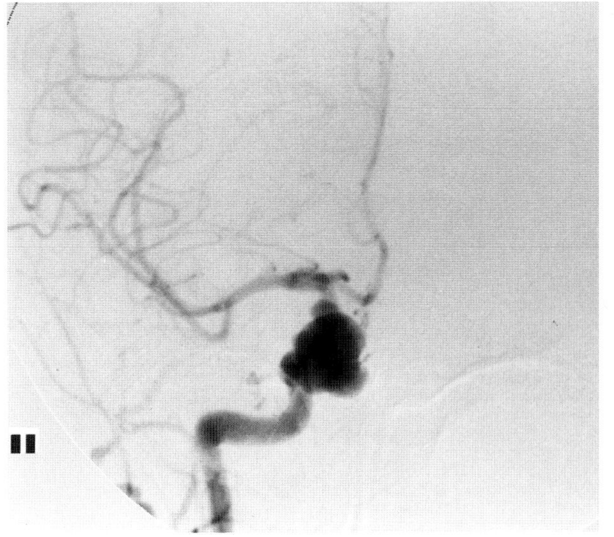

I

The presumptive diagnosis in this unusual case is a connective tissue disorder of unknown type. The advantages and limitations of time-of-flight MRA are well demonstrated by this case. On one hand, the time-of-flight technique gives excellent anatomic detail of the intracranial aneurysm. On the other hand, the saturation effects minimize the length of visualization of the vertebral arteries bilaterally, which could be mistaken for occlusion. Likewise, there are saturation effects that limit the detail of the cervical carotid aneurysm.

CHAPTER 5

# Vascular Malformations

Of the several classifications of vascular malformations of the brain, the most widely accepted is that of McCormick and colleagues.[1,2] This classification consists of five categories: arteriovenous malformation, venous malformation, cavernous malformation, capillary telangectasia, and varices. In the prospective autopsy study of 4069 consecutive brains by Sarwar and McCormick,[2] 165 brains had one or more vascular malformations. The prevalence of venous malformations was 105 (2.6%), capillary telangectasia was 28 (0.69%), arteriovenous malformations was 24 (0.59%), cavernous malformations was 16 (0.39%), and varix malformations was 4 (0.1%). The prevalence of cavernous malformations in this series closely parallels that of a retrospective study performed by Robinson et al,[3] in which the reports of 14,035 MR examinations were evaluated in a 5-year period. In those examinations, there were 76 lesions identified in 66 patients, constituting a prevalence rate of 0.47%.

Intracranial vascular malformations are often identified on the basis of flow or hemorrhage seen on routine spin-echo imaging. Occult vascular malformations are usually detected on the basis of blood by-products present at typical locations in the brain.[4,5] A venous angioma is readily visible as an enlarged vein, usually with a flow void on the T1- or the late echo T2-weighted image.[5] The nidus of an arteriovenous malformation is also generally recognizable on spin-echo images as a central cluster of flow voids within enlarged parenchymal vessels.[6-8] Routine images are also able to detect the parenchymal consequences of hemorrhage, ischemic steal, surgery, embolization, and/or radiation therapy. Nevertheless, preliminary studies indicate that MRA can play a role in this disorder because it may more clearly demonstrate the three-dimensional spatial relationships between the nidus and the feeding arteries and draining veins.[9] In addition, dural fistulae may be imperceptible altogether on spin-echo images unless there is secondary enlargement of cortical veins or dural sinus thrombosis.[10]

Arteriovenous malformations present certain problems to current MRA methods. The vascular nidus and the circle of Willis should be included in the imaging volume to appreciate clinically important vascular relationships, so a large volume of acquisition is often necessary, which can compromise the overall examination time. The three-dimensional time-of-flight sequences can demonstrate the larger afferent arteries reliably because of their relative sensitivity to the rapid flow in these vessels and their resistance to phase dispersion resulting from complex flow. However, the saturation phenomenon in large three-dimensional volume limits visualization of the smaller, slower-flowing afferent arteries (especially in the superior aspect of the volume) and all but the larger efferent veins.[11] Reviewing the individual slices or reconstructing subvolumes may help in defining the vascular malformation because of artifacts inherent to the reconstruction that may hide vessels or artificially narrow vessels resulting from turbulence, flow separation, volume averaging, and background intensity variation.

Two-dimensional time-of-flight techniques may provide a better contrast-to-noise ratio across the imaging volume, improving visualization of the veins and small peripheral arteries.[11] However, the veins inferior to the nidus may be hidden if the rate of slice acquisition (progressing in the same direction—descending) is faster than the venous flow. Portions of the feeding arteries may also be saturated if the flow in these segments is in the same direction as in the slice acquisition (e.g., descending). In addition, the thicker slices and longer echo times of two-dimensional sequences may prevent visualization of the complex flow in the large, tortuous feeding arteries and may obscure aneurysms present in these vessels in up to 10% of cases.[11,12]

The best compromise between two-dimensional and three-dimensional time-of-flight techniques is the use of multiple overlapping thin volumes with intravenous gadolinium.[13] Investigators have demonstrated that the thinner volumes improved arterial visualization, whereas the paramagnetic contrast delineated more of the draining veins in the arteriovenous fistulae.

MR cannot provide the physiologic information shown in conventional angiographic studies (e.g., the arteriovenous circulation time and the degree of shunting). Nevertheless, studies have been able to incorporate limited functional information. Edelman et al[11,14] have added thin saturation slabs in appropriate orientations to eliminate the inflow from potential feeding vessels (e.g. middle cerebral or basilar artery) to assess the contribution of the remaining vascular territories by monitoring the relative intensity of the vascular nidus in a series of two-dimensional acquisitions. For example, if a normal two-dimensional time-of-flight acquisition is compared with one with a saturation slab eliminating the signal in the basilar artery and no intensity difference is appreciated in the vascular nidus, it is concluded that there is little if any contribution from the posterior circulation. These investigators correctly identified the combination of anterior, middle, and/or posterior cerebral arteries as afferent vessels in a preliminary group of 10 patients.

Phase-contrast techniques have an advantage over time-of-flight techniques in that the image is related to flow velocity. Turski et al[9] presented promising results obtained by applying a series of different gradients with a stepwise variation of velocity sensitizations. Two-dimensional projection phase-contrast images can be obtained with different flow-velocity encodings, with the resulting images resembling the arterial and venous phases of an arteriogram. In this fashion it is possible to provide a velocity flow map of the different fistulae components. The rapid flow in the large arterial feeders is seen with the gradients sensitized to higher velocities of 80 to 100 cm/s, the nidus is seen by using the intermediate velocity gradients of 30 to 60 cm/s, and the draining veins are visualized with the gradients sensitized to slower flow such as 10 to 20 cm/s. Further, the slower velocity encoding may help visualize nidal or flow-related aneurysms. Cardiac gating of the phase-contrast study allows display of flow velocity as a function of time. Phase-contrast angiography is thus able to provide not only morphologic information about the vessels, but also information about directional and quantitative flow.[15,16] The evaluation of vascular malformations by phase-contrast techniques may be compromised by higher-order motion, complex vessel geometry, and signal cancellation resulting from vessel overlap.

**REFERENCES**

1. McCormick WF: The pathology of vascular ("arterial venous") malformations, *J Neurosurg* 24:807-816, 1966.
2. Sarwar M, McCormick WF: Intracerebral venous angioma: Case report and review, *Arch Neurol* 35:323-325, 1978.
3. Robinson JR, Awad IA, Little JR: Natural history of the cavernous angioma, *J Neurosurg* 75:709-714, 1991.
4. Gomori JM, Grossman RI, Goldberg HI et al: Occult cerebral vascular malformations: high field MR imaging, *Radiology* 158:707-713, 1986.
5. Atlas S: Intracranial vascular malformations and aneurysms: current imaging applications, *Radiol Clin North Am* 26:821-837, 1988.
6. Kucharczyk W, Lemme-Pleghos L, Uske A et al: Intracranial vascular malformations: MR and CT imaging, *Radiology* 156:383-389, 1985.
7. LeBlanc R, Levesque M, Comair Y, Ethier R: Magnetic resonance imaging of cerebral arteriovenous malformations, *Neurosurgery* 21:15-20, 1987.
8. Noorbehesht B, Fabrikant JI, Enzman DR: Size determination of supratentorial arteriovenous malformations by MR, CT and angiography, *Neuroradiology* 29:512-518, 1987.
9. Turski PA, Partington C, Koresec F et al: *Variable velocity 2-D phase contrast MR angiography for the identification of intracranial slow flow states* (abstract). In Society of Magnetic Resonance in Medicine: *Book of abstracts: SMRM 9th Annual Meeting*. New York, 1990, The Society.
10. DeMarco JK, Dillon WP, Halbach VV, Tsuruda JS: Dural arteriovenous fistulas: evaluation with MR imaging, *Radiology* 175:193-199, 1990.
11. Edelman RR, Wentz KU, Mattle HP et al: Intracerebral arteriovenous malformations: evaluation with selective MR angiography and venography, *Radiology* 173:831-837, 1989.
12. Miyasaka K, Wolpert SM, Prager RJ: The association of cerebral aneurysms, infundibula and intracranial arteriovenous malformations, *Stroke* 1:71-81, 1982.
13. Marchal G, Bosmans H, Van Fraeyenhoven L et al: Intracranial vascular lesions: optimization and clinical evaluation of three-dimensional time-of-flight MR angiography, *Radiology* 175:443-448, 1990.
14. Edelman RR, Mattle HP, O'Reilly GV et al: Magnetic resonance imaging of flow dynamics in the circle of Willis, *Stroke* 21:56-65, 1990.
15. Huston J, Rufenacht DA, Ehman RL et al: Intracranial aneurysms and vascular malformations: comparison of time-of-flight and phase contrast MR angiography, *Radiology* 181:721-730, 1991.
16. Pernicone JR, Siebert JE, Laird TA et al: Determination of blood flow direction using velocity-phase image display with three-dimensional phase contrast MR angiography, *AJNR* 13(5):1435-1438, 1992.

## CASE 80
## PITFALL: VENOUS ANGIOMA NOT SHOWN ON THREE-DIMENSIONAL TIME-OF-FLIGHT STUDY

**History:** 44-year-old with headaches.

**Technique:** axial volume, three-dimensional time-of-flight, 40/7/15, 256 × 256, 64 slices, 60-mm slab, 23-cm field of view, 10:57.

A

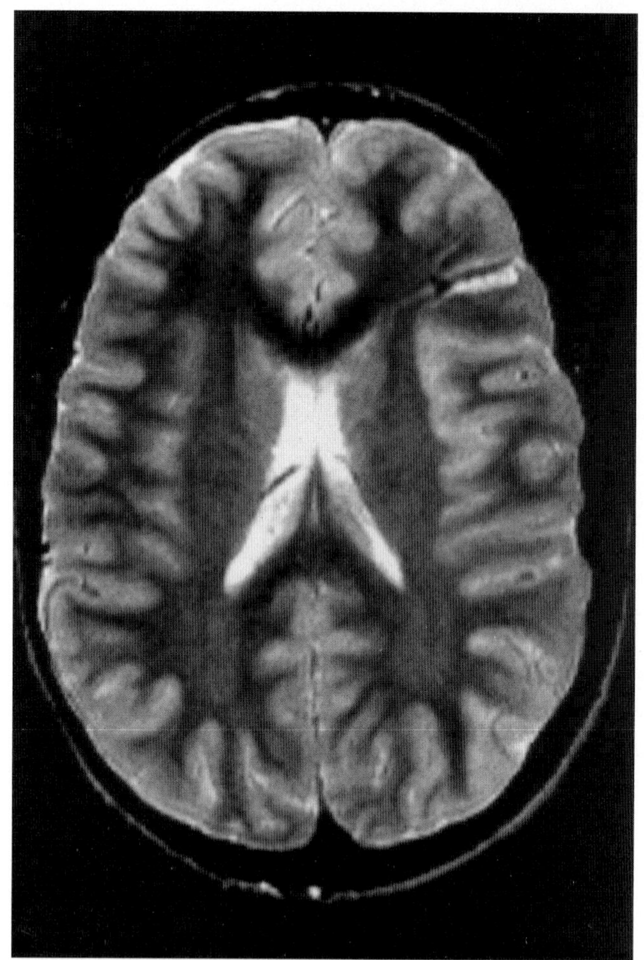

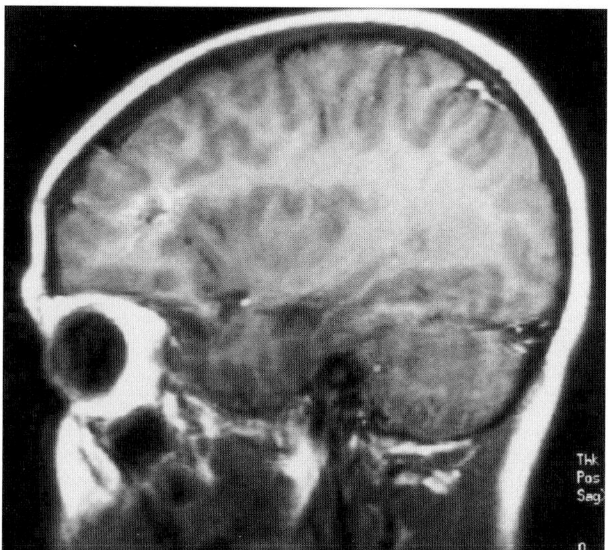


B

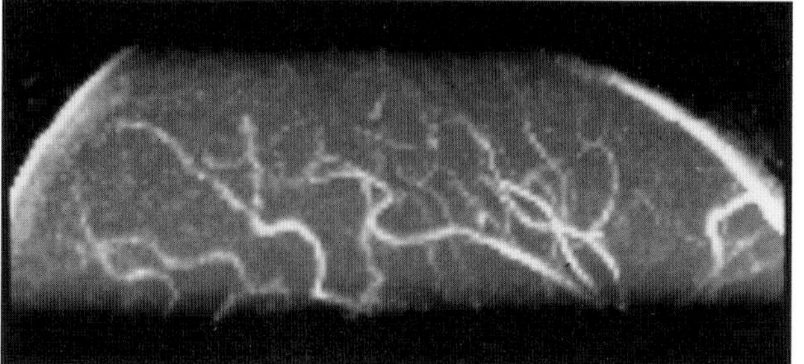

D

C

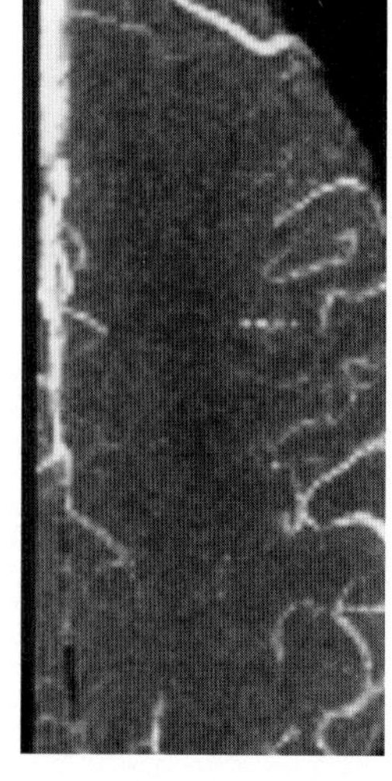

**Axial T2-weighted image (A) demonstrates a linear area of low signal intensity bounded by high signal intensity within the left frontal lobe, which is suspicious for a venous angioma. Sagittal T1-weighted image (B) shows a focal area of flow void within the same region, with a suggestion of a caput medusae radiating from the central vein. The targeted base (C) and lateral maximum intensity projection (D) views of a three-dimensional time-of-flight MRA fail to demonstrate any vascular abnormality within the region of the left frontal lobe.**

The failure of the three-dimensional time-of-flight MRA in identifying an obvious venous angioma is caused by the very flow present within the venous angioma, with concomitant flow saturation on the three-dimensional time-of-flight technique. Contrast administration with repeat imaging, phase-contrast imaging, or two-dimensional imaging would have demonstrated the abnormality.

There is controversy about whether to classify venous angiomas as vascular malformations, venous anomalies, or just normal variants and about to their propensity for intracranial hemorrhage. With the advent of MR, it has become a common occurrence to find a presumably incidental venous angioma on an MR study of the brain, and the tendency is to minimize these lesions as benign venous developmental anomalies. However, cases in which there are parenchymal hemorrhages related to venous angiomas continue to be described. Lupret et al described 11 patients with venous angiomas, 4 with intracerebral hemorrhage and 3 with associated cavernous angiomas.

Venous angiomas are seen as radially oriented dilated medullary veins connecting to a transparenchymal vein, giving rise to the so-called caput medusae sign. The transparenchymal vein may connect to the superficial venous system, dural sinus, or deep venous system. Venous angiomas drain normal brain parenchyma. Hemorrhage appears to be uncommon with venous angiomas, and it has been ascribed to concomitant cavernous angiomas with the venous angioma.

**REFERENCES**

Toro VE, Geyer CA, Sherman JL et al: Cerebral venous angiomas: MR findings, *JCAT* 12:935-940, 1988.

Wilms G, Demaerel P, Marchl G et al: Gadolinium-enhanced MR imaging of cerebral venous angiomas with emphasis on their drainage, *JCAT* 15:199-206, 1991.

Truwit CL: Venous angioma of the brain: History, significance, and imaging findings, *AJR* 159:1299-1307, 1992.

Lupret V, Negovetic L, Smiljanic D et al: Cerebral venous angiomas: surgery as a mode of treatment for selected cases, *Acta Neurochir (Wein)* 120:33-39, 1993.

Kondziolka D, Dempsey PK, Lunsford LD: The case for conservative management of venous angiomas, *Can J Neurol Sci* 18:295-299, 1991.

## CASE 81
## LEFT FRONTAL VENOUS ANGIOMA

**History:** 45-year-old with headaches.

**Technique #1:** two-dimensional phase-contrast, 30/8/20, 512 × 256, eight excitations, 80-mm thick section, 24-cm field of view, 5 minutes.

**Technique #2:** two-dimensional sagittal time-of-flight with the head rotated 15 degrees, 45/9/60, 256 × 128, 1 excitations, 2.5-mm thick sections with 60 total sections with an inferior saturation pulse, 20-cm field of view.

A

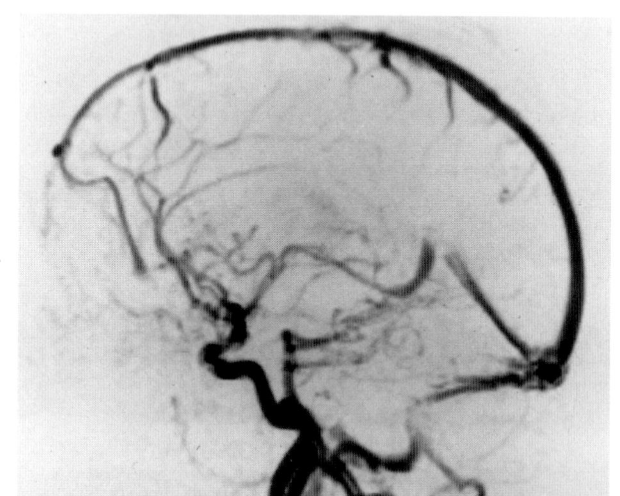

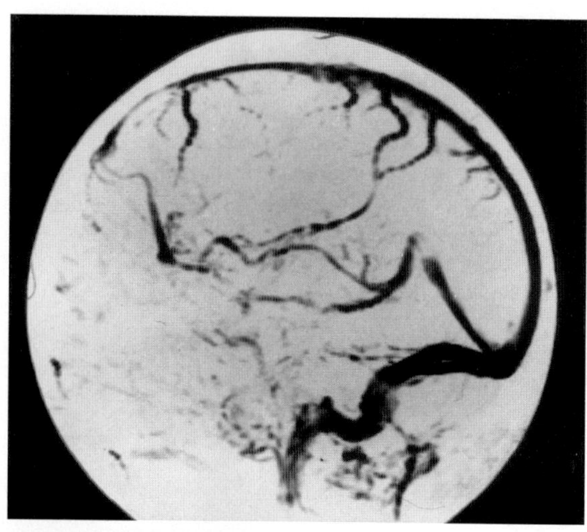

B

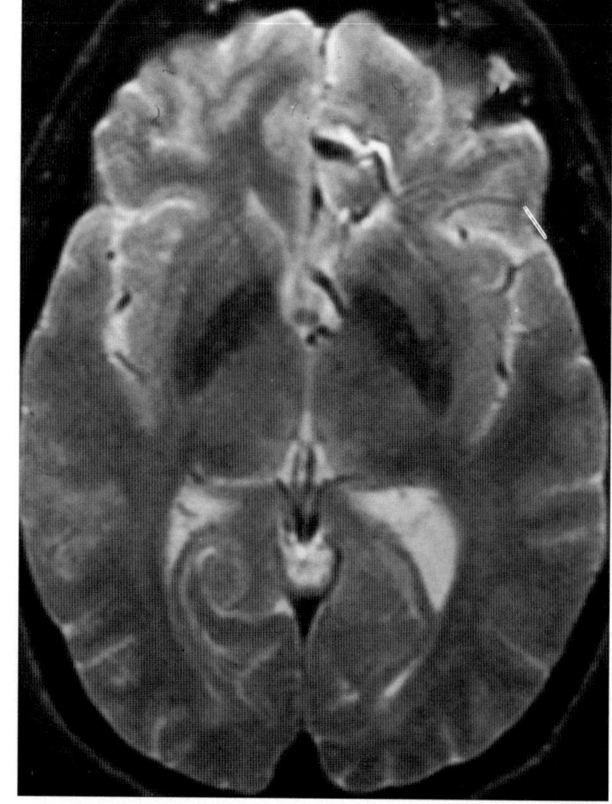

C

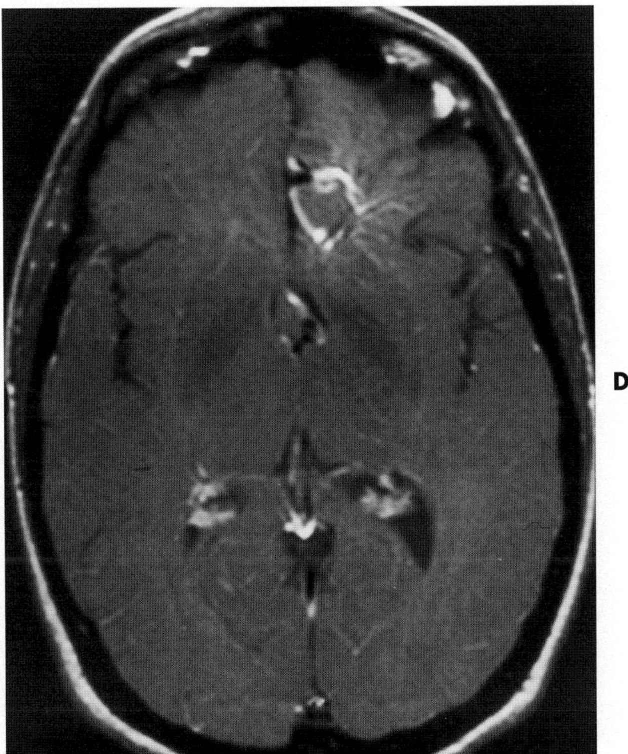


**Lateral maximum intensity projection view of the two-dimensional phase-contrast study (A) demonstrates a curved line of increased signal within the left frontal lobe that extends anteriorly to merge with the anterior aspect of the superior sagittal sinus. This finding is also demonstrated on the lateral maximum intensity projection view of the two-dimensional time-of-flight study (B) with an inferior saturation pulse. The venous angioma is well identified on the conventional T2-weighted spin-echo study (C) as a serpentine area of mixed signal intensity showing spatial mismapping, identifying it as a vascular flow. Faint caput medusae is seen as well. The angioma is more easily identified after administration of contrast material on the axial T1-weighted spin-echo study (D). (Courtesy John Huston, Mayo Clinic, Rochester, Minn.)**

## CASE 82
## VENOUS ANGIOMA OF THE POSTERIOR FOSSA WITH HEMORRHAGE

**History:** 45-year-old with sudden onset of nausea and vertigo.

**Technique:** axial volume, three-dimensional time-of-flight, 40/7/15, 256 × 256, 64 slices, 60-mm slab, 23-cm field of view, 10:57.

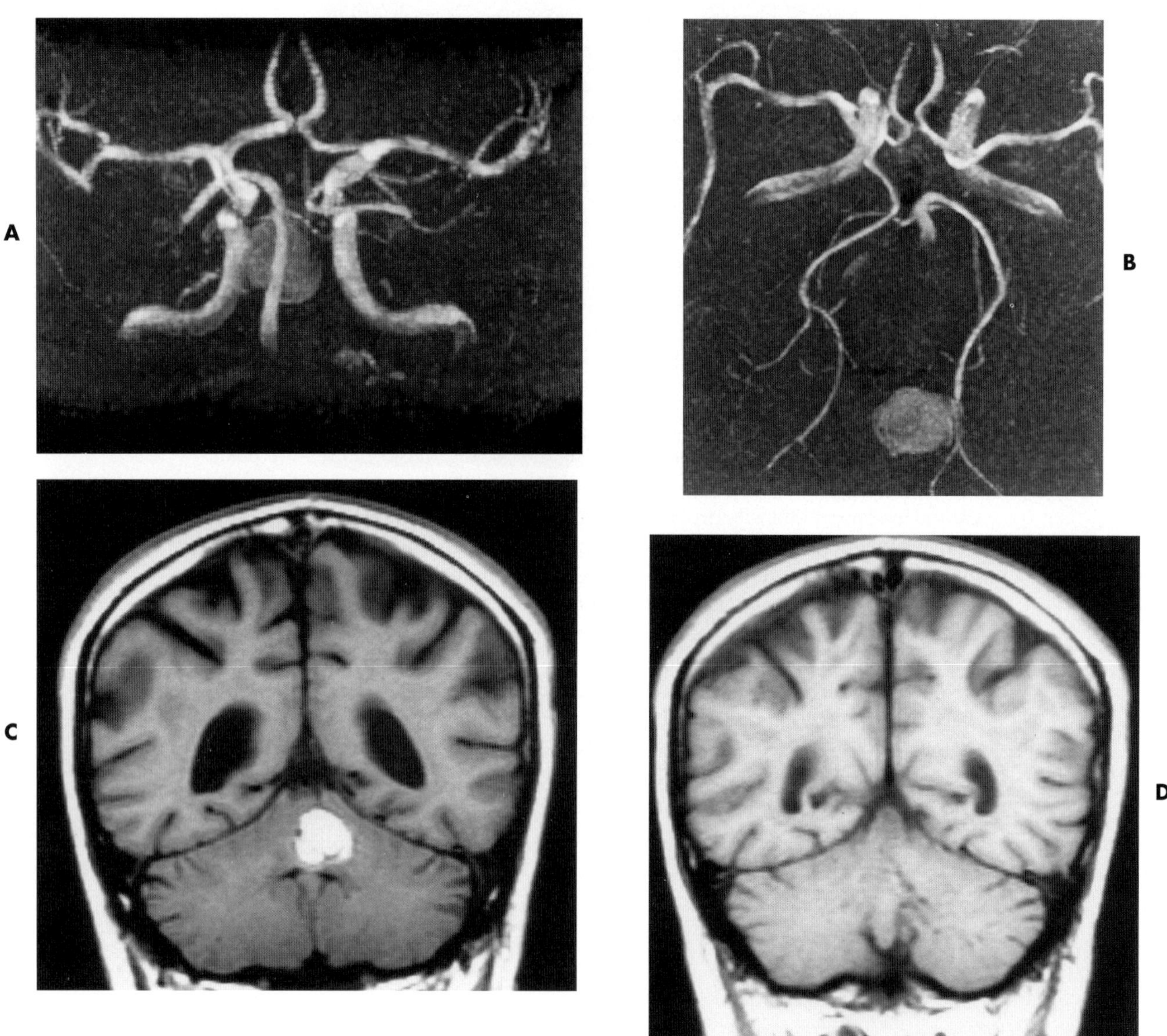

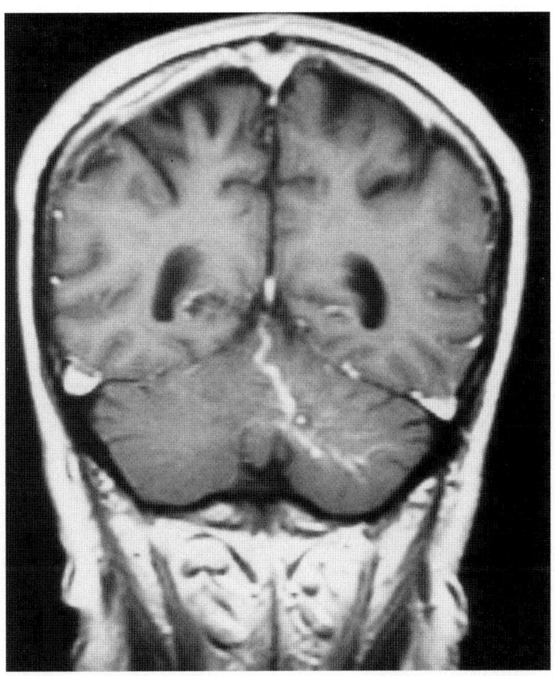

E

**Anteroposterior (A) and base (B) maximum intensity projection views demonstrate a well-defined mass of increased signal intensity that involves the posterior fossa and that is apparently adjacent to the distal branches of the posterior cerebral artery. However, the unenhanced coronal T1-weighted image (C) shows the mass to be well defined and of increased signal intensity, consistent with methemoglobin within a parenchymal hemorrhage. A vague serpentine area of low signal intensity is seen just posterior to the lesion on the unenhanced T1-weighted image just posterior to C (D). This area dramatically enhances in serpentine fashion after contrast administration (E), and the more peripheral aspects of the caput medusae of the venous angioma are also apparent.**

The high signal intensity seen on the MRA relates to T1 shortening of the methemoglobin and does not relate to flow. The slow flow from the enlarged vein is not identified on the three-dimensional time-of-flight MRA because of flow saturation. Phase-contrast or two-dimensional time-of-flight MR venography should be used in these cases, although the diagnosis is easily established by simply giving contrast material. Note the fetal origin of the right posterior cerebral artery.

# CASE 83
## CAVERNOUS ANGIOMA AND VENOUS ANGIOMA OF THE POSTERIOR FOSSA

**History:** 65-year-old with vertigo.

**Technique:** axial volume; three-dimensional time-of-flight; 45/7/20; 256 × 256; 64 slices; 60-mm slab; magnetization transfer background suppression; tilted, optimized nonsaturating excitation radiofrequency pulse; 14-cm field of view; 12:20.

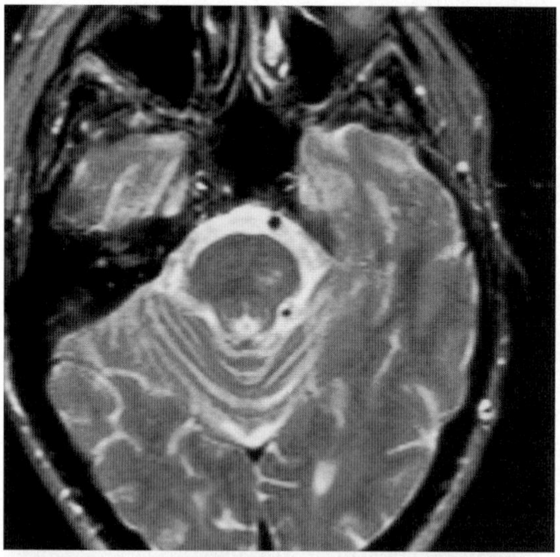

A

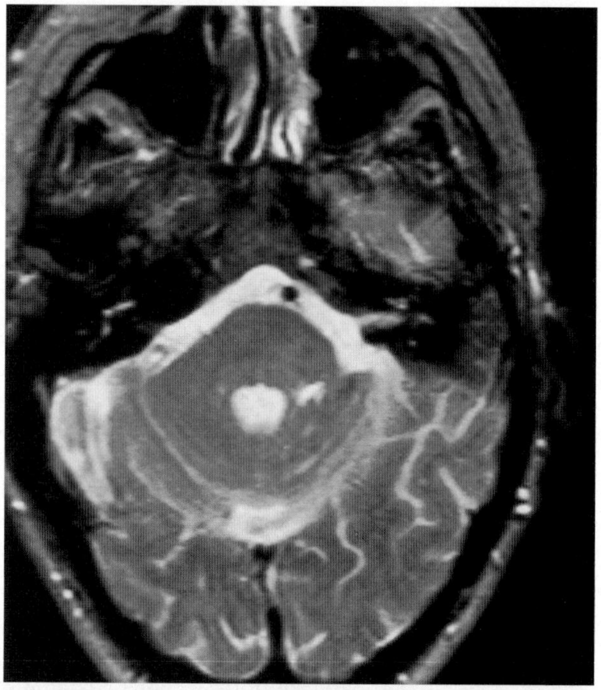

B

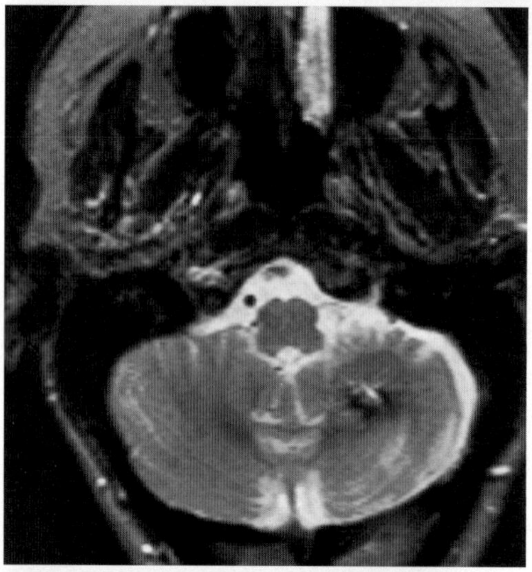

C

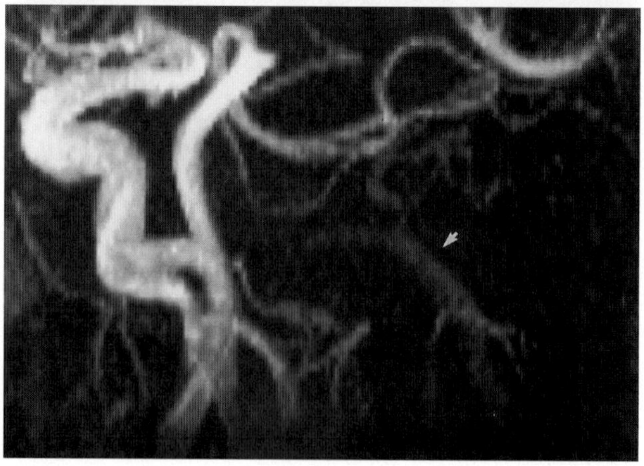

D

E

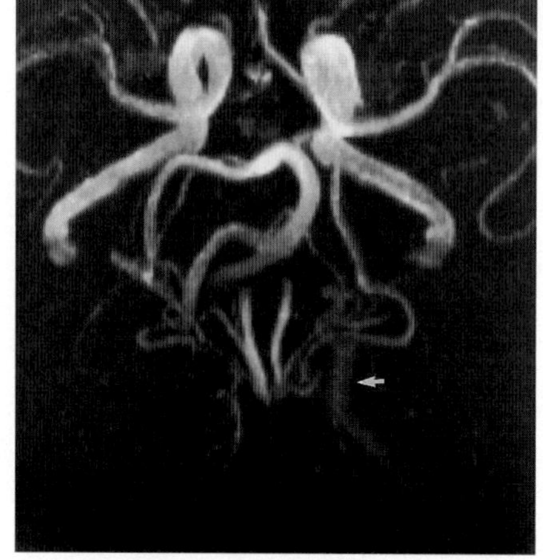

**A series of axial T2-weighted images (A to C) demonstrate an ill-defined area of abnormal low signal intensity within the inferior aspect of the left cerebellar hemisphere. Spiculated high signal intensity is noted within a portion of this, with a linear area of increased signal intensity extending cephalad along the left middle cerebellar peduncle. A prominent vessel is noted within the left circummesencephalic cistern. Lateral (D) and base (E) views from the maximum intensity projection demonstrate a scimitar-shaped area of faint signal intensity extending inferior to cephalid within the left side of the posterior fossa *(arrow)*. The remainder of the intracranial vessels are normal in appearance.**

Findings on the spin-echo study would be consistent with hemosiderin deposition from prior hemorrhage involving a venous angioma that has previously bled or a combination of cavernous angioma and venous angioma. The prominent vessel within the circummesencephalic cistern is the draining vein of the venous angioma. The findings on MRA would also be consistent with the course of the venous portion of the vascular anomaly, which is faintly seen resulting from slow flow saturation. The parenchymal and MRA findings indicate a combination of cavernous hemangioma and venous angioma. The abnormal low signal intensity of the hemosiderin deposition is not visualized on the maximum intensity projection.

Cavernous malformations are hamartomatous lesions composed of enlarged sinusoidal vascular spaces with a single layer of attenuated endothelium, which are devoid of elastin or smooth muscle. The sinusoids are separated from each other by connective tissue, with no intervening neural tissue. The brain parenchyma immediately surrounding the lesion is gliotic and may contain small, slow-flowing arteries and draining veins. In addition, a rim of parenchyma surrounding the lesion is hemosiderin stained.[1-3]

These lesions have frequently been included in a group of arteriovenous malformations of different pathologic characteristics collectively called *angiographically occult vascular malformations.* This is a nonspecific term whose only common feature is the absence of abnormal vascularity on angiography. Morphologically the common feature of all these lesions is slow blood flow. They pathologically comprise thrombosed arteriovenous malformations, capillary telangectasias, cavernous malformations, and venous angiomas.[3,4] Lobato et al[5] summarized hypotheses on the reasons for a frequent lack of angiographic identification of these vascular lesions: (1) compression of the lumen of the cavernous malformation vessel by mass effect from the adjacent hematoma, (2) destruction of the cavernous malformation vessel by macroscopic bleeding, (3) spontaneous thrombosis of the cavernous malformation, (4) thrombosis secondary to a gross hemorrhage, (5) partial thrombosis with sluggish circulation through the remaining patent vessels, (6) posthemorrhagic vascular vasospasm, and (7) dilution of the contrast media in enlarged cavernous vascular spaces of the malformation.

In a retrospective review by Robinson et al,[6] MR images of 76 lesions in 66 patients demonstrated that most intracranial cavernous malformations occur in the frontal and temporal lobes. Approximately 70% of these lesions were in the cerebral hemispheres; approximately 5% were considered deep lesions affecting the diencephalon and septal region. The infratentorial lesions were almost equally split between the cerebellar hemisphere and brainstem locations. The pons is the most common site for brainstem cavernous malformations.[7] In another study of 56 cavernous malformations in 47 patients, 59% of the malformations were supratentorial, the most common locations being the temporal and parietal regions; some 39% of malformations were infratentorial, the most common locations being the pons and the cerebellum.[8] Of significant clinical and therapeutic importance is the association of venous angiomas with cavernous malformations in 5% to 16% of cases, as in the case demonstrated here.[6,9-11] The size of cavernous malformations varies widely, ranging from several millimeters to 4 cm or greater.[6] Pathologic studies have demonstrated that multiple lesions occur in approximately 25% of cases.[3] In an MR imaging–based series, Rigamonti et al[2] demonstrated multiple lesions in approximately 50% of patients. Recent studies by Robinson et al[6] and Requena et al,[8] which were based on the MR imaging diagnosis of cavernous malformations, demonstrated that approximately 11% to 13% of patients had multiple malformations.

## REFERENCES


1. Jellinger K: Vascular malformations of the central nervous system: a morphological overview, *Neurosurg Rev* 9:177-216, 1986.
2. Rigamonti D, Drayer BP, Johnson PC et al: The MRI appearance of cavernous malformations (angiomas). *J Neurosurg* 67:518-524, 1987.
3. Russel DS, Rubenstein LJ: *Pathology of the nervous system,* Baltimore, 1989, Williams & Wilkins.
4. McCormick WF: The pathology of vascular ("arterial venous") malformations, *J Neurosurg* 24:807-816, 1966.
5. Lobato RD, Perez C, Rivas JJ et al: Clinical, radiological, and pathological spectrum of angiographically occult intracranial vascular malformations, *J Neurosurg* 68:518-531, 1988.
6. Robinson JR, Awad IA, Little JR: Natural history of the cavernous angioma, *J Neurosurg* 75:709-714, 1991.
7. McCormick WF, Hardman JM, Boulter TR: Vascular malformations ("angiomas") of the brain, with special reference to those occurring in the posterior fossa, *J Neurosurg* 28:241-251, 1968.
8. Requena I, Arias M, Lopez-Ibor L et al: Cavernomas of the central nervous system: clinical and neuroimaging manifestations in 47 patients, *J Neurol Neurosurg Psychiatr* 54:590-594, 1991.
9. Rigamonti D, Spetzler RF: The association of venous and cavernous malformations: report of four cases and discussion of the pathophysiological, diagnostic, and therapeutic implications, *Acta Neurochir (Wien)* 92:100-105, 1988.
10. Sasaki O, Tanaka R, Koike T et al: Excision of cavernous angioma with preservation of coexisting venous angioma: case report, *J Neurosurg* 75:461-464, 1991.
11. Zimmerman RS, Spetzler RF, Lee KS et al: Cavernous malformations of the brain stem, *J Neurosurg* 75:32-39, 1991.

## CASE 84
## PITFALL: RIGHT PARIETAL ARTERIOVENOUS MALFORMATION WITH THROMBOSED DRAINING VEIN

**History:** 39-year-old complaining of occipital headaches.

**Technique:** axial volume, three-dimensional time-of-flight, 40/7/15, 160 × 256, 128 slices, 140-mm thick slab, 25-cm field of view, 13:41.

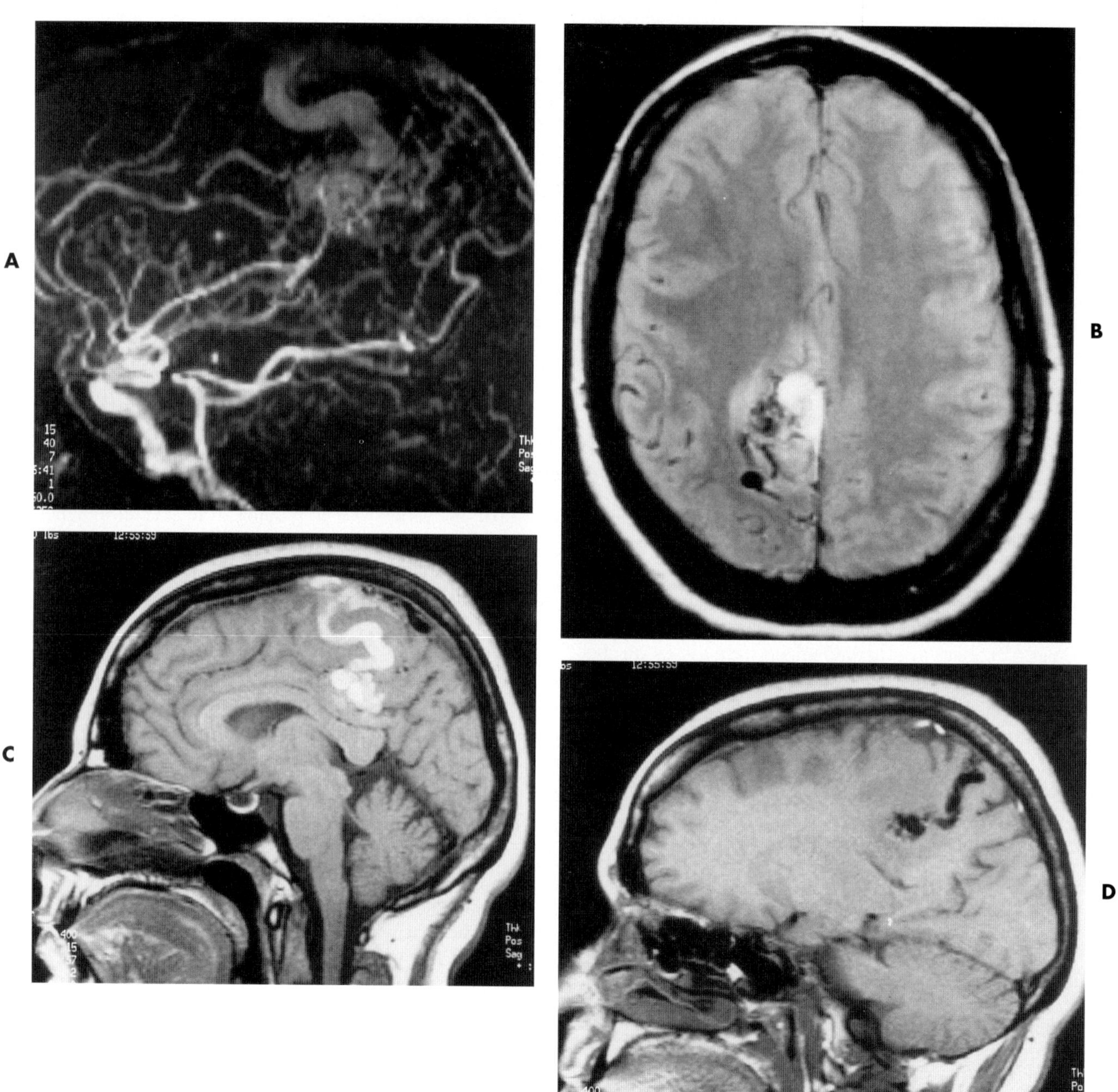

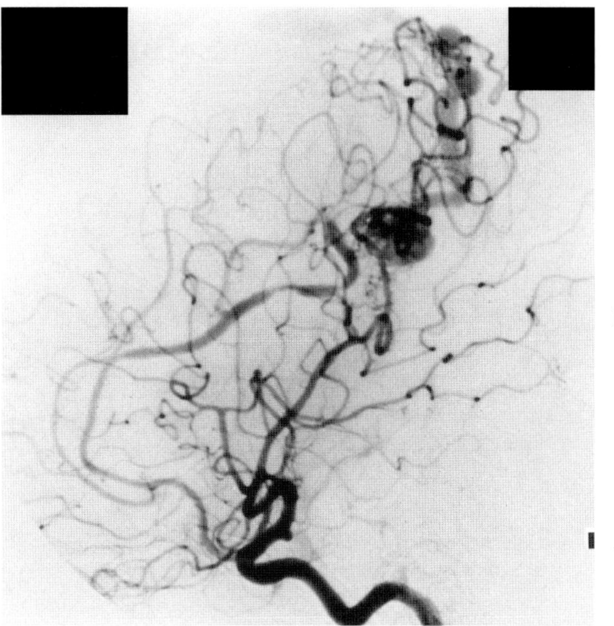


**Lateral maximum intensity projection view (A) shows an arteriovenous malformation in the right parietal lobe with an apparent large draining vein to the superior sagittal sinus. Spin density weighted image (B) shows a well-defined area of increased signal in the mesial right parietal lobe, with serpentine flow voids around the periphery. Sagittal T1-weighted study (C) shows serpentine high signal near the midline, consistent with methemoglobin in a thrombosed draining vein. More laterally on the T1-weighted sequence (D), there is serpentine flow void of a second, nonthrombosed vein. Anteroposterior conventional angiographic view (E) of the right internal carotid injection shows the arteriovenous malformation nidus supplied mainly by an enlarged right pericallosal artery, with only the more lateral patent draining vein being visualized. This vein is not visualized on the time-of-flight MRA because of flow saturation.**

This is yet another example of high signal intensity on the maximum intensity projection views that is unrelated to flowing blood. In this case, the methemoglobin within the thrombosed draining vein mimicked flow on the three-dimensional time-of-flight study. Evaluation of the conventional MR imaging examination allows the distinction between clot and flow.

## CASE 85
## LARGE FRONTAL ARTERIOVENOUS MALFORMATION

**History:** 26-year-old with seizures.

**Technique:** axial volume, three-dimensional time-of-flight, 40/7/15 degrees, 256 × 128, 128 slices, 120-mm slab, 23-cm field of view, 10:57.

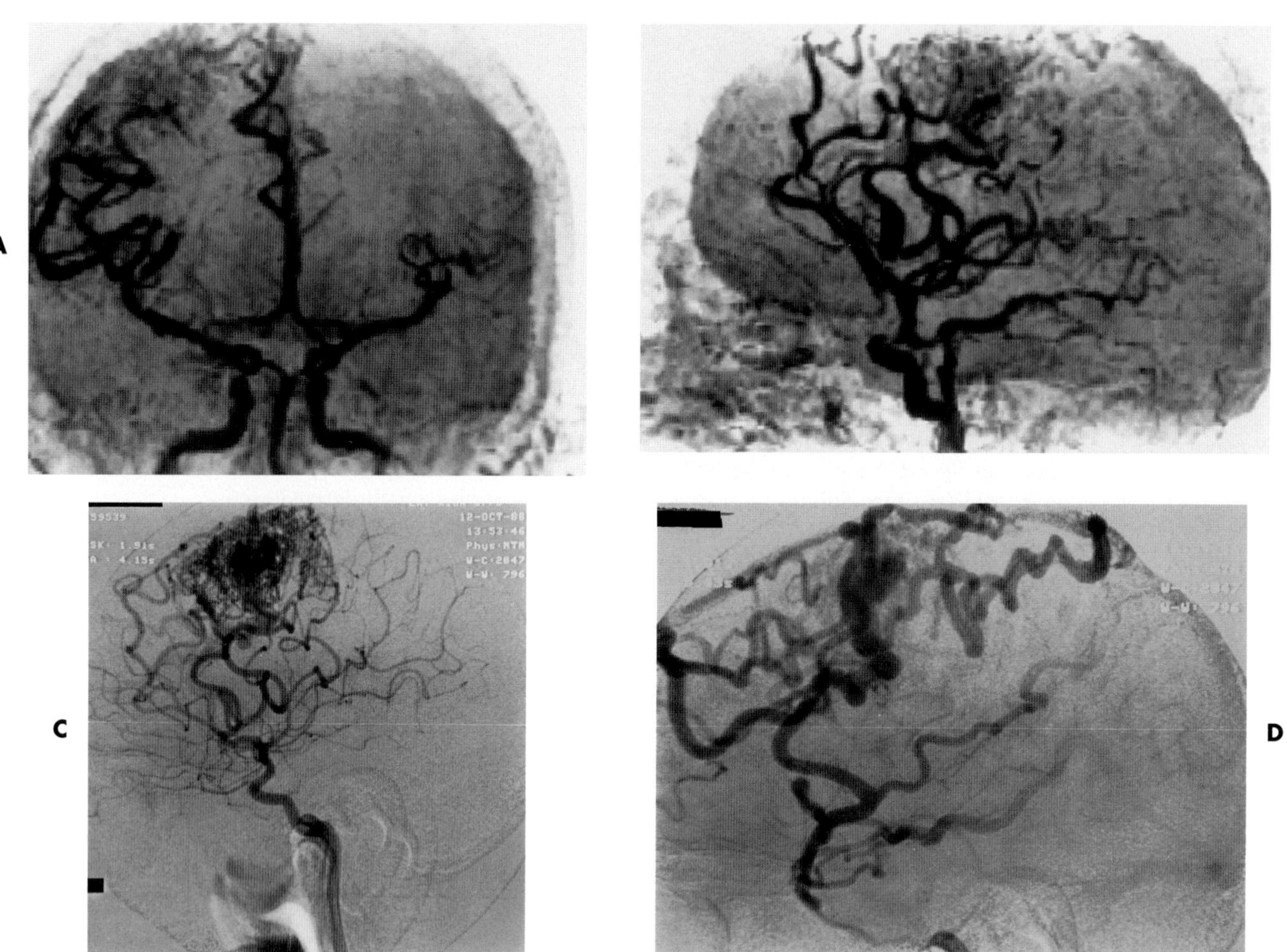


**Anteroposterior (A) and lateral (B) views from a maximum intensity projection demonstrate an ill-defined, large arteriovenous malformation nidus within the posterior right frontal lobe. Feeding vessels appear to arise from the anterior and middle cerebral artery distributions on the right. Arterial (C) and venous (D) lateral views from the conventional angiogram demonstrate the vascular malformation fed from the anterior and middle cerebral artery distributions. The multiple abnormal, enlarged draining veins are not demonstrated on the MRA but are well identified on the conventional lateral view from the angiogram. The veins are not identified because of their slow flow with flow saturation on the three-dimensional time-of-flight study.**

Kauczor et al evaluated 18 patients with intracerebral arteriovenous malformations and followed them after they underwent radiosurgery. They found that MRA detected signs of nidus obliteration earlier and with a higher sensitivity than conventional spin-echo imaging. MRA loss of flow signal within the arteriovenous malformation was related to a reduction in the nidus size. They also saw a decrease in signal intensity of feeding arteries and of the draining veins from the arteriovenous malformation.

MRA provides a great opportunity for follow-up of radiosurgery of arteriovenous malformations, since multiple examinations can be performed to monitor progression of the patient without having to do catheter angiography. The reduction of nidus size after radiosurgery is not necessarily related to occlusion of the arteriovenous malformation. However, it can be regarded as an indirect sign of decreased flow. It appears that a reduction of nidus size indicates scarring, according to signal changes on spin-echo imaging and MRA. Radiation causes intimal proliferation and subsequent reduction in lumen diameter, with eventual fibrosis. The adjacent brain is also irradiated, resulting in ischemia, gliosis, and demyelination with increased signal on T2-weighted spin-echo studies. MRA is more sensitive to transnidal blood flow than the conventional spin-echo study because of this increased signal from adjacent abnormal brain. The size reduction on MRA represents a decrease of patent vessels with flow velocities high enough to be detected by the particular technique used.

As with all three-dimensional time-of-flight techniques, there are some general limitations for using MRA to evaluate radiosurgery changes. These limitations relate to the following: (1) The three-dimensional time-of-flight technique is sensitive to relatively high flow, and the visualization of venous signal and draining veins is limited; (2) the use of the maximum intensity projection by itself results in suppression of very faint flow signals; and (3) the maximum intensity projection is a nonspecific algorithm that shows high signal intensity from many causes of T1 shortening. Therefore different blood breakdown products such as methemoglobin will show up as a high signal intensity. MRA and conventional spin-echo imaging of the brain are complimentary for follow-up evaluation in radiosurgery of arteriovenous malformations. Although the time-of-flight MRA techniques are sensitive to the transnidal blood flow and the overall size of the nidus, the spin-echo sequences (particularly the T2-weighted sequence) is essential for visualizing the side effects of radiosurgery such as edema, demyelination, and encephalomalacia.

## REFERENCES


Kauczor H, Engenhart R, Layer G et al: 3D TOF MR angiography of cerebral AVM after radiosurgery, *JCAT* 17:184-190, 1993.

Ondra SL, Troupp H, George ED, Schwab K: The natural history of symptomatic arteriovenous malformations of the brain: a 24-year follow-up assessment, *J Neurosurg* 73:387-391, 1990.

Spetzler RF, Martin NA: A proposed grading system for arteriovenous malformations, *J Neursurg* 65:476-483, 1985.

Marks MP, Delapaz RD, Fabrikant JI et al: Intracranial vascular malformations: imaging of charged-particle radiosurgery. I. Results of therapy, *Radiology* 168:447-455, 1988.

Marks MP, Delapaz RL, Fabrikant JI et al: Intracranial vascular malformations: imaging of charged-particle radiosurgery. II. Complications, *Radiology* 168:457-462, 1988.

Huston J III, Rufenacht DA, Ehman RL, Wibers DO: Intracranial aneurysms and vascular malformations: comparison of time-of-flight and phase-contrast MR angiography, *Radiology* 181:721-730, 1991.

Edelman RR, Wentz KU, Mattle HP et al: Intracerebral arteriovenous malformations: evaluation with selective MR angiography and venography, *Radiology* 173:831-837, 1989.

Anderson CM, Saloner D, Tsuruda JS et al: Artifacts in maximum-intensity projection display of MR angiograms, *AJR* 154:623-639, 1990.

Nussel F, Wegmuller H, Huber P: Comparison of magnetic resonance angiography, magnetic resonance imaging and conventional angiography in cerebral arteriovenous malformation, *Neuroradiology* 33(1):56-61, 1991.

## CASE 86
## LEFT POSTERIOR PARIETAL ARTERIOVENOUS MALFORMATION WITH BASILAR TIP AND LEFT CAROTID SIPHON ANEURYSMS

**History:** 52-year-old with previous subarachnoid hemorrhage.

**Technique #1:** sagittal or axial two-dimensional phase-contrast, 33/9/20, 256 × 192, eight excitations, 80-mm thick section, velocity encoding of 20, 100 and 200 cm/sec, 24-cm field of view, 4 minutes.

**Technique #2:** axial three-dimensional phase contrast, 26/9/15, 256 × 128, one excitations, 1-mm thick sections with a total of 60 sections, velocity encoding of 30 cm/sec, 18-cm field of view, 13 minutes.

**Technique #3:** sagittal two-dimensional time-of-flight with the head rotated 15 degrees, 45/9/60, 256 × 128, one excitations, 2.5-mm thick slices with 60 total slices, inferior saturation bands, 20-cm field of view.

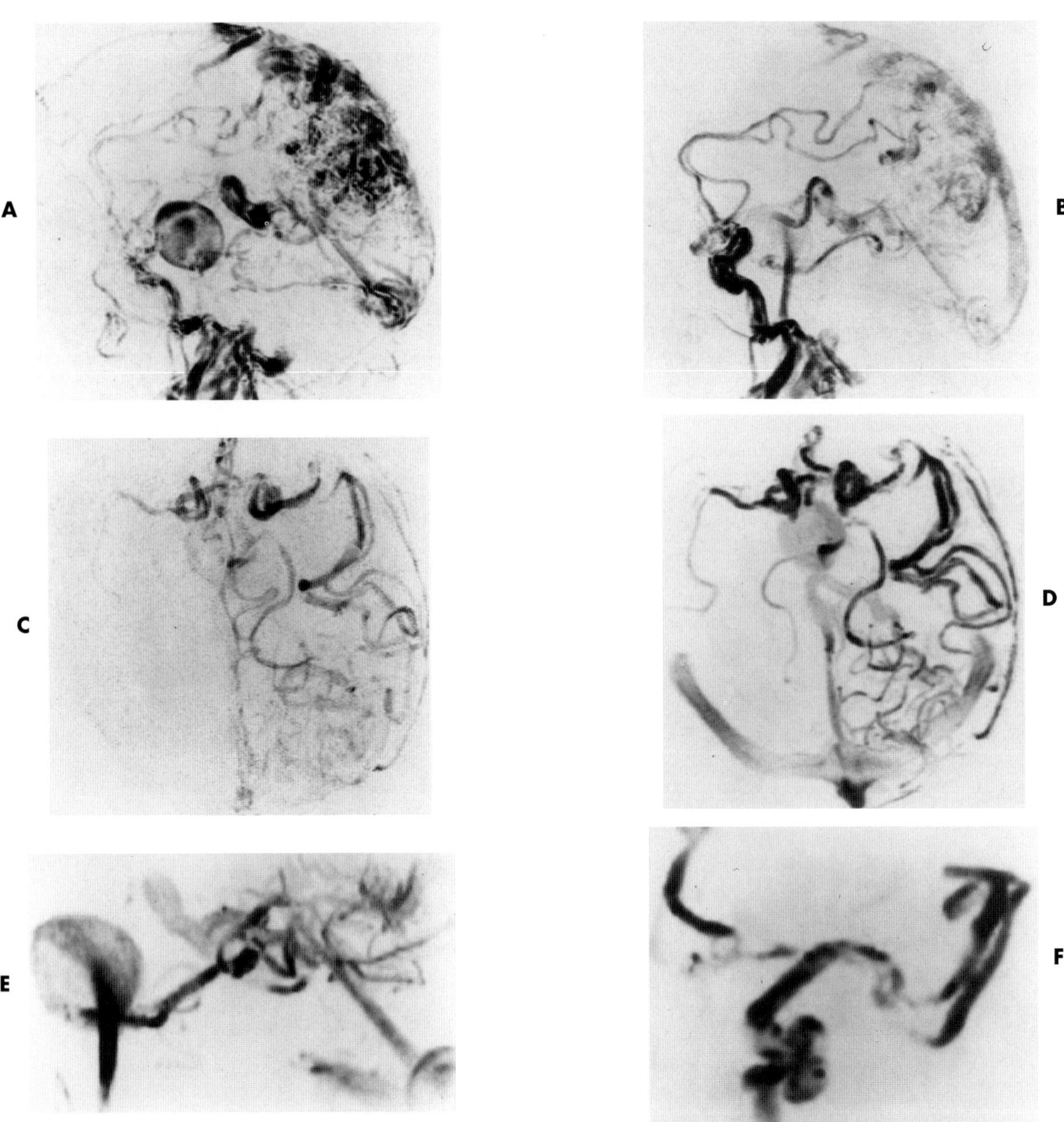

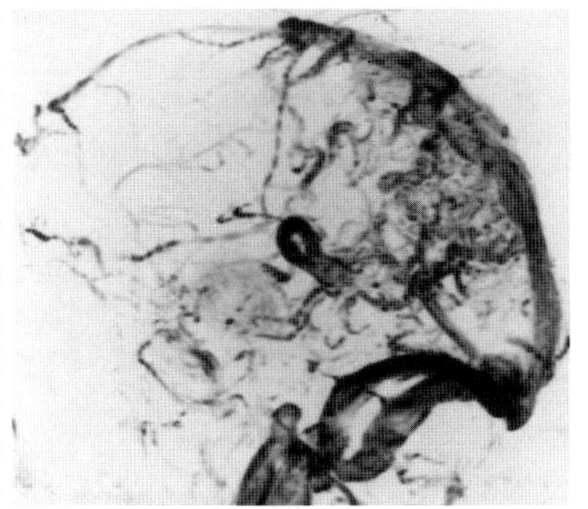

G

**Sagittal two-dimensional phase-contrast study with a velocity encoding of 20 cm/s (A) highlights the relatively slow-flow vessels, such as the serpentine vessels within the arteriovenous malformation nidus, the draining vein of Galen and straight sinus, and the large basilar tip aneurysm. Sagittal two-dimensional phase-contrast study (B) with the velocity encoding at 100 cm/s shows the high-flow regions such as the feeding anterior cerebral vessels and the high-flow portion of the draining veins (e.g., the superior sagittal sinus). The basilar tip aneurysm is very poorly identified at this higher-velocity encoding. Base projection with the velocity encoding at 200 cm/s (C) allows visualization of primarily the arterial flow to the large arteriovenous malformation. Note the supply of the posterior and middle cerebral branches. Very little venous anatomy is depicted with this high-velocity encoding. Axial base view of a three-dimensional phase-contrast angiogram (D) with a 50 cm/s velocity encoding allows visualization of the major arterial feeders to the arteriovenous malformation as well as visualization of the aneurysm involving the basilar artery (3 cm in size) and left carotid siphon (1.5 cm in size). Targeted lateral maximum intensity projection view of the three-dimensional phase-contrast study (E) shows the basilar tip aneurysm and a portion of the draining vein and arteriovenous malformation. Note the jet effect extending from the tip of the basilar artery into the aneurysm. Targeted anteroposterior maximum intensity projection view of the left carotid siphon (F) shows the saccular aneurysm projecting laterally.**
**Contrast A with G, which is a two-dimensional time-of-flight study with a inferior saturation pulse to exclude arterial signal. Slightly greater detail (e.g., the anterior portion of the superior sagittal sinus and the better delineation of the posterior superior sagittal sinus and the arteriovenous malformation nidus) is present in the two-dimensional time-of-flight study. There is nearly complete lack of signal intensity within the arterial structures such as the aneurysms. (Courtesy John Huston, Mayo Clinic, Rochester, Minn.)**

Circulatory breakthrough is a well-known complication of removal of large arteriovenous malformations. *Circulatory breakthrough* is usually defined as severe brain swelling with massive multifocal hemorrhage. These complications may be reduced by staged surgery or by preoperative embolization so that rapid changes in hemodynamics may be avoided.

Pasqualin et al proposed a grading system for arteriovenous malformations defined by several anatomic and physiologic parameters. Arteriovenous malformations with volumes greater than 20 cm$^3$ were associated with significantly higher rates of early and late postoperative complications. Higher morbidity was related to rolandic, inferior limbic, and insular malformations. Deep arterial feeders increased the frequency of circulatory breakthrough complications and morbidity and mortality. The presence of deep venous drainage did not increase the rate of hyperemic complications but did increase the rate of permanent morbidity after removal of the arteriovenous malformation.

Characteristics of arteriovenous malformations positively correlated with intracranial hemorrhage include central venous drainage, a periventricular or intraventricular arteriovenous malformation location, and intranidal aneurysm. The risk of intracranial hemorrhage from arteriovenous malformation is 2% to 3% per year, with the risk of death from the initial bleed being at 10%. The incidence of neurologic deficit is about 50% for each hemorrhagic episode.

**REFERENCES**

Pasqualin A, Barone G, Cioffi F et al: The relavence of anatomic and hemodynamic factors to a classification of cerebral artriovenous malformations, *Neurosurgery* 28:3 370-379, 1991.

Marks MP, Lane B, Steinberg GK, Chang PJ: Hemorrhage in intracerebral arteriovenous malformations: angiographic determinants, *Radiology* 176:807-813, 1990.

Fults D, Kelly DL Jr: Natural history of arteriovenous malformations of the brain: a clinical study, *Neurosurgery* 15:658-662, 1984.

Graf CJ, Perret GE, Torner JC: Bleeding from cerebral arteriovenous malformations as part of their natural history, *J Neurosurg* 58:331-337, 1983.

Wilkins RH: Natural history of intracranial vascular malformations: a review, *Neurosurgery* 16:421-430, 1985.

## CASE 87
## RIGHT PARIETOOCCIPITAL ARTERIOVENOUS MALFORMATION

**History:** 34-year-old with seizures.

**Technique #1:** axial three-dimensional phase-contrast, 26/9/15, 256 × 128, one excitation, 60 slices, 120-mm slab, velocity encoding of 15 cm/sec, 18-cm field of view, 14 minutes.

**Technique #2:** axial three-dimensional time-of-flight, 40/5/20, 256 × 192, one excitation, 60 slices, 120-mm slab, 18-cm field of view, 7:40.

**Technique #3:** sagittal two-dimensional phase contrast, 20/9/30, 256 × 192, six excitations, 80-mm thick section, velocity encoding of 30 and 200 cm/sec, 24-cm field of view, 2 minutes.

**A**

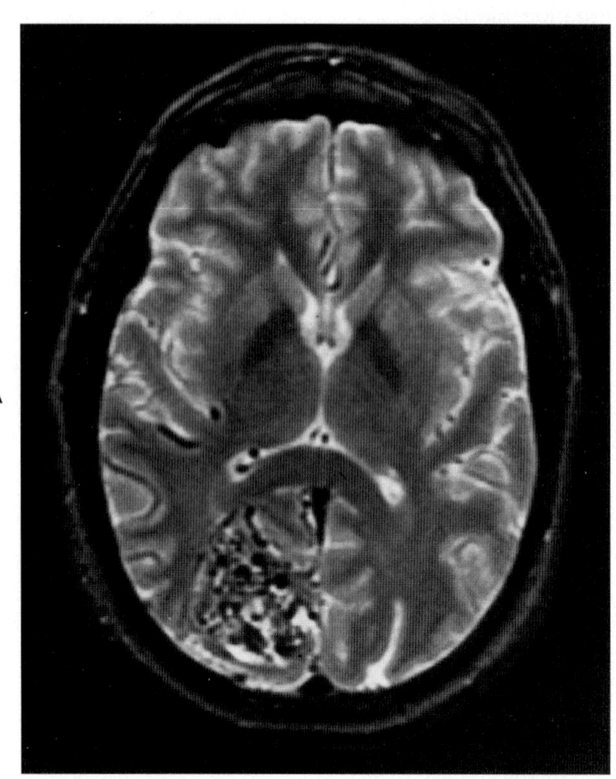

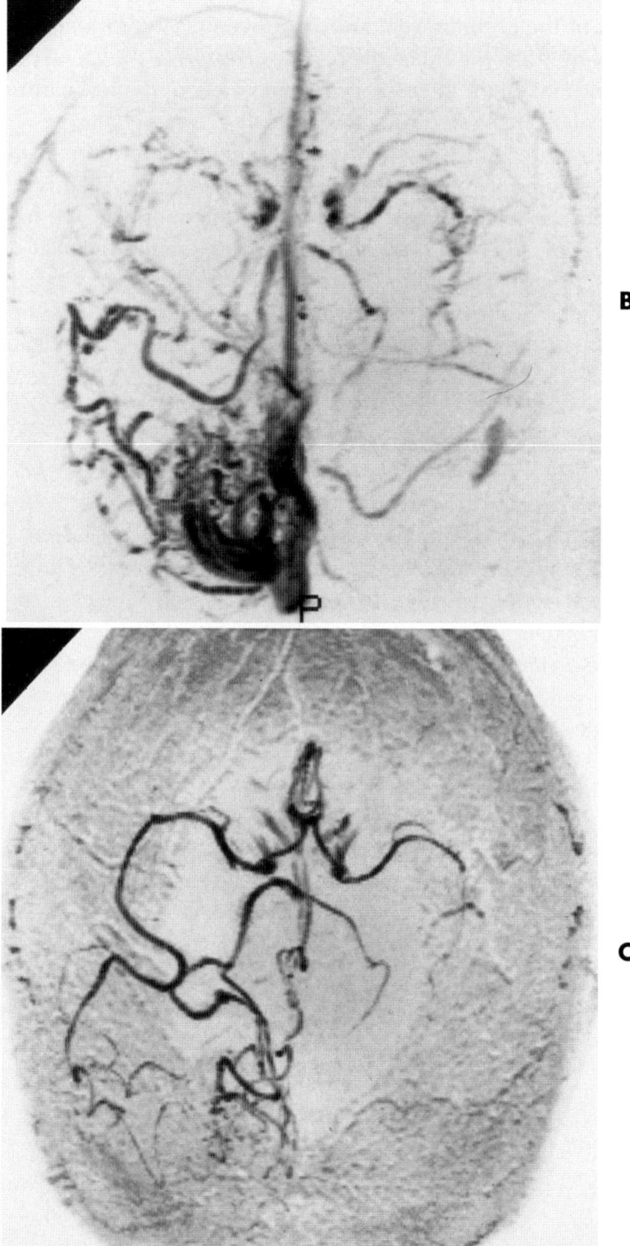


**B**

**C**

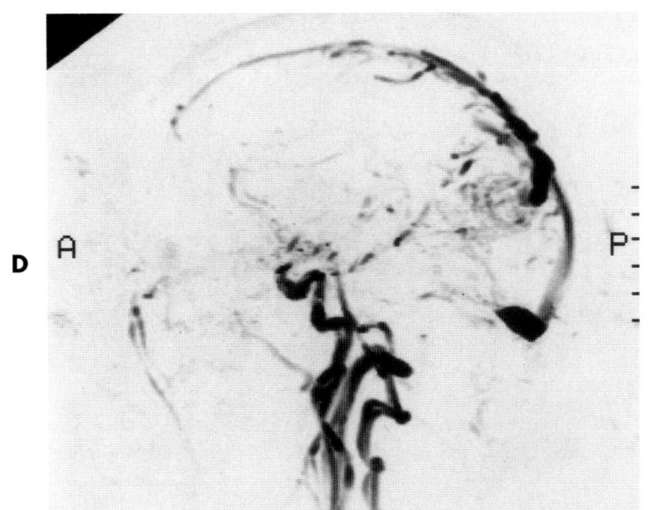


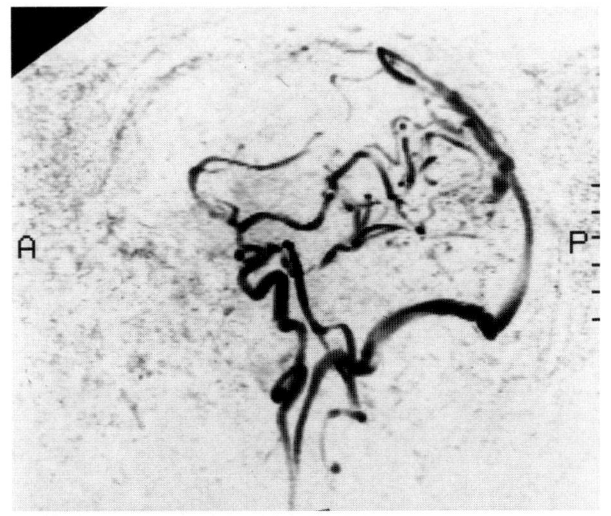


**The right parietal occipital high-flow arteriovenous malformation is evident on the T2-weighted spin-echo image as a well-defined area of serpentine flow voids without edema or hemorrhage (A). The arteriovenous malformation is seen on the base maximum intensity projection view of the three-dimensional phase-contrast MRA (B) using a 15 cm/sec velocity encoding and a three-dimensional time-of-flight sequence (C). Sagittal two-dimensional phase-contrast imaging with velocity encodings of 30 (D) and 200 cm/sec (E) were also performed. (Courtesy John Huston, Mayo Clinic, Rochester, Minn.)**

The time-of-flight and phase-contrast examinations are very complimentary, with the time-of-flight study defining the fast flow-feeding right middle and posterior cerebral arteries and the phase-contrast study demonstrating the nidus and draining veins. The time-of-flight study does not identify the nidus well or the veins, whereas the phase-contrast study does not visualize the feeding high-flow vessels with this velocity encoding. The patient subsequently underwent sagittal two-dimensional phase-contrast imaging with velocity encodings of 30 **(D)** and 200 cm/sec **(E).** The 30 cm/sec encoding depicts the anterior superior sagittal sinus, whereas the higher velocity encoding better depicted the feeding arteries and parts of the draining venous structures consistent with a high-flow state.

Spetzler and Martin have defined a grading system that is widely used for intracranial arteriovenous malformations to predict the operative risks involved. This grading system considers three variables—arteriovenous malformation size, pattern of venous drainage, and eloquence of adjacent brain—and assigns a numerical score to each of these three variables. The size of the arteriovenous malformation is the largest diameter of the nidus on angiography. This is defined as small (smaller than 3 cm = 1 point), medium (3 to 6 cm = 2 points), or large (larger than 6 cm = 3 points). Venous drainage is superficial through the cortical venous system (0 points) or deep through the inferior vena cava and basal veins (1 point). Eloquent regions of the brain are considered as sensory, motor, and language areas; visual cortex; thalamus and hypothalamus; brainstem; internal capsule; cerebellar peduncles; and deep cerebellar nuclei (1 point). The grade of the arteriovenous malformation is therefore the sum of the scores for the three variables, and ranges from grades I to V. Inoperable lesions are considered grade VI. Spetzler and Martin found a good correlation with grade of the arteriovenous malformation and incidence of neurologic complications, with grade V lesions having a 19% incidence of minor deficit and 12% incidence of major deficits.

## REFERENCE

Spetzler RF, Martin NA: A proposed grading system for arteriovenous malformations, *J Neurosurg* 65:476-483, 1986.

## CASE 88
## RIGHT TEMPOROPARIETAL ARTERIOVENOUS MALFORMATION

**History:** 22-year-old with previous subarachnoid hemorrhage.

**Technique #1:** axial three-dimensional phase contrast, 26/9/15, 256 × 128, one excitation, 60 slices, 120-mm slab, velocity encoding of 20 cm/sec, 18-cm field of view, 14 minutes.

**Technique #2:** axial three-dimensional time-of-flight, 40/5/20, 256 × 192, one excitation, 60 slices, 120-mm slab, 18-cm field of view, 7:41.

A

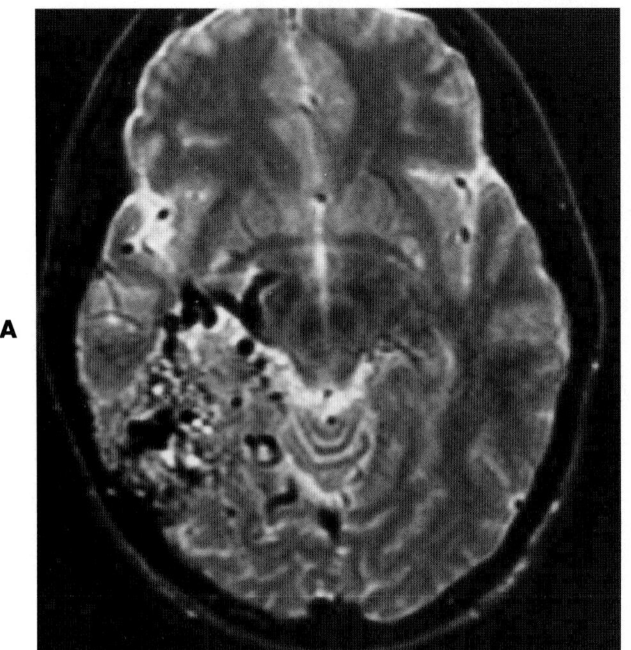

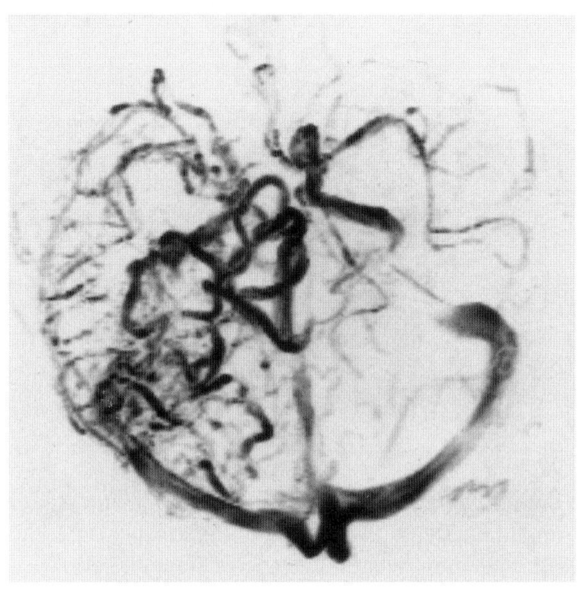

B

C

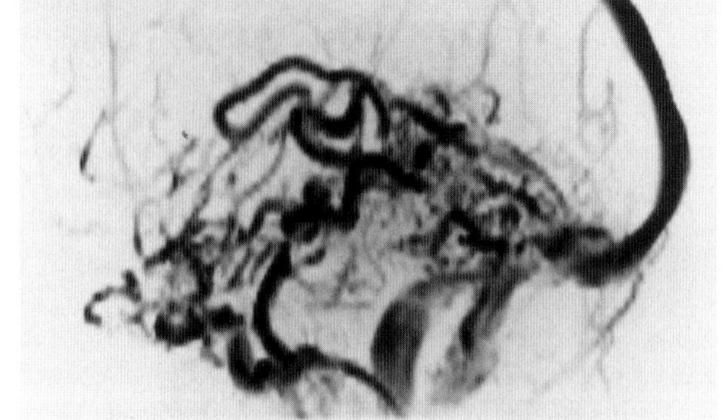

D 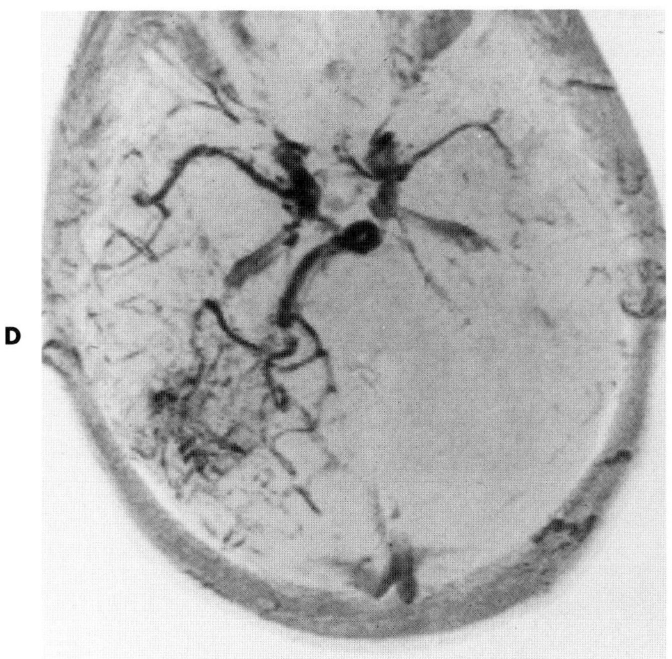

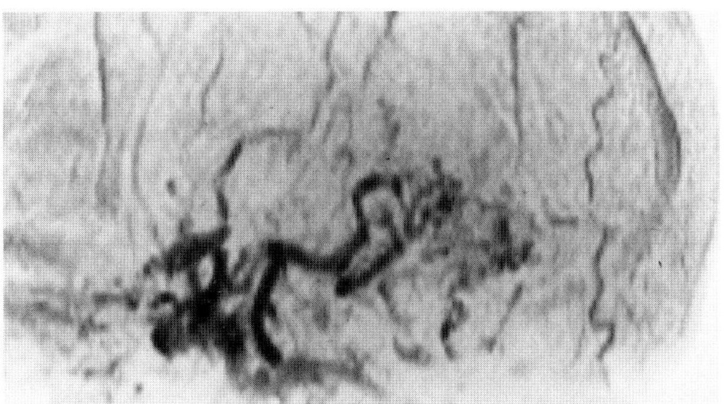 E

**The right temporol parietal arteriovenous malformation is identified on the axial T2-weighted image (A) as a well-defined area of flow voids in the right posterior temporal parietal region. The enlarged basal vein of Rosenthal is easily identified on the T2-weighted images. Base (B) and lateral (C) maximum intensity projection views of the three-dimensional phase-contrast MRA with a 15 cm/sec velocity encoding and the base (D) and lateral (E) maximum intensity projection views of the three-dimensional time-of-flight sequence show complementary information about arterial supply and venous drainage. (Courtesy John Huston, Mayo Clinic, Rochester, Minn.)**

The major feeding arteries off the right posterior cerebral artery are more easily seen on the time-of-flight study, whereas the phase-contrast study defines the nidus and the serpentine, enlarged deep draining veins. There is relatively better visualization of the right middle cerebral artery on the time-of-flight base view **(D)** because of better flow-related enhancement from the arteriovenous malformation.

## CASE 89
## RIGHT TEMPORAL LOBE ARTERIOVENOUS MALFORMATION

**History:** 24-year-old with new onset of left-sided body seizures.

**Technique #1:** enhanced axial three-dimensional phase contrast, 26/9 /15, 256 × 128, one excitation, 60 slices, 120-mm slab, velocity encoding of 20 cm/sec, 18-cm field of view, 14 minutes.

**Technique #2:** enhanced axial three-dimensional time-of-flight, 40/5/20, 256 × 192, one excitation, 60 slices, 120-mm slab, 18-cm field of view, 7:41.

A

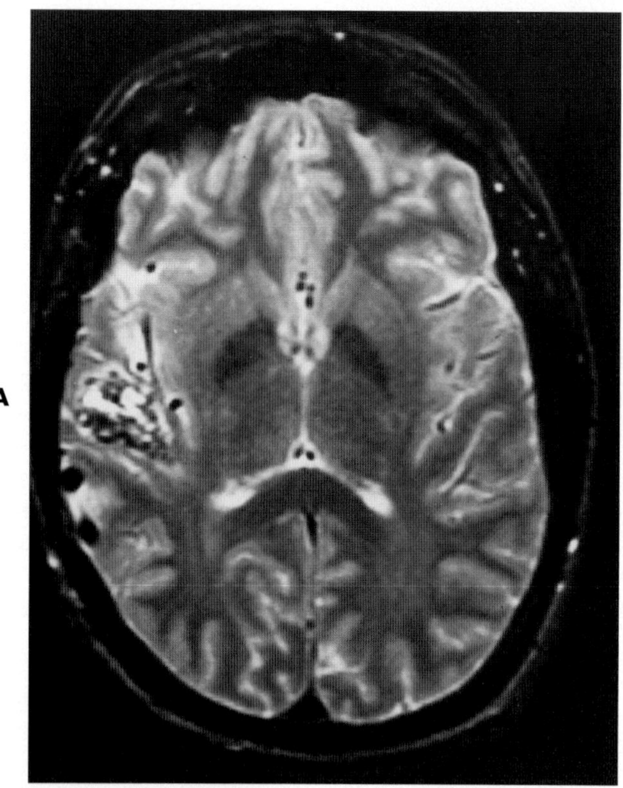

B

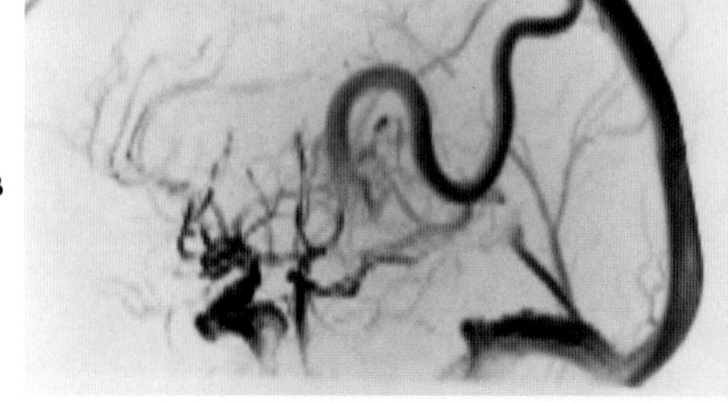

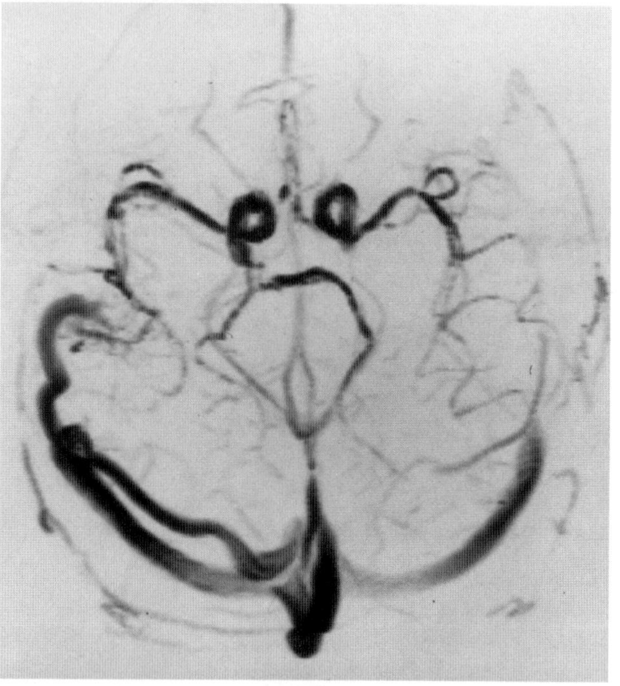

C

D

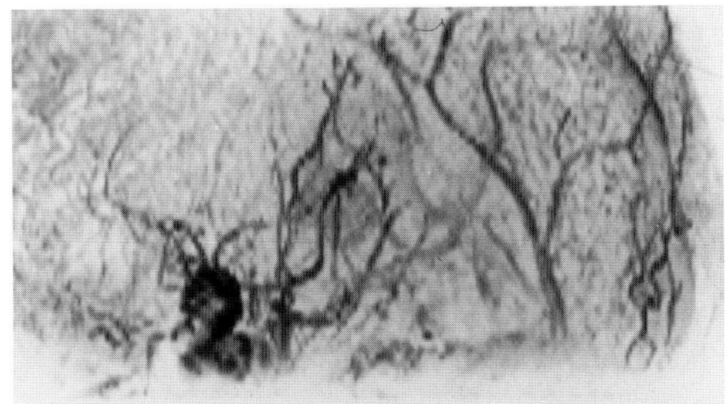

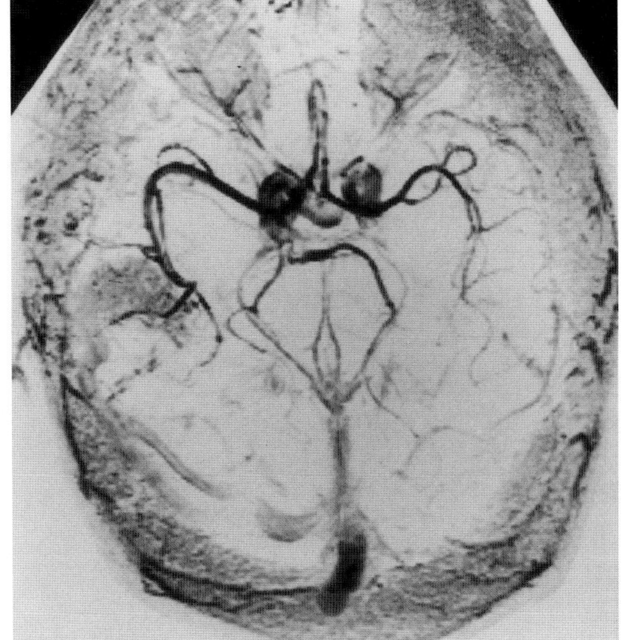

E

F

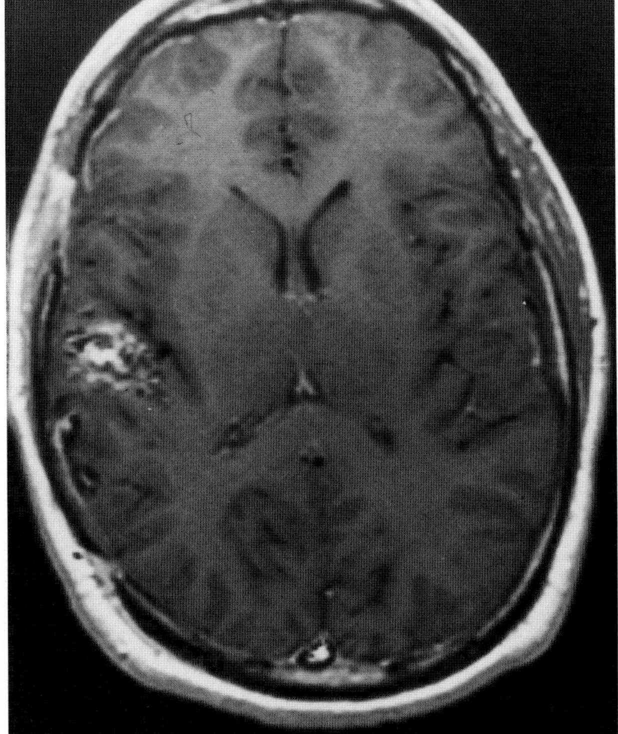

**The right temporal arteriovenous malformation is a well-defined area of heterogeneous flow voids on the T2-weighted spin-echo (A) image. The superficial draining vein going into the superior sagittal sinus is well defined on the lateral (B) and base (C) maximum intensity projection views of the three-dimensional phase-contrast study. The corresponding lateral (D) and base (E) maximum intensity projection views of the contrast-enhanced three-dimensional time-of-flight sequence clearly illustrate the feeding arteries and nidus. (Courtesy John Huston, Mayo Clinic, Rochester, Minn.)**

Three-dimensional time-of-flight and three-dimensional phase-contrast imaging after gadolinium-DPTA shows the relative strengths and weaknesses of the techniques related to arteriovenous malformations. Although the nidus is better visualized after contrast administration on the time-of-flight study because of its enhancement **(F),** the use of gadolinium-DPTA increases the background signal on the three-dimensional time-of-flight sequence.

## CASE 90
## BASAL GANGLIA ARTERIOVENOUS MALFORMATION

**History:** 28-year-old with paresthesias.

**Technique #1:** enhanced axial three-dimensional phase contrast, 26/9/15, 256 × 128, one excitation, 60 slices, 120-mm slab, flow compensation, velocity encoding of 15 cm/sec, 18-cm field of view, 14 minutes.

**Technique #2:** enhanced axial three-dimensional time-of-flight, 40/5/20, 256 × 192, one excitation, 60 slices, 120-mm slab, 18-cm field of view, 7:41.

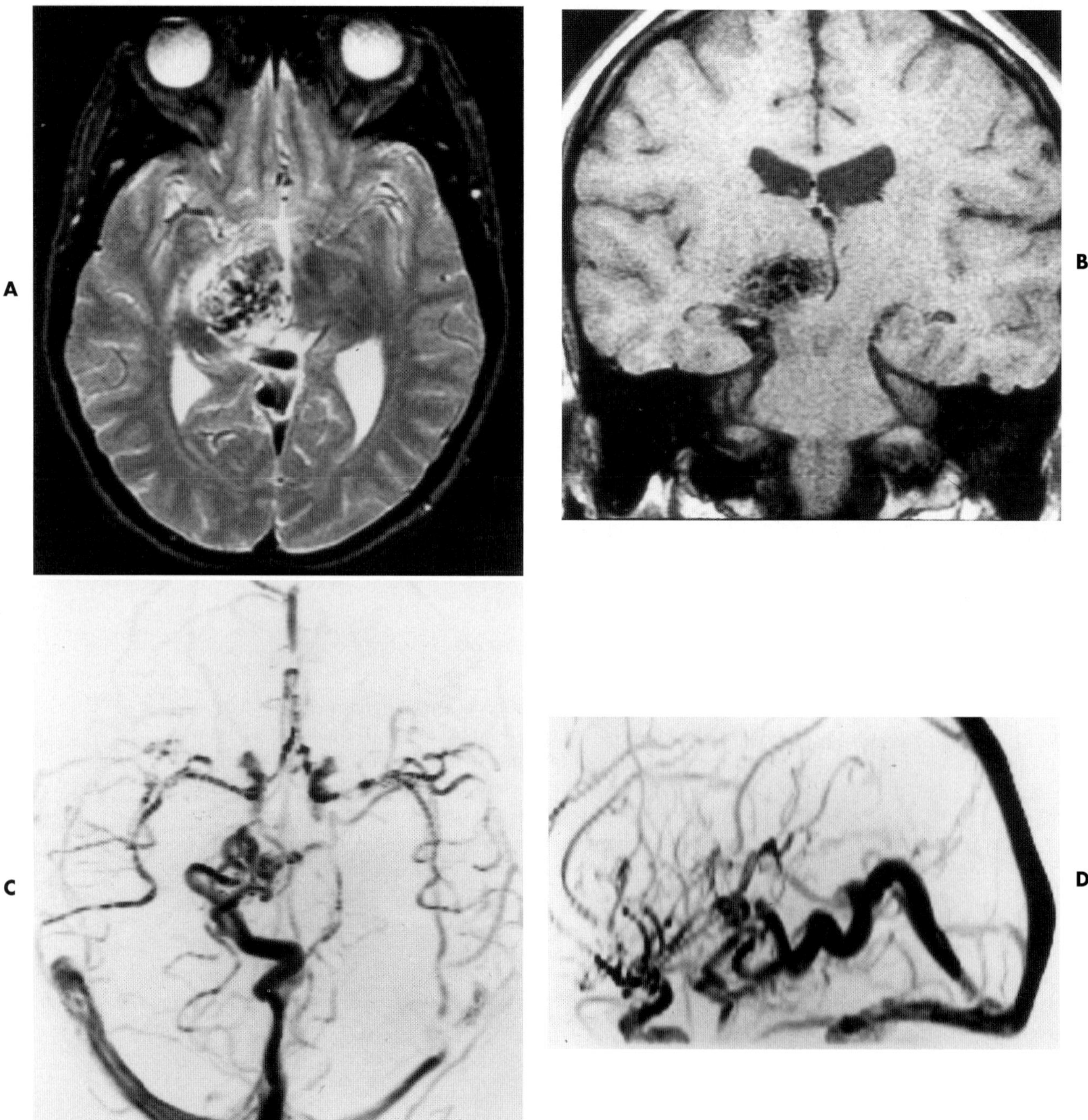

E

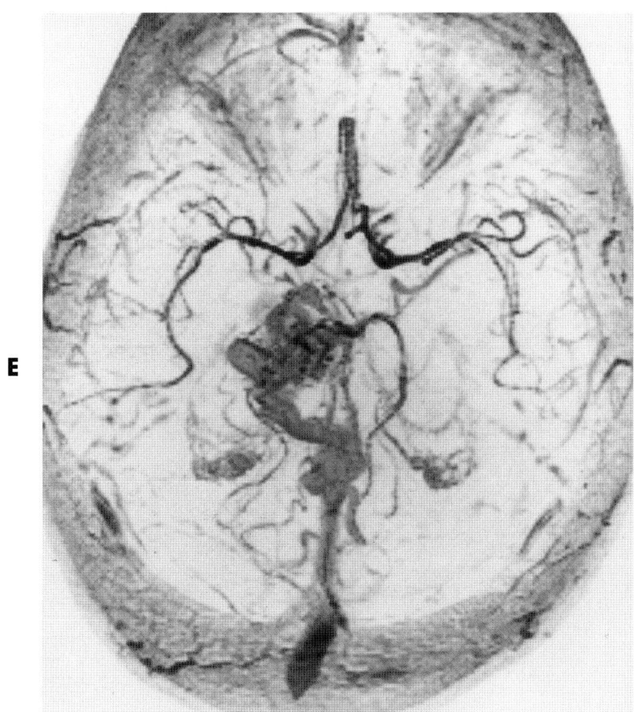

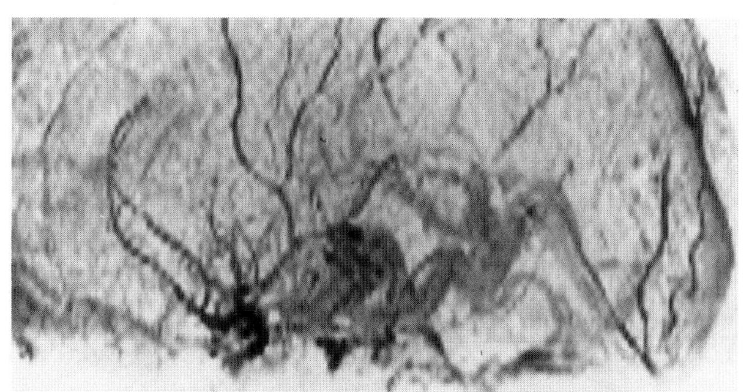

F

**The right basal ganglia and thalamic high flow arteriovenous malformation is seen on T1- (A) and T2-weighted (B) spin-echo MR as multiple punctate areas of flow void, with a slight mass effect on the third ventricle. The arteriovenous malformation is displayed by the base (C) and lateral (D) maximum intensity projection views of a three-dimensional phase-contrast angiogram with a 15 cm/sec velocity encoding and the base (E) and lateral (F) maximum intensity projection views of the three-dimensional time-of-flight MRA. Both three-dimensional sequences were performed after the administration of gadolinium-DPTA. (Courtesy John Huston, Mayo Clinic, Rochester, Minn.)**

There is improved visualization of the draining basal vein into the vein of Galen on the phase-contrast study, in part related to flow saturation on the time-of-flight study but also to the improved background suppression achieved with the phase-contrast technique. This is particularly evident in this case because of the concomitant administration of contrast material, which increases the background signal on the time-of-flight study.

## CASE 91
## PITFALL: DURAL FISTULA NOT VISUALIZED ON TIME-OF-FLIGHT MRA

**History:** 32-year-old with prior cerebellar hemorrhage.

**Technique:** axial volume, three-dimensional time-of-flight, 45/7/20 degrees, 256 × 256, 64 slices, 60-mm slab, 14-cm field of view, 12:20.

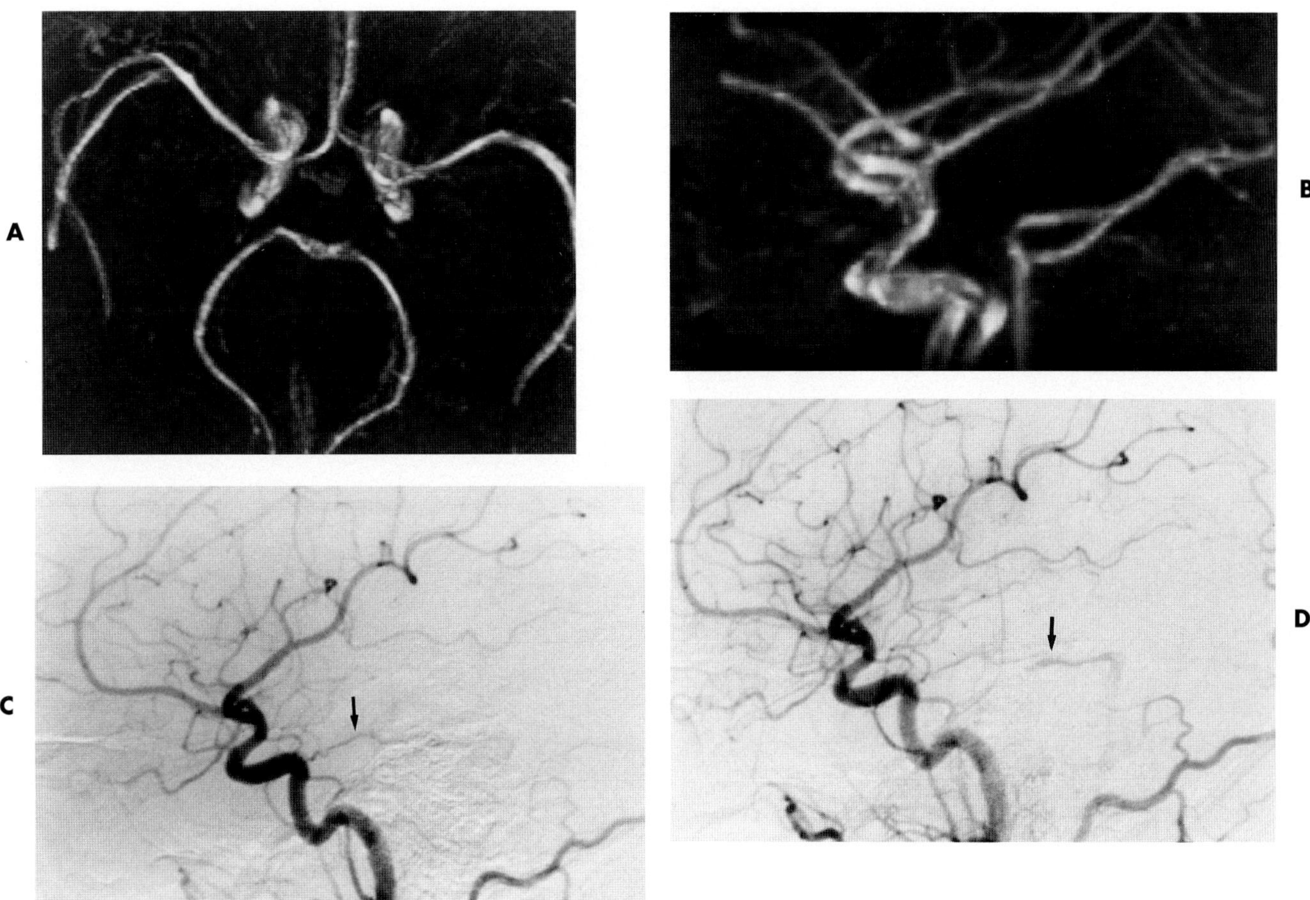


**Base (A) and lateral (B) views from the maximum intensity projection demonstrate a normal-appearing internal carotid and posterior circulation. Conventional left common carotid angiographic injection (C and D) demonstrates normal-appearing carotid and anterior and middle cerebral circulations. However, there is a moderately enlarged meningohypophyseal artery off the internal carotid artery *(arrow)*, which is part of a small tentorial dural fistula with a prominent draining vein *(arrow* on D).**

This case points out the relative insensitivity of three-dimensional time-of-flight techniques to slow flow. Slow flow receives multiple radiofrequency pulses and thus becomes saturated and is not visible on the three-dimensional time-of-flight MRA. In this instance, the dural fistula was an incidental finding and not thought to cause the patient's clinical symptomatology.

## CASE 92
## DURAL CAROTID CAVERNOUS FISTULA

**History:** 27-year-old with painful right-sided ophthalmoplegia.

**Technique:** axial volume; three-dimensional time-of-flight; 45/7/20 degrees; 256 × 256; 64 slices; 60-mm slab; magnetization transfer background suppression; tilted, optimized nonsaturating excitation radiofrequency pulse; 14-cm field of view; 12:20.

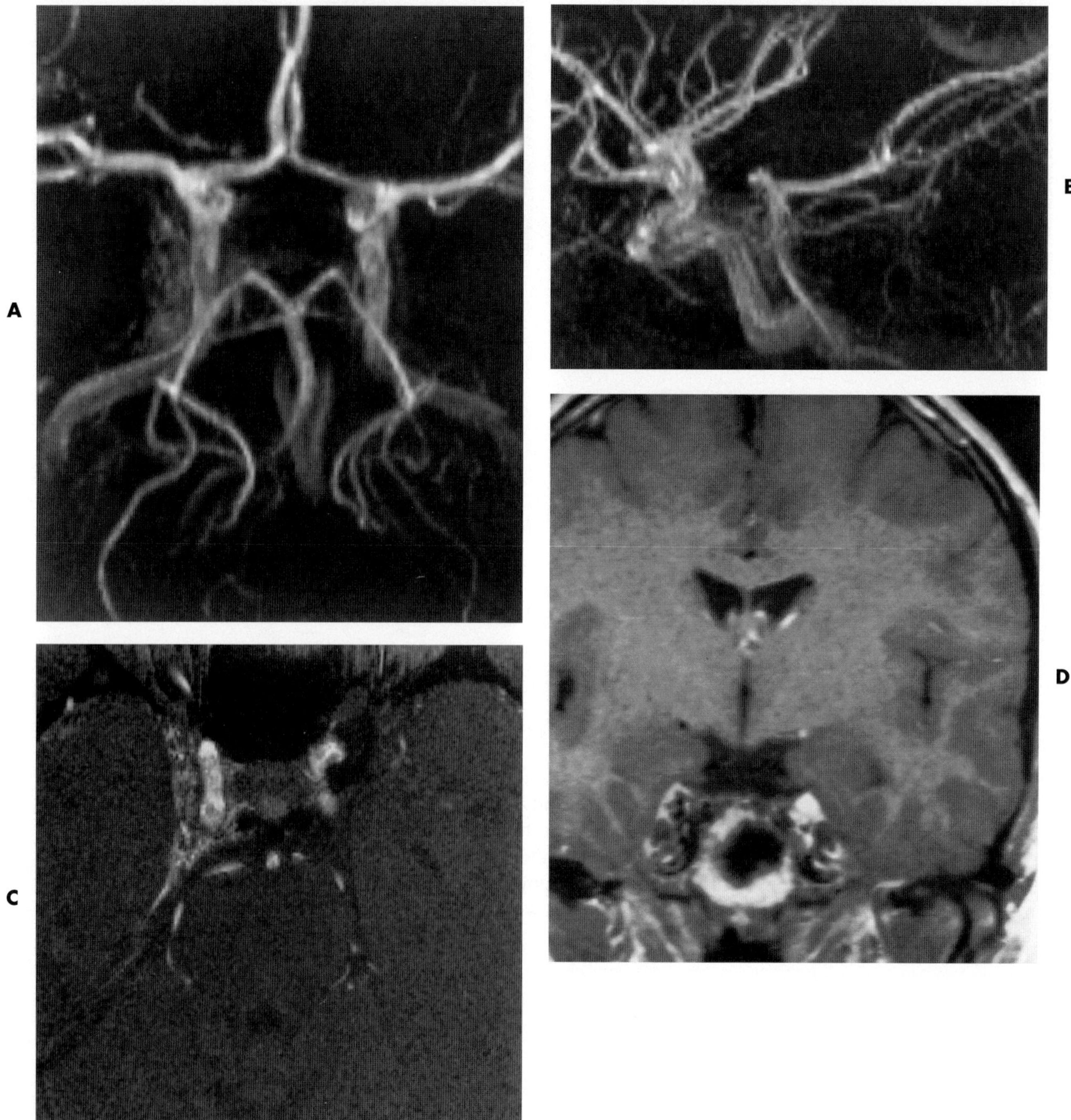

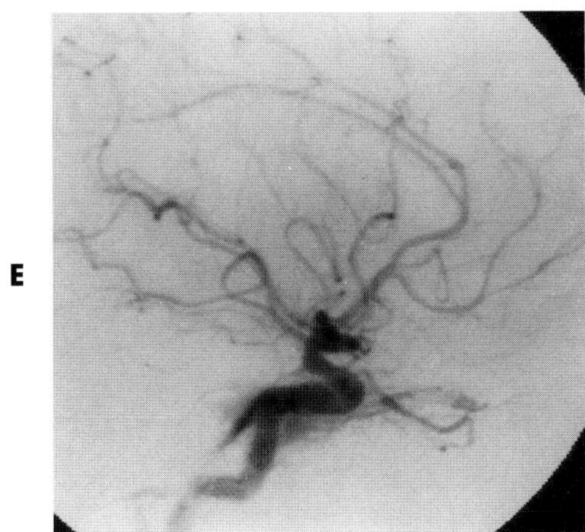
E

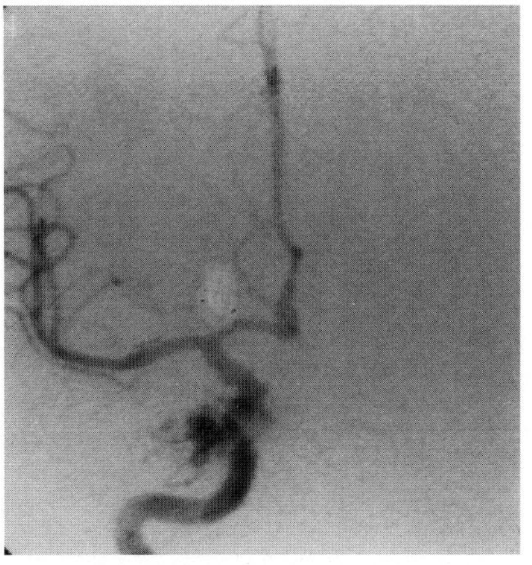
F

**Base (A) and lateral (B) maximum intensity projection views demonstrate an ill-defined "cloud" of increased signal intensity around the distal right internal carotid artery and cavernous carotid artery. Evaluation of the individual MRA slice (C) demonstrates marked asymmetry between the cavernous sinuses. Multiple punctate and serpentine areas of increased signal intensity are seen within the right cavernous sinus and extending along the course of the greater petrosal vein. The left cavernous sinus is normal. The findings are consistent with a dural fistula involving the cavernous sinus. Coronal T1-weighted image with contrast material (D) shows an enlarged right cavernous sinus with abnormally increased punctate flow void within it. Conventional lateral (E) and anteroposterior (F) angiographic views of the right internal carotid artery injection demonstrates the dural cavernous carotid fistula, which drains into the cavernous sinus and petrosal veins. Two dimensional time-of-flight or phase-contrast angiography would also be useful for evaluation of slow flow carotid cavernous fistula.**

Barrow et al classified spontaneous carotid cavernous fistulae into one of four angiographic patterns. Type A are direct shunts between internal carotid artery and cavernous sinus. Types B through C are dural shunts, as in this case. Type B fistulae are fed by the meningeal branches of the internal carotid artery. Type C fistulae are shunts between the meningeal branches of the external carotid. Type D fistulae are shunts from both internal and external carotid arteries. Traumatic carotid cavernous fistulae are nearly always type A, a high-flow direct communication between the internal carotid artery and cavernous sinus. A nontraumatic spontaneous type A fistula could occur with rupture of a intracavernous carotid aneurysm into the cavernous sinus. The patterns of Type B through D fistulae are generally slow flow and idiopathic in nature. Typically, they occur in middle-aged women with glaucoma, proptosis, or injected sclera. Other signs that may be visible on MRA or MR imaging include exophthalmos, enlarged ocular muscles, and an enlarged superior ophthalmic vein. The etiology of these spontaneous dural carotid cavernous fistulae is unknown, with theories ranging from rupture of fragile meningeal branches of the carotid siphon crossing the cavernous sinus to venous thrombosis. Dural carotid cavernous fistulae have a propensity for spontaneous resolution, ranging from 10% to 60%, and may even improve after conventional angiography or air travel. Debrun et al applied the Barrow classification to 132 carotid cavernous fistulae that they treated. They had 100 cases of type A, 28 cases of type D, 4 cases of type C, and no cases of type B. Type D is the most difficult to treat by endovascular therapy because of the multiple feeders involved from one or both of the internal and external carotids.

Hirabuki et al used two-dimensional time-of-flight MRA and spin-echo imaging to follow-up on six patients being treatment for carotid cavernous fistulae. Spin-echo imaging shows resolution of the flow voids, and two-dimensional time-of-flight imaging shows lack of signal from the involved cavernous sinus with successful occlusion.

## REFERENCES


Barrow DL, Spector RH, Braun IF et al: Classification and treatment of spontaneous carotid cavernous sinus fistulas, *J Neurosurg* 62:248-256, 1985.

Newton TH, Hoyt WF: Dural arteriovenous shunts in the region of the cavernous sinus, *Neuroradiology* 1:71-81, 1970.

Slusher MM, Lennington BR, Weaver RG et al: Ophthalmic findings in dural arteriovenous shunts. *Ophthalmology* 86:720-731, 1979.

Debrun GM, Vinuela F, Fox AJ et al: Indications for treatment and classification of 132 carotid-cavernous fistulas, *Neurosurgery* 22(2):285-289, 1988.

Hirabuki N, Fujita N, Hashimoto T et al: Follow-up MRI in dural arteriovenous malformations involving the cavernous sinus: emphasis on detection of venous thrombosis, *Neuroradiology* 34:423-427, 1992.

# CASE 93
# DURAL FISTULA

**History:** 39-year-old being evaluated for tinnitus.

**Technique:** axial volume, three-dimensional time-of-flight, 40/7/15, 256 × 192, 128 slices, 120-mm slab, 25-cm field of view, 16:30.

A

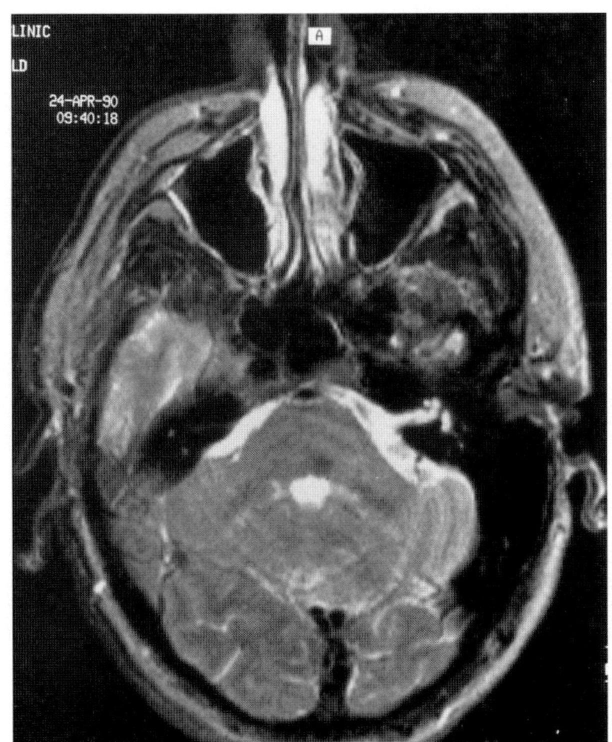


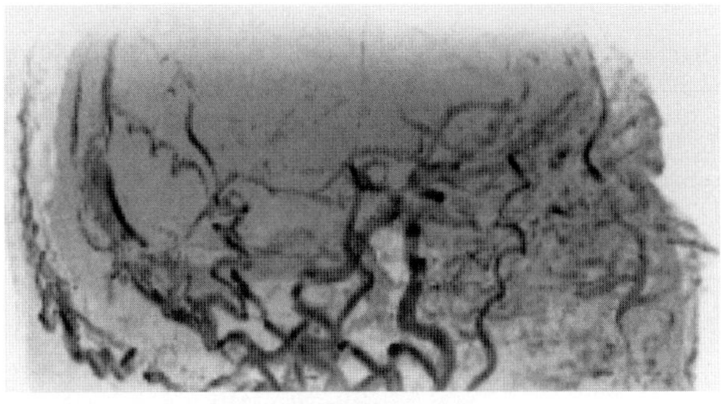

B

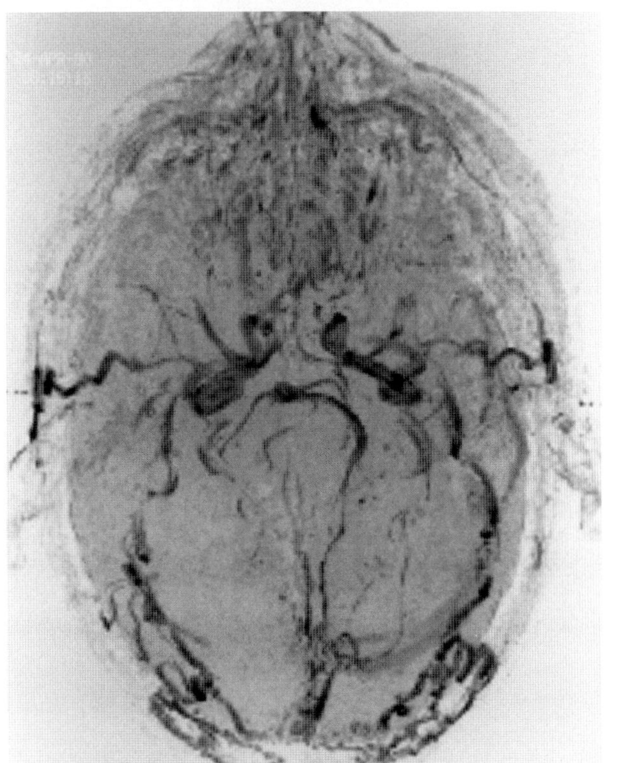

C

**Axial T2-weighted image (A) of the brain is normal. However, the lateral (B) and base (C) maximum intensity projection views of the time-of-flight MRAs are quite dramatic and demonstrate markedly and abnormally enlarged multiple branches of the external carotid arteries bilaterally, which mainly extend over the posterior aspect of the subcutaneous tissues. This enlargement of multiple superficial vessels is consistent with a dural fistula, the nidus of which is not identified specifically on the MRA study. Conventional angiography is necessary to precisely delineate the feeding vessels and their locations.**

## REFERENCES

Chen JC, Tsuruda JS, Halbach VV: Suspected dural arteriovenous fistulas: results with screening MR angiography in seven patients, *Radiology* 183(1):265-271, 1992.

De Marco JK, Dillon WP, Halbach VV et al: Dural arteriovenous fistulas: evaluation with MR imaging, *Radiology* 175:193, 1990.

## CASE 94
## DURAL FISTULA

**History:** 70-year-old with pulsatile tinnitus that has become worse over the previous 3 months.

**Technique:** axial volume, three-dimensional time-of-flight, 40/7/20 degrees, 256 × 256, 64 slices, 60-mm slab, 14-cm field of view, 12:20.

A

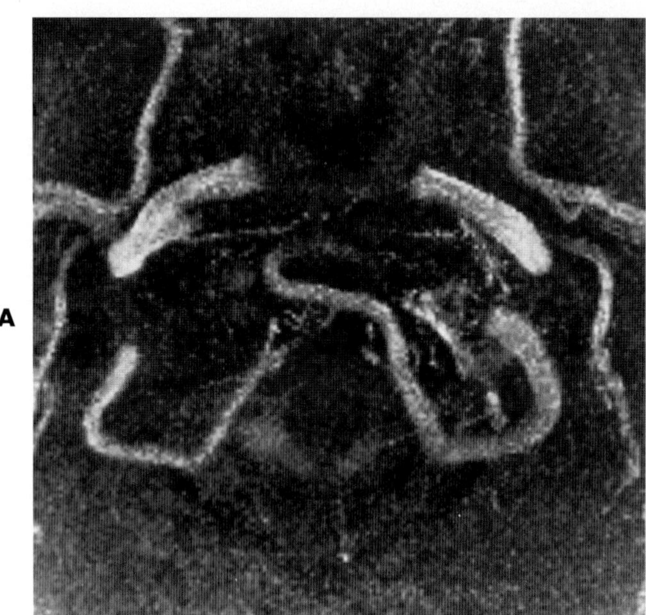

B

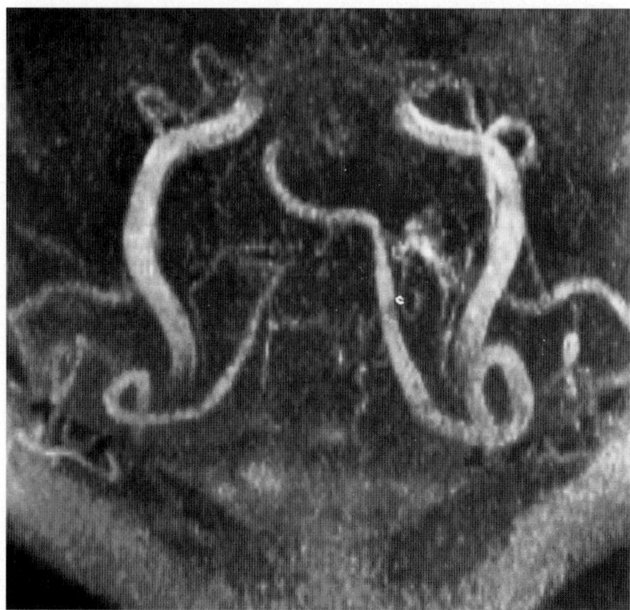

C

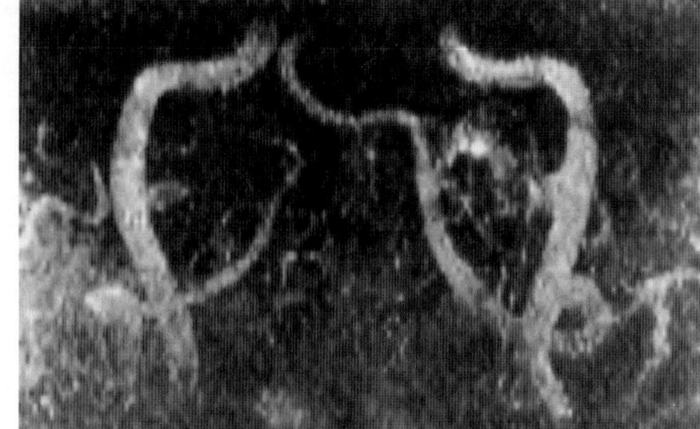

D

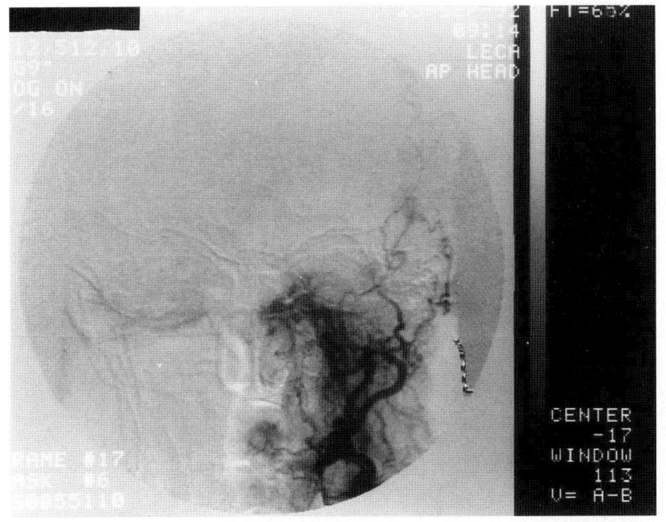


E

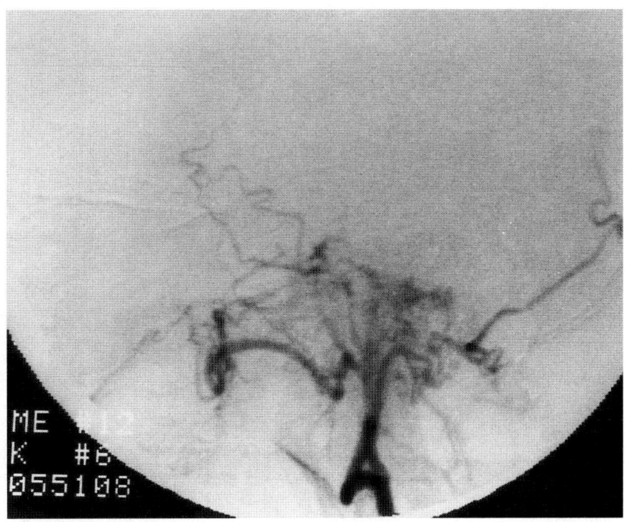


**Two base views (A and B) and an anteroposterior view (C) of the maximum intensity projection centered around the skull base demonstrate an abnormal tangle of signal intensity just lateral to the distal left vertebral artery. There is good overall signal intensity within the left vertebral artery. The right vertebral artery is small and appears to end in a posterior inferior cerebellar artery. The visualized portions of the carotid are normal. Abnormal tangle is consistent with a vascular malformation around the skull base. Conventional anteroposterior (D) and lateral (E) angiographic views of the left external carotid injection demonstrate that the dural fistula is fed not by the left vertebral artery as would be surmised from the MRA, but by multiple small branches of the external carotid artery (occipital and ascending pharyngeal arteries). The number of feeding vessels to these dural malformations are generally underestimated by MRA, and in this case the overall source of the malformation cannot be definitely determined.**

## CASE 95
## DURAL FISTULA OF THE OPHTHALMIC ARTERY

**History:** 28-year-old with left eye pain.

**Technique:** axial volume, three-dimensional time-of-flight, 45/8/20, 256 × 128, 0.9-mm slice thickness, 25-cm field of view, 6.4 minutes.

A

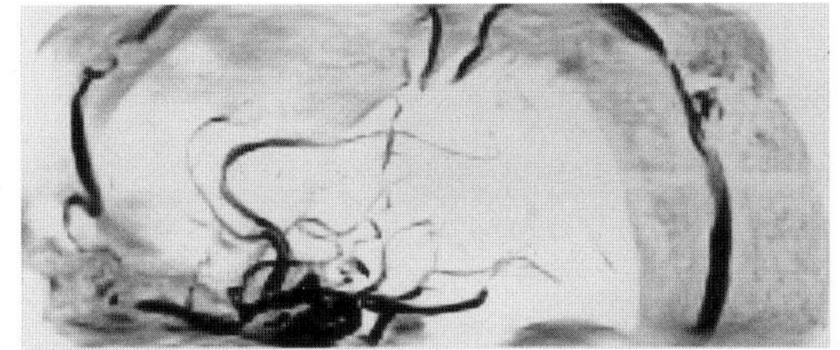

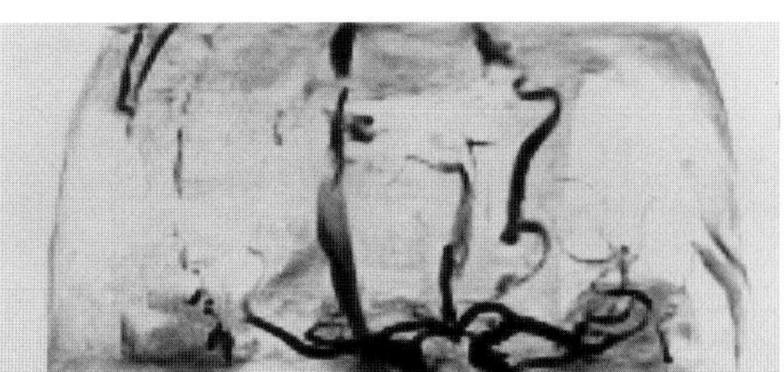

B

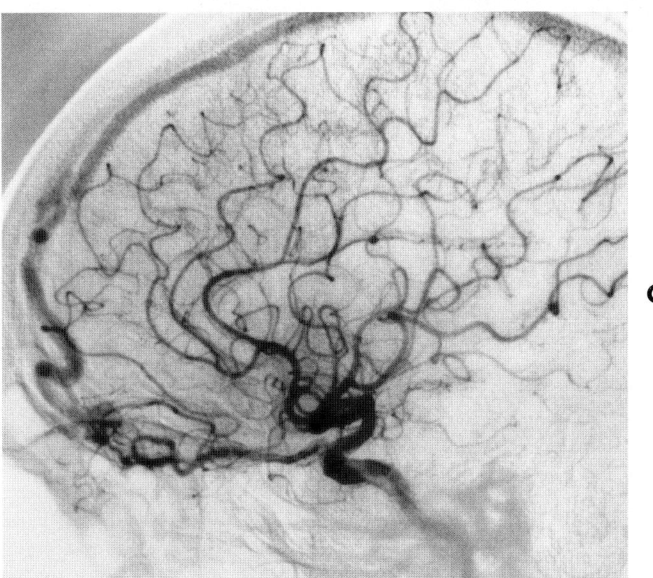

C

**Lateral (A) and oblique (B) maximum intensity projection views of the three-dimensional time-of-flight MRA demonstrate a large serpentine vessel over the anterior convexity in the midline in contiguity with an enlarged ophthalmic artery on the left. Selective injection of the left internal carotid artery on the conventional angiogram (C) shows a dural fistula arising off the enlarged left ophthalamic artery, with shunting of blood into the superior sagittal sinus. (Courtesy John Sherman.)**

## CASE 96
## PETROSAL SINUS FISTULA

**History:** 68-year-old with sudden onset of aphasia.

**Technique:** axial volume; three-dimensional time-of-flight; 45/7/20; 192 × 256; 64 slices; 80-mm slab; magnetization transfer background suppression; tilted, optimized nonsaturating excitation radiofrequency pulse; 14-cm field of view; 9:15.

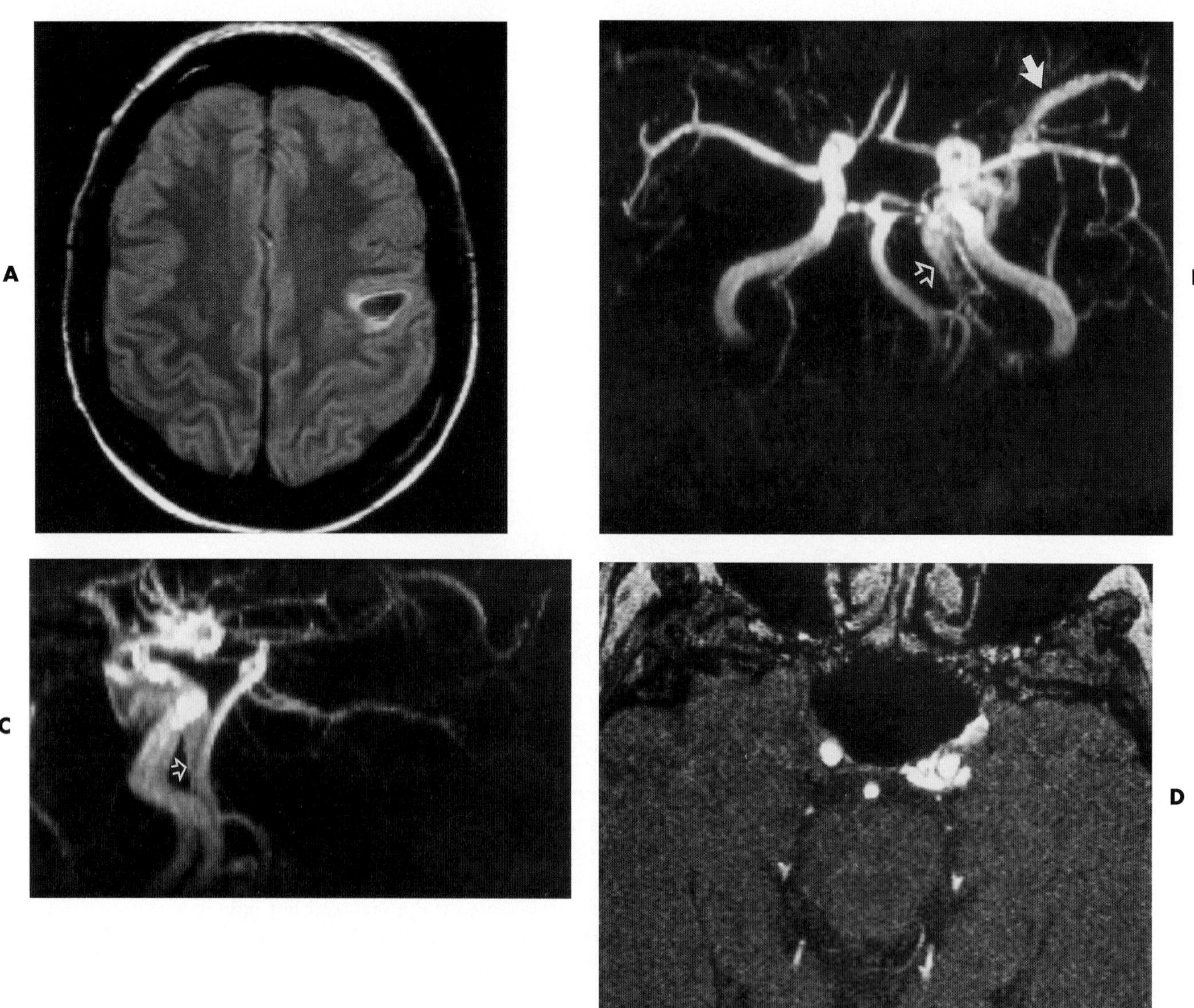

E

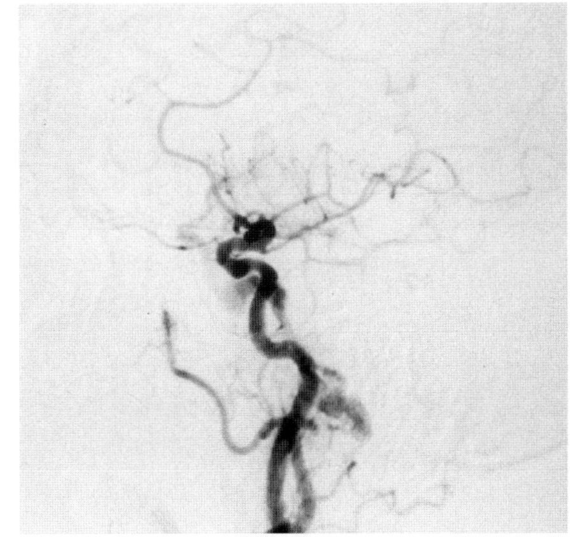

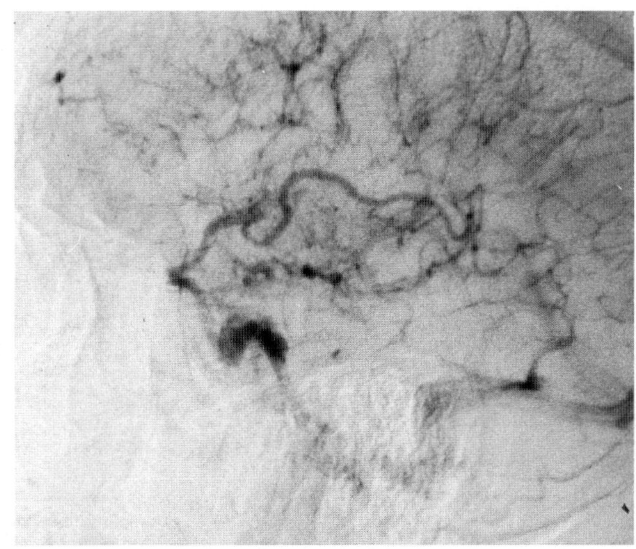

F

**Axial spin density image shows a small parenchymal hemorrhage in the left posterior frontal lobe (A). Water's (B) and lateral (C) maximum intensity projection views of the MRA show increased signal around the inferior cavernous and petrous carotid arteries, with marked enlargement of the left sphenoparietal sinus *(arrow)* and the inferior petrosal sinus (open arrow). Individual slice through the level of the cavernous sinus (D) shows increased signal within the sinus consistent with a dural fistula. Lateral views (E and F) of the conventional angiogram in early and late phases show the dural fistula involving the petrous internal carotid as well as the venous drainage into the petrosal and sphenoparietal sinuses. The parenchymal hemorrhage was presumed secondary to venous hypertension from the fistula.**

# CASE 97
# DURAL FISTULA

**History:** 40-year-old with increasing lump size on the top of the head.

**Technique:** axial volume, three-dimensional time-of-flight, 45/7/15, 192 × 256, 60 slices, 120-mm slab, 20-cm field of view, 9:16.

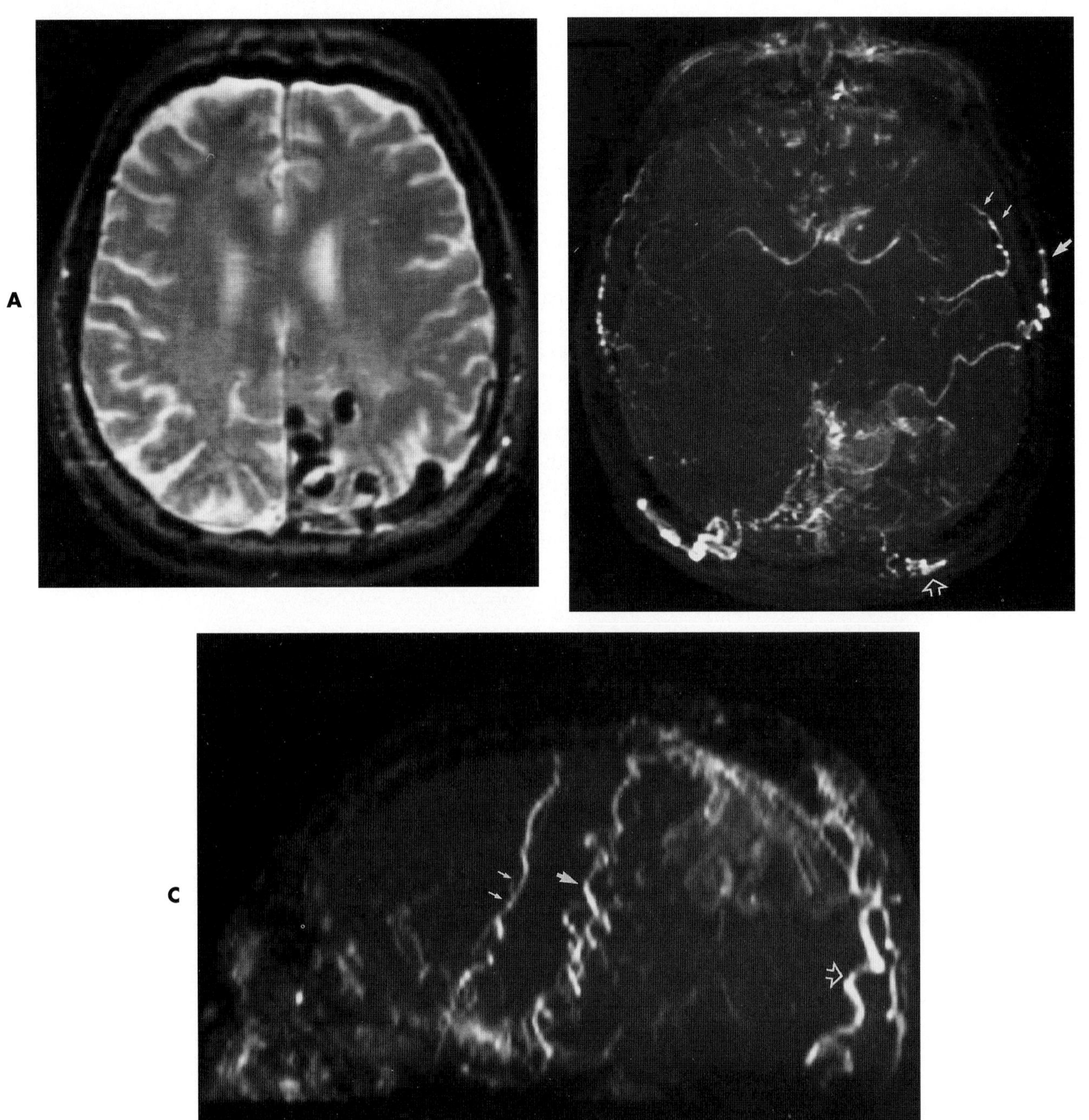

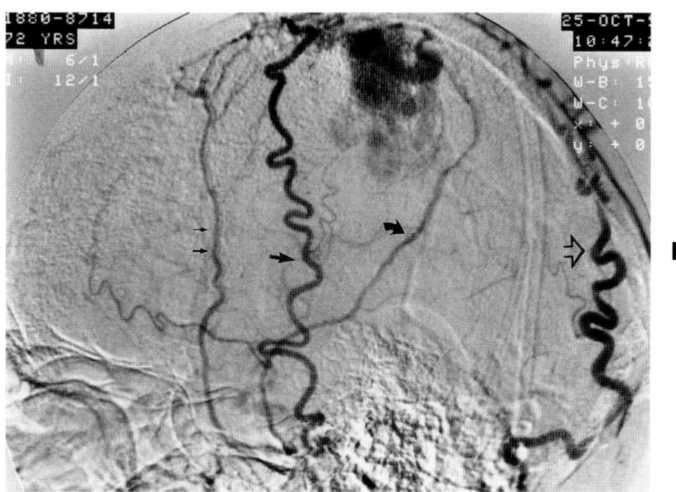


Axial T2-weighted image of the brain (A) shows multiple large flow voids within the left parietal lobe without mass effect or edema and consistent with an arteriovenous malformation. Base (B) and lateral (C) maximum intensity projection views of the three-dimensional time-of-flight MRA show multiple feeding vessels converging of the skull apex, with slight visualization of the dilated draining veins. The feeding vessels can be identified on the MRA as meningeal branches *(small arrows)* as well as the superficial temporal arteries *(arrow)* and occipital arteries *(open arrow)*. Lateral conventional angiographic view of the left external carotid injection (D) shows the feeding meningeal, superficial temporal, and occipital vessels. More feeding vessels are identified on the conventional angiographic view than are seen on the MRA. In particular, there is a large posterior branch of the middle meningeal artery *(curved arrow)* that is not seen on the MRA.

# CHAPTER 6

# Intracranial Stenosis and Occlusion

Intracranial arterial occlusions may be classified as thrombotic (primary occlusions) or embolic strokes, whereas interruptions of the smaller penetrating arteries fall under the category of lacunar infarction. Thrombotic infarction frequently occurs during sleep or may be preceded by transient ischemic symptoms, with a stuttering onset and gradual evolution. Embolic infarction typically occurs with an apoplectic onset of symptoms commonly traced to the middle cerebral artery distribution. MRA techniques are quite capable of demonstrating the major intracranial vessels. However, visualization of the normal lenticulostriate and thalamoperforating vessels is currently beyond the spatial resolution of even the most sophisticated MRA techniques. The inherent technical limitations of the technique as well as specific machine and manufacturer differences must always be kept in mind when using MRA for the evaluation of ischemic disease.

For the most part, radiologists have relied on indirect signs on spin-echo imaging to diagnose vasoocclusive disease. These include parenchymal changes suggesting an infarct or signal intensity changes within a vessel suggesting slow flow, occlusion, or thrombosis.[1,2] In practice, patients with suspected cerebrovascular occlusive disease are often evaluated with multiple modalities to assess the integrity of vascular structures and the brain parenchyma. Because MRA can directly visualize vascular occlusions and large vessel stenoses, it can be used to complement the spin-echo examination and provide a vascular and parenchymal assessment at the same sitting; it may obviate the need for invasive angiography or direct, more aggressive interventional therapies.

The accuracy of MRA for large vessel occlusive disease has been shown in pediatric and adult populations.[3-5] MRA has been used to monitor infants who had previously undergone extracorporeal membrane oxygenation for life-threatening respiratory failure. In these infants, the right common carotid artery and internal jugular vein had been interrupted. MRA was able to confirm the occlusion and document patency of the right internal carotid artery proximal to the ophthalmic artery origin in 9 of 16 patients. Good cross-filling was demonstrated intracranially via the circle of Willis in all but 1 infant, as evidenced by symmetric flow to the anterior circulation.

Children with sickle cell disease are known to have a higher incidence of thrombotic cerebral infarcts as a result of stenosis and/or occlusion of the internal carotid arteries.[6-8] MRA is able to identify large vessel occlusive disease. This ability may translate into a useful clinical screening test for patients at high risk. The detection of large vessel occlusive disease in this population would mandate a change in therapy: These patients might profit from prophylactic exchange transfusions.[9-11]

The ability to identify large vessel disease can also be extended to the adult population. The brain parenchyma and intracranial circulation can be monitored by MR in patients after Hunterian occlusion of an internal carotid artery or external carotid–internal carotid artery bypass procedure. MRA findings can alert the clinician to the nature and location of the occlusive disease, and a more definitive conventional angiographic study may then be performed to delineate the full extent of pathology before the initiation of medical or surgical treatment. A negative study might obviate the need for angiography. This rationale is appropriate for evaluating patients suspected of posterior fossa ischemia in whom the risk of angiography is increased.

In the preliminary studies that reported using a three-dimensional time-of-flight technique, it was possible to detect intracranial stenoses, although this was limited to relatively large vessels such as the juxtasellar and supraclinoid internal carotid artery or the horizontal middle cerebral artery.[3,4] This limitation is in part attributable to the spatial resolution of these sequences and the small vessel caliber of the cerebral vasculature. Flow rates also impose restrictions because only the larger arteries of the circle of Willis have flow rapid enough to cause the flow-related enhancement to reliably "opacify" the vessel distal to the stenosis. This limitation is not shared by phase-contrast techniques. Also, just as in cases of extracerebral carotid artery stenoses, more severe intracranial stenoses tend to be exaggerated because of higher-order motion terms at and immediately distal to the stenoses. Reviewing individual three-dimensional slices for flow voids helps distinguish true stenoses from the commonly seen filling defects or variations of signal intensity across the lumen in normal vessels from turbulence, tortuosity, or adjacent paranasal sinuses. The use of very short echo times and small voxels reduces this dephasing related to motion and local field inhomogeneities. As techniques have improved, the confidence and ability to see more peripheral stenoses have likewise increased. Rother et al[12] evaluated time-of-flight MRA for vertebrobasilar ischemia in 41 patients. MRA correctly identified all occlusions and stenoses seen on conventional intraarterial angiography (sensitivity of 97% and specificity of 98.9%). However, these authors found the degree of stenosis difficult to evaluate by MRA because of the problem of collateral flow, as might occur with a midbasilar occlusion with retrograde flow to the distal basilar artery via the posterior communicating artery. Heiserman et al[13] assessed MRA in the characterization of intracranial occlusion and stenosis in 29 patients. They correctly graded 97% of the normal vessels and 100% of the occlusions compared with grading using conventional angiography. Both overestimation and underestimation of stenoses occurred with MRA compared with estimation using conventional angiography. They concluded that MRA allows a more complete evaluation of the patient with symptoms of ischemia when coupled with MR imaging.

Cross-filling between vascular territories can have a significant impact on the initial clinical presentation and subsequent therapeutic decisions. MRA studies have been designed in non-selective and selective fashions to assess the degree of intracranial collateral flow.[3,14] In a patient with an acute occlusion of the internal carotid artery, MRA is able to confirm the lack of opacification of the involved vessel and the cross-filling from the posterior circulation and contralateral anterior circulation. At the same time, the corresponding spin-echo images can evaluate the brain parenchyma for infarction distal to the occlusion. The relative contributions from the other vascular territories can be evaluated through the use of saturation pulses to eliminate the inflow from any one or any combination of the remaining feeding vessels.[14] This can be important not only for the right-to-left flow of the anterior circulation, but also for the anterior-to-posterior circulation collateral flow for the basilar artery with occlusion. Phase images can also be examined to document flow rates and direction in the arterial segments providing collateral flow (e.g., A1 segment of the ipsilateral anterior cerebral artery in a patient with an occluded internal carotid artery).

Time-of-flight or phase-contrast techniques may be used to evaluate posterior fossa atherosclerotic disease. Care must be taken in interpretation of three-dimensional time-of-flight MRA because of the relatively slow flow seen in most of these lesions (e.g., dolichoectasia, dissection, incomplete thrombosis).[15,16] Although these lesions can frequently be discovered on spin-echo images, the appearance may be confusing at times, and additional confirmation of inflow in these vascular segments using time-of-flight techniques can be quite helpful.[2] With partial or complete thrombosis, the presence of methemoglobin may result in false-negative time-of-flight studies (the high intensity of methemoglobin is similar to that of flow-related enhancement). Using a phase-contrast MRA technique or reconstructing the phase images from the original dataset avoids this pitfall.

## REFERENCES

1. Brant-Zawadski M: Routine MR imaging of the internal carotid artery siphon: angiographic correlation with cervical carotid lesions, *AJNR* 11:467-471, 1990.
2. Schwaighofer BW, Klein MV, Lyden PD, Hesselink JR: MR imaging of vertebrobasilar vascular disease, *JCAT* 14:895-904, 1990.
3. Wiznitzer M, Ruggieri PM, Masaryk TJ et al: Diagnosis of cerebrovascular disease in sickle cell anemia by magnetic resonance angiography, *J Pediatr* 117:551-555, 1990.
4. Wiznitzer M, Masaryk TJ: Cerebrovascular abnormalities in pediatric stroke: diagnosis using magnetic resonance angiography, *Ann Neurol* 26:440-441 (abstract), 1989.
5. Lewin JS, Masaryk TJ, Modic MT et al: Extracorporeal membrane oxygenation in infants: angiography and parenchymal evaluation of the brain with MR imaging, *Radiology* 173:361-365, 1989.
6. Sydenstricker VP, Mulherin WA, Houseal RW: Sickle cell anemia, *Am J Dis Child* 26:143-154, 1923.
7. Bridgers WH: Cerebrovascular disease accompanying sickle cell anemia, *Am J Pathol* 15:353-361, 1939.
8. Rothman SM, Fulling KH, Nelson SJ: Sickle cell anemia and central nervous system infarction: a neuropathological study, *Ann Neurol* 20:346-350, 1986.
9. Lusher JN, Haghight M, Khalifa AS: A prophylactic transfusion program for children with sickle cell anemia complicated by CNS infarction, *Am J Hematol* 1:265-273, 1976.
10. Schmalzer E, Chien S, Brown AK: Transfusion therapy in sickle cell disease, *Am J Pediatr Hematol Oncol* 4:395-406, 1982.
11. Bogousslavsky U, Regli R: Borderzone infarctions distal to internal carotid artery disease, *Ann Neurol* 20:346-350, 1986.
12. Rother J, Wentz K, Rautenberg W et al: Magnetic resonance angiography in vertebrobasilar ischemia, *Stroke* 24(9):1310-1315, 1993.
13. Heiserman JE, Drayer BP, Keller PJ, Fram EK: Intracranial vascular stenosis and occlusion: evaluation with three-dimensional time-of-flight MRA, *Radiology* 185:667-673, 1992.
14. Edelman RR, Mattle HP, O'Reilly GV et al: Magnetic resonance imaging of flow dynamics in the circle of Willis, *Stroke* 21:56-65, 1990.
15. Dumoulin CL, Souza SP, Walker MF, Wagle W: Three-dimensional phase contrast angiography, *Magn Reson Med* 9:139-149, 1989.
16. Keller PJ, Drayer BP, Fram EK et al: MRA with two-dimensional acquisition and three-dimensional display, *Radiology* 173:527-532, 1989.

## CASE 98
## PITFALL: CAROTID SIPHON SIGNAL LOSS

**History:** 8-year-old with headaches.

**Technique:** axial volume, three-dimensional time-of-flight, 45/8/20, 256 × 256, 64 slices, 60-mm slab, 15-cm field of view, 12:19.

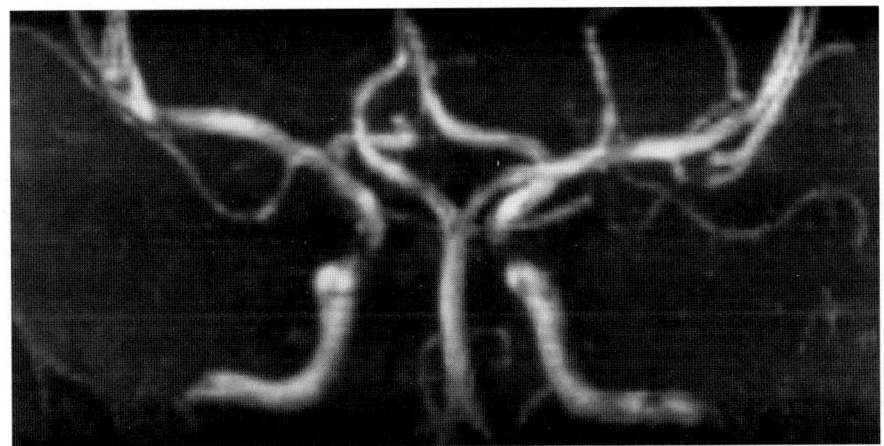

A

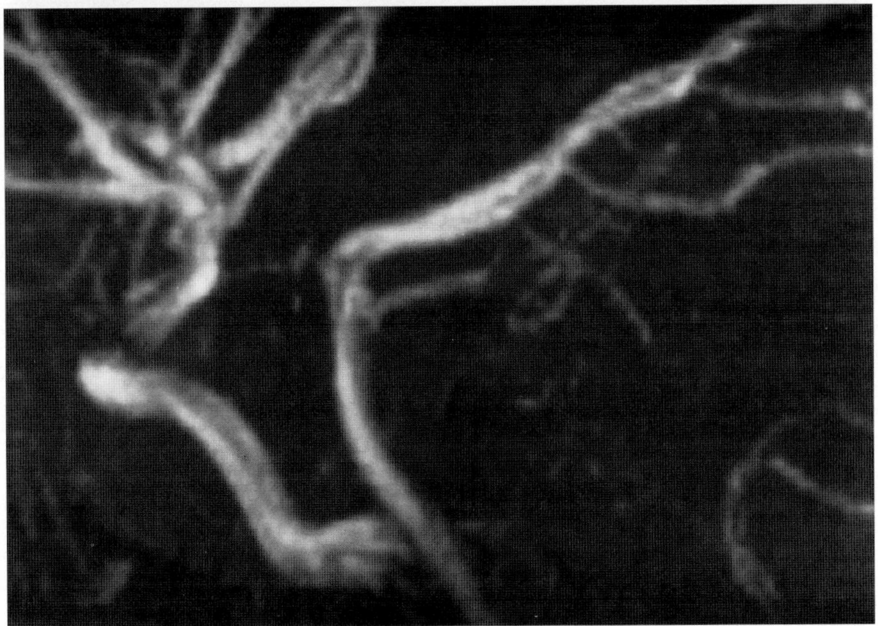

B

**Anteroposterior (A) and lateral (B) maximum intensity projection views show marked loss of signal involving both carotid siphons, which begins just distal to the siphon's anterior bend. The remainder of the vessels are normal in appearance.**

This signal loss is due to spin dephasing related to complex and accelerated flow around the carotid siphon bend, which is not completely compensated for on this MRA (velocity compensation in read and slice-select directions). This finding is particularly common in young people (age 20 and under) and usually occurs superior to the anteriormost carotid siphon bend. Distinction from pathologic narrowing as in sickle cell, Takayasu's arteritis, or atherosclerosis can be difficult. Distinction is made with correlation to the spin-echo parenchymal examination, and the presence of excellent flow-related enhancement of the distal middle cerebral branches, which would not be expected to occur if there were severe stenoses of the carotid siphons.

## CASE 99
## PITFALL: SIGNAL LOSS ON TIME-OF-FLIGHT MRA RELATED TO LOW CARDIAC OUTPUT

**History:** 82-year-old with aphasia and atrial fibrillation.

**Technique #1:** axial volume, three-dimensional time-of-flight, 45/8.5/20, 128 × 256, 60 slices, 60-mm slab, 18-cm field of view, 6:09.

**Technique #2:** coronal two-dimensional phase-contrast, 33/8.9/20, 192 × 256, eight excitations, one slice, 60-mm thick, 22-cm field of view, 3:25.

A

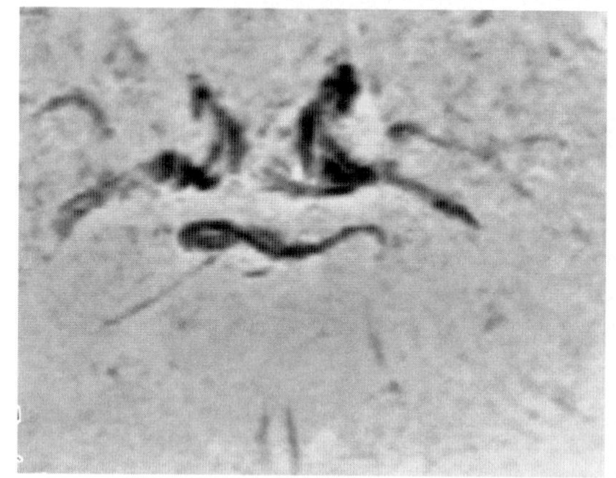

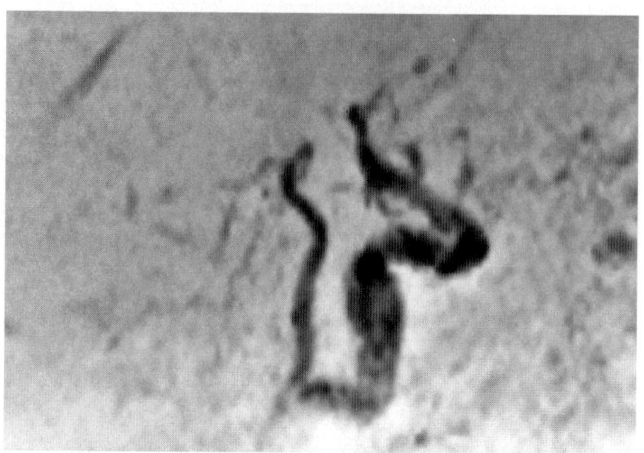

B

C

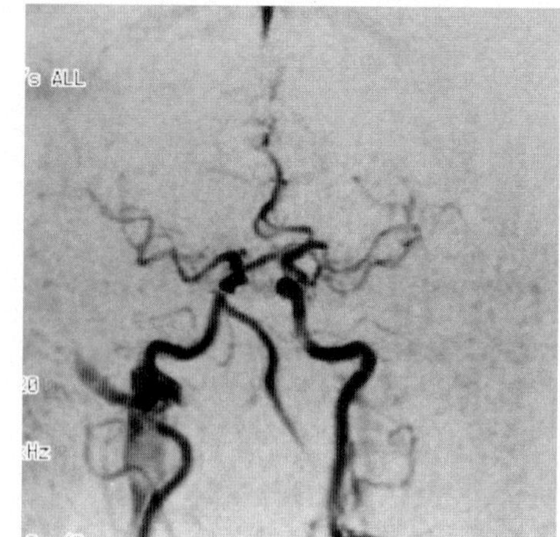

**Base (A) and lateral (B) maximum intensity projection views of the time-of-flight MRA show a study of very poor quality without visualization of the intracranial circulation beyond the carotid siphons and basilar artery. The thick-slice two-dimensional phase-contrast study (C) shows good signal from the middle cerebral and anterior cerebral branches bilaterally.**

In patients with poor cardiac output, there is slowed flow to the intracranial circulation, which causes increased saturation effects on the time-of-flight MRA. This is most severe for the distal branches because of (1) the slower flow of the smaller branches and (2) their position deeper in the imaging volume, which causes them to experience more radiofrequency pulses and thus have more saturation. The phase-contrast study showed that the vessels were patent with the relatively low velocity encoding of 30 cm/sec.

## CASE 100
## PITFALL: OVERESTIMATION OF MIDDLE CEREBRAL ARTERY STENOSIS

**History:** 72-year-old with left hemispheric transient ischemic attacks.

**Technique #1:** axial volume, three-dimensional time-of-flight, 45/7/20, 256 × 256, 64 slices, 60-mm slab, 15-cm field of view, 12:19.

**Technique #2:** axial volume, three-dimensional time-of-flight, 45/8.5/20, 256 × 256, 64 slices, 60-mm slab, 15-cm field of view, 12:19.

A

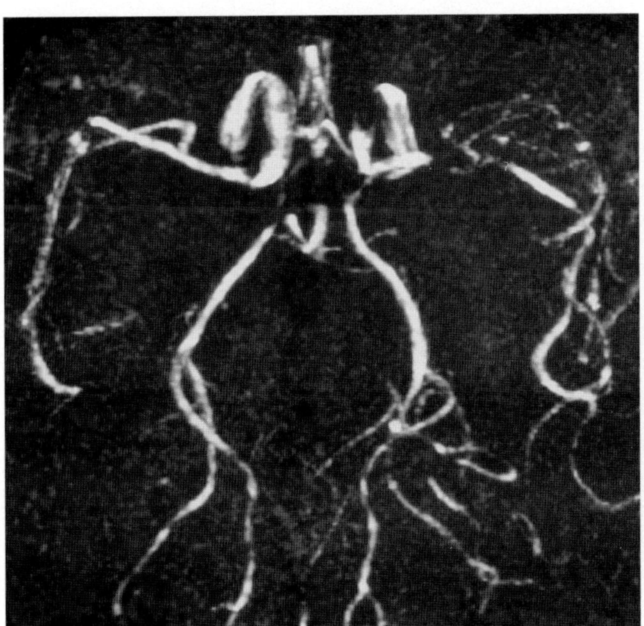

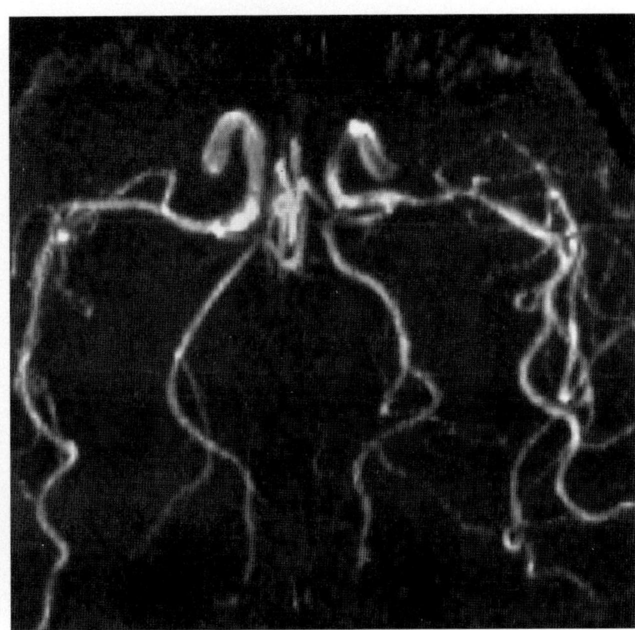

B

**Base maximum intensity projection view of the three-dimensional time-of-flight angiogram (A) with an echo time of 8.5 msec shows marked loss of signal from the left M1 segment, which is consistent with marked stenosis. There is good signal distal to this region, which makes the possibility of occlusion much less likely. The same view from an MRA with a 1.5-msec shorter echo time (B) now shows a moderate stenosis of the left M1 segment, which was grossly overestimated with only a slightly longer echo time.**

A small increase in echo time can exert a powerful negative effect on overall image quality. In general for time-of-flight techniques, the shortest opposed-phase echo time should be used with velocity compensation for the highest quality MRA. If image quality is still not sufficient, an even shorter echo time may be obtained by going more in-phase. However, in these instances, additional peripheral saturation slabs must be placed to minimize the high signal intensity that will occur from the scalp and orbital fat and limiting the volume of maximum intensity projection reconstruction to the area of interest is mandatory.

## CASE 101
## PITFALL: MOYAMOYA DISEASE WITH FALSE-POSITIVE RESULTS INDICATING STENOSIS

**History:** 41-year-old with headaches and paresthesias.

**Technique:** axial volume, three-dimensional time-of-flight, 43/6/20, 512 × 256 matrix, one excitation, 60 slices, 60-mm slab, 18-cm field of view, 11:00.

A

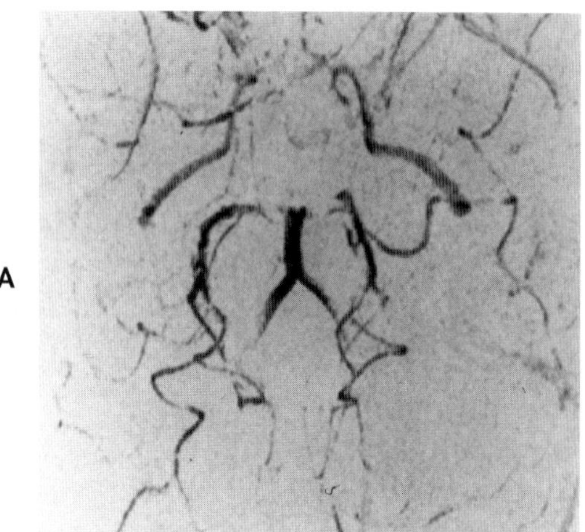

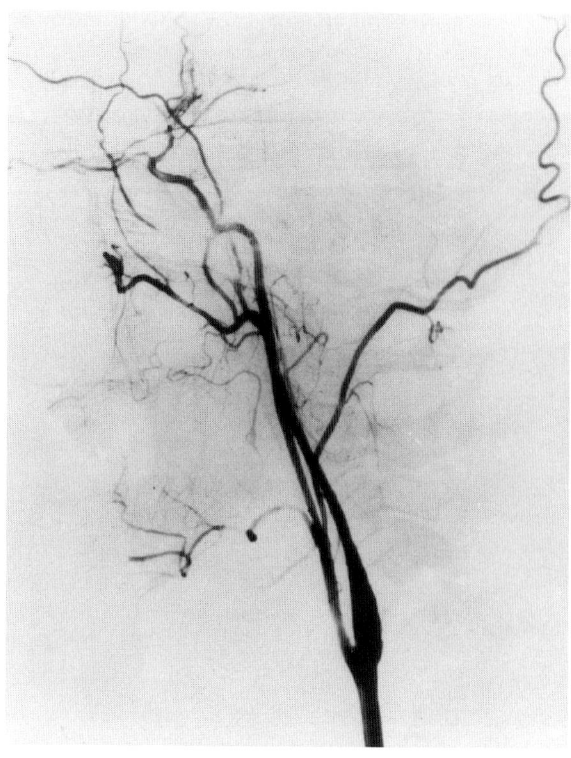

B

C

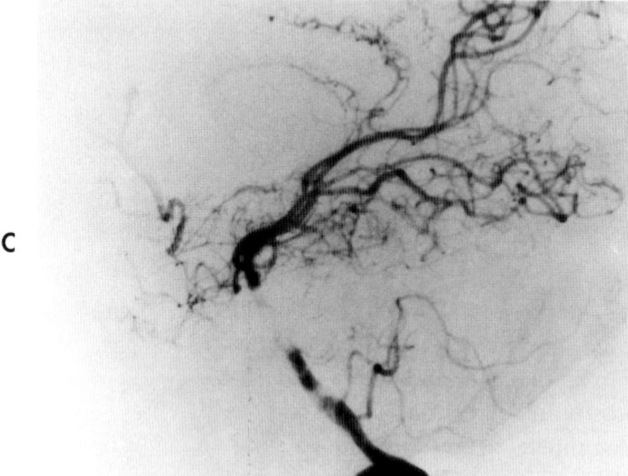

**Base maximum intensity projection view of the three-dimensional time-of-flight MRA (A) demonstrates marked narrowing of the distal internal carotid arteries bilaterally and striking paucity of branches of the middle cerebral arteries. There is also an apparent stenosis involving the P1 segments bilaterally. Lateral view of the left common carotid injection (B) demonstrates the narrowing of the supraclinoid internal carotid artery, with a few moyamoya-like vessels extending superiorly. There is essentially no filling of the middle cerebral distribution. Lateral conventional angiographic view of a right vertebral injection (C) demonstrates mild narrowing involving the P1 segments bilaterally, but no significant narrowing is demonstrated, as is seen on the three-dimensional time-of-flight MRA. On the lateral angiographic view, there is significant collateral flow through the posterior communicating arteries to the anterior cerebral artery. (Courtesy John Huston, Mayo Clinic, Rochester, Minn.)**

---

The false-positive stenosis with loss of signal in the P1 segments on the MRA relates to retrograde flow through the posterior communicating arteries, with subsequent turbulence flow and phase dispersion. (See Case 125 for discussion of moyamoya disease.)

## CASE 102
## PITFALL: DESTRUCTIVE INTERFERENCE ON A TWO-DIMENSIONAL PHASE-CONTRAST STUDY

**History:** 30-year-old healthy volunteer.

**Technique:** sagittal, two-dimensional phase-contrast, 30/8/20, 512 × 256, eight excitations, 80-mm thick slice, 24-cm field of view, 5 minutes.

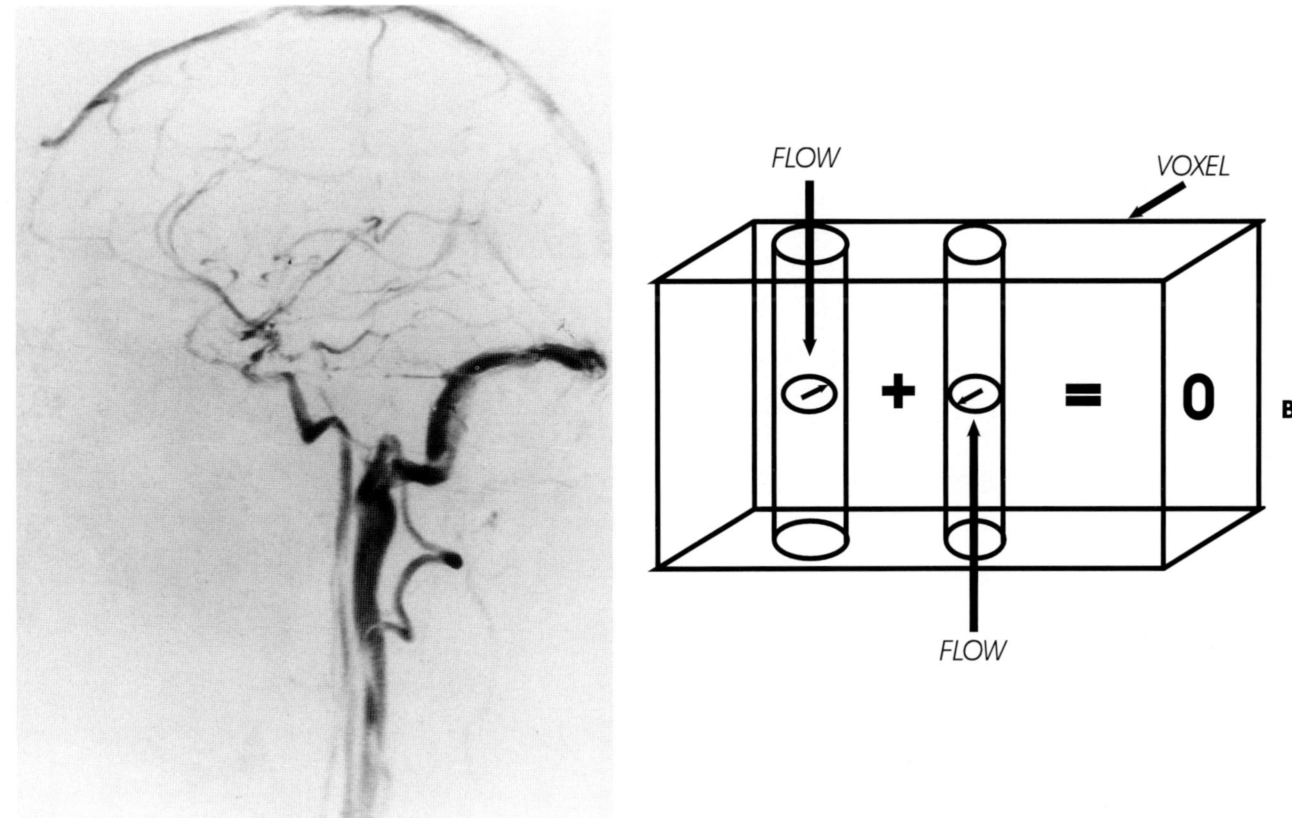


**A single sagittal thick-slice two-dimensional phase-contrast study (A) with a 30 cm/sec velocity encoding centered over the left carotid artery, cerebral artery, and jugular vein shows prominent signal loss involving the inferior portion of the left jugular vein and left vertebral artery. (A courtesy John Huston, Mayo Clinic, Rochester, Minn.)**

The signal loss in this instance is due to overlap of the superiorly flowing vertebral artery and inferiorly flowing jugular vein, causing destructive interference. This is a nonspecific phenomenon that can occur when any vessels with different flow directions are within the same slice or slab on a phase-contrast study.

Destructive interference occurs between the phases of spins within separate vessels within a voxel **(B).** Signal loss occurs in the vessels when multiple phases occur within a single voxel, some of which cancel each other out. This would be particularly prone to occur when the voxel size is very large (anisotropic), as in a two-dimensional thick-slice phase-contrast technique.

## CASE 103
## PITFALL: OCCLUSION OF THE LEFT SUPRACLINOID INTERNAL CAROTID ARTERY, WITH COLLATERAL FLOW FROM THE RIGHT SUPRACLINOID INTERNAL CAROTID ARTERY MASKING THE OCCLUSION

**History:** 70-year-old with left hemispheric transient ischemic attacks.

**Technique:** axial volume, three-dimensional time-of-flight, 34/10/15, 256 × 256, 64 slices, 60-mm slab, 25-cm field of view, 9:20.

A

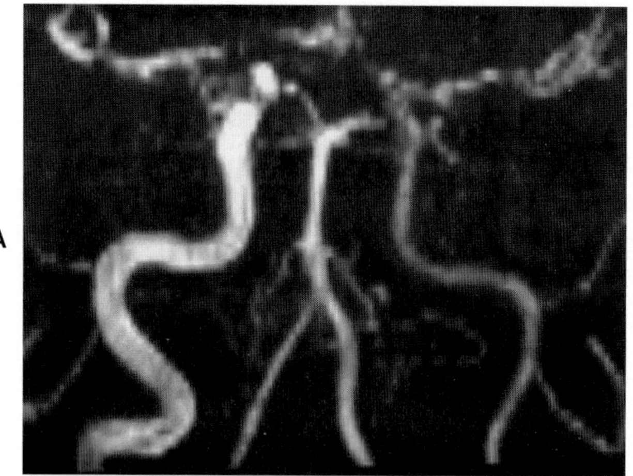

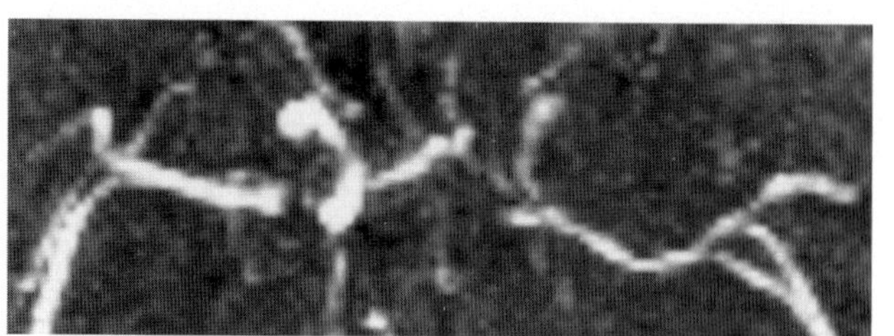

B

C

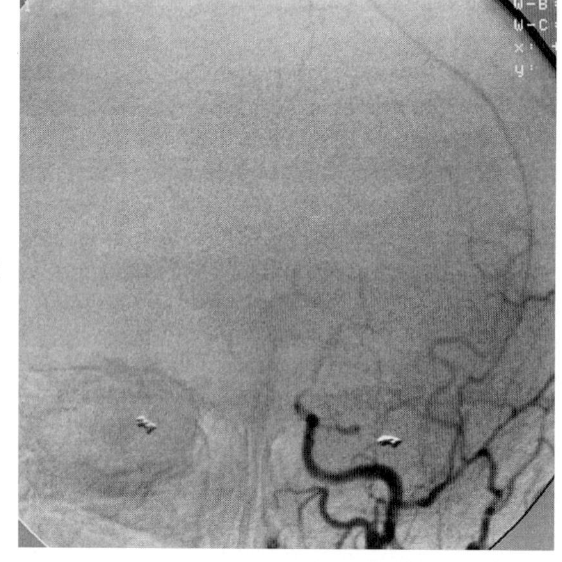

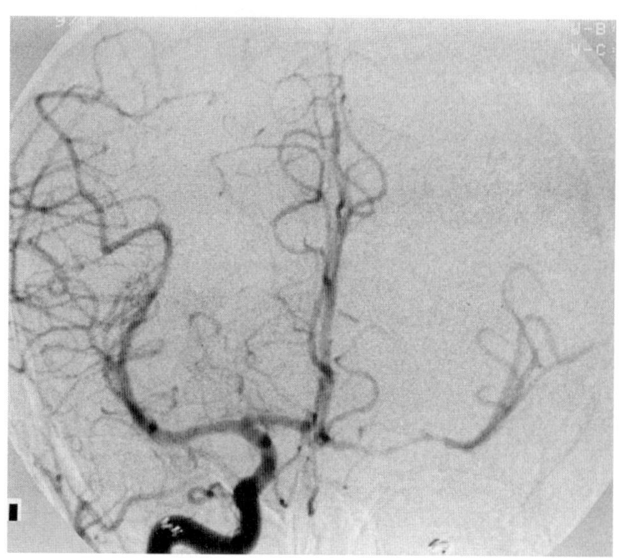

D

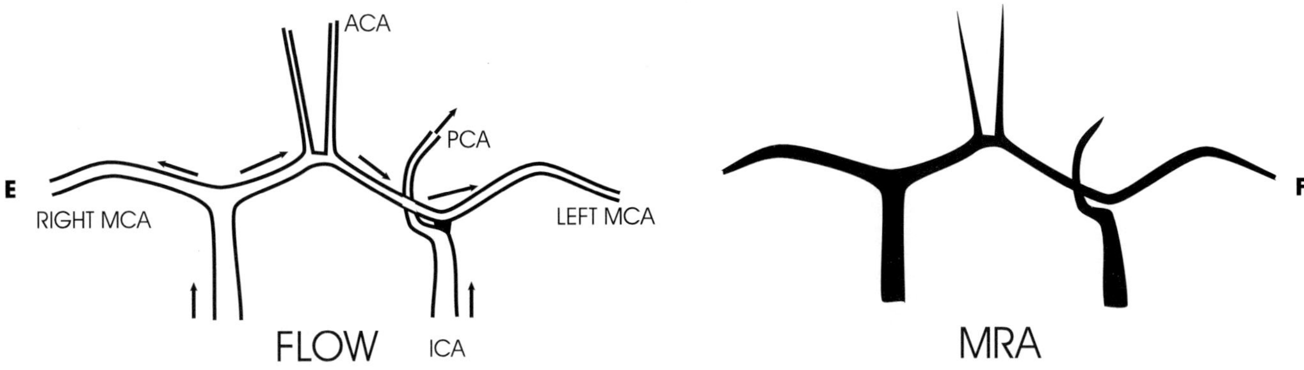


**Anteroposterior (A) and base (B) maximum intensity projection views show decreased signal from the left internal carotid artery, which is suspicious for a severe carotid bifurcation stenosis producing slowed flow (resulting from saturation). There is also loss of signal in the proximal right M1 and A1 segments, which is suspicious for at least moderate stenosis. The basilar artery is widely patent. The conventional angiogram (left common carotid injection) (C) shows occlusion of the supraclinoid internal carotid artery with filling of only the left posterior cerebral artery. Injection of the right common carotid artery shows cross-filling to the left anterior and middle cerebral arteries (D).**

The time-of-flight MRA missed the occlusion of the distal left internal carotid artery because of the cross-filling from the opposite side via the A1 and M1 segments that masked the signal loss of the distal internal carotid occlusion **(E** and **F).**

**E** shows the flow with the occlusion of the left distal internal carotid artery, with filling of only the left posterior cerebral artery from the left. The left anterior cerebral and middle cerebral arteries are filled by cross-flow from the right internal carotid artery. **F** shows the MRA appearance of this anatomy and flow conditions. The limited spatial resolution of the MRA and the small area of distal internal carotid artery occlusion combine to hide the separation of the distal internal carotid artery from the A1 and M1 origins.

## CASE 104
## LEFT INTERNAL CAROTID ARTERY OCCLUSION WITH COLLATERAL FLOW VIA THE ANTERIOR COMMUNICATING ARTERY

**History:** 70-year-old with right-sided hemiplegia.

**Technique #1:** intracranial/axial volume, three-dimensional time-of-flight, 40/7/15, 256 × 256, 64 slices, 60-mm slab, 25-cm field of view, 10:57.

**Technique #2:** carotid/axial volume, three-dimensional time-of-flight, 45/7/20, 256 × 192, 64 slices, 60-mm slab, 20-cm field of view, 9:20.

A

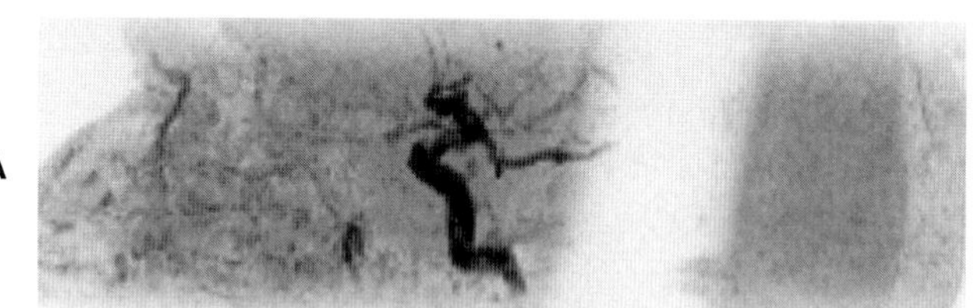

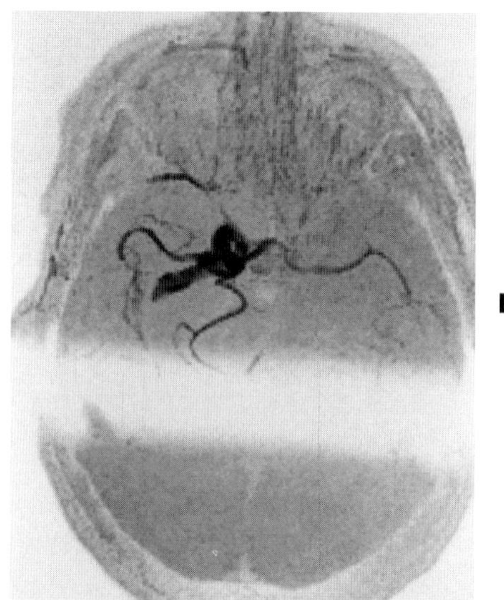

B

C

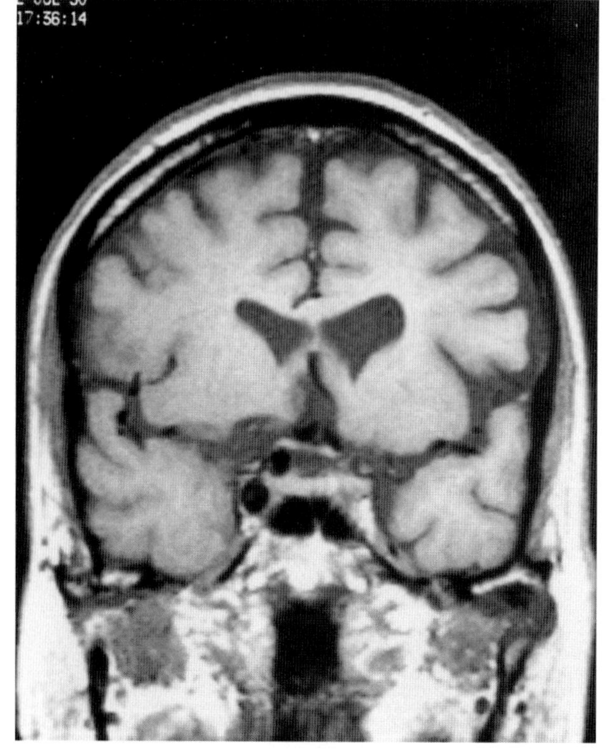


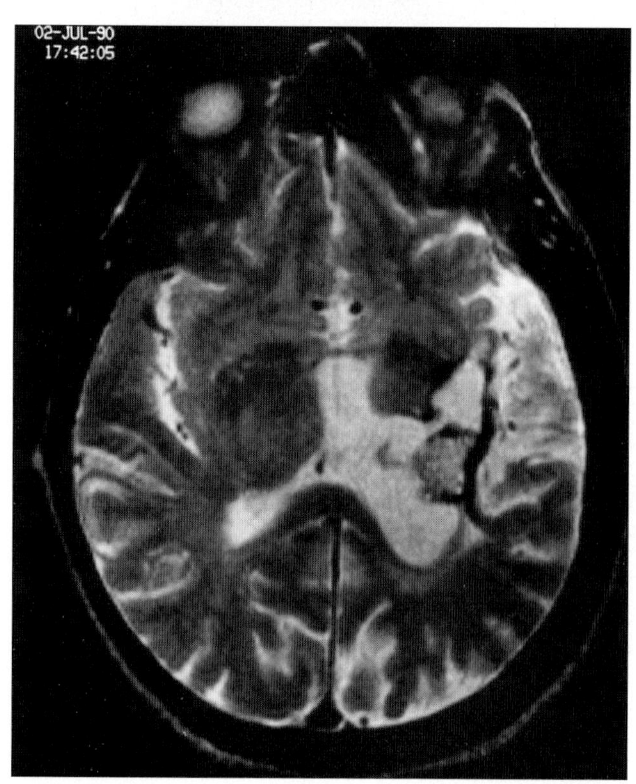


D

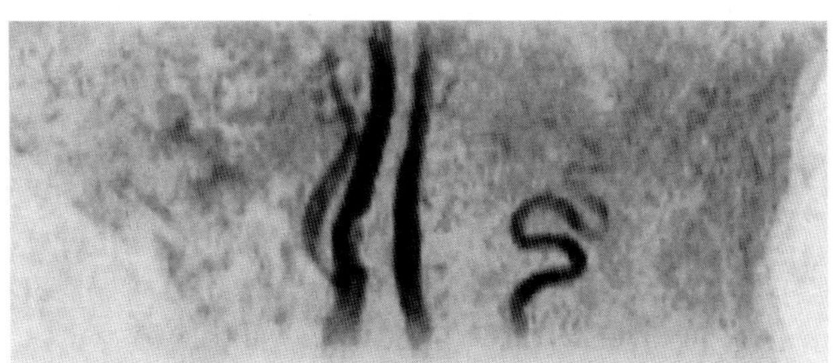

E

**Lateral view from the maximum intensity projection (A) shows placement of an oblique saturation pulse through the region of the posterior circulation. Placement of the saturation pulse removes any signal from the intracranial vasculature that may relate from flow through the basilar artery. Base view from the maximum intensity projection (B) demonstrates a patent distal right internal carotid circulation, as well as the right anterior and middle cerebral circulations. Signal intensity is also noted within the left middle cerebral circulation. The left internal carotid artery shows no signal intensity and is thus occluded. Because of the placement of the saturation pulse over the posterior circulation, the signal intensity present within the left middle cerebral artery must result from cross-filling from the right internal carotid artery distribution. Coronal T1-weighted image of the head (C) shows lack of the usual flow void within the left carotid siphon, which is consistent with the occlusion. T2-weighted axial image of the head (D) shows parenchymal volume loss within the left middle cerebral distribution and the remote hemorrhagic infarct involving the insular cortex and the left thalamus. Oblique view of the maximum intensity projections of the carotid bifurcation (E) demonstrate the occluded left internal carotid artery, with only the external carotid being widely patent. There is a moderate stenosis involving the origin of the right internal carotid artery, seen as a broad-based plaque along the posterior wall of the origin of the internal carotid. There is also severe stenosis involving the origin of the external carotid artery.**

Furst et al performed selective MRA of the carotid and vertebrobasilar territory by presaturation of up to three brain-supplying arteries at the level of the middle and lower neck using angle presaturation slabs. Sensitivity of selective MRA for intracranial collateral circulation via the anterior and posterior communicating arteries was 95% and 97%. They noted the visibility of the posterior communicating artery that MRA predicted for pathologic collateral flow via this vessel in all cases. They considered MRA of the cerebral arteries a powerful evasive method of demonstrating collateral circulation via the basal communicating arteries.

Another method of flow-supply definition is analogous to bolus tracking and may be used to define early vs late venous drainage as shown by Pernicone et al. They saturated the arterial system below a questionable arteriovenous malformation with a large basal vein of Rosenthal, which could not be distinguished as drainage of an arteriovenous malformation or a venous angioma. Transmission of the saturated blood to the basal vein was demonstrated, thus inferring that the basal vein was involved in early venous drainage of the arteriovenous malformation.

A simple alternative method of determining direction of flow would be the selective use of two-dimensional phase-contrast study. In this instance, flow through the anterior communicating artery could be defined by a few two-dimensional slices with flow sensitivity along the right-to-left direction.

## REFERENCES

Pernicone JR, Siebert JE, Potchen EJ: Demonstration of an early draining vein by MRA. *JCAT* 15(5):829-831, 1991.

Furst G, Steinmetz H, Fisher H et al: Selective MRA in Intercranial Collateral Blood Flow, *JCAT* 17:178-183, 1993.

## CASE 105
## SEVERE CAROTID BIFURCATION STENOSIS WITH DECREASED INTRACRANIAL SIGNAL

**History:** 65-year-old with previously documented left-sided occipital stroke.

**Technique #1:** intracranial/axial volume, three-dimensional time-of-flight, 40/7/15, 256 × 256, 64 slices, 60-mm slab, 25-cm field of view, 10:57.

**Technique #2:** carotid/axial volume, three-dimensional time-of-flight, 45/7/20, 256 × 192, 64 slices, 60-mm slab, 18-cm field of view, 9:20.

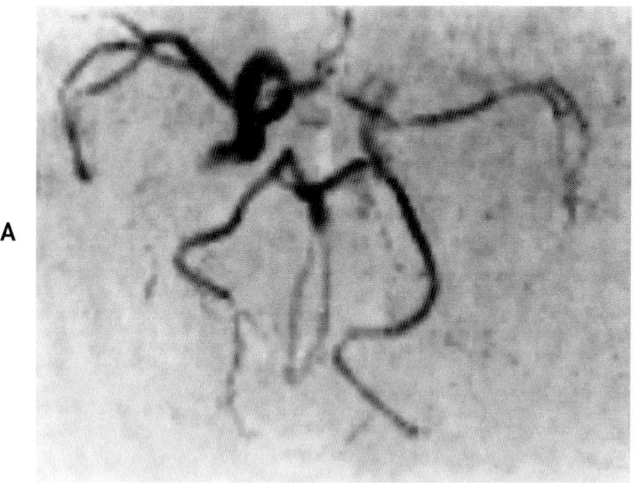

A

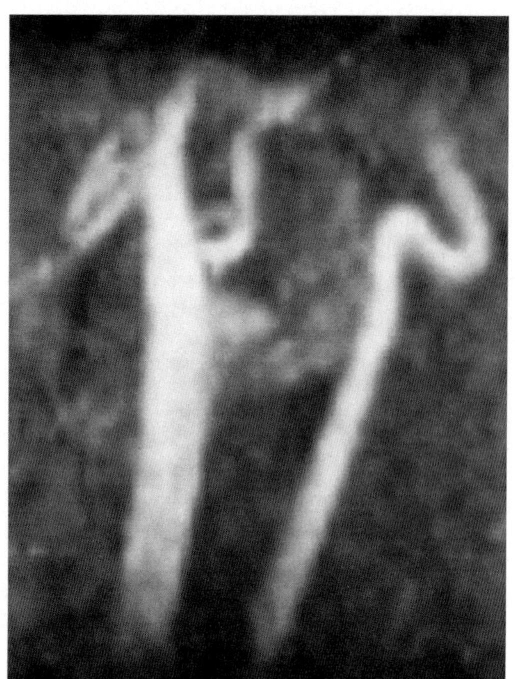

B

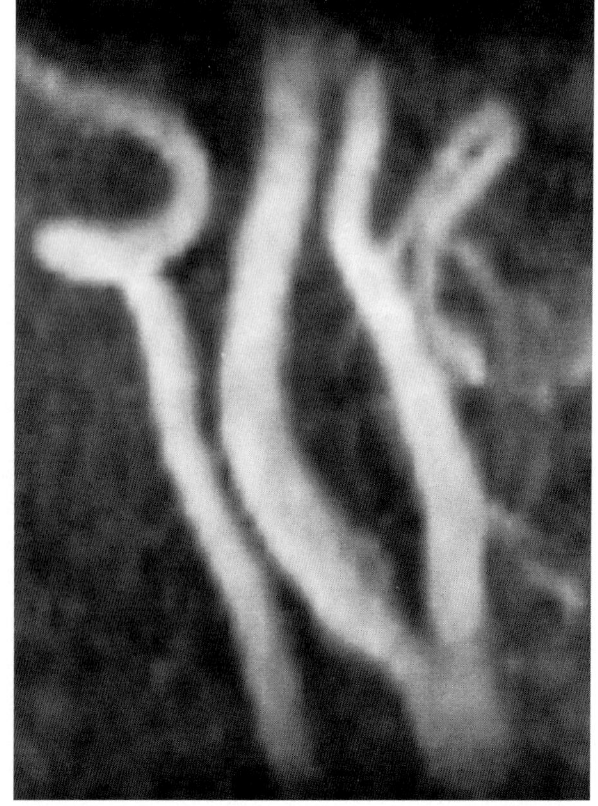

C

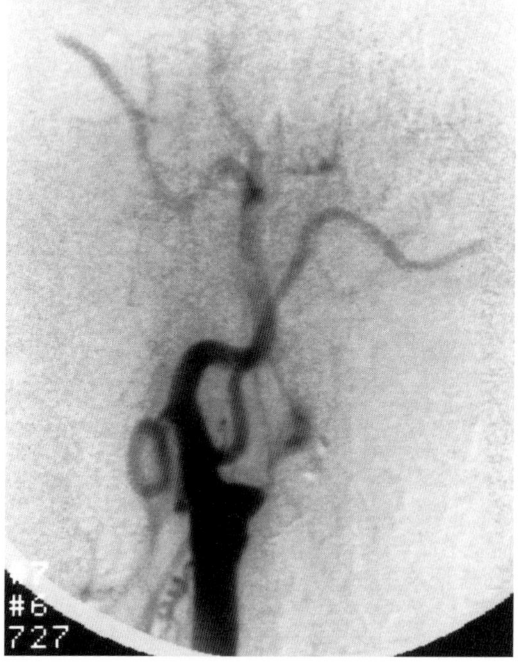


D

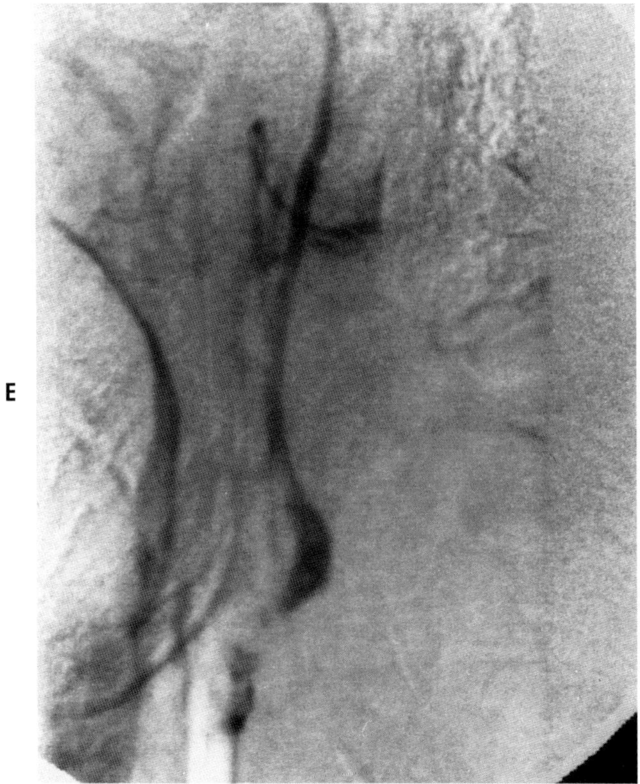

E

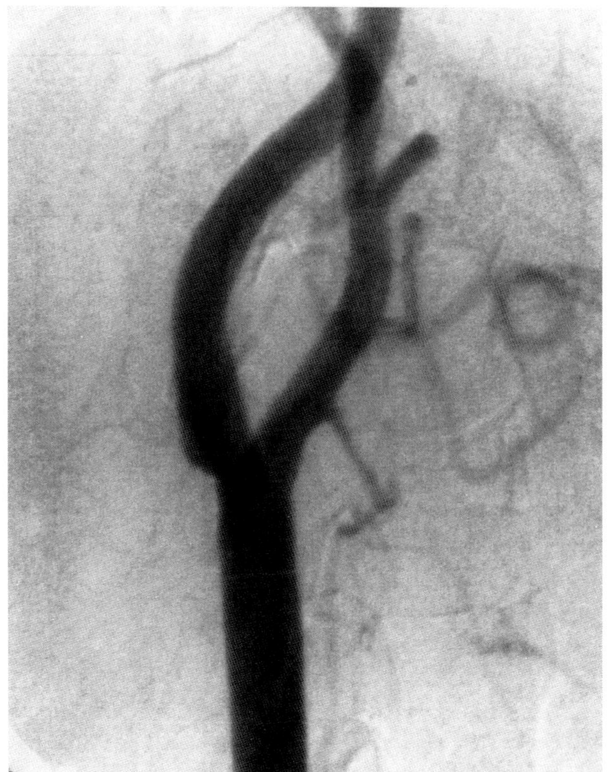

F

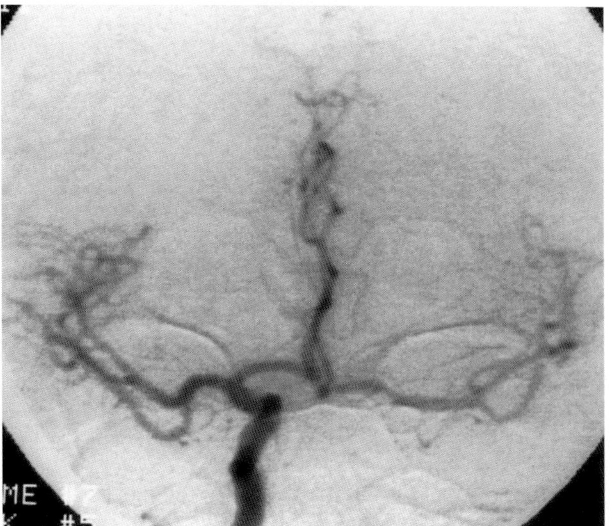

G

**Base maximum intensity projection view of the time of flight MRA demonstrates a small distal left internal carotid artery with decreased signal intensity (A). The left middle cerebral artery is also small and threadlike in appearance. The lateral targeted maximum intensity projection view of the left internal carotid artery bifurcation (B) shows an ill-defined area of triangular signal intensity off the posterior margin of the distal left common carotid artery, which is apparently at the stub of an occluded internal carotid artery. No definite signal intensity is seen within the more distal internal carotid artery. The right carotid bifurcation lateral targeted maximum intensity projection view (C) shows a mild narrowing involving the origin of the right internal carotid artery. Conventional intraarterial angiography demonstrates a near occlusion of the internal carotid artery on the left with markedly slowed distal flow (D and E). Lateral angiographic view of the right carotid bifurcation (F) shows the mild stenosis at the origin of the internal carotid artery, with the anteroposterior intracranial view (G) demonstrating cross-filling from right to left, further confirming the decreased flow to the left middle cerebral circulation.**

The MRA findings of attenuated signal from the left internal carotid and left middle cerebral arteries could result from diffuse atherosclerotic narrowing of the internal carotid and middle cerebral vessels, but this would be an unusual pattern of unilateral involvement. These findings are also seen on time-of-flight MRA with a proximal stenosis of the cervical internal carotid artery, with resultant flow saturation of the slowly flowing blood within the internal carotid artery and middle cerebral branches. Thus the slowed, saturated flow gives an artificial appearance of vessel caliber reduction resulting from vessel pathology. Similarly, the false-positive MRA for left carotid occlusion occurs because of slow flow with a critical stenosis with a slowed distal flow and saturation effects.

## CASE 106
## SEVERE DISTAL INTERNAL CAROTID STENOSIS

**History:** 62-year-old man with left-sided hemispheric transient ischemic attacks.

**Technique:** axial volume; three-dimensional time-of-flight; 45/7/20; 256 × 256; 64 slices; 60-mm slab; magnetization transfer background suppression; tilted, optimized nonsaturating excitation radiofrequency pulse; 14-cm field of view; 12:20.

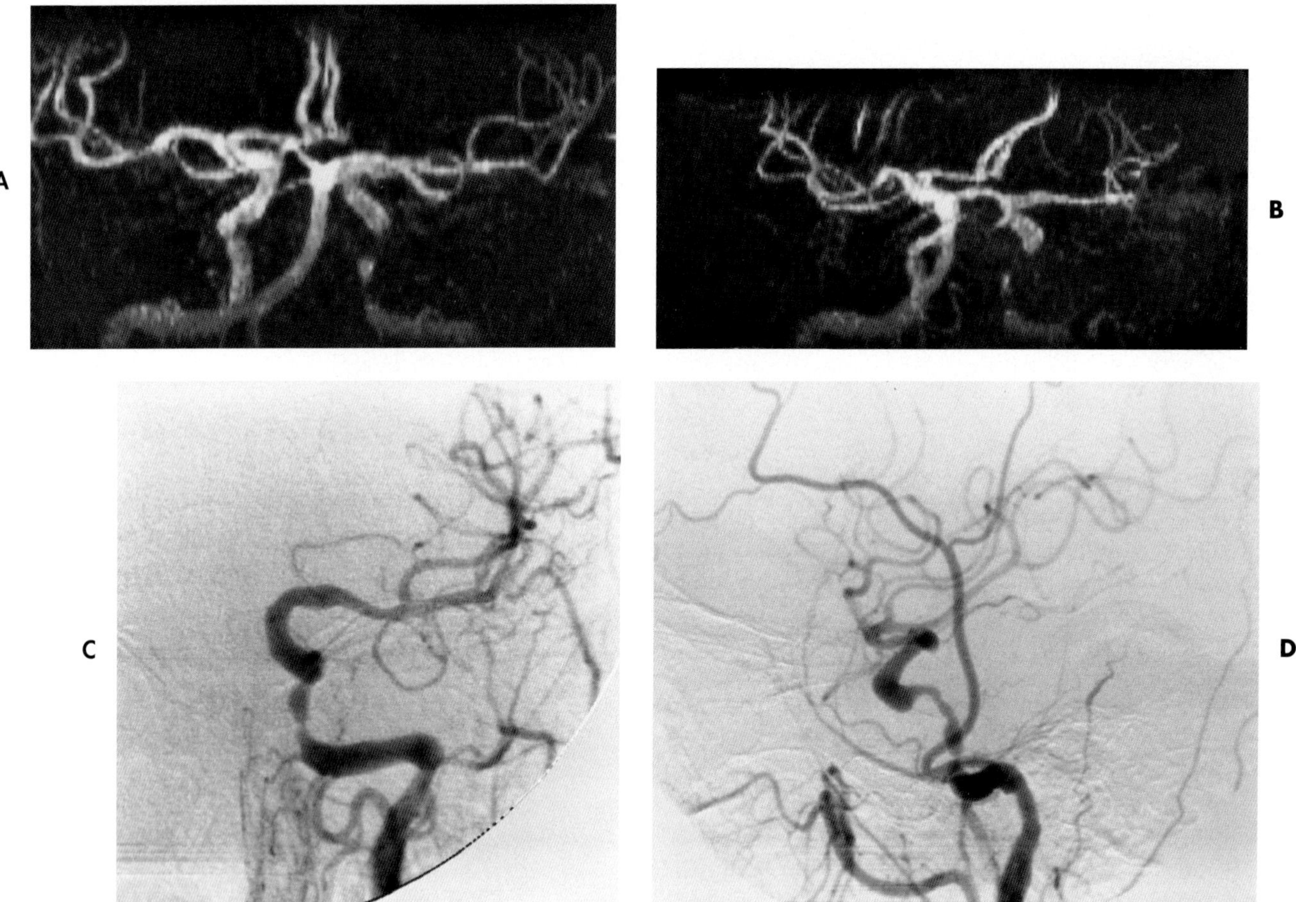

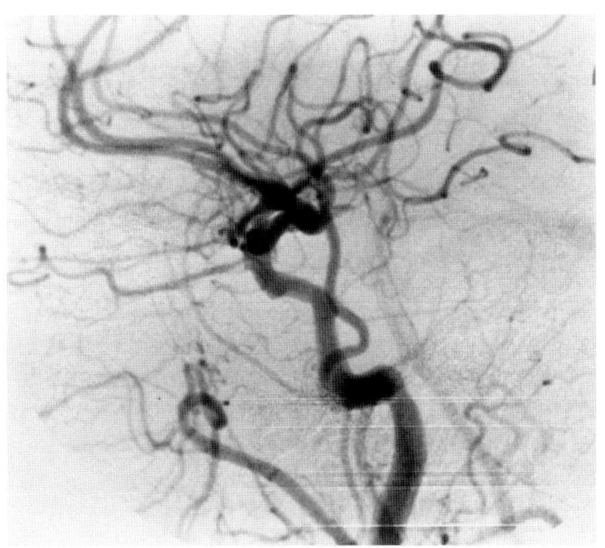

E

**Anteroposterior (A) and oblique (B) maximum intensity projection views show marked irregularity and signal loss throughout the distal petrous and cavernous portions of the left carotid internal carotid, with maintained flow and signal in the most distal left internal carotid artery. Although there are areas of complete signal loss on the maximum intensity projection in the distal left internal carotid artery, this represents overestimation of stenosis resulting from turbulent or slow flow and not occlusion. This is because there is signal in the most distal internal carotid artery that would not be present with occlusion of the siphon. There is also mild narrowing along the inferior aspect of the right carotid siphon. Anteroposterior (C) and lateral (D) conventional intraarterial digital subtraction angiographic views of the left common carotid injection confirm the severe stenosis with marked irregularity. Right common carotid injection (E) shows the mild narrowing of the right siphon. Incidentally noted is the absent left A1 segment on the right anterior oblique maximum intensity projection (B), which is also confirmed on the conventional angiogram (C).**

## REFERENCE

Heiserman JE, Drayer BP, Keller PJ, Fram EK: Intracranial vascular stenosis and occlusion: evaluation with three-dimensional time-of-flight MRA, *Radiology* 185:667-673, 1992.

## CASE 107
## ACUTE MIDDLE CEREBRAL ARTERY OCCLUSION

**History:** 45-year-old with acute onset left-sided hemiplegia.

**Technique:** axial volume; three-dimensional time-of-flight; 45/7/20; 256 × 256; magnetization transfer background suppression; tilted, optimized non-saturating excitation radiofrequency pulse; 14-cm field of view; 12:20.

A

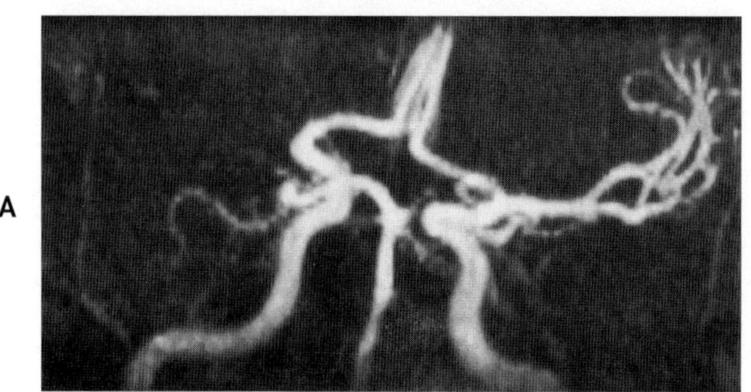

B

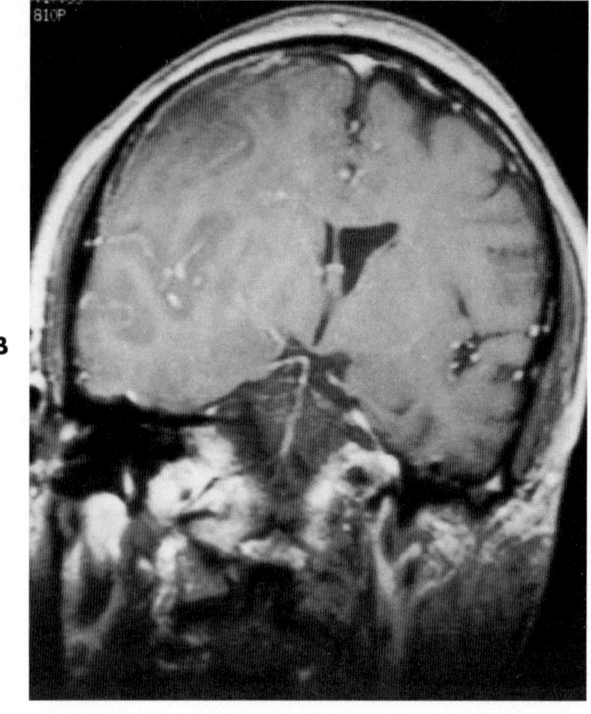

C

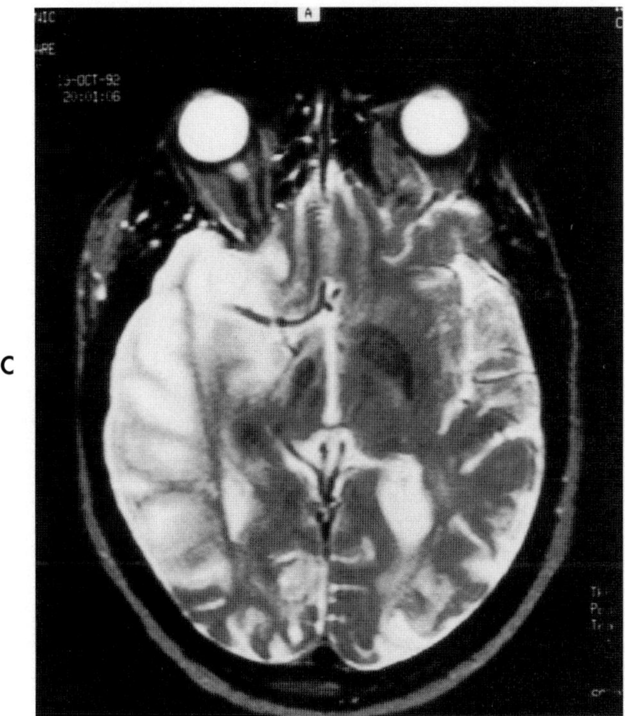

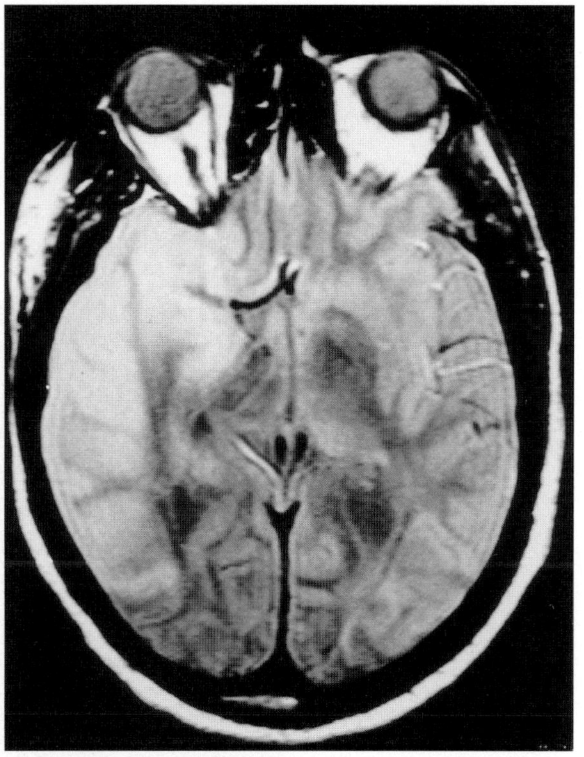

D

**Anteroposterior maximum intensity projection view (A) demonstrates an occluded right middle cerebral artery, with no signal from the middle cerebral distribution. There is normal signal intensity from the internal carotids bilaterally, as well as the anterior and middle cerebral distributions on the left. There is also a fetal origin of the left posterior cerebral artery from the left internal carotid artery. T1-enhanced coronal image of the brain (B) shows right hemispheric edema, with mild shift of the midline to the left. There is abnormal leptomeningeal enhancement related to slowed flow and collateral flow. Axial T2-weighted image of the brain (C) demonstrates a large area of abnormal increased signal intensity involving gray and white matter in the right middle cerebral artery distribution. There is low signal intensity within the proximal middle cerebral artery. However, the M1 segment shows higher signal intensity than the A1 segment on the spin-density image (D). This abnormal increased signal on the spin density, which drops in signal intensity on the T2-weighted image represents thrombus in the M1 segment.**

---

**REFERENCE**

Warach S, Li W, Ronthal M, Edelman R: Acute cerebral ischemia: evaluation with dynamic contrast-enhanced MR imaging and MRA, *Radiology* 182:41-47, 1992.

## CASE 108
## ACUTE MIDDLE CEREBRAL ARTERY INFARCT WITH PERIPHERAL VESSEL SIGNAL LOSS

**History:** 69-year-old with acute onset right-sided hemiplegia and aphasia.

**Technique:** axial volume; three-dimensional time-of-flight; 45/7/20; 256 × 256; magnetization transfer background suppression; tilted, optimized non-saturating excitation radiofrequency pulse; 14-cm field of view; 12:20.

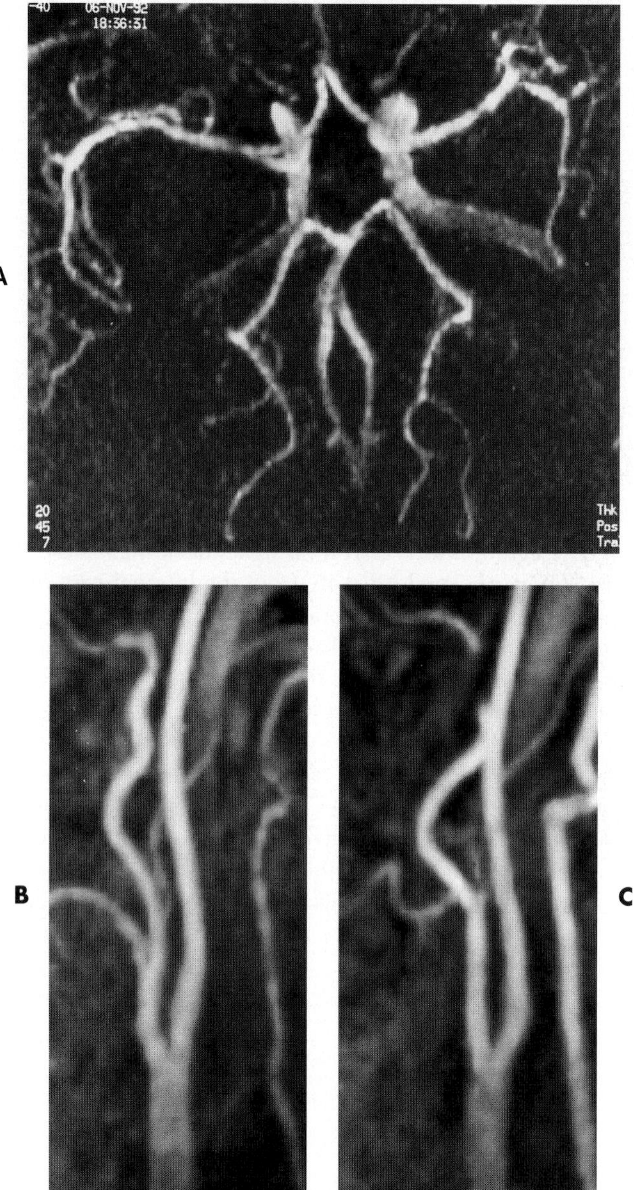

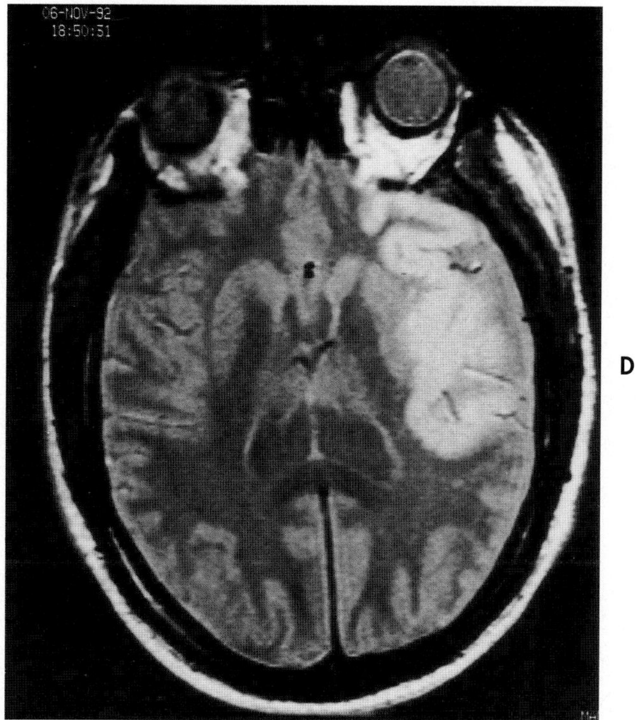


D

**Base maximum intensity projection view of the time-of-flight MRA (A) shows attenuation of the more peripheral branches of the left middle cerebral artery. No definite focal stenosis or large branch occlusion is identified. Lateral maximum intensity projection views of the carotid bifurcations (B and C) demonstrates normal-appearing right and left bifurcations. Axial spin-density image of the head shows a large left middle cerebral artery infarct (D).**

The pruning of the peripheral branches of the left middle cerebral artery on the time-of-flight MRA relates to absent or slowed flow in the infarcted territory. Slowed flow results in increased saturation with signal loss on the three-dimensional time-of-flight study.

#### REFERENCE

Warach S, Li W, Ronthal M, Edelman R: Acute cerebral ischemia: evaluation with dynamic contrast-enhanced MR imaging and MRA, *Radiology* 182:41-47, 1992.

## CASE 109
## MIDDLE CEREBRAL ARTERY STENOSIS

**History:** 64-year-old with left hand numbness and weakness.

**Technique:** axial volume, three-dimensional time-of-flight, 40/7/15, 256 × 256, 64 slices, 60-mm slab, 25-cm field of view, 10:57.

A

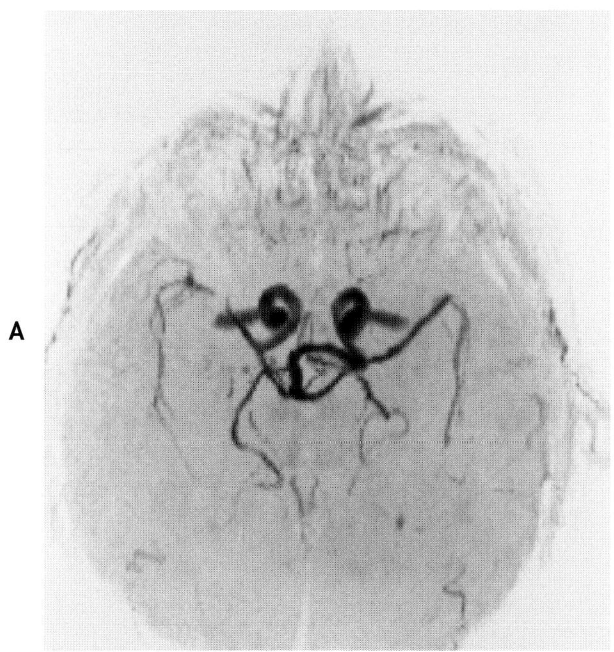

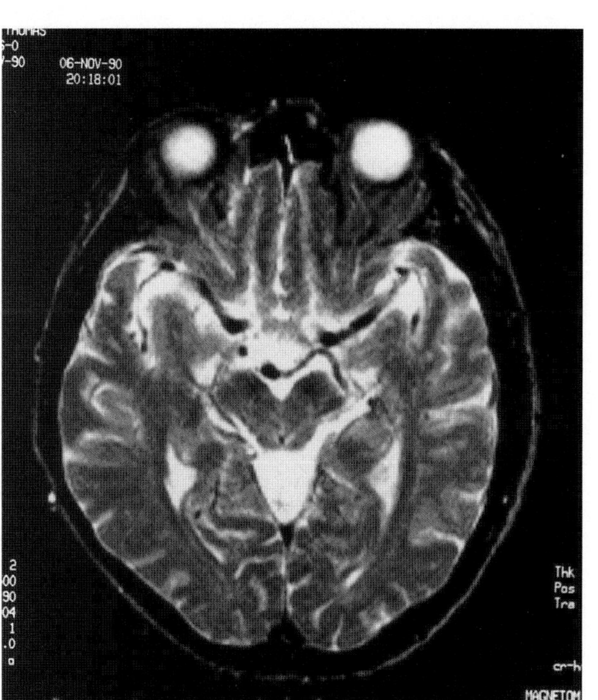


B

**Base maximum intensity projection view (A) demonstrates a focal area of signal loss involving the distal right middle cerebral artery (M1 segment). Because there is good signal intensity from the more peripheral branches of the middle cerebral artery, this is not consistent with an occlusion but would relate to dephasing effects and signal loss related to severe (greater than 70%) stenosis. T2-weighted image through the brain (B) shows normal-appearing right hemisphere and middle cerebral arteries. Anteroposterior view from the conventional intraarterial angiogram (C) demonstrates a severe stenosis involving the middle portion of the right middle cerebral artery with moderate irregularity.**

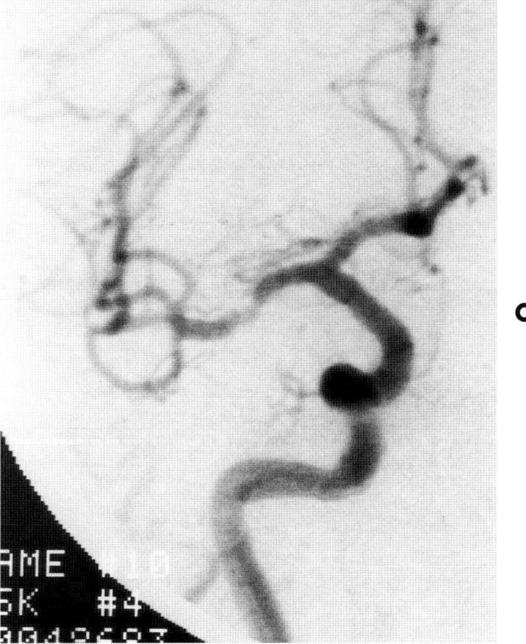

C

Although there is good correlation of the MRA findings and the arteriographic findings in this case, caution must be exercised in evaluating stenoses occurring within the in-plane direction on three-dimensional time-of-flight studies. The in-plane direction is not the optimal orientation for maximizing flow-related enhancement, and dephasing effects can accentuate the degree of stenosis.

## CASE 110
## SUPERFICIAL TEMPORAL ARTERY TO MIDDLE CEREBRAL ARTERY BYPASS

**History:** 53-year-old with an occluded left internal carotid artery.

**Technique #1:** axial three-dimensional time-of-flight, 43/6/20, 512 × 256, one excitation, 1.5-mm slices, 90-mm slab, 18-cm field of view, 11:00.

**Technique #2:** two-dimensional phase-contrast coronal, 30/8/20, 512 × 256, eight excitations, 80-mm thick section, 24-cm field of view, 5 minutes.

**Technique #3:** axial three-dimensional phase-contrast, 26/9/15, 256 × 128, one excitation, 1.5-mm slices, 90-mm slab, velocity encoding of 30 cm/sec, 18-cm field of view, 14 minutes.

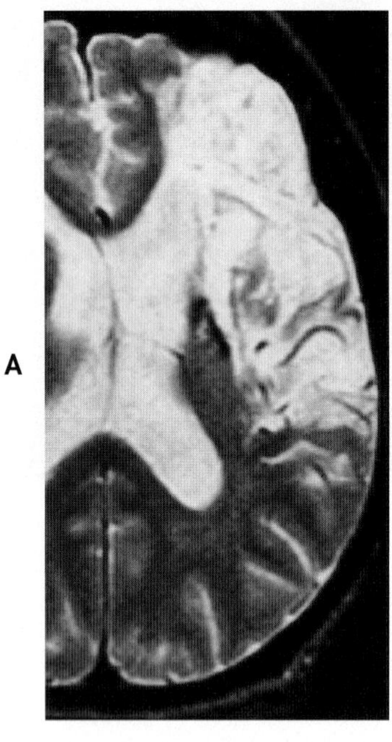
A

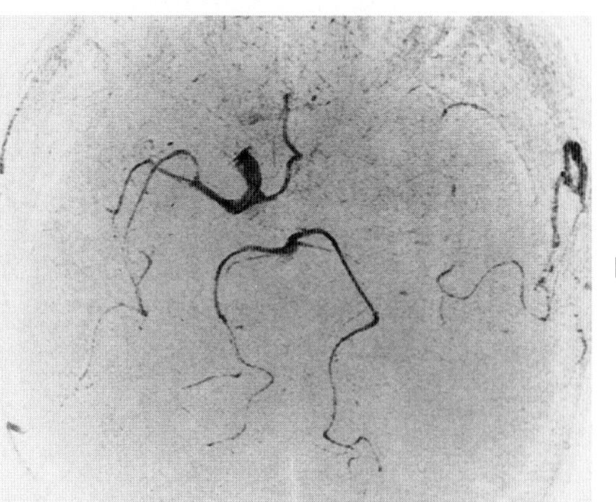
B

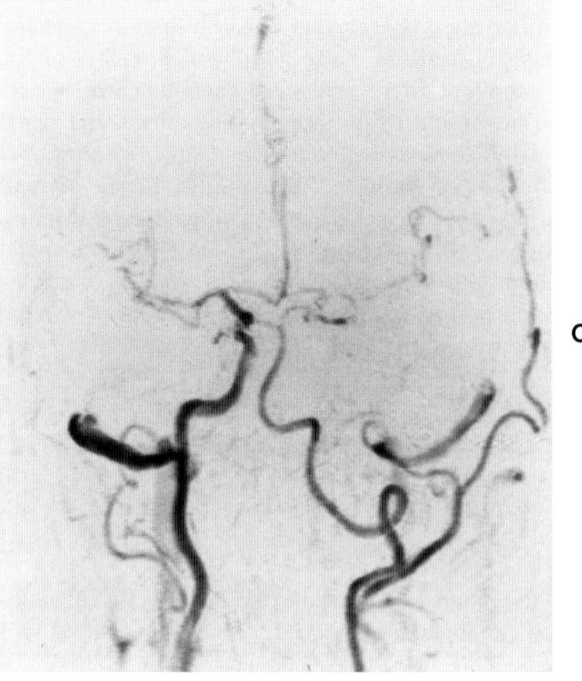
C

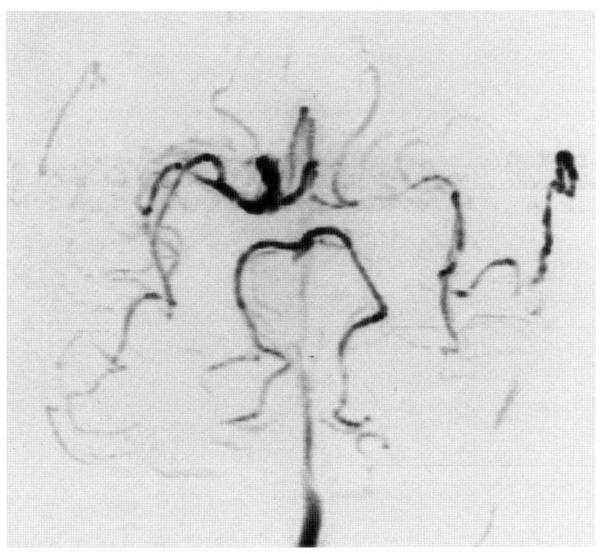


**The well-defined area of increased signal on the T2-weighted image in the left middle cerebral distribution represents a remote hemorrhagic infarct with macrocystic and microcystic encephalomalacia (A). The base maximum intensity projection view of the three-dimensional time-of-flight MRA (B) demonstrates very little flow in the left middle cerebral artery distribution resulting from slow flow and saturation effects, although the left superficial temporal artery is visualized. The coronal two-dimensional phase-contrast study with a 30 cm/sec velocity encoding (C) and the base maximum intensity projection views of the three-dimensional phase-contrast study with a 30 cm/sec velocity encoding (D) successfully demonstrates flow within the left middle cerebral artery distribution and the bypass graft. (Courtesy John Huston, Mayo Clinic, Rochester, Minn.)**

The first extracranial to intracranial bypass was performed in 1967 and was widely applied over the next decade. However, its use does not benefit patients with symptomatic atherosclerotic disease of the internal carotid artery, as shown by the report of the EC/IC Bypass Study Group. In this study, 1377 patients with recent hemisphere strokes, retinal infarction, or transient ischemic attacks were randomly assigned to medical therapy or medical therapy plus superficial temporal artery to middle cerebral artery bypass. Nonfatal and fatal stokes occurred more frequently and earlier in the operated patients.

Extracranial/intracranial bypass is not an effective method of preventing cerebral ischemia in patients with atherosclerosis of the carotid and middle cerebral vessels.

**REFERENCE**

The EC/IC Bypass Study Group: Failure of extracranial-intracranial arterial bypass to reduce the risk of ischemic stroke, *New Engl J Med* 313(19):1191-1200, 1985.

## CASE 111
## REMOTE LEFT POSTERIOR CEREBRAL ARTERY OCCLUSION WITH INFARCT

**History:** 51-year-old with left-sided hemiparesis.

**Technique:** three-dimensional time-of-flight, 40/7/15, 256 × 256, 64 slices, 60-mm slab, 25-cm field of view, 10:57.

A

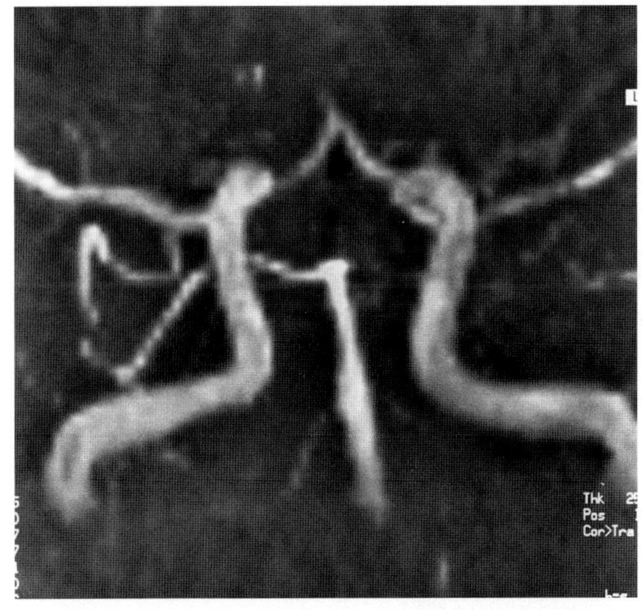


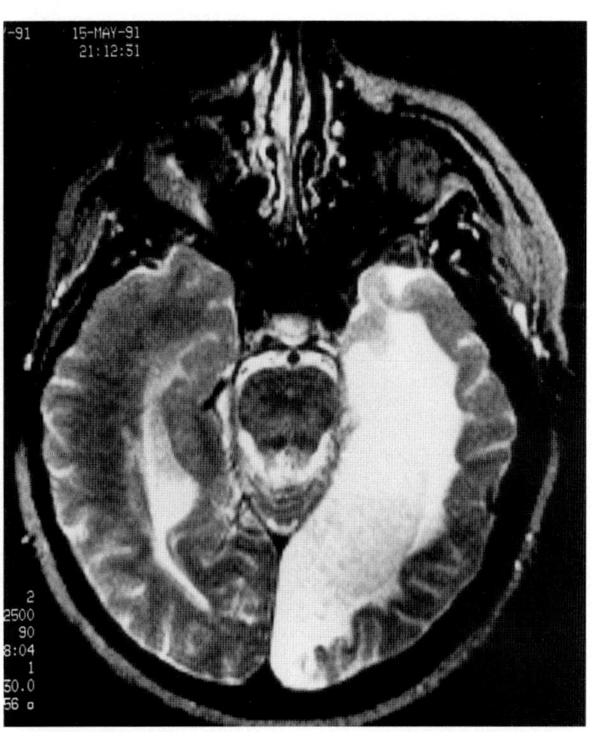


B

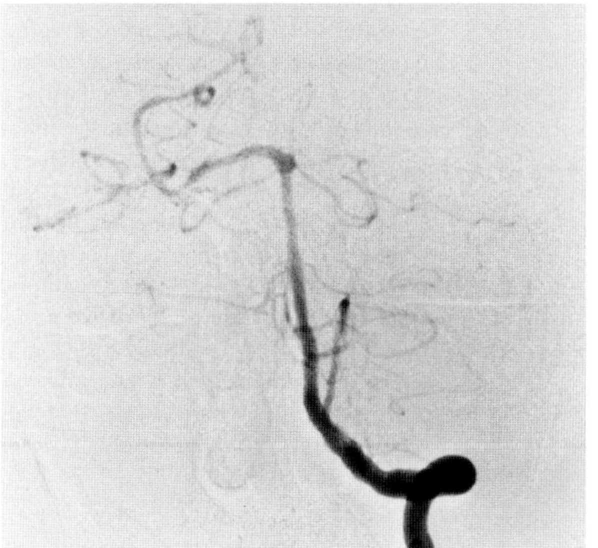

C

**Anteroposterior view of the maximum intensity projection (A) shows no signal within the region of the left posterior cerebral artery, which represents an occlusion. The right posterior cerebral artery is well identified, as is the normal-appearing basilar artery. Axial T2-weighted spin-echo image (B) demonstrates an old left posterior cerebral artery distribution infarct, with dilatation of the left lateral ventricle and marked volume loss. Conventional angiographic anteroposterior view of the left vertebral artery injection (C) confirms the occlusion of the left posterior cerebral artery at its origin.**

A similar appearance to the distal basilar artery on the anteroposterior maximum intensity projection view might also occur when there is a prominant posterior communicating artery or fetal origin of the posterior cerebral artery from the internal carotid artery, which supplies the posterior cerebral artery distribution. In these instances, examination of the base maximum intensity projection view allows identification of the normal variants.

## CASE 112
## DISTAL VERTEBRAL ARTERY STENOSIS

**History:** 56-year-old with right-sided facial numbness and right-sided hearing loss.

**Technique:** axial volume; three-dimensional time-of-flight; 45/7/20; 256 × 256; 64 slices; 60-mm slab; magnetization transfer background suppression; tilted, optimized nonsaturating excitation radiofrequency pulse; 12-cm field of view; 12:20.

A

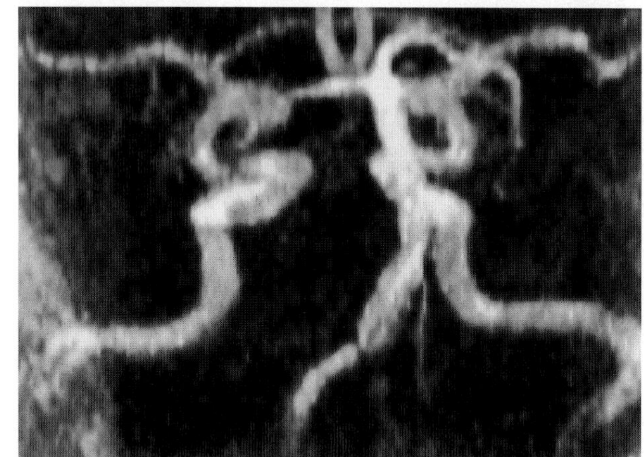

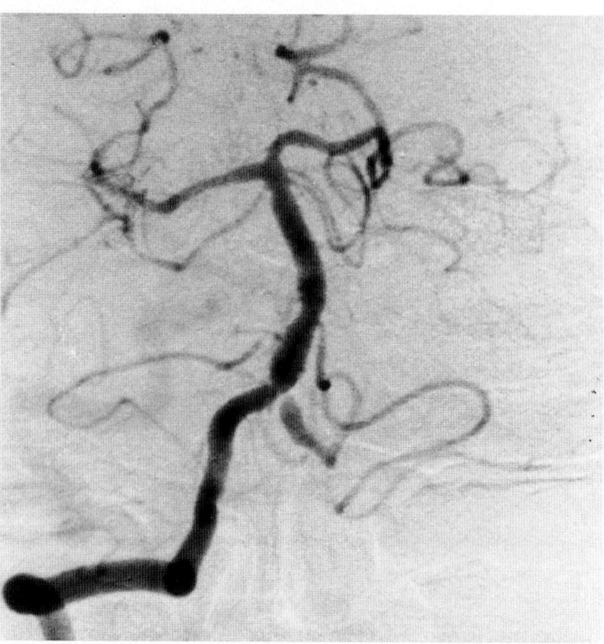

B

**Water's-like maximum intensity projection view (A) demonstrates a shelflike severe stenosis involving the junction of the right vertebral artery and the basilar artery. The remainder of the basilar artery is widely patent. A large inferior cerebellar artery is present on the left. A small amount of signal is seen within the distal left vertebral artery, which is consistent with severe stenosis at the junction of the left vertebral and the basilar arteries. This small amount of signal could be manifested by slow antegrade flow within the left vertebral artery or retrograde flow from the right vertebral artery. The anteroposterior view of a right vertebral artery injection (B) demonstrates severe stenosis involving the junction of the right vertebral and basilar arteries as well as a severe stenosis of the distal left vertebral artery. There is retrograde flow from the right vertebral artery down the left vertebral artery and subsequent filling of the left posterior inferior cerebellar artery. There is sufficient saturation effects on the MRA that the patent left posterior inferior cerebellar artery is not visualized.**

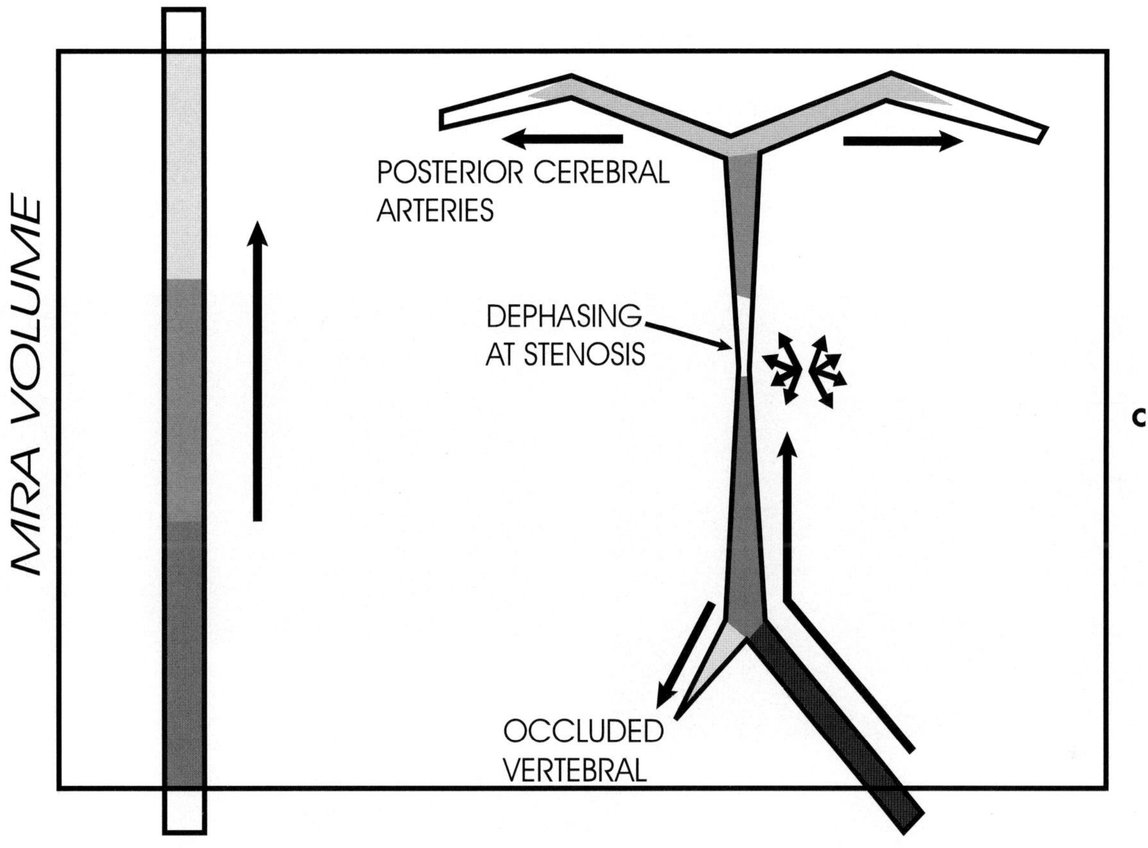


**Saturation effects (C). The normal signal intensity of a vessel traveling perpendicular to an axial time-of-flight volume MRA gradually decreases because of saturation effects (left side). With the posterior circulation, the anatomy makes this effect more complex (right side). Occlusion of a vertebral artery may allow retrograde filling, which would increase the saturation effects on this segment. A stenosis of the basilar may decrease vascular signal enough to obscure or limit the amount of flow-related enhancement of the posterior cerebral arteries, limiting their visibility.**

## CASE 113
## BASILAR ARTERY STENOSES

**History:** 74-year-old with vertigo.

**Technique:** axial volume; three-dimensional time-of-flight; 45/7/20; 256 × 256; magnetization transfer background suppression; tilted, optimized non-saturating excitation radiofrequency pulse; 12-cm field of view; 12:20.

A

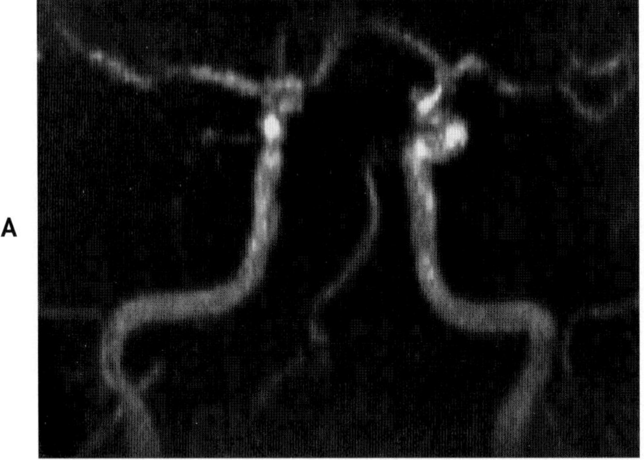

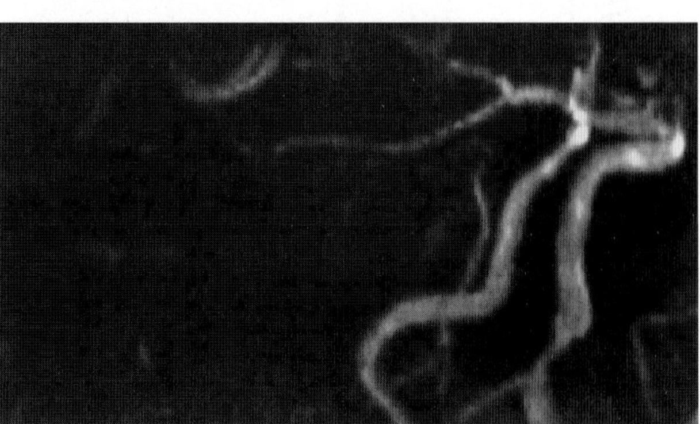

B

C

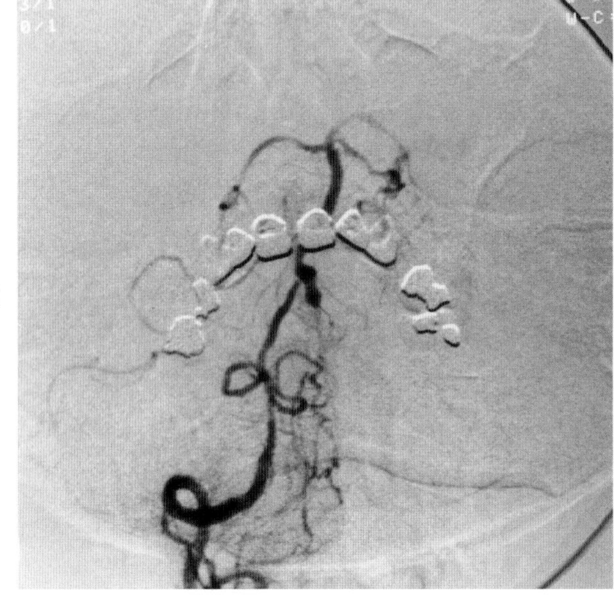

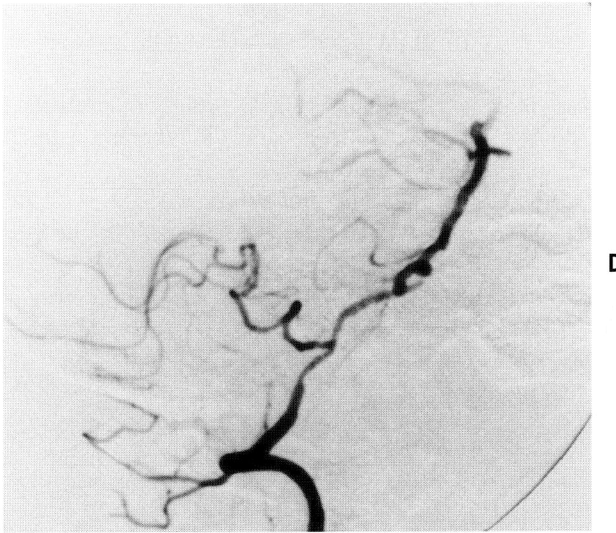


**Anteroposterior (A) and lateral (B) views from the maximum intensity projection demonstrate a markedly narrowed and irregular vertebrobasilar system. There is no flow seen within the left vertebral artery. The right vertebral artery is quite small, and there is a severe stenosis at the junction of the right vertebral and the basilar arteries. The basilar artery itself is very small. No appreciable flow is seen extending into the posterior cerebral arteries. Anteroposterior (C) and lateral (D) angiographic views from a right vertebral artery injection confirm the severe stenosis at the junction of the right vertebral artery and the basilar artery, as well as occlusion of the left vertebral artery. There is slight retrograde flow down the most distal aspect of the left vertebral artery. The basilar artery is diffusely small. There is marked irregularity of the proximal P1 segments bilaterally, which is not visualized on the MRA because of flow saturation.**

The time-of-flight MRA technique is pushed to the limits of its ability in cases such as this, with long segments of diffuse and more focal stenoses. The diffuse nature of the disease produces slowed flow, which allows flow saturation and signal loss. This flow saturation is the reason that the posterior cerebral arteries are not visualized.

## CASE 114
## FOCAL BASILAR STENOSIS

**History:** 78-year-old with incapacitating ataxia, posterior circulation transient ischemic attacks, and maximal anticoagulation therapy with coumadin.

**Technique:** axial volume; three-dimensional time-of-flight; 45/7/20; 256 × 256; magnetization transfer background suppression; tilted, optimized nonsaturating excitation radiofrequency pulse; 14-cm field of view; 12:20.

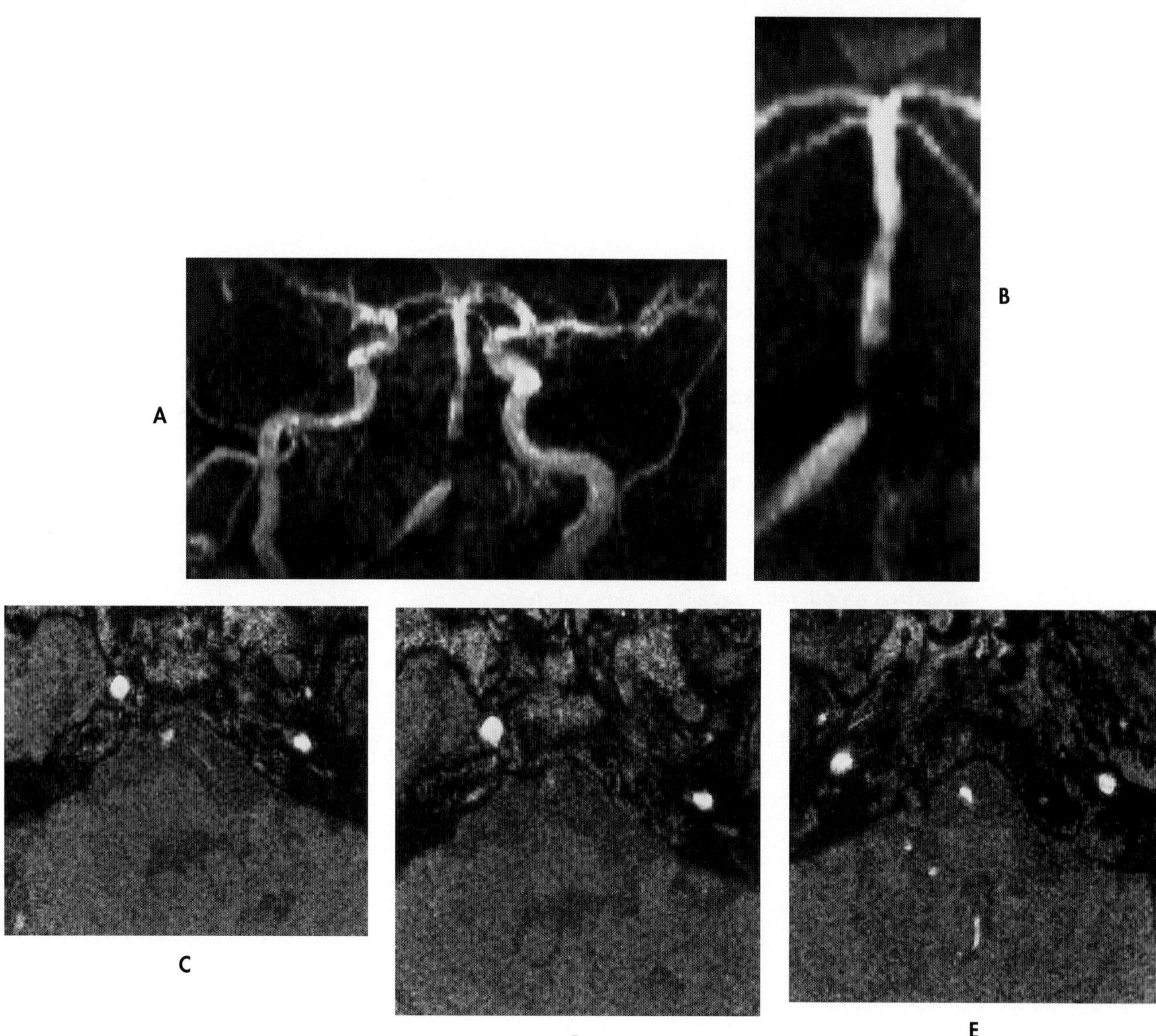

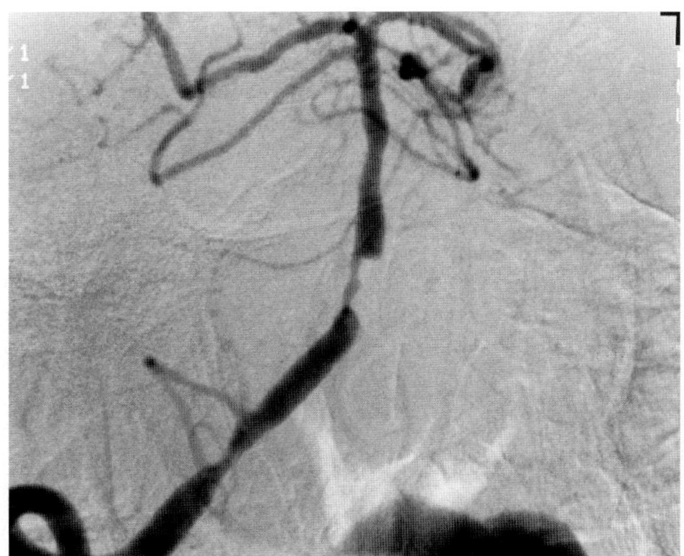

F

**Whole head maximum intensity projection (A) shows an absent left vertebral artery, severe stenosis of the right vertebral artery, and apparent discontinuity of the proximal basilar artery. Targeted anteroposterior maximum intensity projection shows that this is a severe eccentric stenosis with a threadlike lumen (B). Individual slices from the MRA also demonstrate the severity of the stenosis with good vascular signal above (C) and below (E) the focal stenosis but with loss of signal at the level of the severe stenosis (D). Conventional angiogram, right anterior oblique view from a right vertebral injection (F) demonstrates a concentric stenosis of the right vertebral artery and eccentric stenosis of the basilar artery. The left vertebral artery (not shown) was occluded, as shown in the MRA. The patient underwent basilar artery angioplasty with a good clinical result, which is demonstrated on the follow-up MRA 2 days after angioplasty (G).**

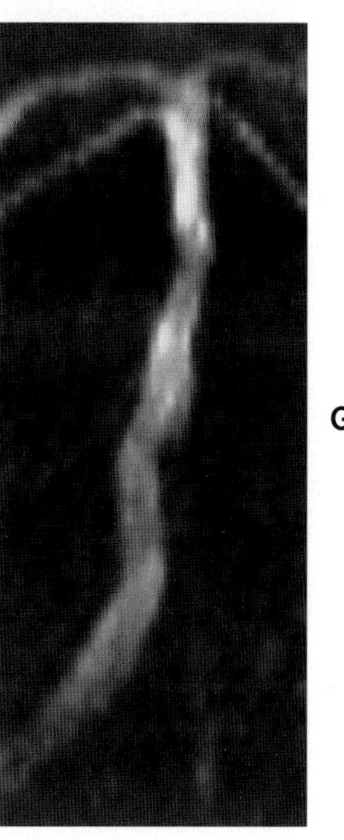

G

MRA is an easy and noninvasive means of follow-up in patients who have undergone interventional vascular procedures, as seen here. MRA was able to precisely define the severe stenosis in this patient and maintain a good signal-to-noise ratio, despite the acceleration of flow that must occur across this stenosis.

#### REFERENCE

Ahuja A, Guterman LR, Hopkins LN: Angioplasty for basilar artery atherosclerosis, *J Neurosurg* 77:941-944, 1992.

## CASE 115
## BASILAR ARTERY STENOSIS

**History:** 62-year-old with vertigo.

**Technique:** axial volume, three-dimensional time-of-flight, 45/7/20, 512 × 160, 64 slices, 60-mm slab, 24-cm field of view (rectangular), 7:43.

A

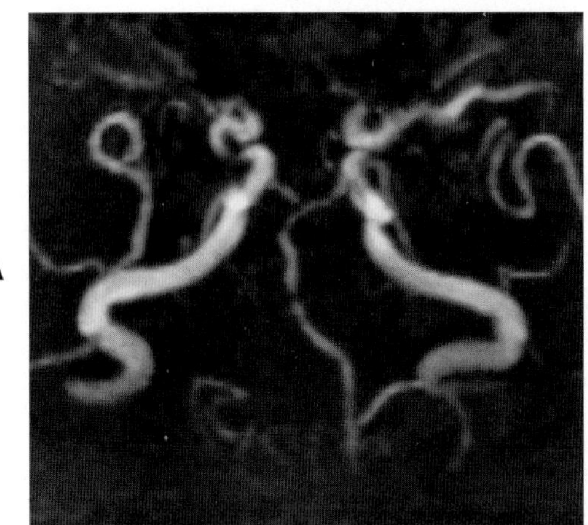

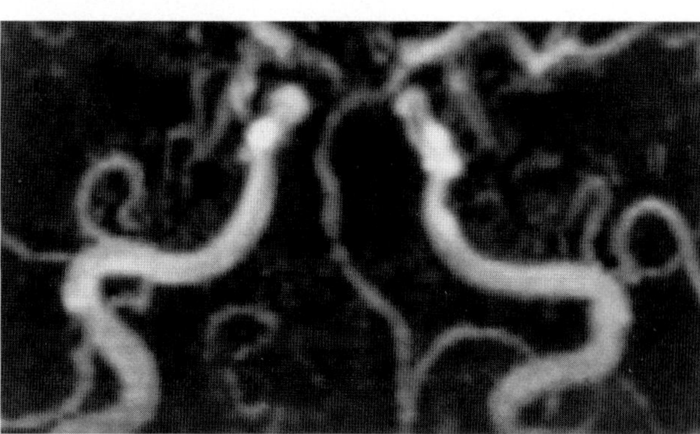

B

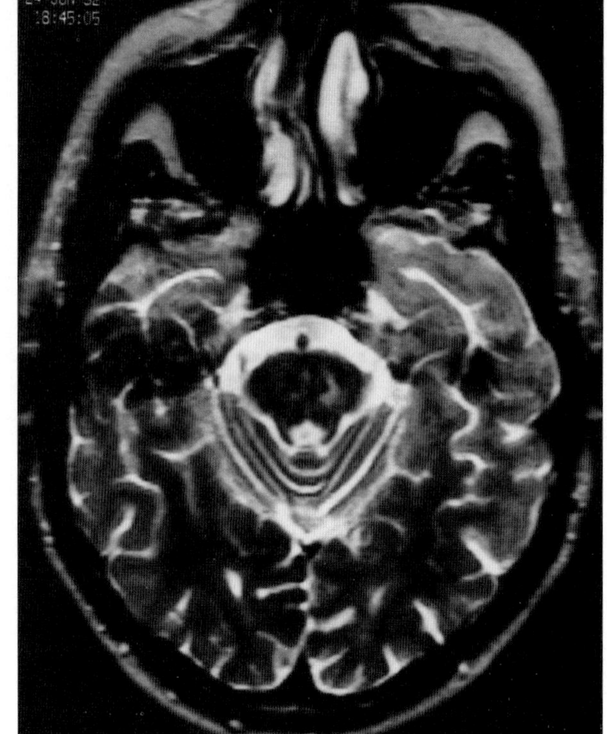


C

**Base (A) and anteroposterior (B) maximum intensity projection views demonstrate diffuse atherosclerotic change in the anterior and posterior circulations. Of particular significance, given the clinical history, is the diffusely small and irregular vertebrobasilar system with threadlike distal basilar and posterior cerebral arteries. Severe narrowing is also seen within both carotid siphons. The diminished signal intensity within the right middle cerebral artery is related to the edge of the MRA volume and not to stenosis or slowed flow. Axial T2-weighted image of the brain (C) shows a small infarct within the left side of the pons.**

The patient was placed on anticoagulation therapy and did well, and the conventional angiogram was not requested. The prognosis of vertebrobasilar stroke is related to the location and nature of the vascular abnormality, which reflects the particular vascular anatomy present. For instance, acute basilar thrombosis has a poor prognosis because of thrombus in the basilar artery that may propagate or fragment, causing extensive infarction. A pontine lacunar infarct has a more benign outcome, since it reflects a completed stroke involving only one perforating vessel. Gillilan described four anatomic zones in the brainstem, based on the microvascular anatomy of penetrating vessels: (1) median, (2) paramedian, (3) lateral, and (4) dorsal. These terminal distributions tend to be quite constant from brain to brain compared to the wider variability of the larger vessels such as posterior cerebral arteries. For example, since the motor pathways are confined to near the midline, brainstem motor symptoms generally involve the median zone except for the top of the basilar infarctions, which have characteristic features. *Top-of-the-basilar syndrome* was a name coined by Caplan to distinguish as a separate clinical group the ischemic changes of the rostal basilar artery. The clinical signs include a variety of visual, oculomotor, and behavioral abnormalities, with motor disturbances being less prominent. Caplan postulated embolic occlusion as a major cause of the syndrome.

Nadeau et al classified 57 vertebrobasilar strokes into three groups based on computed tomographic and clinical findings: single-zone, multizone, and top-of-the-basilar groups. They looked at survival rates. Single-zone and top-of-the-basilar strokes had a relatively benign prognosis, with 71% to 73% having 3-year survival rates and 64% of the multizone patients dying within 2 months of ictus. Other studies (Currier et al) have also shown that single-zone infarcts, such as lateral medullary infarcts, have a benign early course (77% having a 2-year survival rate).

#### REFERENCES


Gillilan LA: The correlation of the blood supply to the human brain stem with clinical brainstem lesions, *J Neuropathol Exp Neurol* 23:73-108, 1964.

Caplan LR: Top of the basilar syndrome, *Neurology* 30:72-79, 1980.

Barkhof F, Valk J: Top of the basilar syndrome: a comparison of clinical and MR findings, *Neuroradiology* 30:293-298, 1988.

Currier RD, Giles CL, Westerberg MR: The prognosis of some brainstem vascular syndromes, *Neurology* 8:664-668, 1958.

Nadeau S, Jordon J, Mishra S: Clinical presentation as a guide to early prognosis in vertebrobasilar stroke, *Stroke* 23(2):165-170, 1992.

## CASE 116
## BASILAR ARTERY STENOSIS WITH POSTERIOR CIRCULATION INFARCTS

**History:** 68-year-old with right-sided homonymous hemianopsia.

**Technique:** axial volume, three-dimensional time-of-flight, 45/7/20, 512 × 160, 64 slices, 60-mm slab, 24-cm field of view (rectangular), 7:43.

A

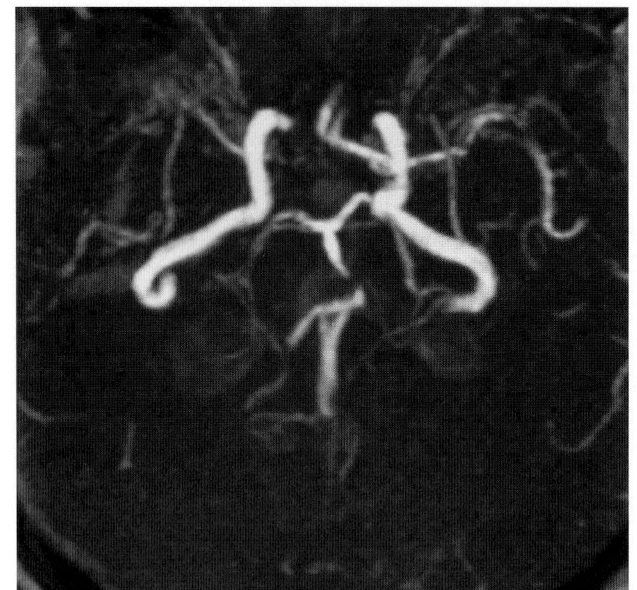

B

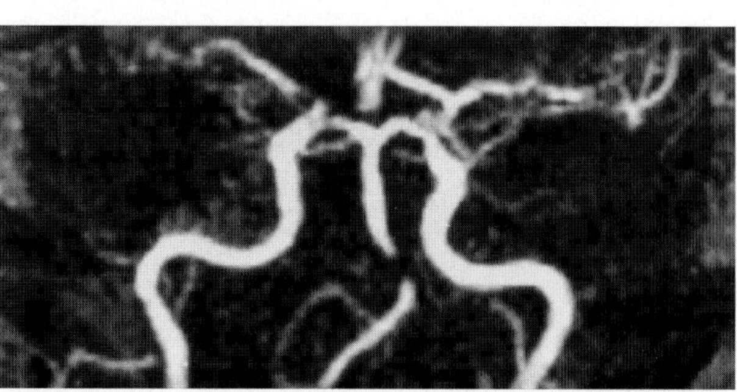

C

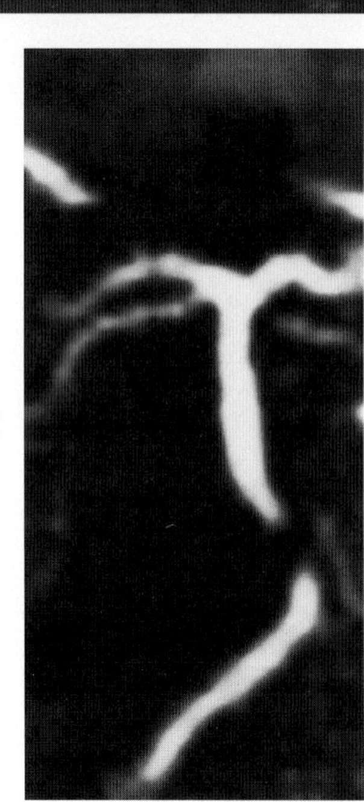

D

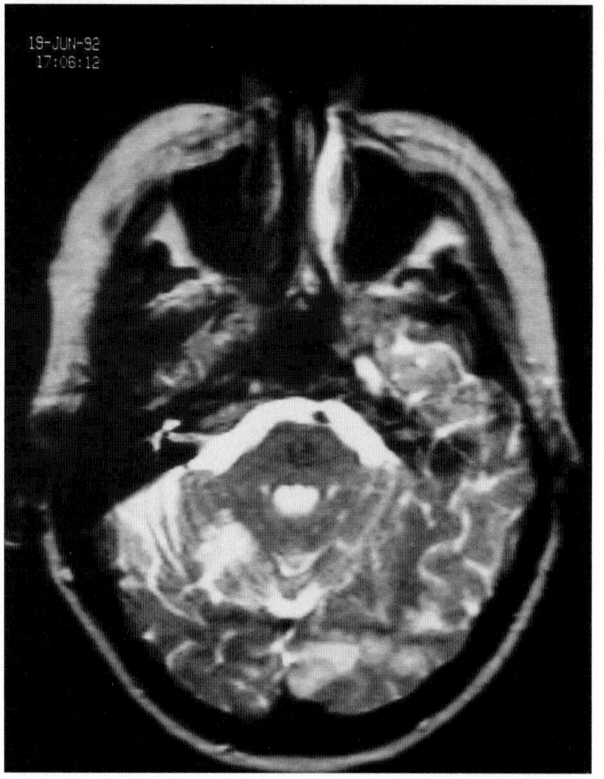


**Base (A) and anteroposterior (B) views from the maximum intensity projection demonstrate a severe focal stenosis involving the junction of the right vertebral and the basilar arteries. The left vertebral artery is occluded. The distal basilar artery shows good signal intensity, as do the posterior cerebral arteries. The targeted maximum intensity projection view shows the basilar stenosis to better advantage (C). Axial T2-weighted image (D) demonstrates an infarct involving the left posterior cerebral distribution (left occipital lobe) and the right superior cerebellar artery distribution.**

Cerebellar infarction represents only 1.5% of strokes. Cerebellar infarctions tend to present with two clinical presentations depending on the vascular distribution involved. Posterior inferior cerebellar artery infarcts present with a triad of vertigo, headache, and gait imbalance and produce mass effect and hydrocephalus. This postinfarct mass effect may lead to brainstem compression and death in approximately 20% of cases. The "classic" superior cerebellar artery syndrome results from infarction of the superior cerebellum and lateral tegmental pons and consists of ipsilateral limb ataxia, Horner's syndrome, and choreic dyskinesia with contralateral thermoanalgesia. However, this complete type of infarct is quite uncommon, and most superior cerebellar artery infarcts are partial. These partial infarcts produce predominantly gain and limb ataxia and vertigo and headaches less commonly and have a rather benign course. Poor outcome with these infarcts usually relates to accompanying brainstem infarcts from distal basilar occlusion or the presence of multiple supratentorial and infratentorial infarcts.

**REFERENCES**

Kase CS, Norrving B, Levine SR et al: Cerebellar infarction: clinical and anatomic observations in 66 cases, *Stroke* 24:76-83, 1993.

Amarenco P, Hauw JJ: Cerebellar infarction in the territory of the superior cerebellar artery: a clinicopathologic study of 33 cases, *Neurology* 40:1383-1390, 1990.

Macdonell RAL, Kalnins RM, Donnan GA: Cerebellar infarction: natural history, prognosis, and pathology, *Stroke* 18:849-855, 1987.

## CASE 117
## BASILAR STENOSIS

**History:** 56-year-old with intermittent dizziness and nystagmus.

**Technique:** axial volume; three-dimensional time-of-flight; 45/7/20; 256 × 256; magnetization transfer background suppression; tilted, optimized non-saturating excitation radiofrequency pulse; 14-cm field of view; 12:20.

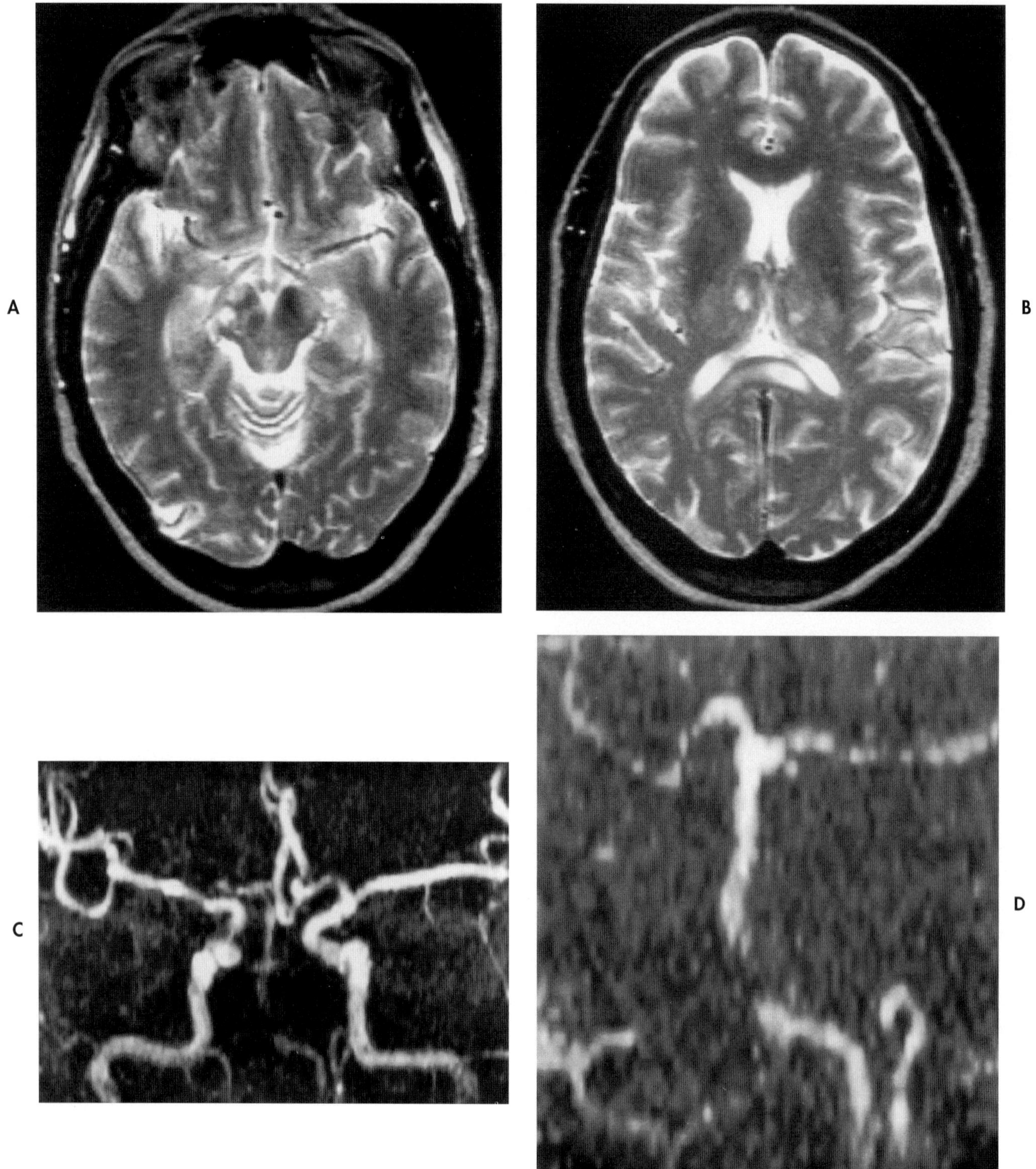

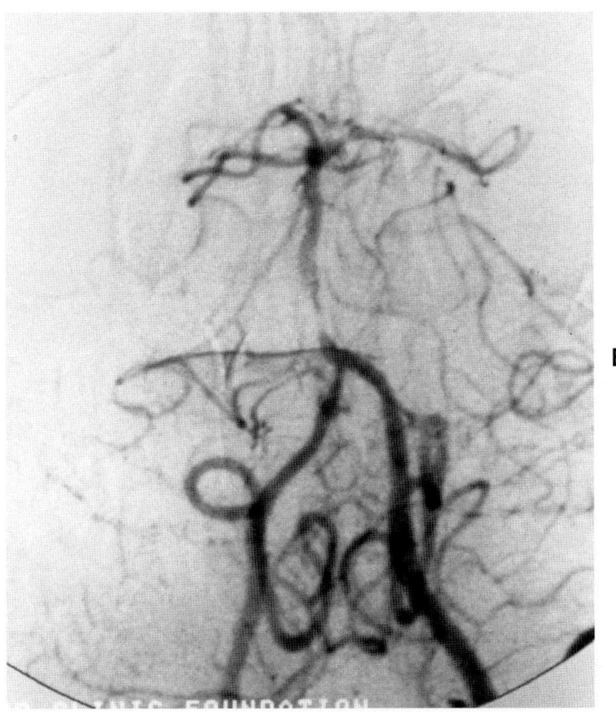

E

**Axial T2-weighted images of the brain show small infarcts involving the thalami, the right cerebral peduncle, and the splenium of the corpus callosum (A and B). Whole head anteroposterior maximum intensity projection (C) demonstrates an extremely small and irregular-appearing vertebral basilar system. Targeted maximum intensity projection (D) also shows a very small distal right vertebral artery and a severe stenosis involving the junction of the vertebral and basilar arteries. This is a marked stenosis, since there is complete loss of signal intensity at the stenotic site. Conventional angiographic Water's view of the left vertebral artery injection (E) confirms the severe stenosis involving the proximal basilar artery, with slow distal flow. There is pronounced retrograde filling of the distal right vertebral artery related to proximal right vertebral stenosis (not shown).**

The right vertebral artery appears small on the MRA because of flow saturation effects resulting from the long course that the spins are taking, antegrade up the left vertebral artery and then retrograde down the right vertebral artery. Complex, turbulent and accelerated flow at the site of the basilar stenosis causes the slight overestimation on the MRA.

# CASE 118
# BASILAR ARTERY OCCLUSION

**History:** 67-year-old with ataxia and dysarthria.

**Technique:** axial volume, three-dimensional time-of-flight, 40/7/15, 256 × 256, 64 slices, 60-mm slab, 25-cm field of view, 10:57.

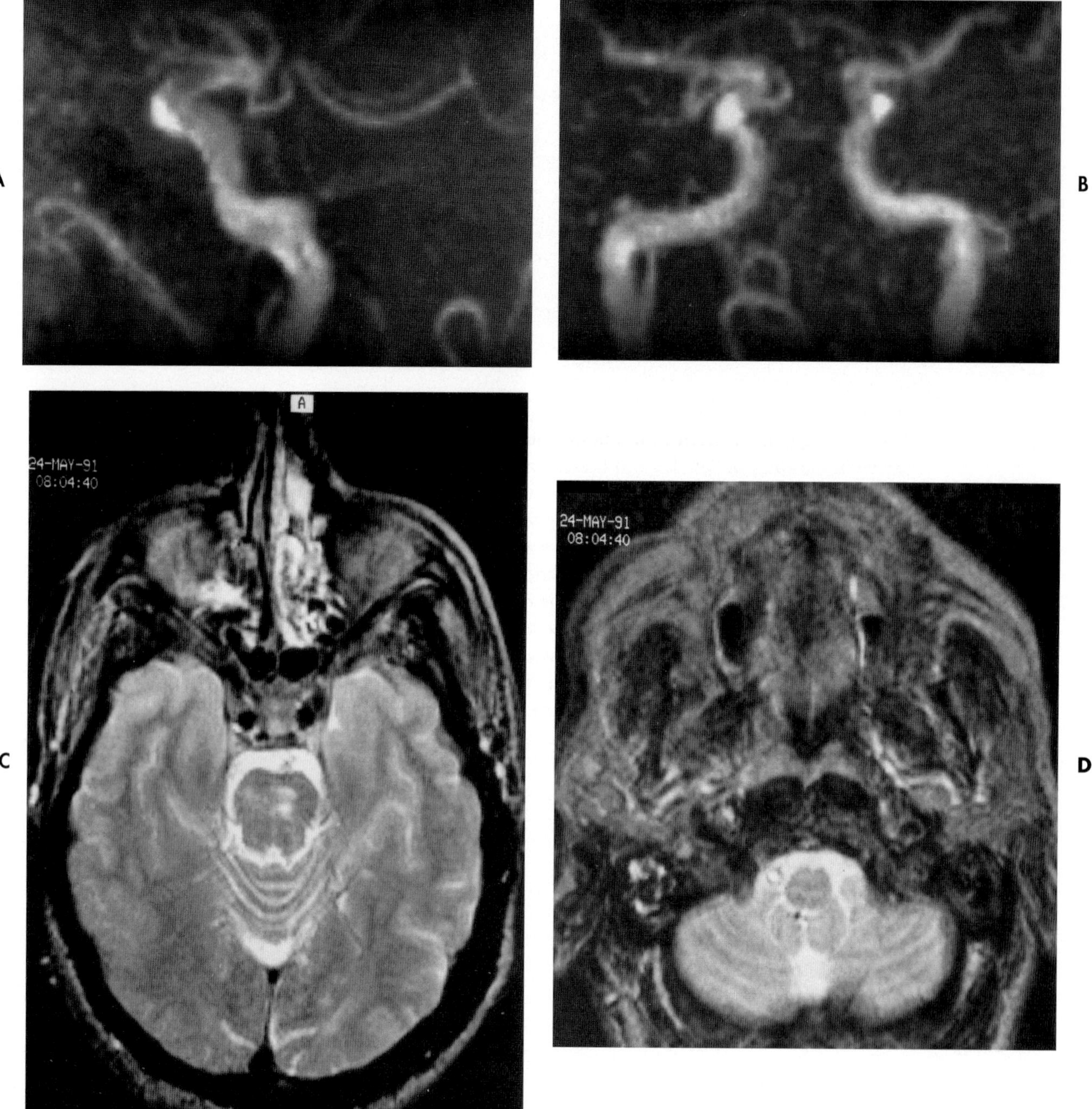

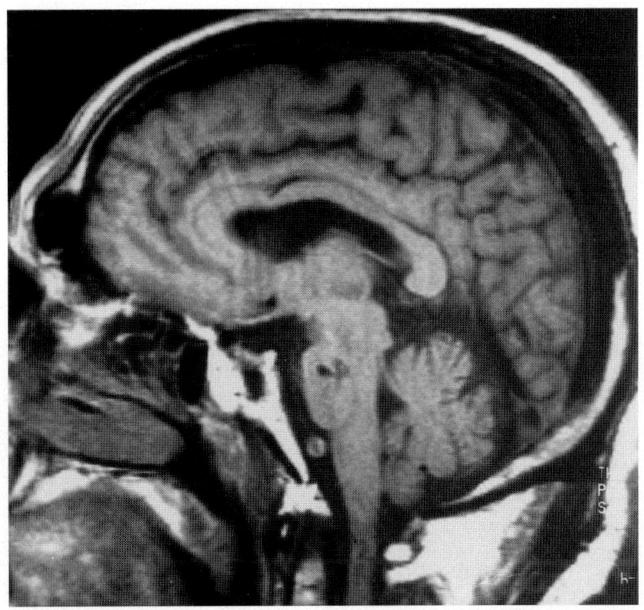

E

**Lateral (A) and anteroposterior (B) views from the maximum intensity projection demonstrate essentially no signal intensity from the basilar or right vertebral arteries. The internal carotid arteries appear widely patent bilaterally, and flow is seen through the posterior communicating arteries to the posterior cerebral arteries. Occlusion of the right vertebral and basilar arteries is further confirmed by the axial T2-weighted images of the brain (C). At the level of the carotid siphons, there is no flow void involving the basilar artery. Note also the infarct involving the upper pons. A more caudal T2-weighted image (D) shows abnormal high signal intensity within the occluded right vertebral artery. An additional sagittal T1-weighted image (E) shows abnormal increased signal intensity thrombus within the inferior basilar artery. The infarct within the upper pons is again identified.**

The clinical signs of basilar artery occlusion and stenosis may be identical, and because of this, MR imaging and MRA are ideally suited to make that diagnostic distinction. Caplan reported six patients who survived basilar artery occlusion and noted that the outcome of basilar occlusion is variable. Some patients survive with little or no neurologic deficit, whereas others are severely disabled or die. Most infarctions are preceded by transient ischemic attack symptoms within 1 month of the final stroke. Outcome appears to critically depend on the development of adequate collateral circulation and the presence of distal embolization as well as location.

### REFERENCE

Caplan LR: Occlusion of the vertebral or basilar artery: follow up analysis of some patients with benign outcome, *Stroke* 10:277-282, 1979.

## CASE 119
## BASILAR OCCLUSION AND INCIDENTAL ABERRANT INTERNAL CAROTID ARTERY

**History:** 41-year-old with transient left-sided weakness.

**Technique:** axial volume; three-dimensional time-of-flight; 45/7/20; 512 × 160; magnetization transfer background suppression; tilted, optimized non-saturating excitation radiofrequency pulse; 24-cm field of view (rectangular); 7:42.

A

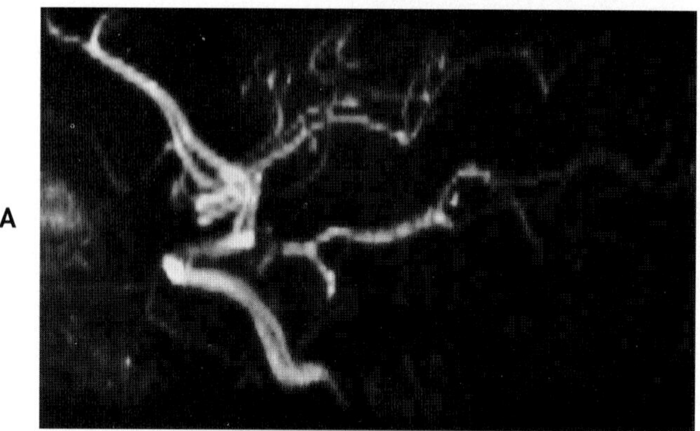

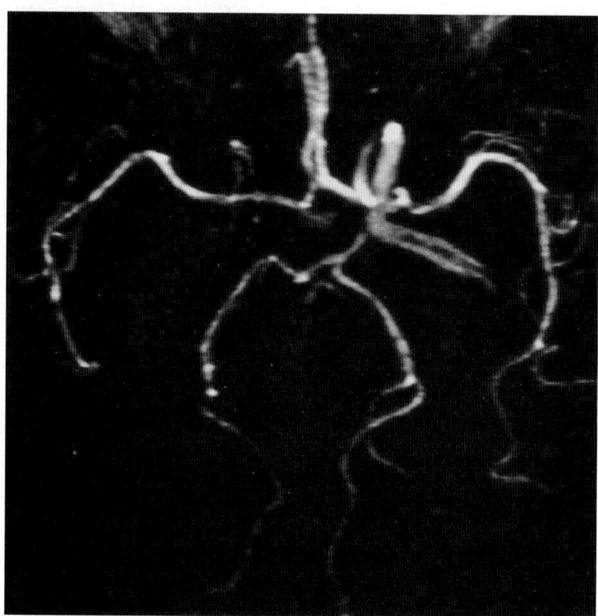

B

C

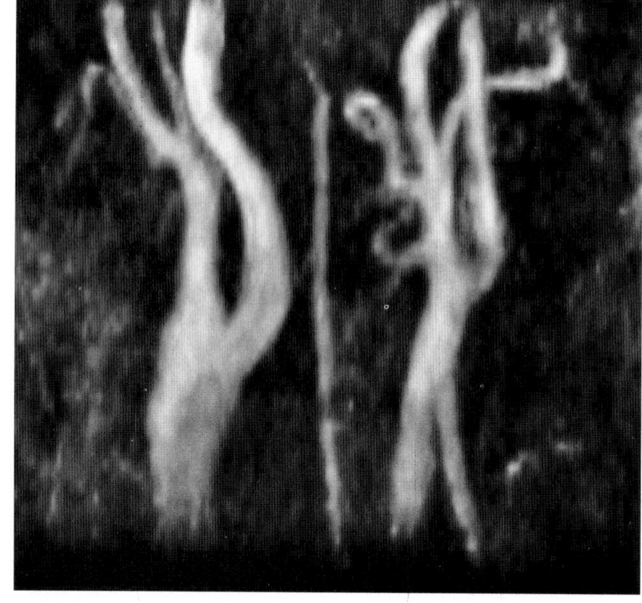

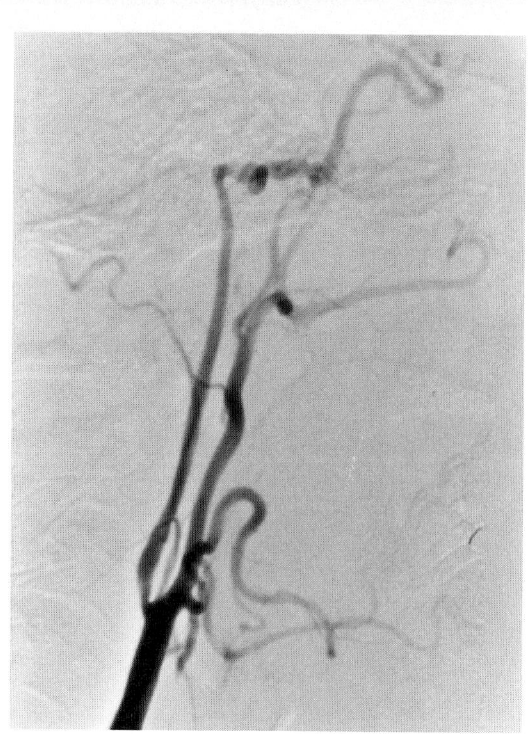

D

E

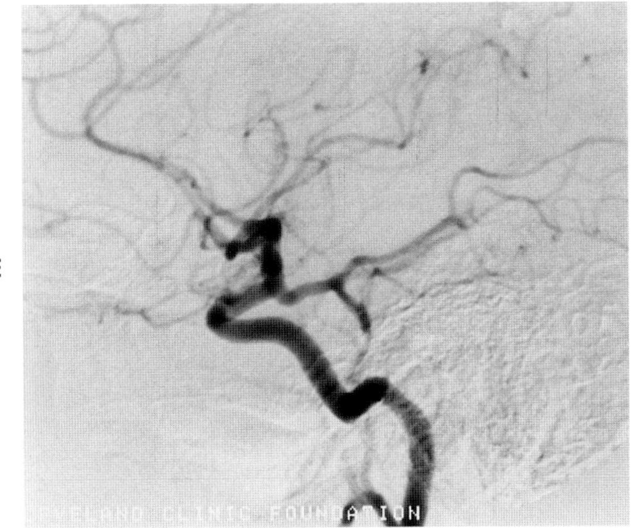

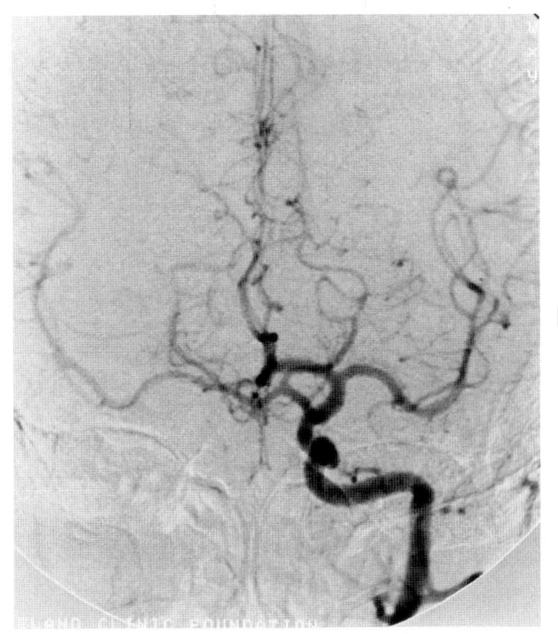

F

**Lateral (A) and base (B) maximum intensity projection views show that the proximal basilar and distal vertebral arteries are not visualized and that the posterior circulation is supplied by a large left posterior communicating artery with good flow signal intensity within the proximal basilar and posterior cerebral arteries bilaterally. This pattern is due to occlusion of the proximal basilar artery, with collateral flow being supplied via the posterior communicating artery from the anterior circulation. In addition, there is markedly decreased signal from the right internal carotid artery. This finding is suspicious for a proximal severe stenosis of the carotid bifurcation, with resultant flow saturation related to slow distal internal carotid artery flow. Oblique maximum intensity projection view of the carotid bifurcation (C) demonstrates a marked disparity in size between the normal-sized left carotid bifurcation and the small right bifurcation.**

These confusing findings are due to a congenitally aberrant and slightly hypoplastic right internal carotid artery, which simulates the appearance of a string sign on the intracranial three-dimensional time-of-flight study when combined with the occlusion of the inferior basilar artery. Conventional angiography of the right common carotid artery in the neck **(D)** and left common carotid artery anteroposterior **(E)** and lateral **(F)** intracranial views demonstrate the findings of an aberrant right internal carotid artery and occlusion of the basilar artery. There is filling of the basilar tip and posterior circulation via the posterior communicating artery. (See also Cases 28 and 29).

## CASE 120
## BASILAR ARTERY THROMBOSUS

**History:** 67-year-old with right hemiparesis and diplopia.

**Technique:** axial volume, three-dimensional time-of-flight, 40/7/15, 256 × 160, 64 slices, 60-mm slab, 20-cm field of view (rectangular), 6:53.

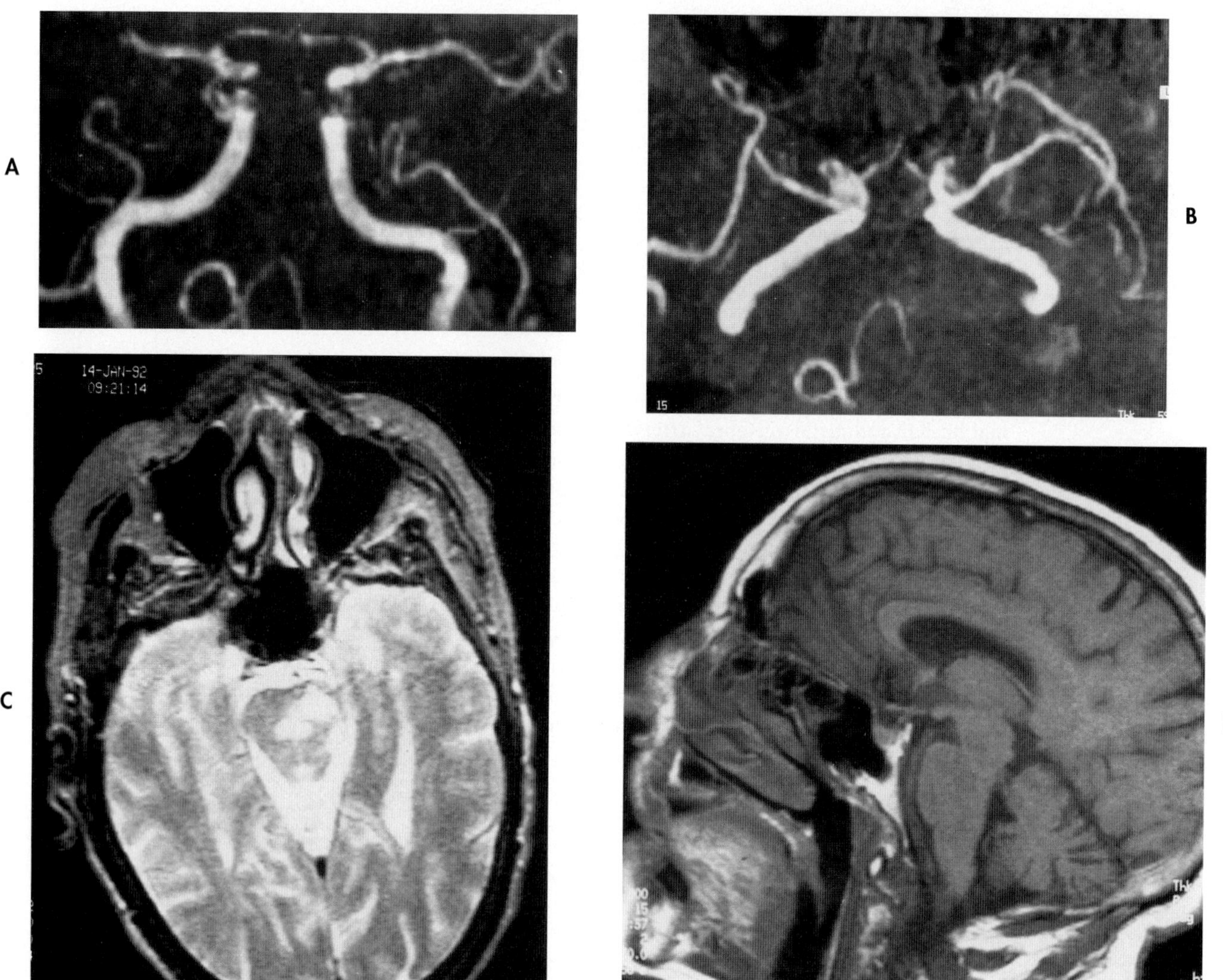

E 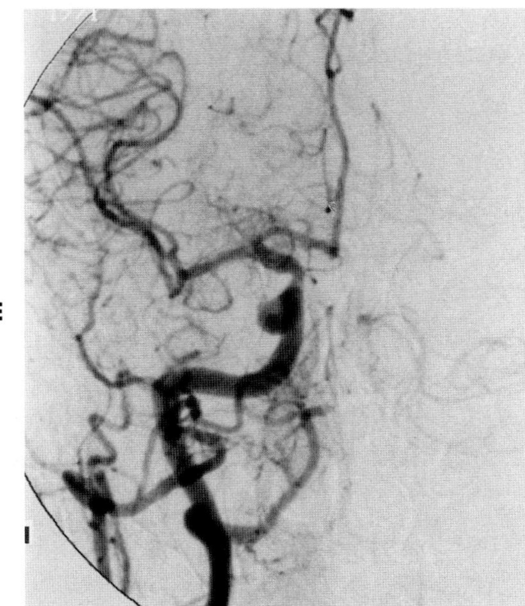

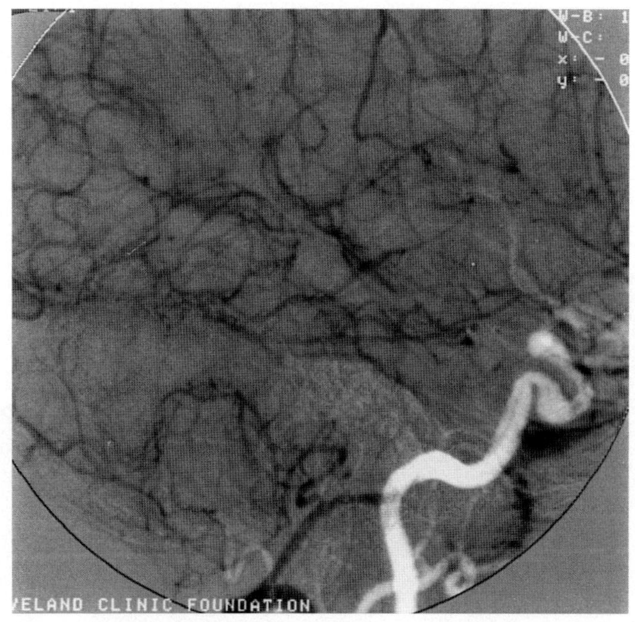

F

**Anteroposterior (A) and base maximum intensity projection (B) views demonstrate no signal within the left vertebral and basilar arteries because of occlusion. A large right posterior inferior cerebellar artery is identified. The lack of signal within the right middle cerebral artery relates to cutoff of the artery at the superior aspect of the imaging volume and does not represent a true occlusion. T2-weighted spin-echo image of the brain (C) demonstrates a large infarct involving the pons, with abnormal increased signal intensity thrombus seen within the basilar artery. Basilar artery thrombosis is further confirmed on the sagittal T1 image (D), which shows diffuse increased signal intensity throughout the basilar artery. Anteroposterior (E) and lateral (F) views of the conventional intraarterial angiogram demonstrate the patent right vertebral artery and the right posterior inferior cerebellar artery. There is no filling of the basilar artery, even on the delayed image, in the lateral projection. On the lateral view (F) the early arterial phase is displayed in white overlying the late arterial phase in black.**

## CASE 121
## VASCULITIS AND EARLY MOYAMOYA DISEASE

**History:** 7-year-old with previous left-sided hemorrhagic stroke.

**Technique:** axial volume, three-dimensional time-of-flight, 40/6/15, 256 × 160, 64 slices, 60-mm slab, 20-cm field of view (rectangular), 6:53.

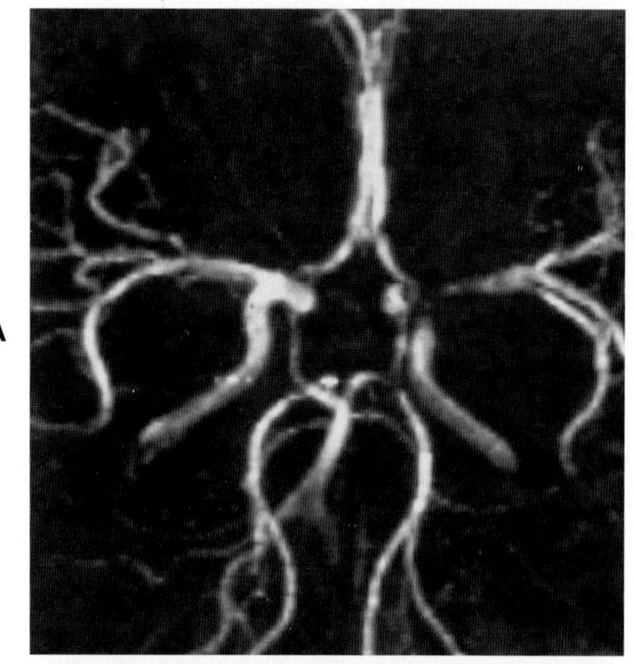

**A**

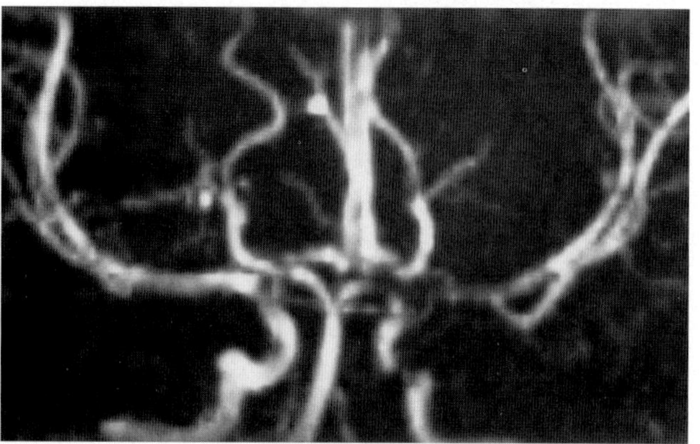

**B**

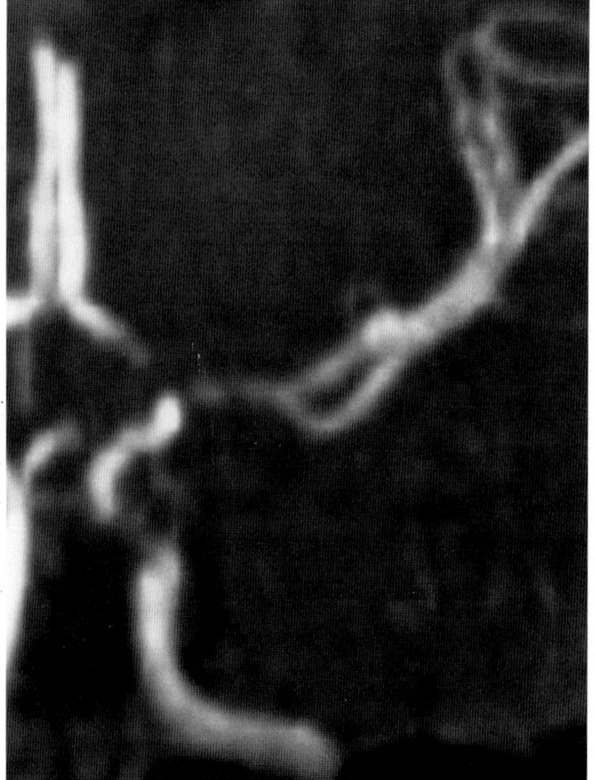

**C**

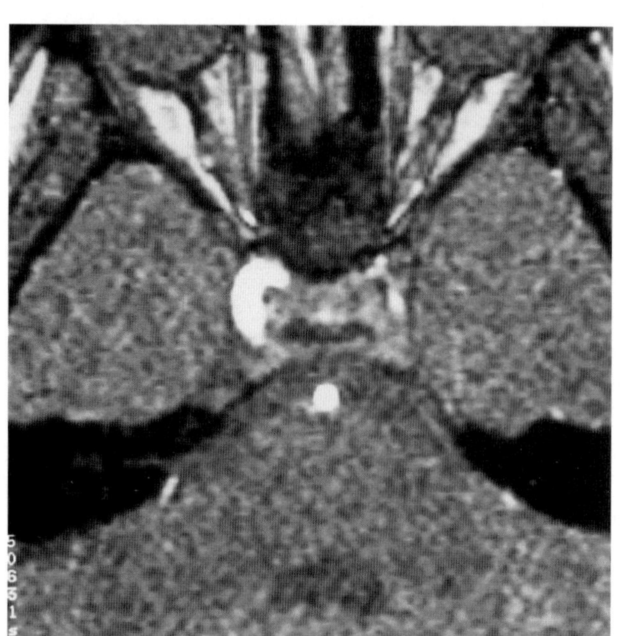

**D**

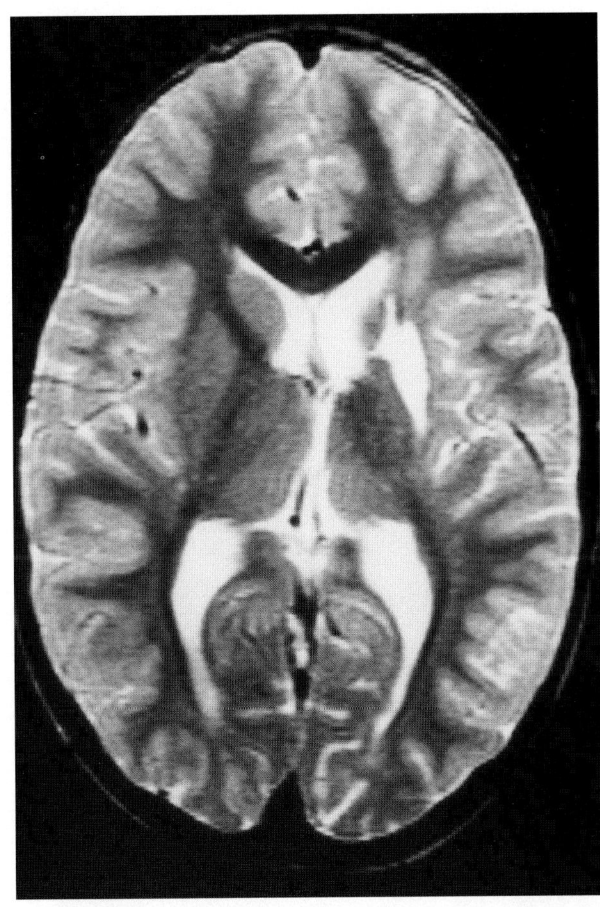


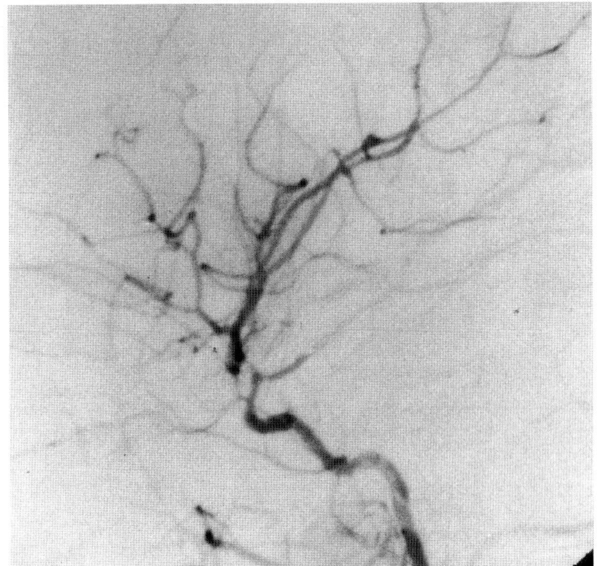


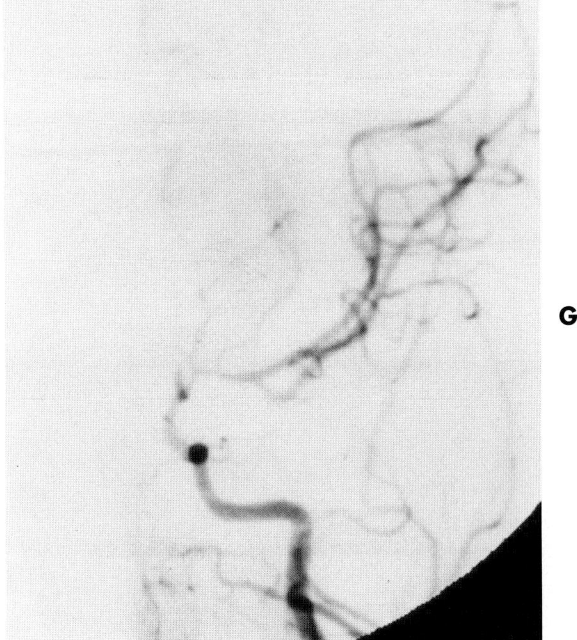


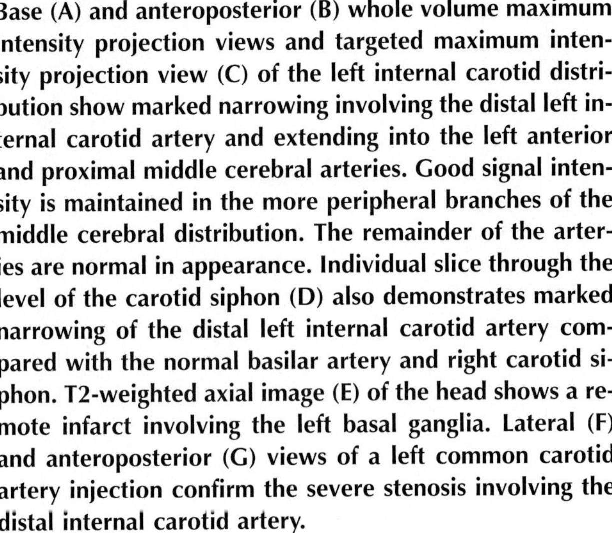
**Base (A) and anteroposterior (B) whole volume maximum intensity projection views and targeted maximum intensity projection view (C) of the left internal carotid distribution show marked narrowing involving the distal left internal carotid artery and extending into the left anterior and proximal middle cerebral arteries. Good signal intensity is maintained in the more peripheral branches of the middle cerebral distribution. The remainder of the arteries are normal in appearance. Individual slice through the level of the carotid siphon (D) also demonstrates marked narrowing of the distal left internal carotid artery compared with the normal basilar artery and right carotid siphon. T2-weighted axial image (E) of the head shows a remote infarct involving the left basal ganglia. Lateral (F) and anteroposterior (G) views of a left common carotid artery injection confirm the severe stenosis involving the distal internal carotid artery.**

The MRA has overestimated the degree of distal internal carotid and proximal middle cerebral stenosis. This occurs secondary to acceleration of blood flow through areas of stenoses, which is not compensated for by these sequences that have velocity compensation but not acceleration compensation. Additional dephasing occurs because of inplane flow and turbulent flow (i.e., higher-order motion terms). (See Case 125 for discussion of moyamoya disease.)

# CASE 122
# BASILAR ARTERY VASCULITIS

**History:** 40-year-old with headaches.

**Technique:** axial volume, three-dimensional time-of-flight, 27/7/15, 256 × 192, 128 slices, 120-mm slab, 20-cm field of view, 11:06.

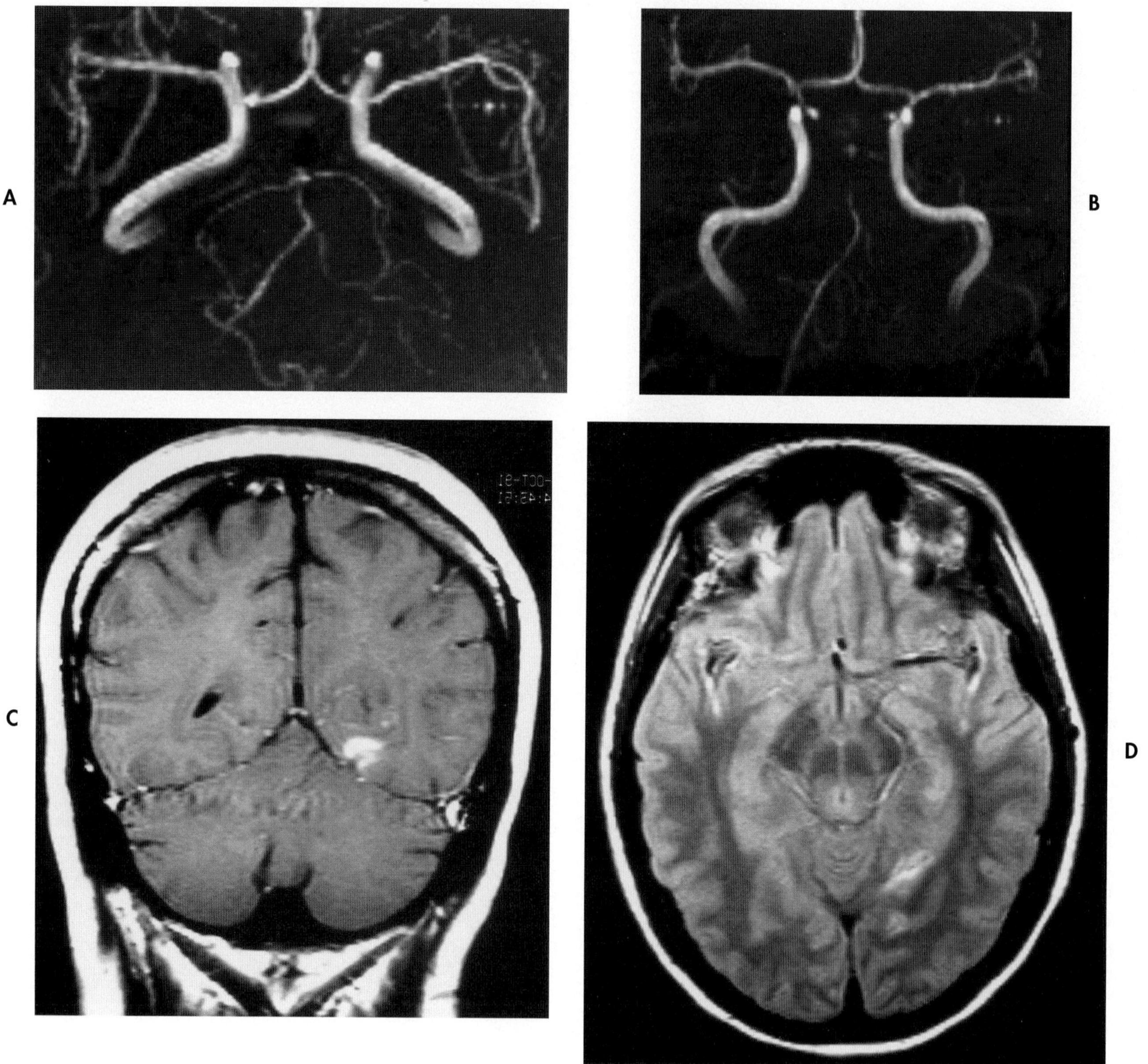

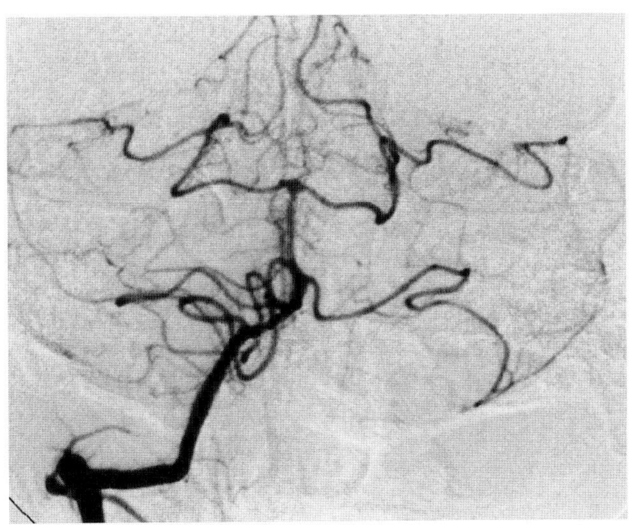


**Base (A) and Water's (B) maximum intensity projection views show marked narrowing involving the vertebral basilar system in a diffuse pattern. The most severe stenosis occurs in the distal third of the basilar artery. Note the apparent marked narrowing involving the origins of the posterior cerebral arteries bilaterally. Coronal enhanced T1-weighted image of the brain (C) and the axial spin-density image (D) show an enhancing small infarct involving the left posterior cerebral artery distribution. However, the conventional intraarterial angiogram (E) demonstrates that, although there is severe diffuse narrowing of the basilar artery concordant with the MRA findings, the arteries arising off the basilar tip are in fact the superior cerebellar arteries and not the posterior cerebral arteries (which are occluded). Blood supply to the posterior circulation was through leptomeningeal collaterals.**

The correct diagnosis of failure to visualize the posterior cerebral arteries on the MRA is possible by paying careful attention to the position of the pseudobasilar tip, which is positioned too inferior for normal anatomy.

### REFERENCE

Greenan TJ, Grossman RI, Goldberg HI: Cerebral vasculitis: MR imaging and angiographic correlation, *Radiology* 182:65-72, 1992.

## CASE 123
## VASCULITIS

**History:** 46-year-old with recent onset of debilitating headaches previously diagnosed as "cluster" type.

**Technique:** axial volume; three-dimensional time-of-flight; 45/7/20; 256 × 256; 64 slices; 60-mm slab; magnetization transfer background suppression; tilted, optimized nonsaturating excitation radiofrequency pulse; 14-cm field of view; 12:20.

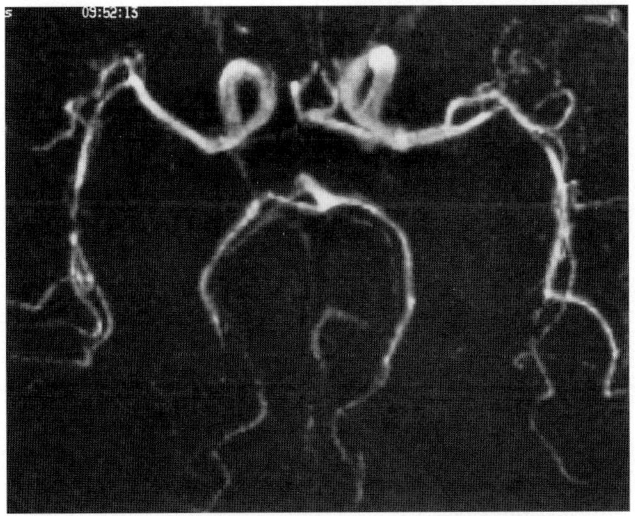


A

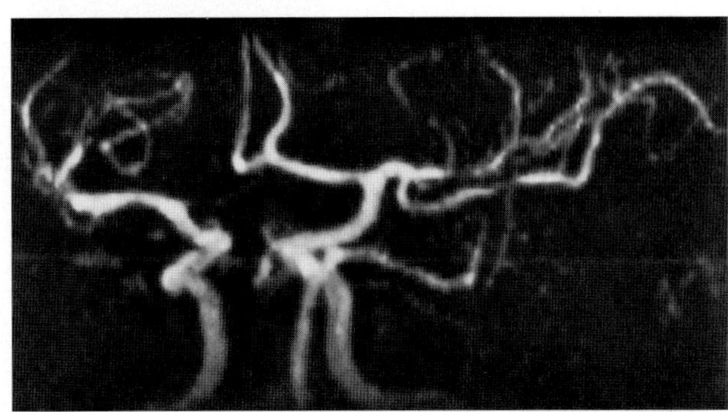

B

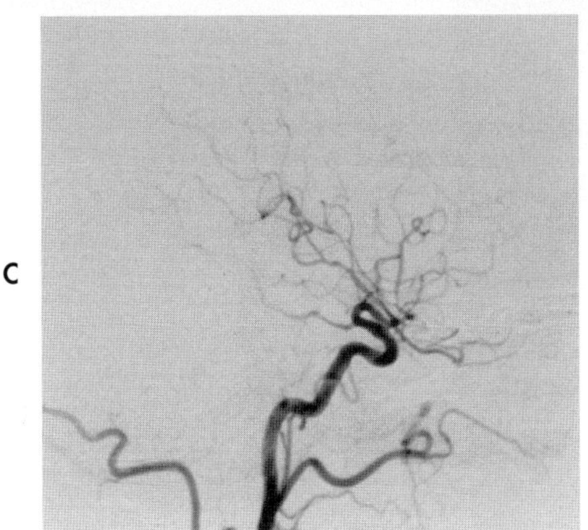

C

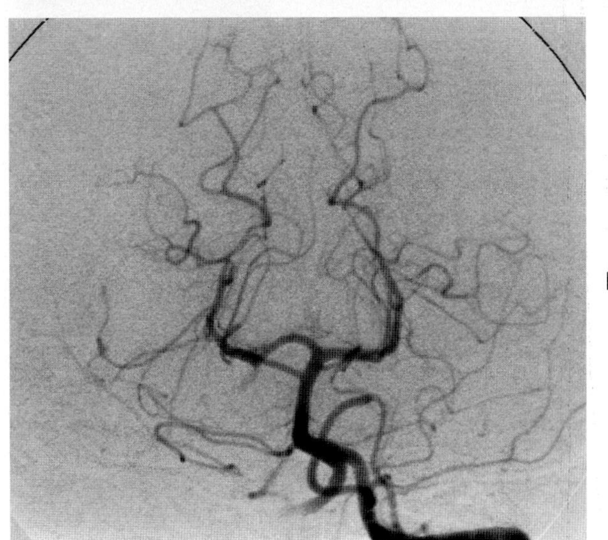

D

**Base (A) and right anterior oblique (B) maximum intensity projection views show narrowing of a branch of the middle cerebral artery on the right and an area of signal loss from the right posterior cerebral artery with "reconstitution" of signal from the more distal aspect. Conventional angiographic lateral view of a right common carotid injection (C) shows smooth concentric narrowing of a posterior middle cerebral branch. Town's view of a left vertebral artery injection (D) shows smooth concentric narrowing of the right distal posterior cerebral artery.**

The conventional angiographic findings are typical for vasculitis. However, the resolution of MRA is currently unable to depict subtle details of the morphologies of smaller vessel stenoses. For instance, in this case the MRA identified the areas of abnormality and directed the patient workup toward conventional angiography for a definitive diagnostic procedure. However, the MRA is incapable of distinguishing the appearance of intracranial atherosclerosis from that of vasculitis (i.e, focal and eccentric vs. smooth and concentric or "beaded").

## CASE 124
## DISTAL INTERNAL CAROTID STENOSIS RESULTING FROM VASCULITIS

**History:** 44-year-old being evaluated for right hemipheric transient ischemic attacks.

**Technique:** three-dimensional time-of-flight; 45/7/20 degrees; 256 × 256; magnetization transfer background suppression; tilted, optimized nonsaturating excitation radiofrequency pulse; 12-cm field of view; 12:20.

A

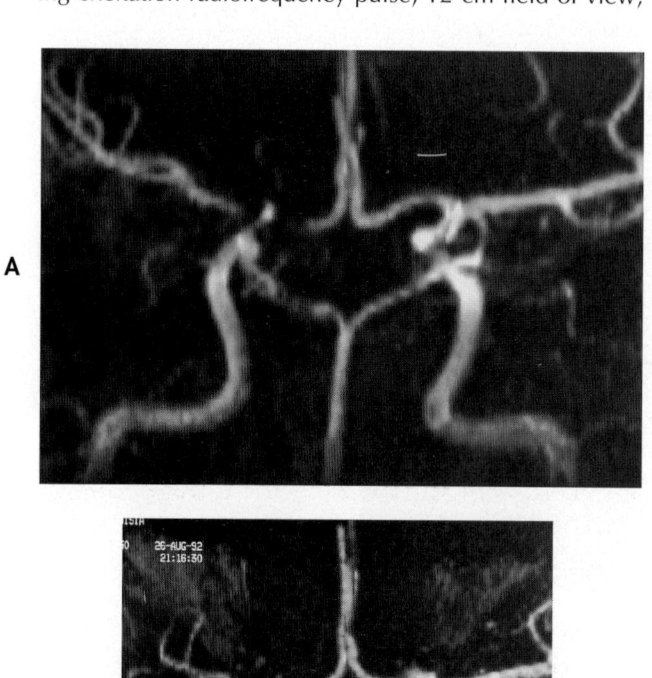

B

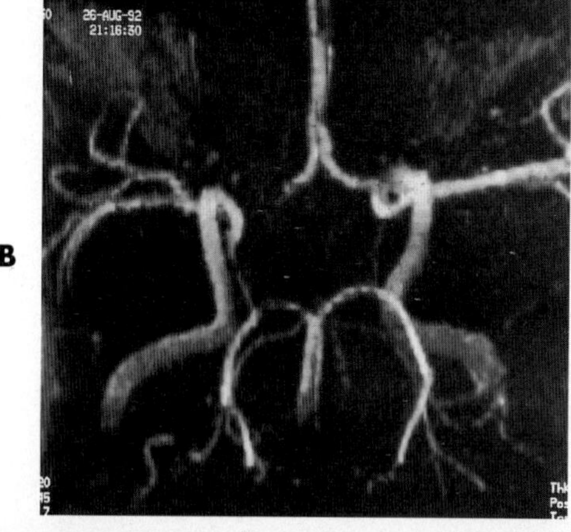


C

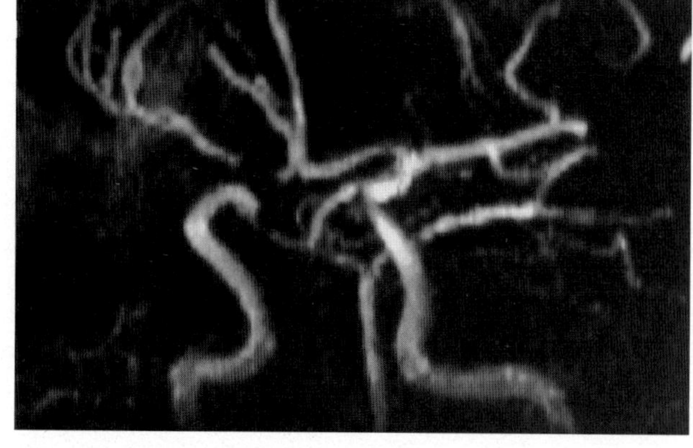

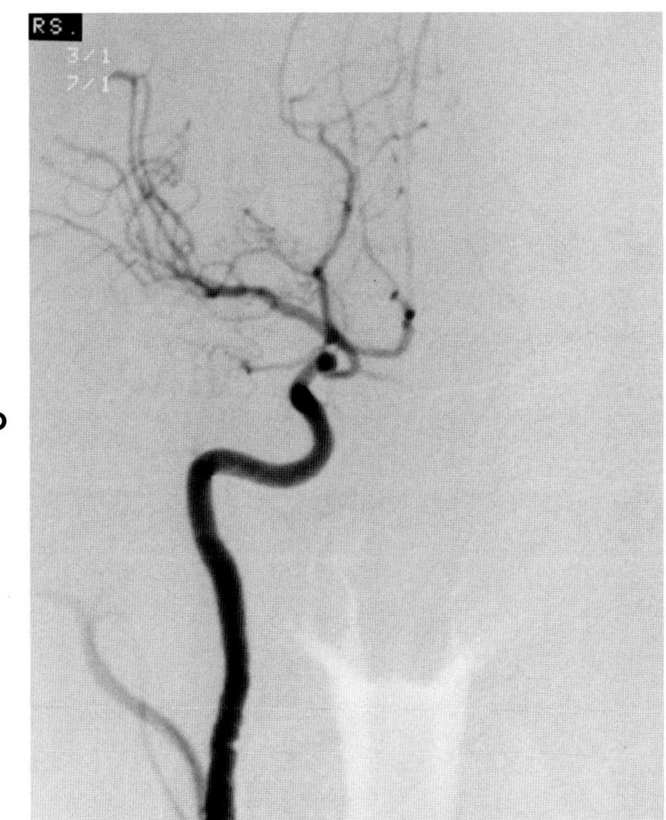


D

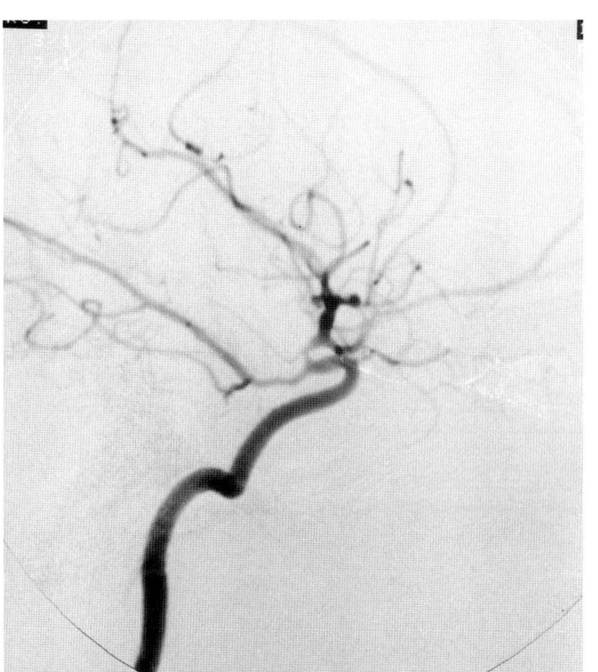

E

**Anteroposterior (A), base (B), and left anterior oblique (C) maximum intensity projection views demonstrate lack of signal intensity involving the distal right internal carotid artery, which extends to involve the A1 and M1 segments. Anteroposterior (D) and lateral (E) conventional angiographic images demonstrate the severe stenosis involving the distal internal carotid artery as well as the proximal anterior and middle cerebral arteries in this patient with vasculitis.**

Because of the relatively good signal intensity involving the more peripheral branches of the right anterior and middle cerebral arteries, the signal loss involving the distal right internal carotid artery is most consistent with severe stenosis and not total occlusion. It would be very unusual for leptomeningeal collateral flow to provide such a good depiction of vascular signal intensity.

## CASE 125
## MOYAMOYA DISEASE

**History:** 10-year-old with headaches and a 5-year history of "spells" associated with staring.

**Technique #1:** axial volume; three-dimensional time-of-flight; 45/7/20; 256 × 256; magnetization transfer background suppression; tilted, optimized nonsaturating excitation radiofrequency pulse; 14-cm field of view; 12:20.

**Technique #2:** axial slice, two-dimensional phase-contrast, 32/10.9/30, 256 × 192, eight excitations, 40-mm thick, velocity encoding of 10 cm/sec, flow encoding in all directions, 20-cm field of view, 3:17.

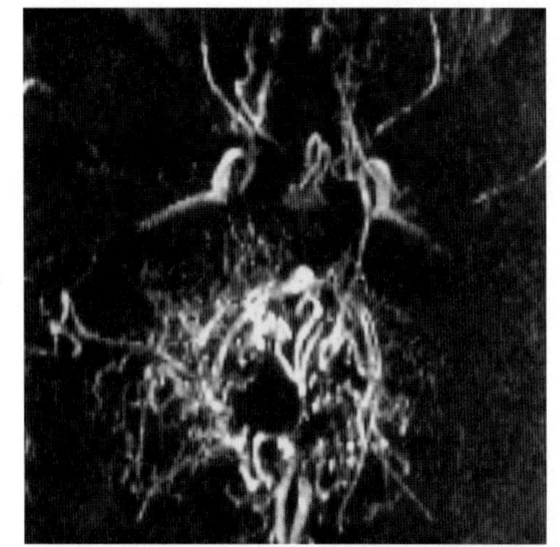

A

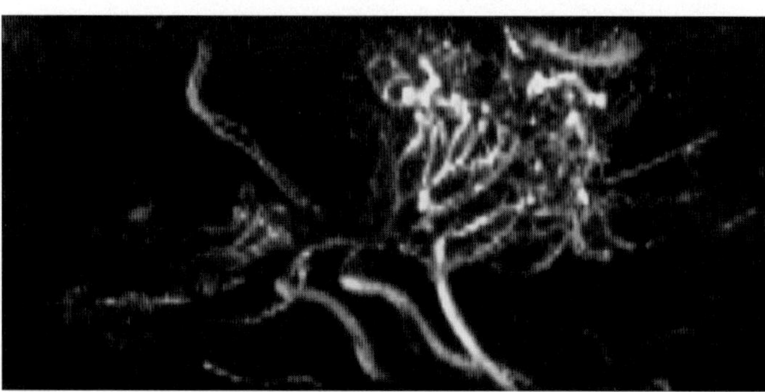

B

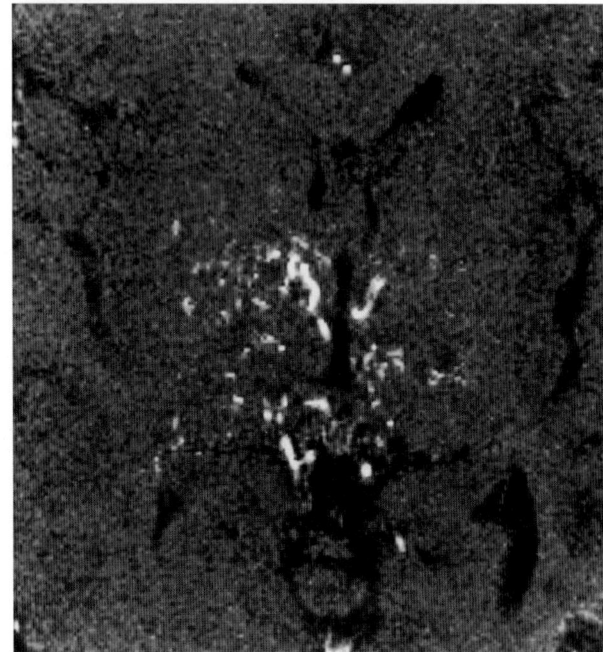

C

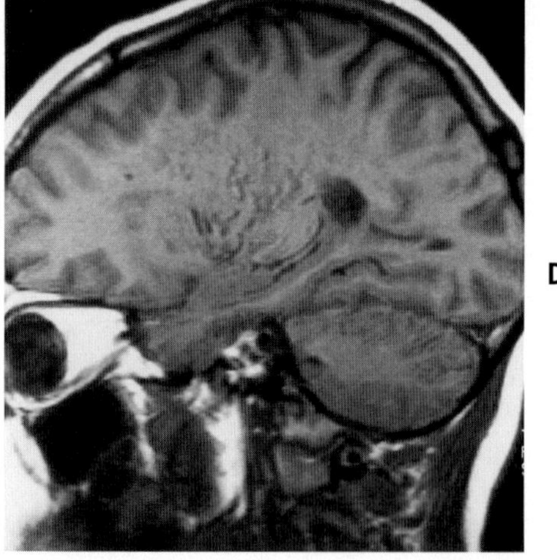

D

**Base (A) and oblique (B) maximum intensity projection views show loss of signal involving the distal internal carotid arteries bilaterally and extending into the proximal anterior cerebral arteries. No signal is seen in the middle cerebral distributions bilaterally. There is a prominent tangle of serpentine vessels extending superiorly from the region of the basilar artery into the region of the thalami and parietal lobes. Individual slice from the MRA data set shows the multiple collateral vessels extending into the thalami and basal ganglia bilaterally (C). Sagittal T1-weighted image (D) shows multiple linear flow voids in the left basal ganglia. Axial T2-weighted image (E) shows an infarct in the left occipital lobe and left subinsular cortex. Thick-slab two-dimensional phase-contrast study also shows the multiple small moyamoya vessels (F).**

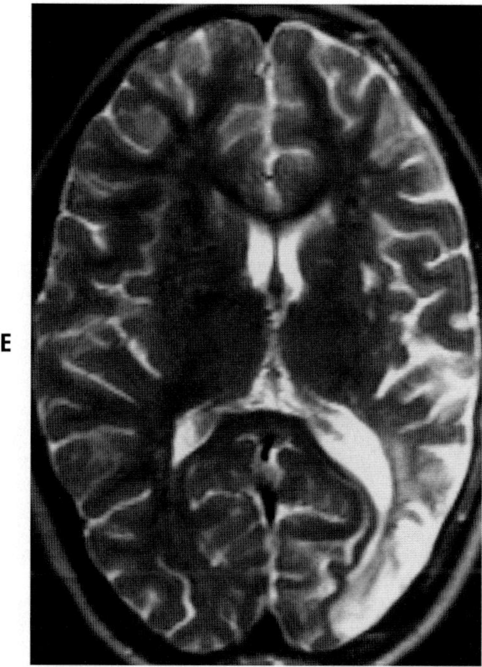

E

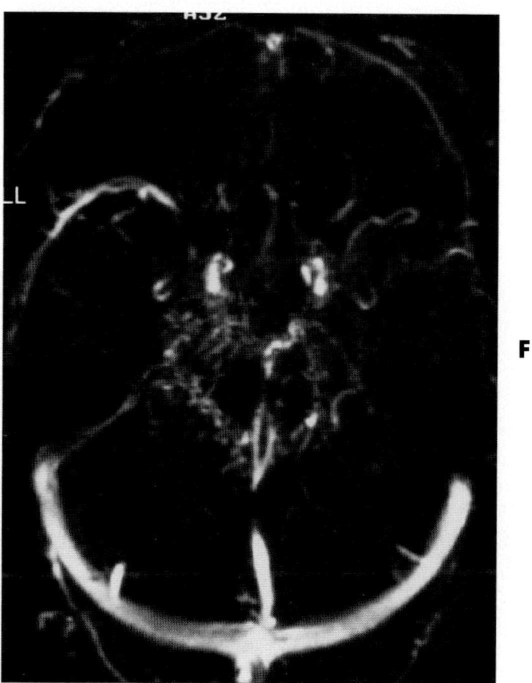

F

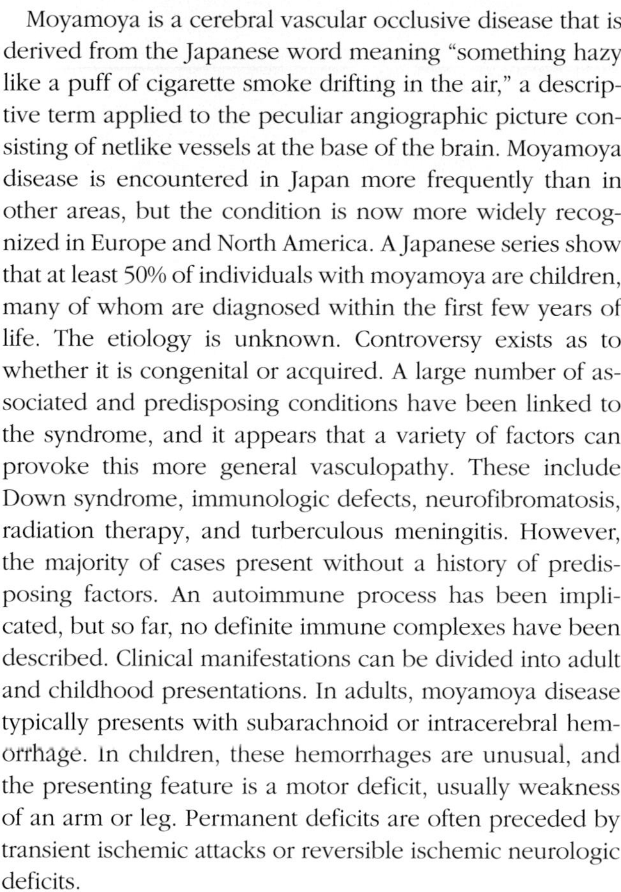

Moyamoya is a cerebral vascular occlusive disease that is derived from the Japanese word meaning "something hazy like a puff of cigarette smoke drifting in the air," a descriptive term applied to the peculiar angiographic picture consisting of netlike vessels at the base of the brain. Moyamoya disease is encountered in Japan more frequently than in other areas, but the condition is now more widely recognized in Europe and North America. A Japanese series show that at least 50% of individuals with moyamoya are children, many of whom are diagnosed within the first few years of life. The etiology is unknown. Controversy exists as to whether it is congenital or acquired. A large number of associated and predisposing conditions have been linked to the syndrome, and it appears that a variety of factors can provoke this more general vasculopathy. These include Down syndrome, immunologic defects, neurofibromatosis, radiation therapy, and turberculous meningitis. However, the majority of cases present without a history of predisposing factors. An autoimmune process has been implicated, but so far, no definite immune complexes have been described. Clinical manifestations can be divided into adult and childhood presentations. In adults, moyamoya disease typically presents with subarachnoid or intracerebral hemorrhage. In children, these hemorrhages are unusual, and the presenting feature is a motor deficit, usually weakness of an arm or leg. Permanent deficits are often preceded by transient ischemic attacks or reversible ischemic neurologic deficits.

The disease process involves the supraclinoid portion of the internal carotid extending to the proximal portions of the anterior and middle cerebral arteries. Posterior cerebral arteries are occasionally involved. Autopsy cases have shown narrowing of the main trunks of the intracranial skull base arteries, many abnormal small vessels originating from the circle of Willis, undifferentiated small arteries, and veins in the subarachnoid space and cerebral parenchyma. It appears that the amplification of these perforating vessels at the base of the brain is a nonspecific response to gradual occlusion of the larger feeding vessels. Leptomeningeal anastomoses between cortical branches of the posterior circulation and internal carotid systems and transdural external-to-internal carotid anastomoses also provide additional sources of collateral circulation. Thus sources of collateral circulation would include the perforators extending into the basal ganglia, as well as the so-called ethmoidal moyamoya, which has its collateral pathways via the opthalmic artery through the ethmoidal arteries and supplies collateral circulation to the frontal basal region. In addition, transdural anastomoses, which have been called *rete mirabile* or *vault moyamoya,* may occur. The arteries that contribute to these collateral supplies are the anterior falcal, middle meningeal, ethmoidal, occipital, tentorial, and superficial arteries.

### REFERENCES

Suzuki J, Kodama N: Moyamoya disease: a review, *Stroke* 14:104-109, 1983.

Suzuki J, Takaku A: Cerebrovascular "Moyamoya" disease, *Arch Neurol* 20:288-299, 1969.

Yonekawa Y et al: *Moyamoya disease: clinical review and surgical treatment,* In Fein JM, Flalm ES: *Cerebrovascular surgery,* vol 2, New York, 1985, Springer-Verlag.

Vogl TJ, Balzer JO, Stemmler J: MRA in children with cerebral neurovascular diseases: findings in 31 cases, *AJR* 159:817-823, 1992.

## CASE 126
## MOYAMOYA DISEASE

**History:** 8-year-old with episodic right-extremity weakness.

**Technique:** axial volume, three-dimensional time-of-flight, 35/8/13, 512 × 256, 64 slices, 60-mm slab, 22-cm field of view, 9:3.

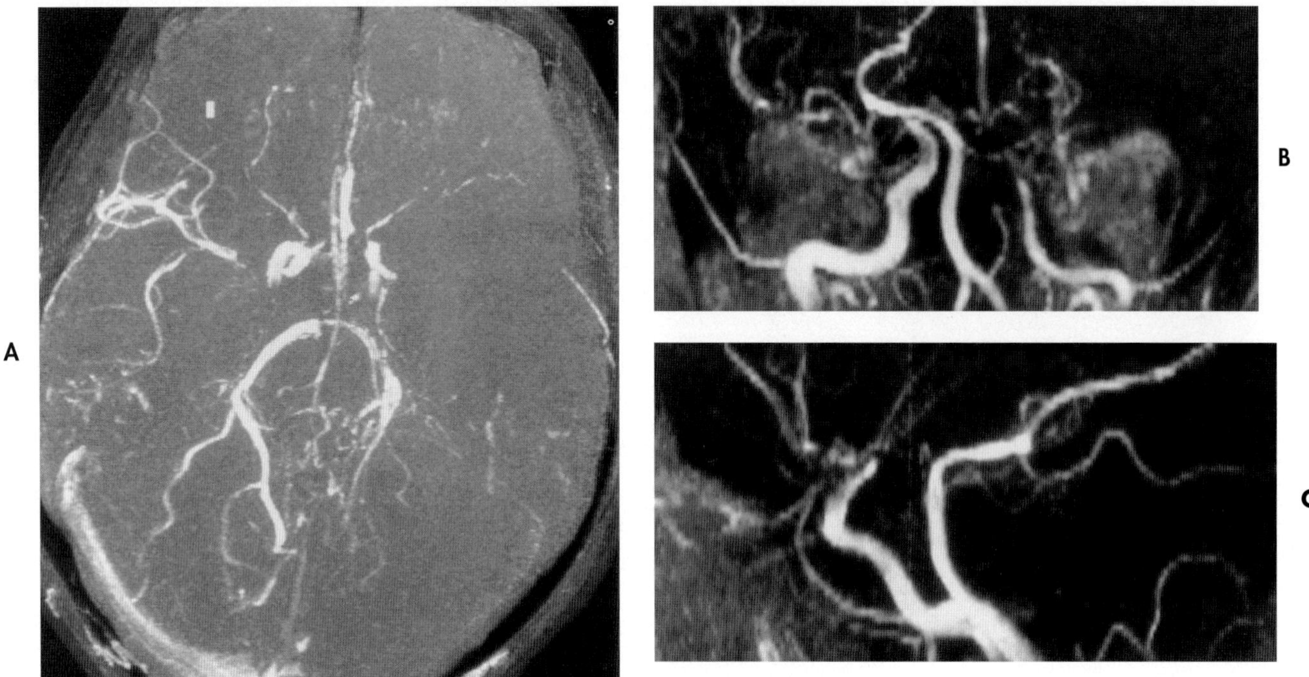

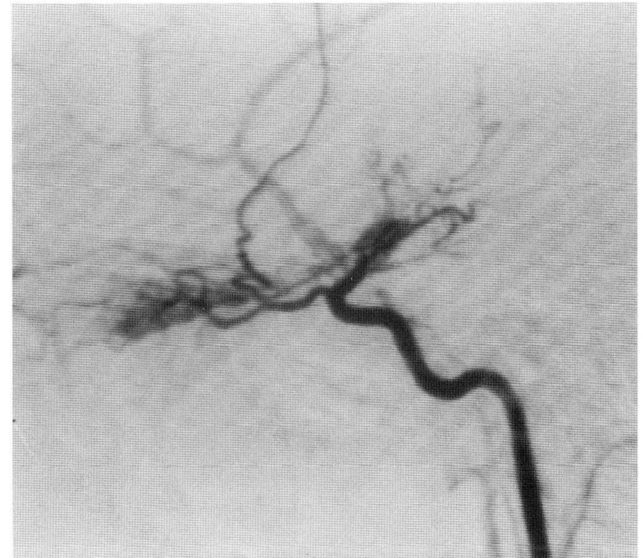


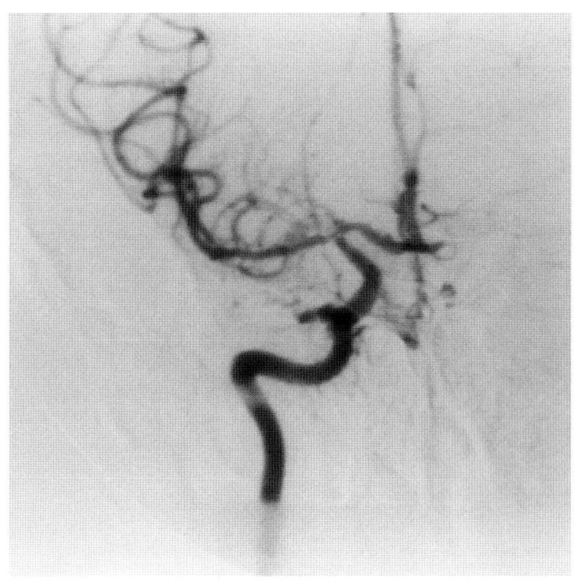


**Whole head base (A), anteroposterior (B), and lateral (C) maximum intensity projection views demonstrate the marked loss of signal involving the distal left internal carotid artery and the left anterior and middle cerebral artery branches. There appears to be a severe stenosis involving the distal right internal carotid artery, with a small amount of signal from the peripheral middle cerebral artery branches. The right posterior cerebral artery is normal, as is the basilar artery. The left posterior cerebral artery is not identified. Lateral view from the left internal carotid artery injection (D) and anteroposterior view from the right internal carotid artery injection (E) demonstrate the severe stenosis involving the distal right internal carotid artery as well as narrowing of the M1 and A1 segments on the right. The lateral view from the left injection demonstrates occlusion of the supraclinoid internal carotid artery, with no flow noted in the middle cerebral artery branches and a puff-of-smoke appearance from the supraclinoid collateral moyamoya vessels. (Courtesy Alison S. Smith, Aultman Hospital, Canton, Ohio.)**

Suzuki et al classified the progression of moyamoya disease as six phases: (1) stenosis of intracranial bifurcation of the internal carotid, (2) appearance of moyamoya (with dilatation of the intracerebral arteries), (3) increasing moyamoya (with decreasing size of middle and anterior cerebral arteries), (4) finer formation of moyamoya with disappearance of the posterior cerebral arteries, (5) decrease in size of the moyamoya vessels with continued disappearance of the intracerebral arteries, and (6) disappearance of moyamoya with collateral circulation supplied only by external carotid branches.

Treatment of moyamoya has been primarily by a surgical means. In general, the procedures are a form of bypass, the idea of which is to give additional collateral flow to the ischemic brain to prevent or minimize irreversible brain damage on progression of the disease. Types of bypass have included superficial temple artery to middle cerebral artery bypass, encephalomyosynangiosis in which a partially freed flap of temporalis muscle is directly laid on the cortical surface, and encephaloduroarteriosynangiosis in which an uninterrupted superficial temporal arteries is approximated to the cerebral cortical surface.

Fujisawa et al described the MR findings in 11 patients with moyamoya disease. They noted that occlusion or stenosis of the terminal portion of the internal carotid artery was clearly demonstrated on the spin-echo images. MR was quite sensitive to the ischemic changes of infarction, atrophy, and ventricular dilatation in these patients.

## REFERENCES

Suzuki J, Kodama N: Moyamoya disease: a review, *Stroke* 14:104-109, 1983.

Fujisawa I, Asato R, Nishimura K et al: Moyamoya disease: MR imaging, *Radiology* 164:103-105, 1987.

## CASE 127
## SICKLE CELL VASCULOPATHY WITH MOYAMOYA DISEASE

**History:** 3½-year-old child with sickle cell anemia who was in sickle crisis with left hemiplegia and was being treated via transfusion therapy.

**Technique:** axial volume; three-dimensional time-of-flight; 45/7/20; 256 × 256; 64 slices; 60-mm slab; magnetization transfer background suppression; tilted, optimized nonsaturating excitation radiofrequency pulse; 14-cm field of view; 12:20.

A

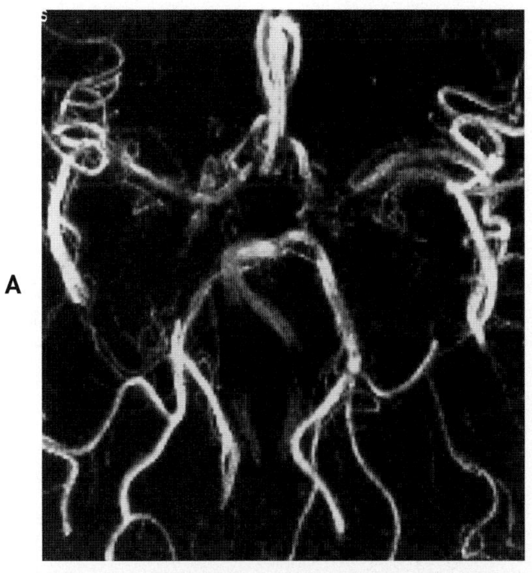

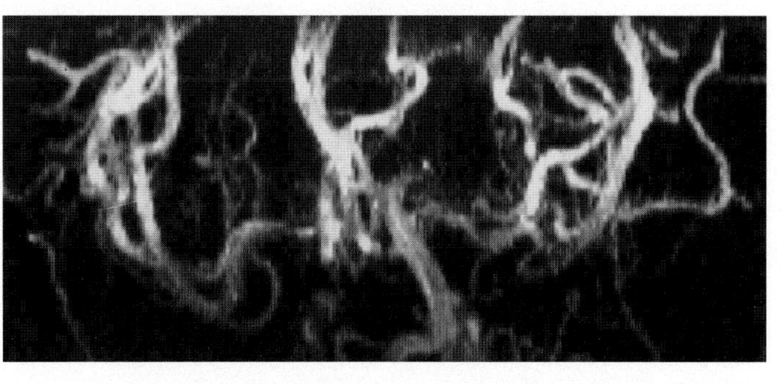

B

C

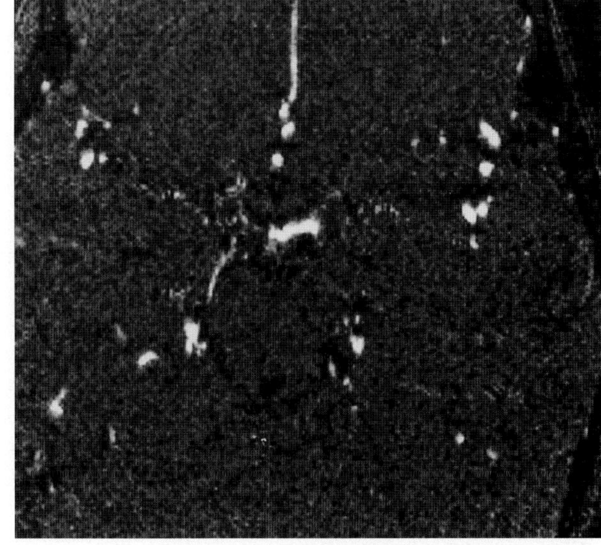

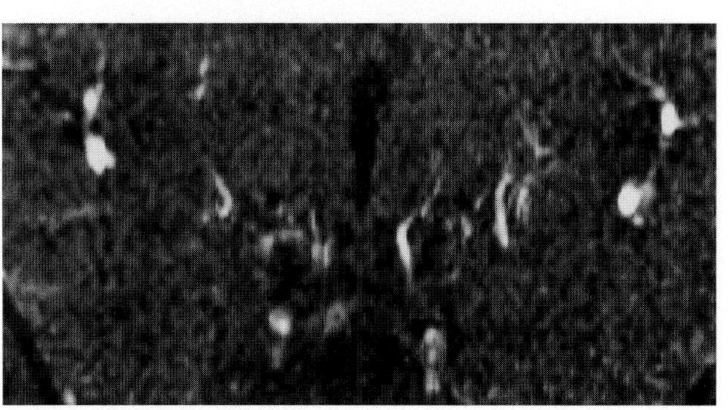

D

**Base (A) and anteroposterior (B) maximum intensity projections show lack of signal from the internal carotids bilaterally and the proximal M1 segments. There are multiple prominent perforating vessels extending into the basal ganglia bilaterally. The basilar artery is widely patent. Axial individual slice (C) and coronal reformat (D) also show the abundant collateral vessels supplying the basal ganglia. (See Case 128 for discussion of sickle cell disease.)**

## CASE 128
## SICKLE CELL DISEASE WITH LARGE VESSEL OCCLUSIVE DISEASE

**History:** 8-year-old with sickle cell disease.

**Technique #1:** intracranial/axial volume, three-dimensional time-of-flight, 50/13/20, 256 × 128, 64 slices, 60-mm slab, 23-cm field of view, 6:50.

**Technique #2:** carotid/three-dimensional time-of-flight, 50/13/20, 256 × 128, 64 slices, 60-mm slab, 18-cm field of view, 6:50.

A

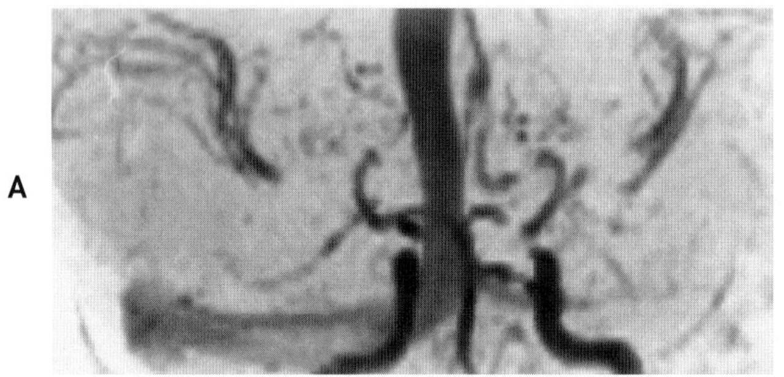

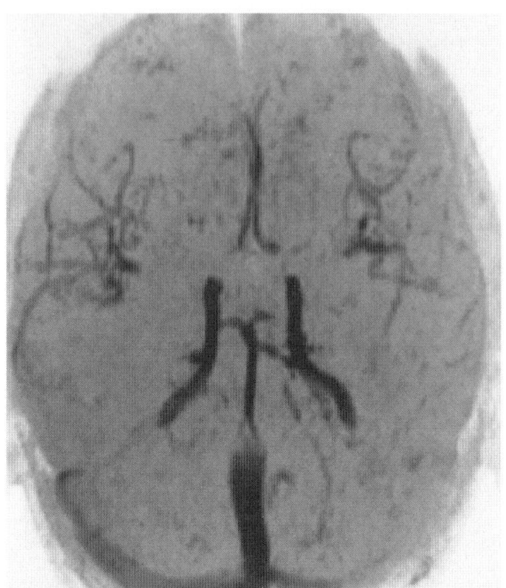

B

C

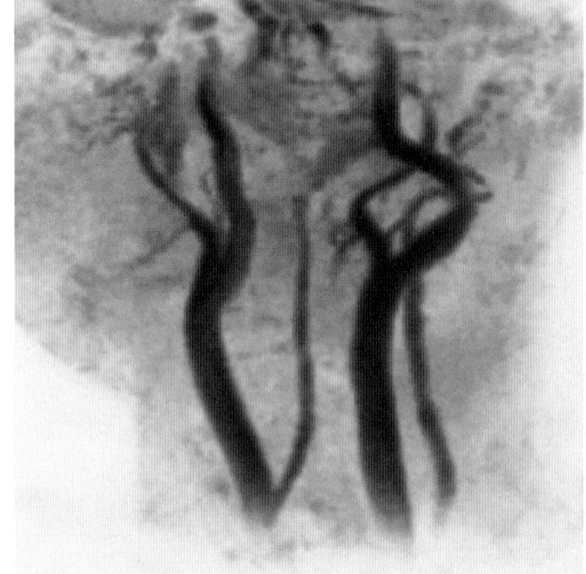

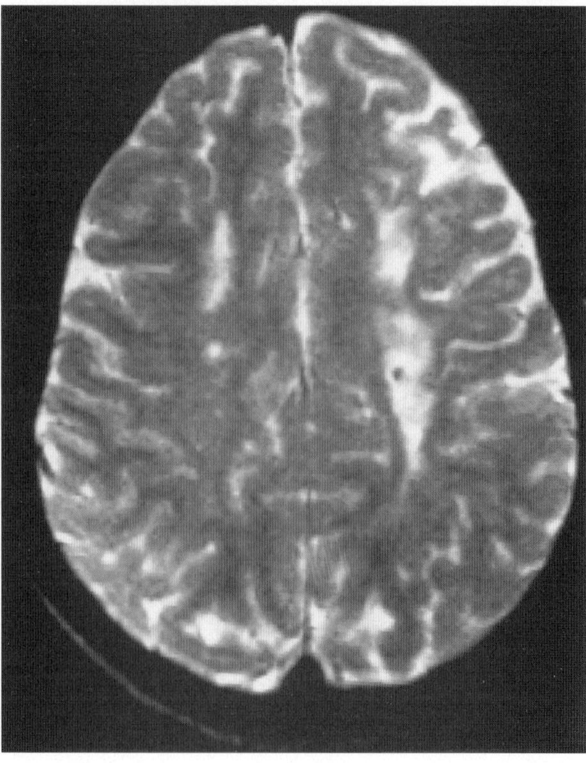

D

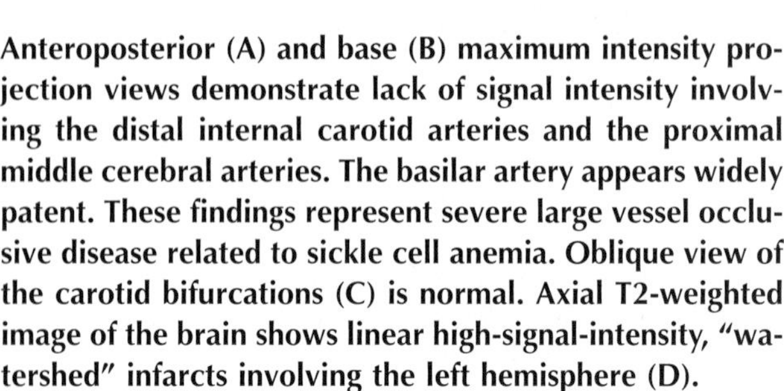

**Anteroposterior (A) and base (B) maximum intensity projection views demonstrate lack of signal intensity involving the distal internal carotid arteries and the proximal middle cerebral arteries. The basilar artery appears widely patent. These findings represent severe large vessel occlusive disease related to sickle cell anemia. Oblique view of the carotid bifurcations (C) is normal. Axial T2-weighted image of the brain shows linear high-signal-intensity, "watershed" infarcts involving the left hemisphere (D).**

Approximately 25% of sickle cell patients develop cerebrovascular complications. Although intravascular sickling is thought to play a role in some sickle cell neurologic complications, these are a minority. The development of large vessel occlusive disease in sickle cell patients, now known to be related to intimal proliferation, appears to be of more importance. Infarcts often occur most extensively in territory supplied by distal branches of the internal carotid artery, particularly the regions of the anterior/middle cerebral artery border zones. These findings are identified on the T2-weighted axial image **(D)** showing linear abnormal high signal intensity at the watershed regions of the anterior and middle cerebral arteries. This evaluation has led to the use of chronic prophylactic transfusion therapy in patients who have cerebral infarction or occlusion. Periodic blood transfusions can decrease the recurrence of strokes from 90% to 10%, according to Russell et al. Transfusion therapy also appears to halt the progression of the large vessel occlusive disease and decreases the irregularity of luminal surfaces.

Although cerebrovascular disease in children is an uncommon problem, its overall incidence is higher than that of pediatric brain tumors (2.52 cases per 100,000 vs. 2.17 cases per 100,000, respectively [per Schoenberg]). These numbers are after excluding causes related to infection and trauma. The causes of stroke in children are legion, with the most common causes related to sickle cell disease, homocystinuria, heart disease with embolic events, disseminated intravascular coagulation and leukemia. A more complete list is given in the box.

**STROKES IN CHILDREN**

1. Congenital heart disease
2. Acquired heart disease: rheumatic, dysrhythmias, prosthetic valves
3. Hematologic: sickle cell, anemia, disseminated intravascular coagulation, leukemia
4. Hypotension
5. Metabolic: homocystinuria, diabetes
6. Infection: viral condition, bacterial condition, tuberculosis
7. Vascular: arteriovenous malformation, aneurysm, fibromuscular disease, moyamoya disease, neurocutaneous syndromes
8. Collagen vascular disease
9. Trauma
10. Drug abuse
11. Migraine

## REFERENCES


Witznitzer M, Ruggieri PM, Masaryk TJ: Diagnosis of cerebrovascular disease in sickle cell anemia by magnetic resonance angiography, *J Pediatr* 117(4):551-555, 1990.

Stockman JA, Nigro MA, Mishkin MM et al: Occlusion of large cerebral vessels in sickle-cell anemia, *New Engl J Med* 287 846-849, 1972.

Huttenlocher PR, Mohr JW, Johns L et al: Cerebral blood flow in sickle cell cerebrovascular disease, *Pediatrics* 73:155-181, 1984.

Schoenberg BS, Mellinger JF, Schoenberg DG: Cerebrovascular disease in infants and children: a study of incidence, clinical features, and survival, *Neurology* 28:763-768, 1978.

Schoenberg BS, Schoenberg DG, Christine BW: The epidemiology of primary intracranial neoplasms of childhood: a population study. *Mayo Clin Proc* 51:51-56, 1976.

Ausman JI, Diaz FG, M SH et al: Cerebrovascular occlusive disease in children: a survey, *Acta Neurochir (Wien)* 94:117-128, 1988.

Russell MO, Goldberg HI, Hodson A et al: Effect of transfusion therapy on arteriographic abnormalities and on recurrence of stroke in sickle cell disease, *Blood* 63:162, 1984.

## CASE 129
## TAKAYASU'S ARTERITIS WITH SUBCLAVIAN STEAL

**History:** 33-year-old woman with an acute onset of left-sided hemiparesis.

**Technique #1:** intracranial/axial volume; three-dimensional time-of-flight; 45/7/20; 256 × 256; magnetization transfer background suppression; tilted, optimized nonsaturating excitation radiofrequency pulse; 14-cm field of view; 12:20.

**Technique #2:** cervical carotid/three-dimensional time-of-flight axial volume; 34/6/20; 128 × 256; 140-mm thick; 128 slices; tilted, optimized nonsaturating excitation pulse; 20-cm field of view (rectangular); 9:19.

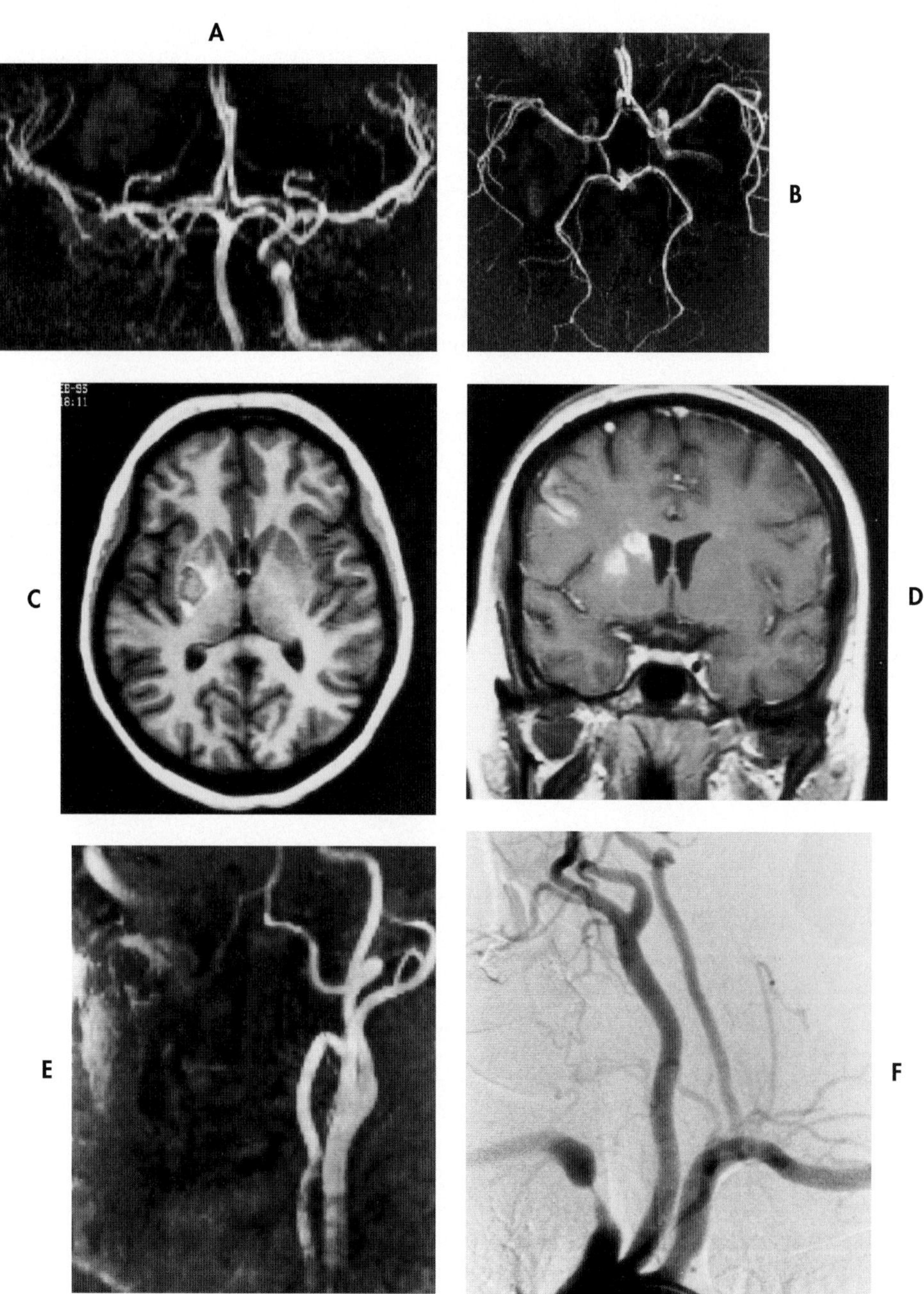

G

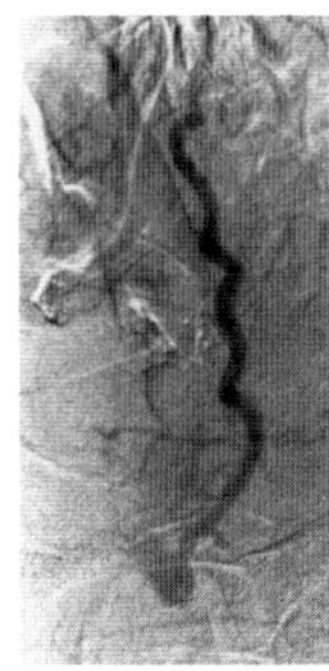

H

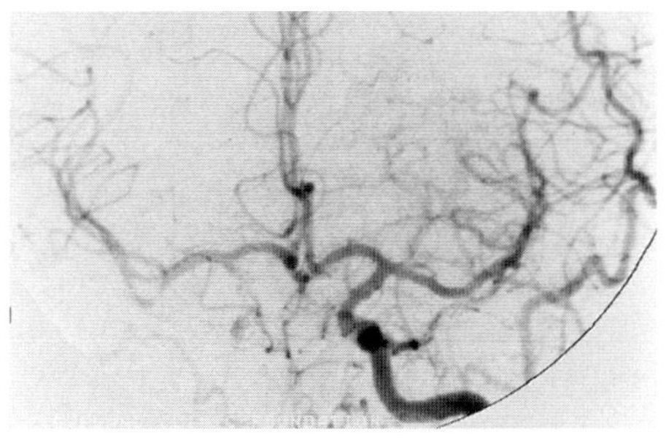

I

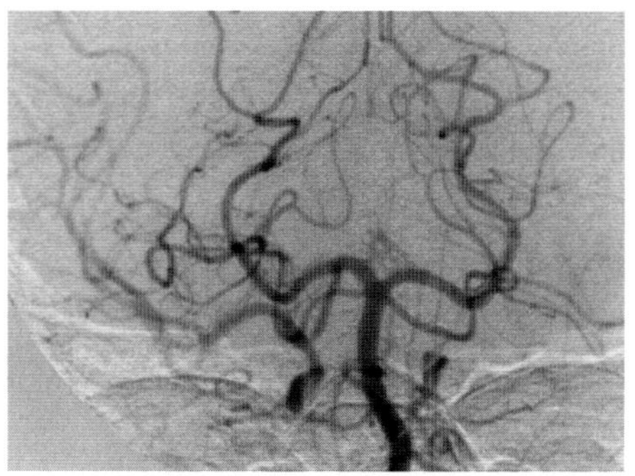

**Anteroposterior (A) and base (B) maximum intensity projection views of the intracranial circulation demonstrate lack of signal from the right internal carotid artery, with only faint signal from the right carotid siphon. The remainder of the intracranial vessels appear normal, with the exception of slight loss of signal from the peripheral middle cerebral branches on the right (slow flow-related saturation effect). Globular faint area of increased signal is seen in the region of the right basal ganglia. Axial T1-weighted gradient-echo image (C) shows a hemorrhagic infarction in the right basal ganglia, which accounts for the increased parenchymal signal on the maximum intensity projection views. T1-weighted coronal image after contrast (D) shows gyriform enhancement of the right middle cerebral distribution infarct and enhancement of the caudate head infarct. There is a normal flow void in the left carotid siphon. Whole volume anteroposterior maximum intensity projection view from the neck MRA (E) shows no signal in the right common carotid distribution. The left carotid is normal. The left vertebral artery is normal, with faint signal in the distal right vertebral artery.**

On this three-dimensional time-of-flight study, this could represent either a proximal vertebral occlusion with retrograde flow or subclavian steal. A single axial gradient-echo image low in the neck could differentiate these possibilities, since occlusion would show no signal and flow in either direction would show high signal. Alternatively, a phase-contrast MRA would show the signal in the vertebral artery, since a phase-contrast image is not as sensitive to flow saturation and it would give the direction of flow. Conventional arch **(F** and **G),** left carotid **(H),** and vertebral **(I)** angiograms show occlusion of the right common carotid, with a severe stenosis of the proximal subclavian artery. A delayed image shows the retrograde flow in the right vertebral artery with subsequent filling of the right subclavian artery **(G).**

Takayasu's arteritis, or "pulseless disease," is a chronic inflammatory disease of unknown etiology that primarily involves the aorta and its major branches. It produces stenoses, occlusions, dilatations, and aneurysms. It is typically a disease affecting young Oriental women, but the disease has a worldwide distribution.

Involvement has been divided into four types. Type I is involvement localized to the aortic arch and its branches. Type II involves the decending thoracic aorta and branches. Type III involves the abdominal aorta and branches, and type IV is extensive involvement of the entire aorta. An additional type, in which pulmonary arteries are involved, has also been suggested.

Two stages of the disease process are generally recognized: (1) the "prepulseless" stage with nonspecific inflammatory features such as fever, night sweats, arthralgia, myalgia, and rash; and (2) the chronic or "burned-out" stage with vascular stenoses. The histology of the acute phase is a granulomatous arteritis, with inflammatory cells in the media and adventitia attack (lymphocytes and plasma cells). Sclerosing arteritis is characterized by fibrous intimal hyperplasia, medial degeneration, and adventitial fibrosis. The angiography pattern is helpful in the differential diagnosis. Takayasu's arteritis generally shows an alternating pattern of stenosis and occlusion (often bilateral and involving multiple proximal branches of the aorta). Temporal arteritis can cause similar changes in the subclavian and axillary arteries.

The American College of Rheumatology criteria for classification include age of onset of less than 40 years, claudication of an extremity, a decreased brachial artery pulse, a bruit over the subclavian arteries or aorta, and arteriographic evidence of narrowing or occlusion of the aorta, branches, or major arteries.

## REFERENCES


Arend WP, Michel BA, Bloch DA et al: The American College of Rheumatology 1990 criteria for the classification of Takayasu arteritis, *Arthritis Rheumatism* 33(8):1129-1133, 1990.

Lupi HE, Seoane M: *Takayasu's arteritis.* In Lande A, Berkman YM, McAllister HA Jr, ed: *Aortitis: clinical, pathologic, and radiographic aspects,* New York, 1986, Raven Press.

Yamato M, Lecky J, Hiramatsu K, Kohda E: Takayasu arteritis: radiographic and angiographic findings in 59 patients, *Radiology* 161:329-334, 1986.

Park JH, Han MC, Kim SH et al: Takayasu arteritis: angiographic findings and results of angioplasty, *AJR* 153:1069-1074, 1989.

Oneson SR, Lewin JS, Smith AS: MRA of Takayasu arteritis, *JCAT* 16(3):478-480, 1992.

## CASE 130
## TAKAYASU'S ARTERITIS

**History:** 30-year-old woman with headaches, left upper extremity paresthesias, and left arm weakness.

**Technique:** axial volumes, three-dimensional time-of-flight with multiple overlapping slabs (multiple overlapping thin-slab acquisition technique), 57/8/20, 180 × 180, 1.7-mm slice thickness, 30-cm field of view, 11:58.

A

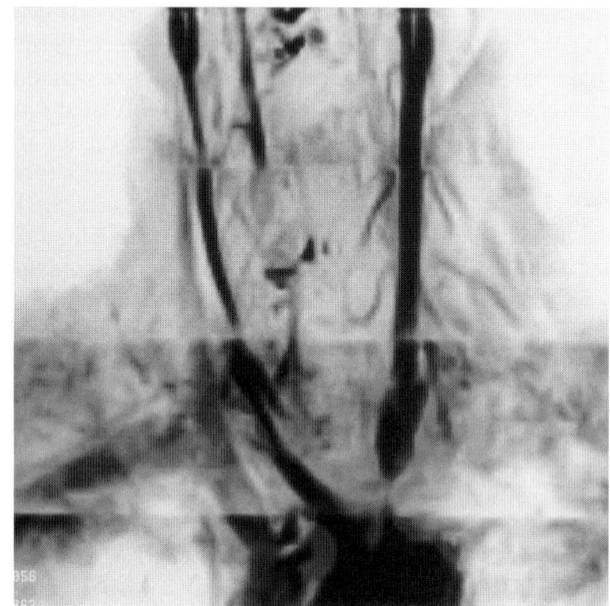

B C

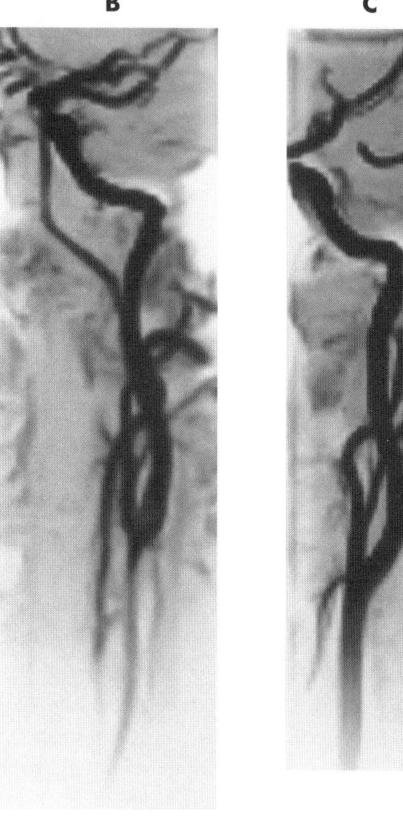

D

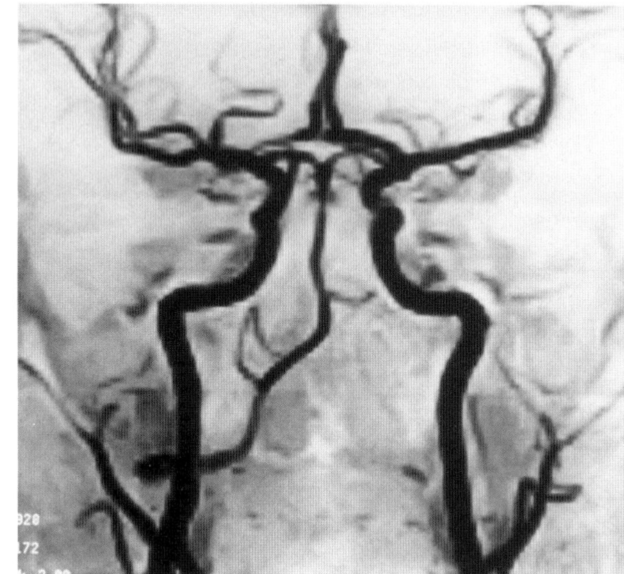

**Anteroposterior maximum intensity projection view of the multislab MRA (A) demonstrates a long segment of stenosis of the right common carotid artery and its origin to the bifurcation. There is also a severe focal stenosis of the proximal left common carotid artery, with poststenotic dilatation. Neither subclavian artery is visualized. There is a long segment of stenosis involving the right vertebral artery, which is then reconstituted distally and is more normal in caliber. The left vertebral artery is not seen. Lateral targeted maximum intensity projection views of the carotid arteries demonstrate the severe stenosis involving the right common carotid artery (B) in contrast with the normal-appearing distal left common carotid artery (C). The intracranial carotid distribution and the basilar artery are normal (D). (See Case 129 for discussion of Takayasu's arteritis.) (Courtesy John L. Sherman, Colorado Springs, Colo.)**

# CHAPTER 7

# Tumors and Vascular Loops

MRA has been applied to a limited extent in the evaluation of intracranial neoplasms.[1,2] The more common uses include evaluation of an extraaxial mass lesion to confirm that it is not an aneurysm or to identify a vascular loop that is compressing cranial nerves.[3] Occasionally, it may also be necessary to evaluate the extent of vascular involvement by skull base neoplastic processes. This is most efficiently done with the individual slices from a three-dimensional time-of-flight acquisition, as opposed to the maximum intensity projection views. In this situation, evaluating the individual slices or multiplanar reconstructions of the volume data is helpful to demonstrate the intricate brain/cranial nerve/vessel/mass relationships that may not be apparent on the reconstructed MRA images or the corresponding spin-echo study. Although the MRA images can diagnose vessel displacement or encasement, only conventional angiographic studies can provide the spatial resolution, dynamic capability, and selectivity needed for complete preoperative evaluation.[1] Furthermore, only selective angiography can clearly demonstrate neurovascularity, arteriovenous shunting, and dominant afferent vessels.

Although the use of intravenous gadolinium may help by improving the visualization of veins and smaller peripheral arteries,[2] it has definite disadvantages as well. The contrast-enhanced mass may simulate the appearance of an abnormal cluster of vessels. Likewise, the enhancing mass or the enhancing surrounding normal structures, such as the nasopharynx, may degrade or obscure the visualization of flowing spins because of the similar high intensities of those tissues. In such cases it may be possible to exclude potentially confusing, normally enhancing structures from the data to be reconstructed by limiting or targeting the maximum intensity projection views or confining the region of reformatting. In such cases in which the imaging concern is the relationship of vessel to brain parenchyma or tumor, the time-of-flight sequence should *not* include additional methods of background suppression. In particular, magnetization transfer suppression should not be implemented, since the suppression of brain parenchyma may be so effective that the determination of relationships between brain and vessel is impossible.

### REFERENCES


1. Masaryk TJ, Modic, MT, Ross JS et al: Intracranial circulation: preliminary clinical results with three-dimensional (volume) MR angiography, *Radiology* 171:793-799, 1989.
2. Creasy JL, Price RR, Presbey T et al: Gadolinium-enhanced MR angiography, *Radiology* 175:280-283, 1990.
3. Adler CH, Zimmerman RA, Savino PJ et al: Hemifacial spasm: evaluation by magnetic resonance imaging and magnetic resonance tomographic angiography, *Ann Neurol* 32:502-506, 1992.

## CASE 131
## SELLAR MENINGIOMA

**History:** 42-year-old with mass discovered on computed tomography obtained for the evaluation of headaches.

**Technique:** axial volume, three-dimensional time-of-flight, 50/13/20, 256 × 128, 64 slices, 72-mm slab, 23-cm field of view, 6:50.

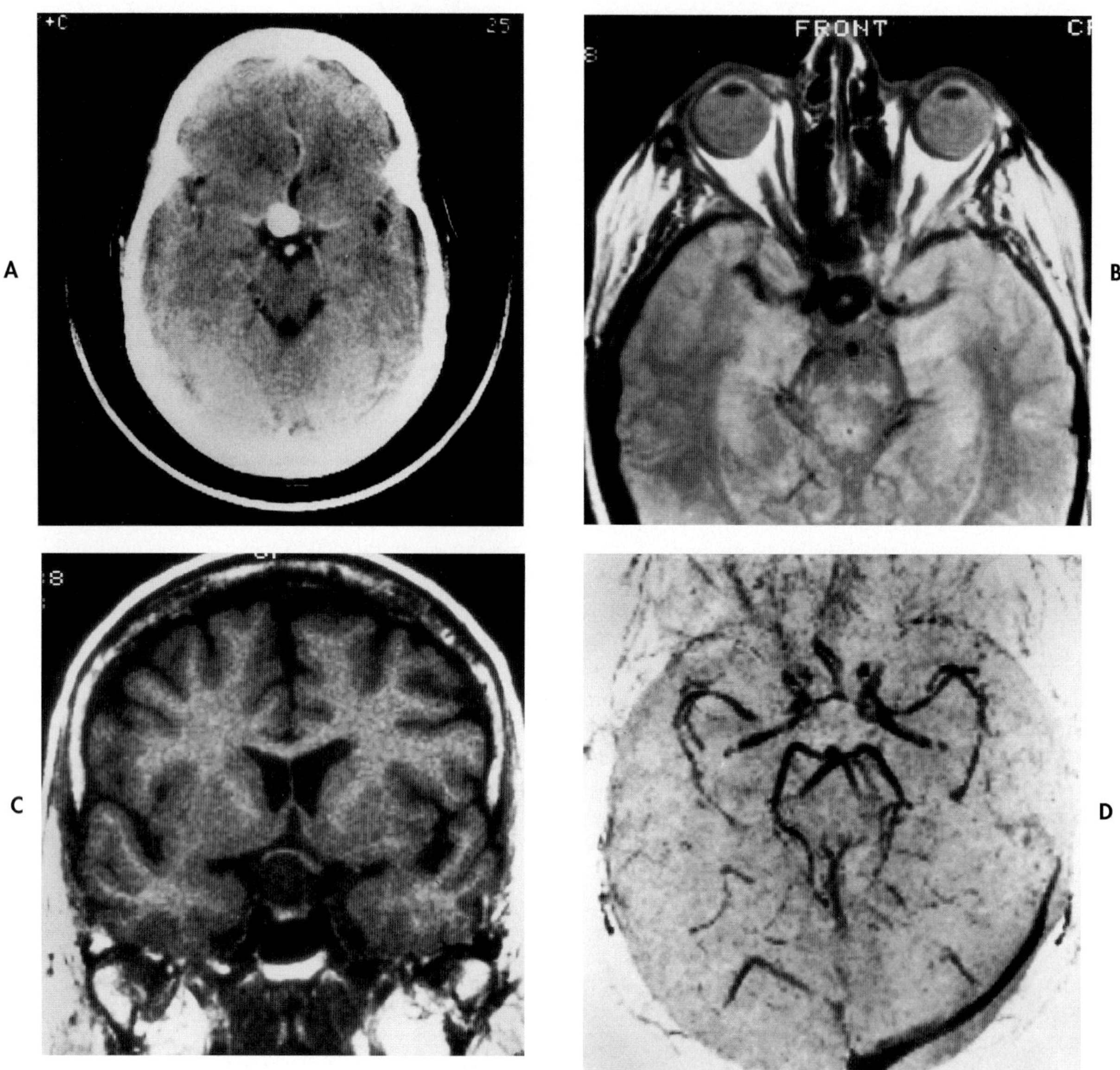


**Contrast-enhanced computed tomographic scan of the brain (A) shows a rounded area of increased attenuation involving the suprasellar cistern. Axial spin-density-weighted (B) and coronal T1-weighted images (C) of the brain demonstrate a rounded mass of predominately low signal intensity with elevation of the optic chiasm. Base maximum intensity projection view of the MRA (D) demonstrates no signal intensity within the region of the suprasellar cistern.**

The differential diagnosis on the computed tomography and MR imaging would be that of a large aneurysm vs. a calcified lesion, such as a meningioma. The MRA effectively excludes the possibility of an aneurysm with a patent lumen, making clear the diagnosis of a calcified meningioma.

## CASE 132
## CLIVAL CHORDOMA

**History:** 43-year-old with progressing cranial nerve palsies.

**Technique:** axial volume, three-dimensional time-of-flight, 40/7/15 degrees, 256 × 256, 64 slices, 80-mm slab, 25-cm field of view, 10:50. In cases in which vascular anatomy in relation to the brain parenchyma is important, it is critical that the MRA technique not include magnetization transfer background suppression. Magnetization transfer background supppression can decrease the signal of the brain to such a degree that the vessel-to-brain relationships cannot be appreciated.

A 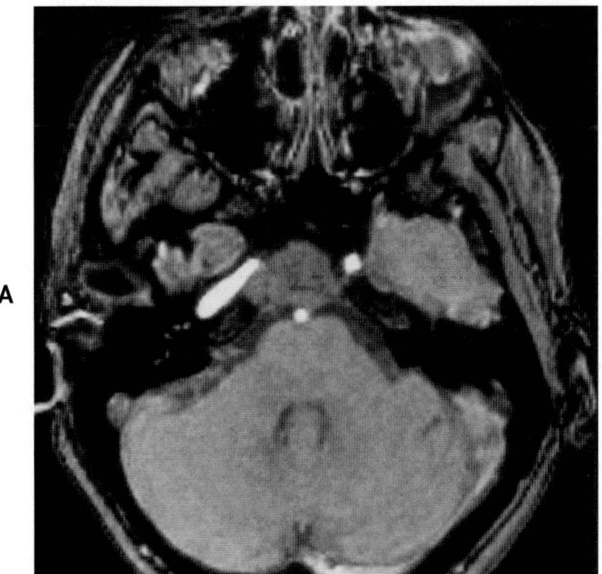

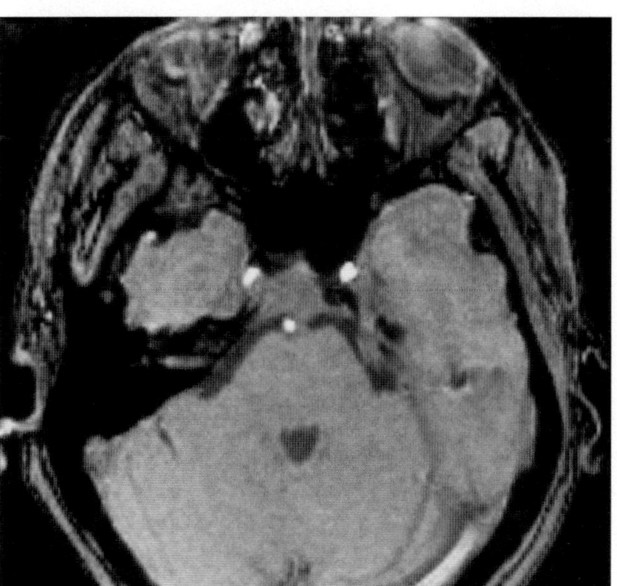 B

**A series of two individual slices from the three-dimensional time-of-flight MRA data set (A and B) demonstrates a clival chordoma involving the skull base, with extension into the right petrous apex. The mass extends up adjacent to the petrous carotid and abuts the basilar artery anteriorly and to the left.**

Chordomas are histologically benign, locally aggressive tumors of notochordal derivation affecting 20- to 40-year-old patients. Approximately 35% of these tumors involve the skull base, predominately the clivus. The tumors have a very high recurrence rate after surgical excision and are radioresistant. The tumors are slightly decreased in signal on T1-weighted images and increased signal on T2-weighted images. Low signal areas related to calcification and cystic areas may occur.

### REFERENCES

Sze G, Uichanco LS III, Brant-Zawadzki MN et al: Chordomas: MR imaging, *Radiology* 166:187-191, 1988.

Oot RF, Melville GE, New PFJ et al:The role of MR and CT in evaluating clival chordomas and chrondrosarcomas, *AJR* 151:567-575, 1988.

Ginsberg LE: Neoplastic diseases affecting the central skull base: CT and MR imaging, *AJR* 159:581-589, 1992.

## CASE 133
## PITUITARY ADENOMA ENCASING THE INTERNAL CAROTID ARTERY

**History:** 61-year-old with a pituitary adenoma.

**Technique:** axial volume, three-dimensional time-of-flight, 45/6.9/20 degrees, 256 × 256 matrix, 60 slices, 72-mm slab, 15-cm field of view, 12:19.

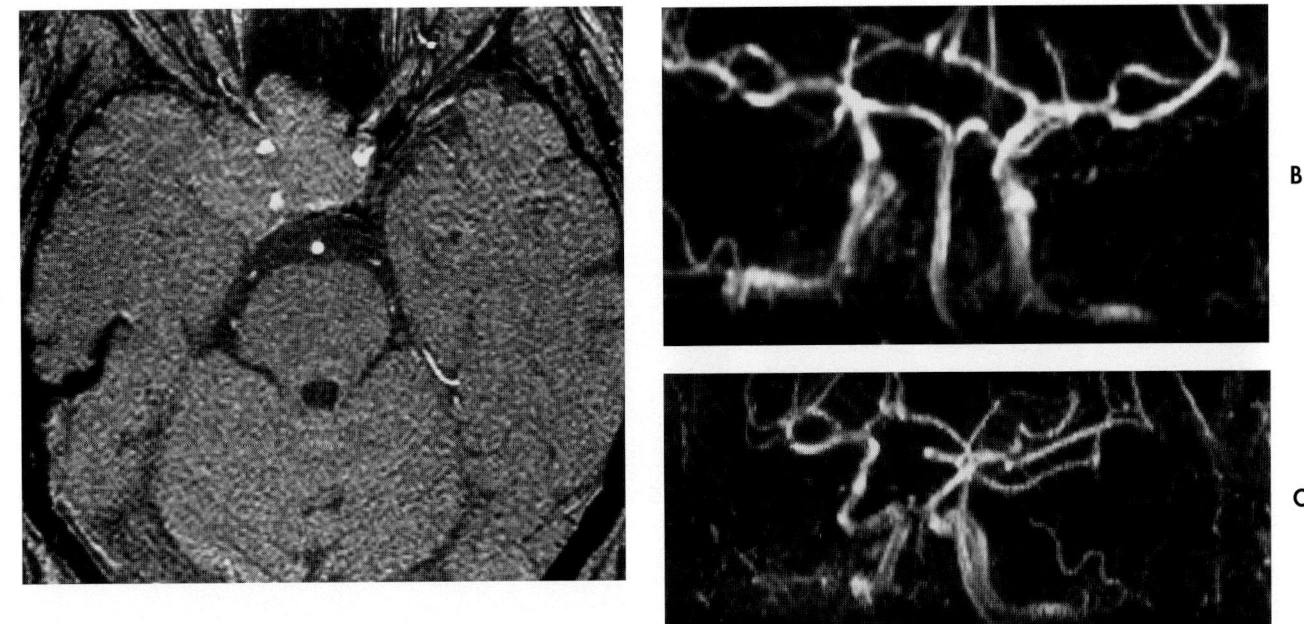


**A large pituitary adenoma extends out of the pituitary fossae into the suprasellar cistern and encases the distal right internal carotid artery on the individual slices from the MRA (A). The internal carotid is not significantly narrowed by the circumferential tumor. Anteroposterior (B) and oblique (C) maximum intensity projection views demonstrate the mass effect of the tumor by (1) straightening and slight lateral displacement of the right internal carotid, 2) splaying or opening of the right carotid siphon, (3) elevation of the right A1 segment, and (4) elevation and straightening of the right P1 and P2 segments.**

## CASE 134
## RIGHT TUBERCULUM SELLAE MENINGIOMA AND RIGHT POSTERIOR COMMUNICATING ARTERY ANEURYSM

**History:** 67-year-old after motor vehicle accident with computed tomographic scan of the head showing a suprasellar mass.

**Technique:** axial volume, three-dimensional time-of-flight, 45/6.9/20 degrees, 256 × 256 matrix, 60 slices, 72-mm slab, 15-cm field of view, 12:19.

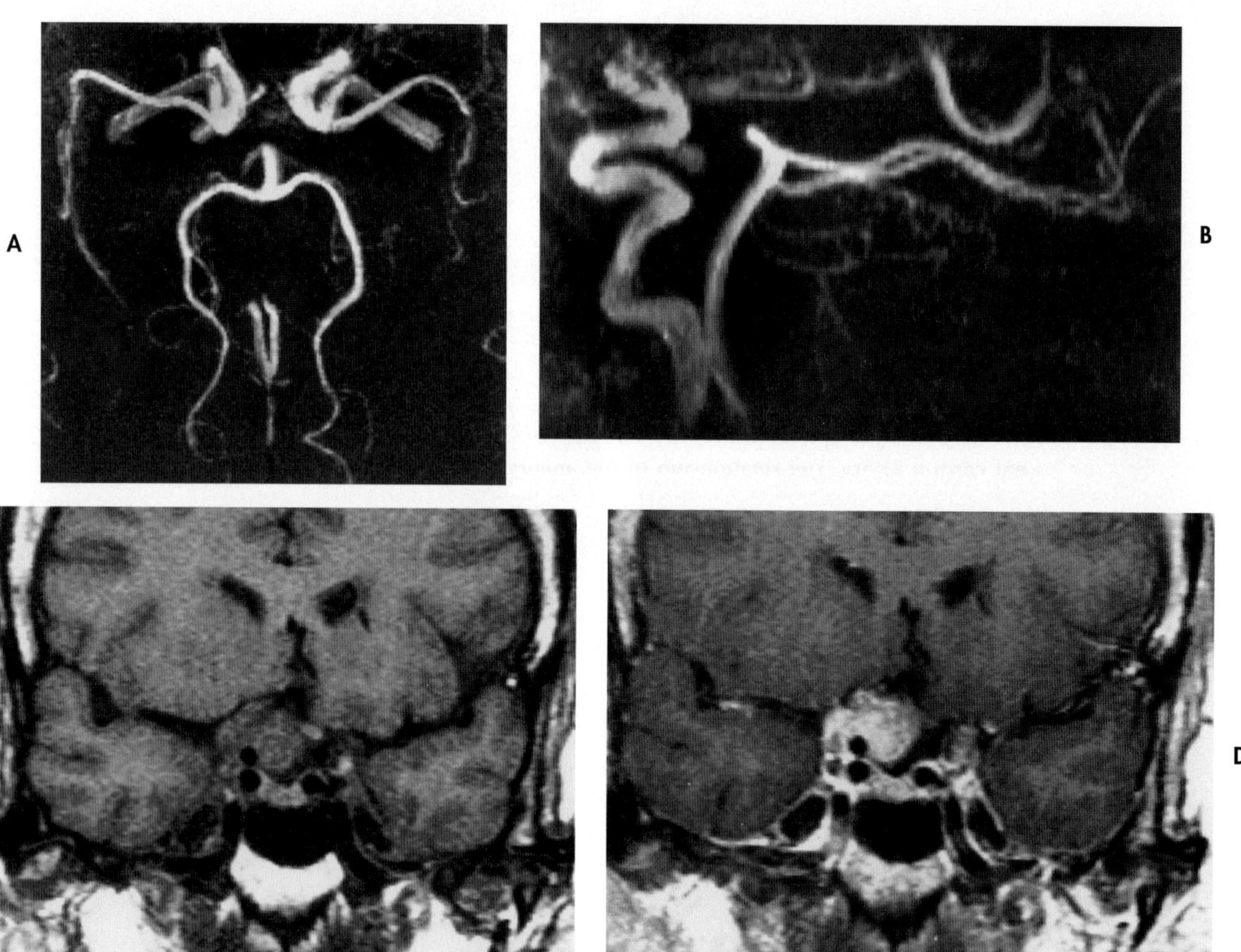

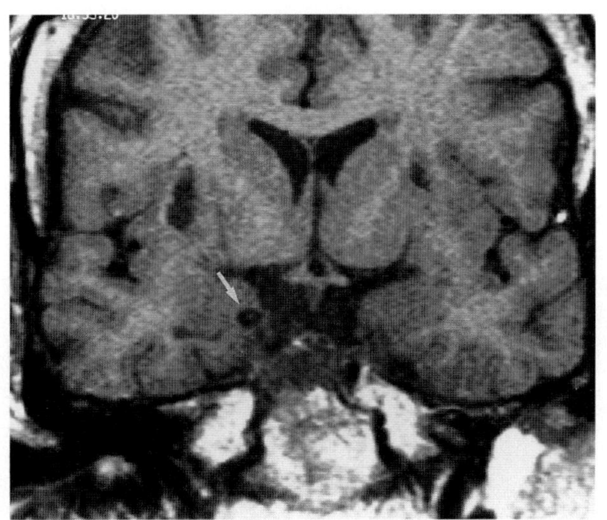

E

**Base (A) and lateral (B) maximum intensity projection views of the time-of-flight MRA show a well-defined aneurysm arising off the distal right internal carotid in the region of the posterior communicating artery. Coronal spin-echo images without (C) and with (D) contrast demonstrate a well-defined homogeneously enhancing mass arising off the right side of the tuberculum sellae and extending toward the right optic chiasm and posterior and medial arteries to the right distal internal carotid artery. The relationship of the aneurysm to the meningioma is seen best on the T1-weighted coronal spin-echo examination in which the flow void of the laterally projecting aneurysm is separate from the area of the tumor (E) *(arrow),* making access to the aneurysm possible, since it is separate from the tumor, and allowing clipping of the aneurysm neck.**

## CASE 135
## LEFT TENTORIAL AND JUXTASELLAR MENINGIOMA

**History:** 58-year-old with a new onset of left temporal lobe seizures.

**Technique:** axial volume, three-dimensional time-of-flight, 45/6.9/20 degrees, 256 × 256 matrix, 60 slices, 72-mm slab, 15-cm field of view, 12:19.

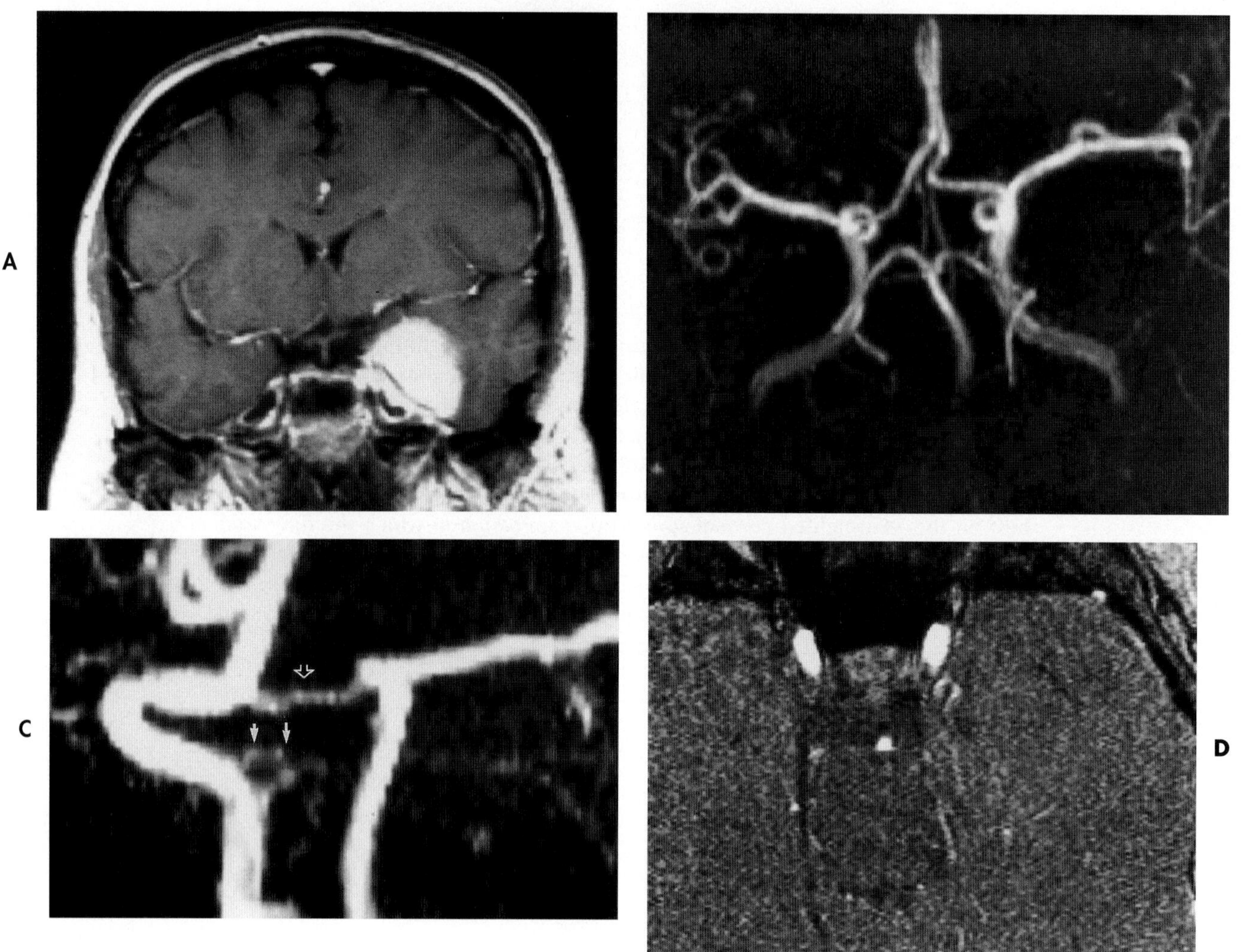

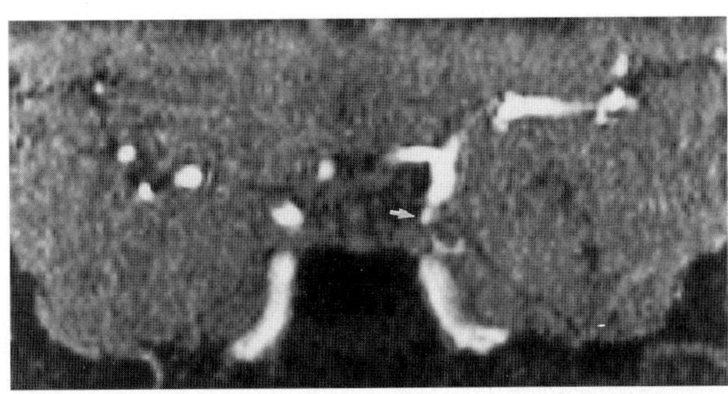


Contrast-enhanced coronal spin-echo T1-weighted image (A) demonstrates a large, well-defined homogeneously enhancing meningioma involving the greater sphenoid wing and left cavernous sinus and extending posteriorly along the margin of the tentorium. Whole volume Water's (B) and targeted lateral (C) maximum intensity projection views of the MRA data demonstrate upward bowing of the left middle cerebral artery and a small tangle of vessels rising off the region of the meningohypophyseal artery *(arrows),* a typical location for arterial supply for this tentorial meningioma. Note the more cephalad origin of the normally positioned posterior communicating artery *(open arrow)* in relationship to the meningohypophyseal artery. Axial individual slice from the MRA data set (D) shows the ill-defined tangle of vessels arising off the meningohypophyseal artery on the left. The meningohypophyseal artery is seen on the coronal reformat (E). Again, the meningohypophyseal is seen arising more inferiorly off the internal carotid artery and extending slightly laterally to where the tumor is. The posterior communicating artery is more superior and extends posteriorly towards the P1-P2 junction *(arrow).*

## CASE 136
## LARGE MENINGIOMA

**History:** 43-year-old with headache.

**Technique:** axial volume, three-dimensional time-of-flight, 40/8/15, 256 × 128, 128 slices, 128-mm slab, 25-cm field of view, 10:56.

A

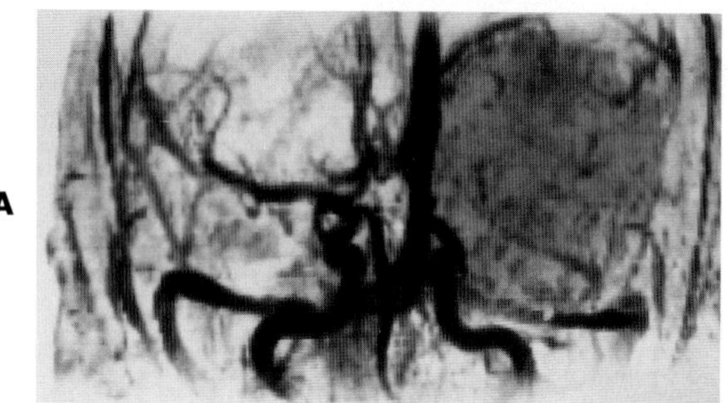

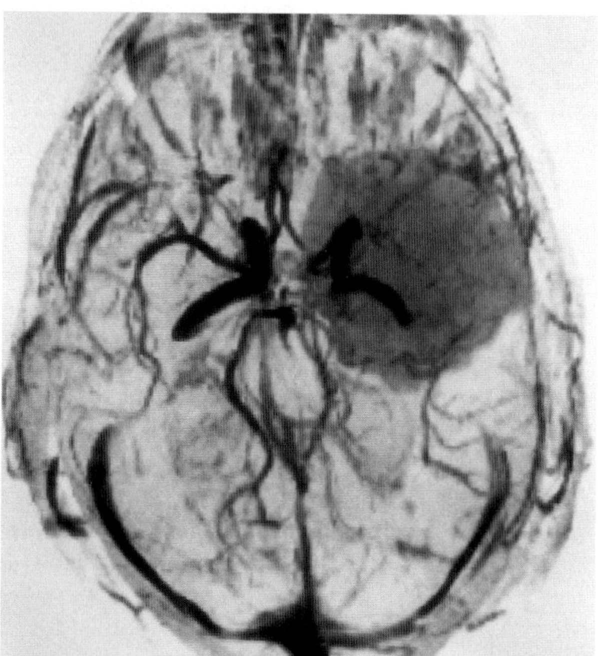

B

C

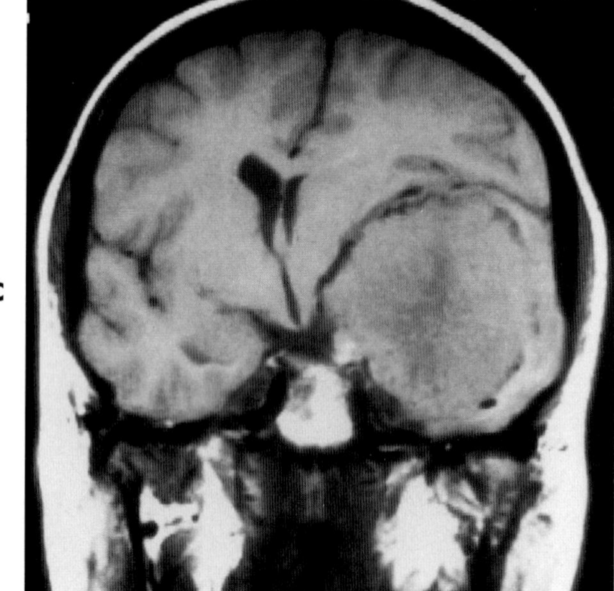

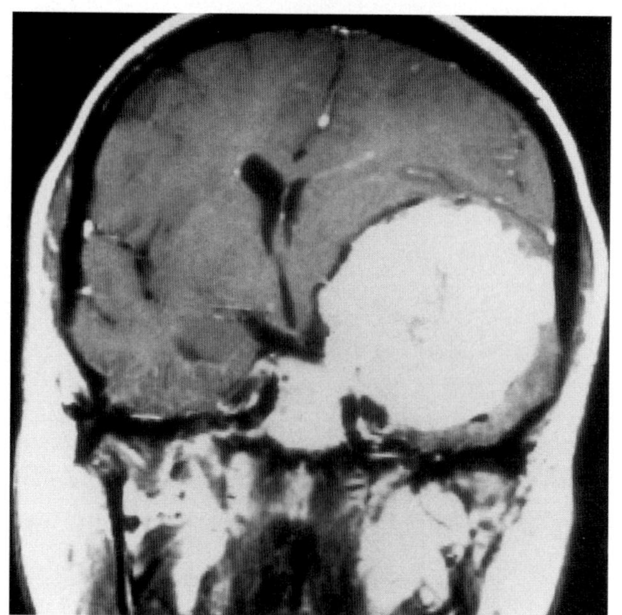

D

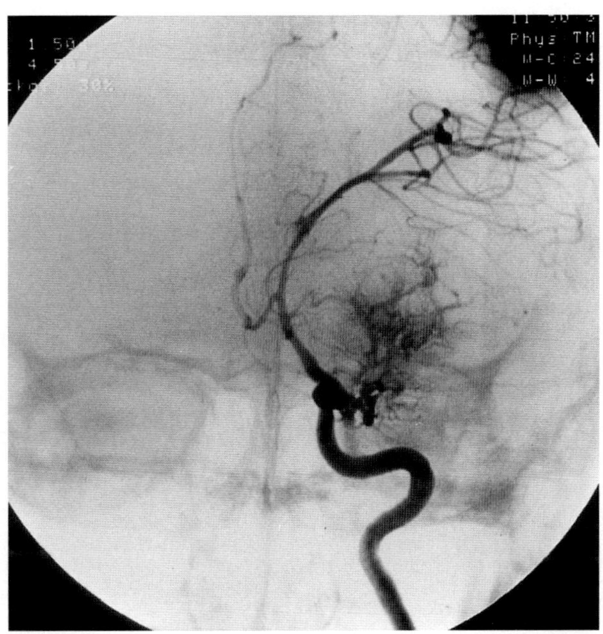

E

**Anteroposterior (A) and base (B) maximum intensity projection views after contrast administration demonstrate a well-defined mass within the region of the left middle fossa, with marked elevation of the left middle cerebral artery. Coronal T1-weighted spin-echo images before (C) and after (D) contrast administration show marked enhancement of the large meningioma. Anteroposterior view from the left internal carotid artery injection (E) demonstrates the bowing and elevation of the left middle cerebral artery and the distal internal carotid artery. The tumor blush is pronounced on the conventional angiogram but is not evident on the MRA images. On the base maximum intensity projection view, the superiorly elevated left middle cerebral artery is not visible; it is obscured by the enhancing meningioma. (From Masaryk TJ, Ross JS: *MR angiography: clinical applications.* In Atlas S: *Magnetic resonance imaging of the brain and spine,* New York, 1991, Raven.)**

## CASE 137
## LARGE POSTERIOR FOSSAE MENINGIOMA WITH OCCIPITAL SINUS

**History:** 44-year-old with ataxia.

**Technique:** contrast-enhanced, axial volume, three-dimensional time-of-flight, 40/8/15, slice thickness 0.9-mm, 206 × 180, 22-cm field of view, 7.3 minutes.

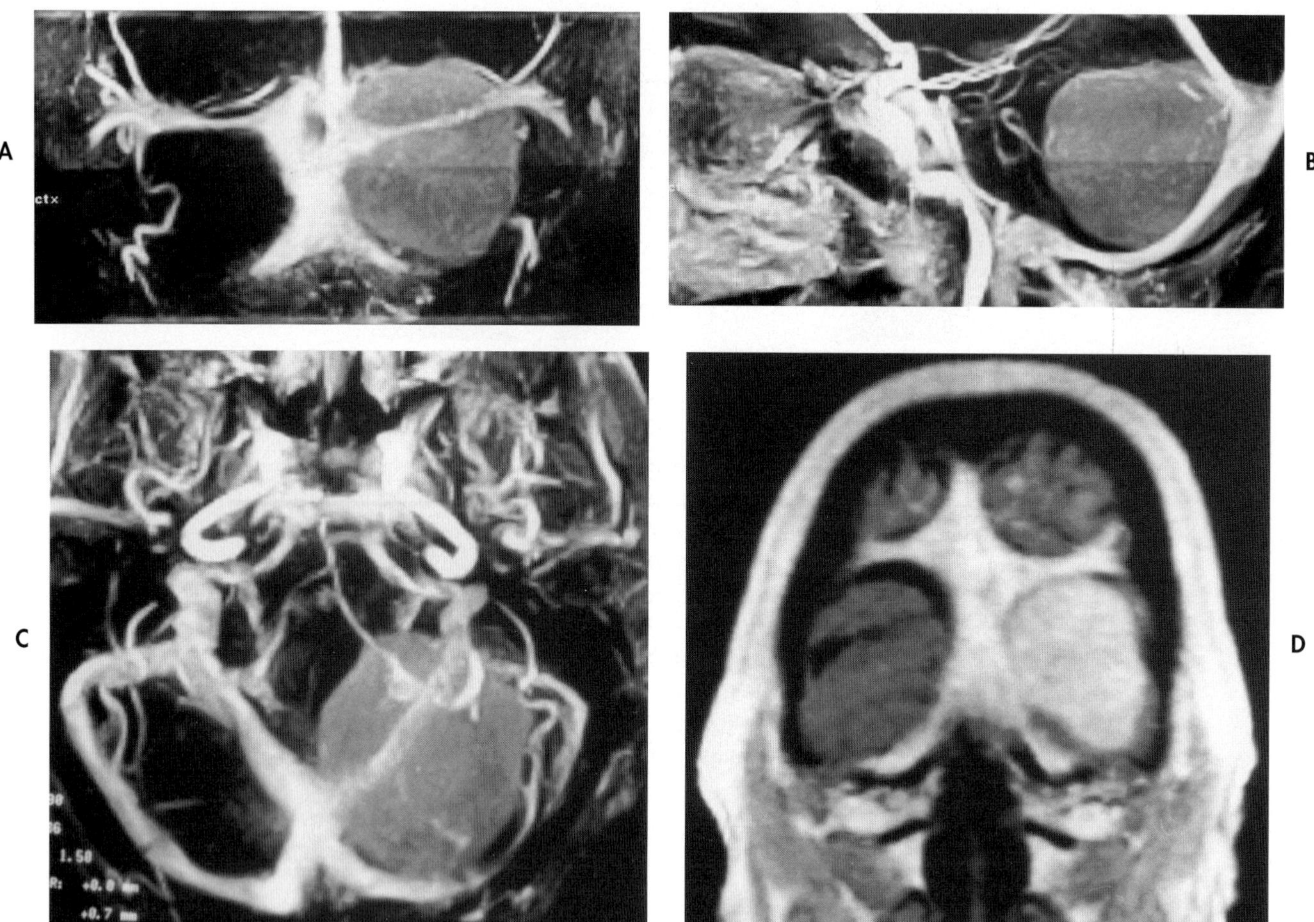


**Anteroposterior (A), lateral (B), and base (C) maximum intensity projection views of three-dimensional time-of-flight MRA demonstrate homogeneous enhancement of a large posterior fossa meningioma. Of particular interest is the venous anatomy, which in addition to the usual transverse sinus, straight sinus, and torcula, there is the presence of an occipital sinus in the inferior midline of the posterior fossa. This is also demonstrated on the coronal T1-weighted enhanced image (D) showing the separation of the meningioma from the occipital sinus. (Courtesy John L Sherman, Colorado Springs, Colorado.)**

The occipital sinus is a midline venous channel connecting the torcula to the marginal sinus surrounding the foramen magnum. It is usually not visualized on conventional angiography. The importance of this variant obviously lies in its recognition as normal venous structure and avoiding it if posterior fossae surgery is contemplated.

### REFERENCE

Newton TH, Potts DG: *Radiology of the skull and brain,* vol 2, Great Neck, NY, 1966, Medibooks.

## CASE 138
## MELANOMA METASTASIS WITH MASS EFFECT ON THE MIDDLE CEREBRAL ARTERY

**History:** 45-year-old with melanoma and right-sided paresthesia.

**Technique:** axial volume, three-dimensional phase-contrast, 24/8.9/20, 256 × 128, velocity encoding of 40 cm/sec, 60 slices, 90-mm slab, 20-cm field of view, 13:08.

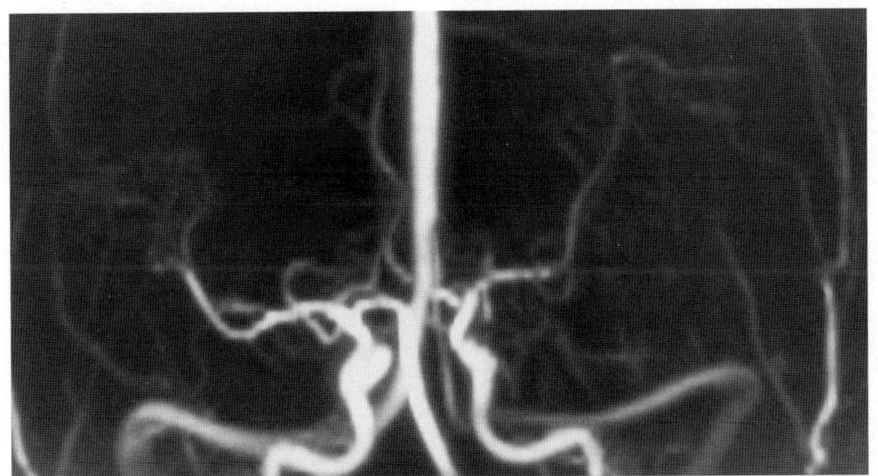

A

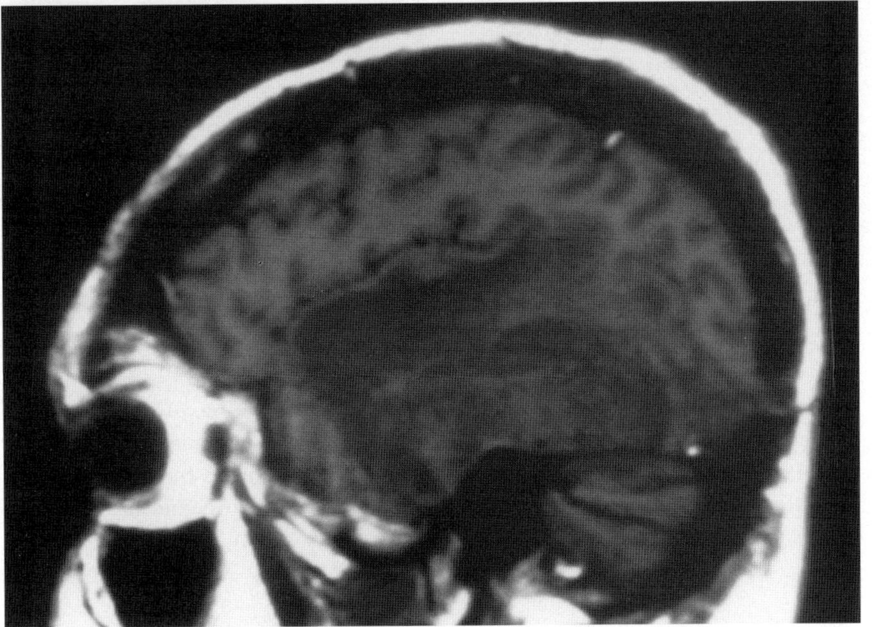

B

**Anteroposterior maximum intensity projection view of the three-dimensional phase-contrast study (A) demonstrates marked superior elevation of the left middle cerebral branches and the angular point, which is consistent with a middle fossa mass. The mass is identified on the sagittal T1-weighted (B) study as melanoma metastasis to the left temporal lobe. There is marked vasogenic edema and marked elevation of the left sylvian fissure.**

# CASE 139
# EXOPHYTIC BRAINSTEM GLIOMA

**History:** 4-year-old with left ptosis and facial droop.

**Technique:** axial volume, three-dimensional time-of-flight, 45/8/20, 256 × 256, 60 slices, 72-mm slab, 15-cm field of view, 12:19.

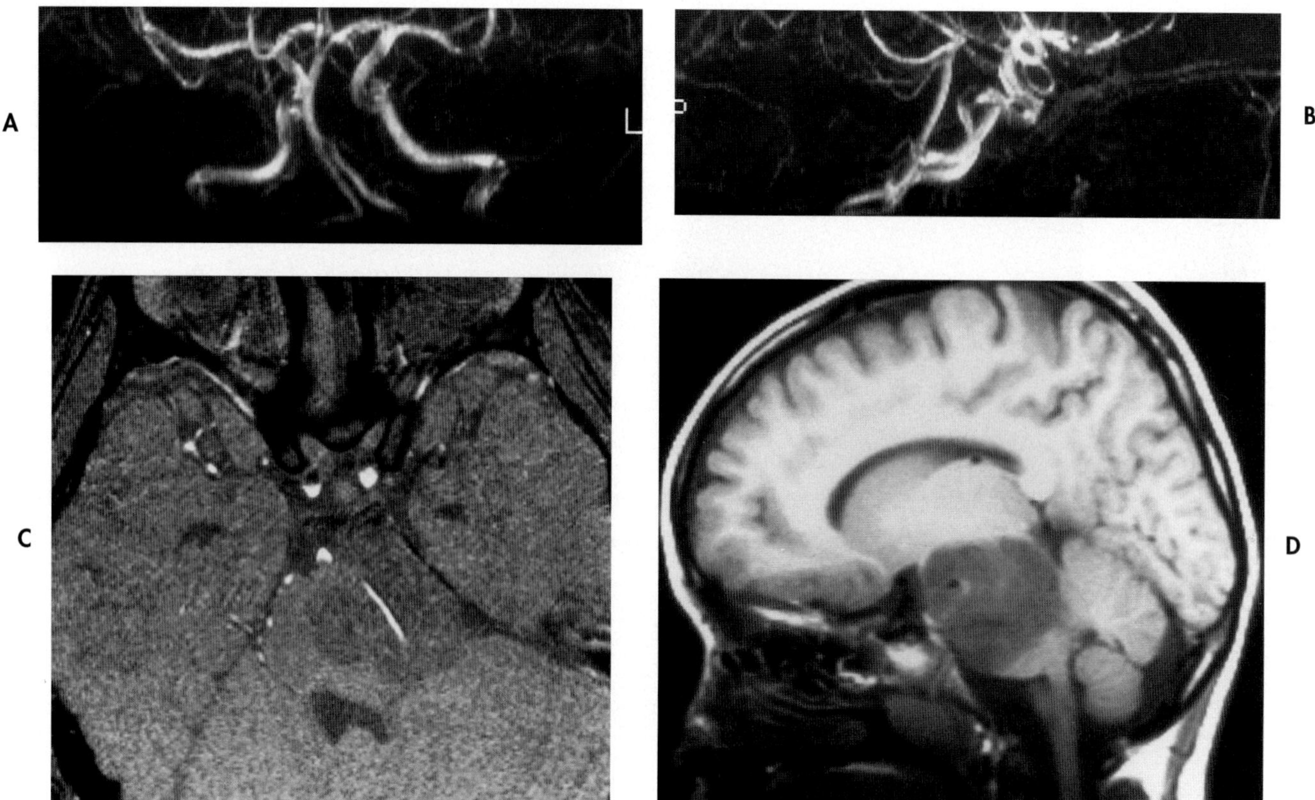


**Anteroposterior (A) and lateral (B) maximum intensity projections show a bowed and displaced basilar artery to the right. Individual slices from the MRA data set (C) show encasement of the left superior cerebellar artery by a tumor arising off the left side of the brainstem, which is slightly decreased in signal compared with signal of the normal brain. Encasement is further supported by the sagittal T1-weighted spin-echo image showing the punctate dot of flow void of the left superior cerebellar artery within the tumor mass (D).**

# CASE 140
# RIGHT OCCIPITAL MENINGIOMA

**History:** 55-year-old with visual disturbance and new seizures.

**Technique:** axial volume, three-dimensional time-of-flight, 40/13/15, 256 × 256, 64 slices, 64-mm slab, 25-cm field of view, 10:57.

A

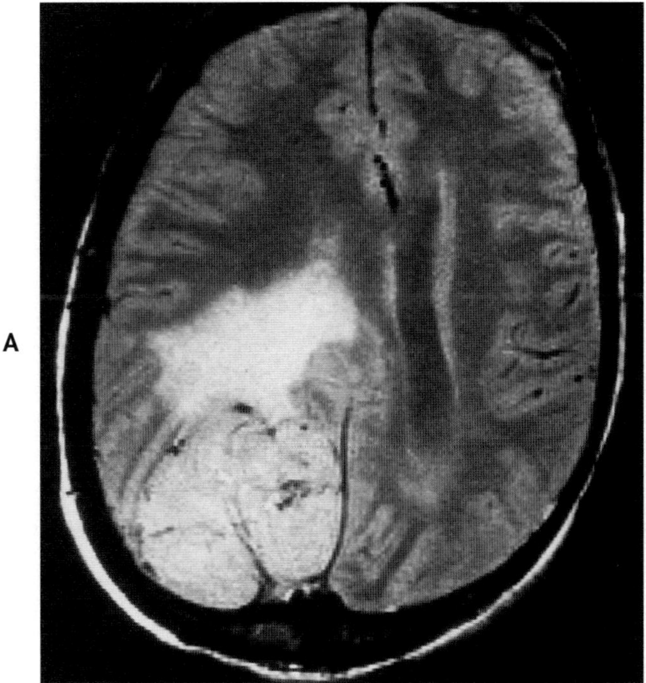

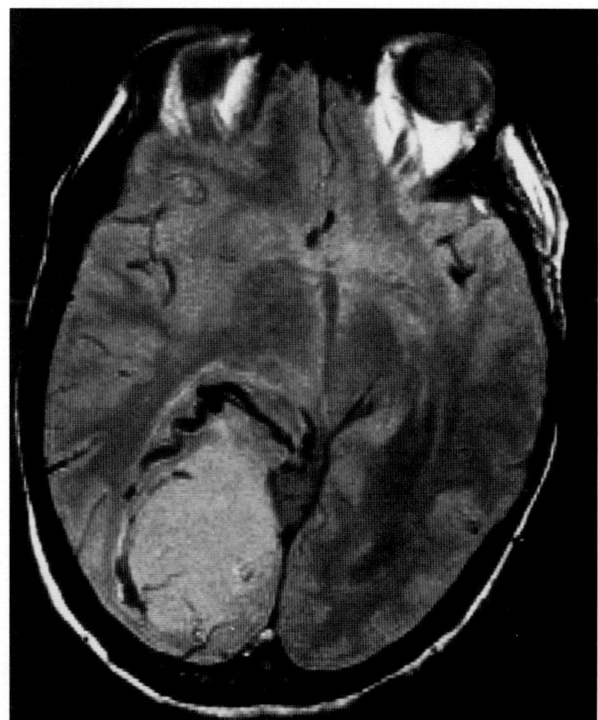

B

**Axial spin-density images of the brain (A and B) demonstrate a large, homogeneous mass that is dura based within the right occipital region. There are multiple serpiginous vessels along the anterior aspect of the mass, with central penetrating vessels along the posterior medial aspect of this meningioma. Base maximum intensity projection view of the MRA (C) demonstrates the serpiginous vessels along the anterior margin, fed off of the leptomeninges. The central posterior penetrating vessels off of the external carotid supply are also visualized.**

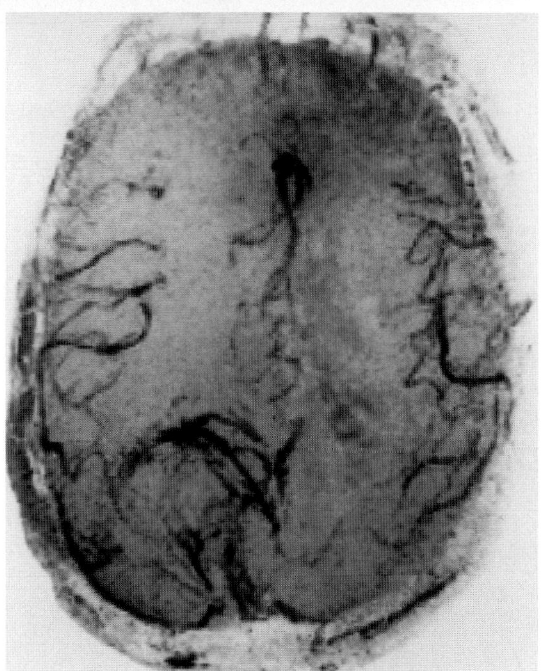

C

## CASE 141
## CAROTID BODY TUMOR

**History:** 45-year-old with a neck mass.

**Technique:** multiple axial volumes (multiple overlapping thin-slab acquisition), three-dimensional time-of-flight, 33/7/20, 256 × 128, one excitation, 64 slices, 64-mm slab, 20-cm field of view, 9:07.

A
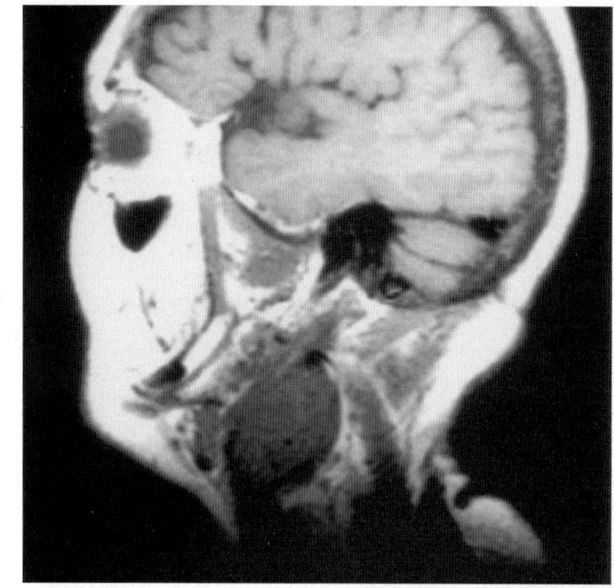

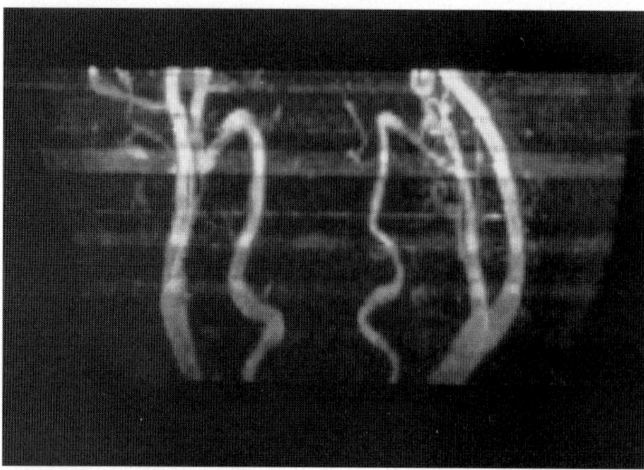
B

C
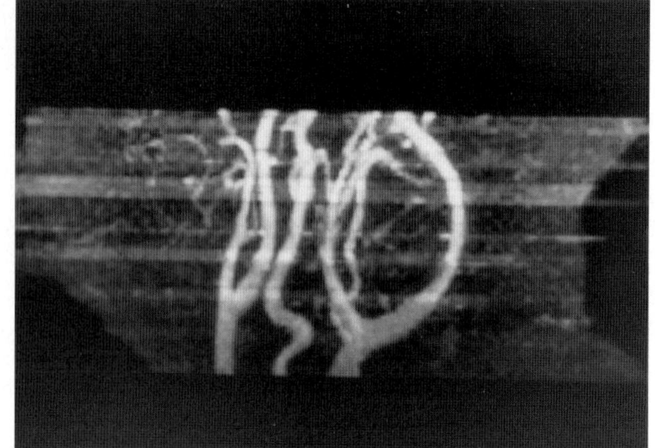

**Sagittal T1-weighted spin-echo MR image (A) demonstrates a left neck mass with a few punctate areas of low signal intensity within it. Anteroposterior (B) and oblique (C) maximum intensity projection views of the three-dimensional time-of-flight MRA show wide separation of the left external and internal carotid arteries by the mass. The right carotid bifurcation is normal. (Courtesy Walter Kucharczyk, Toronto, Canada.)**

Carotid body tumors arise from the carotid body, which is derived from neural crest tissue. Thus the carotid body is found in the amine precursor uptake decarboxylase classification. The carotid body lies in the adventitia of the carotid artery, usually posteromedially at the bifurcation of the common carotid artery. It derives its blood supply through the origins of the external carotid artery and ascending pharyngeal artery. These tumors are also called *chemodectomas* or are described as *nonchromaffin paragangliomas* to differentiate them from the positive chromaffin reaction that would characterize pheochromocytoma. However, studies have demonstrated chromaffin-positive secretory granules, suggesting that the carotid body can secrete catecholamines. There are reports of hypertension resulting from carotid body tumors. Other chemodectomas would include the glomus jugulare, glomus tympanicum, and glomus vagale. The incidence of multicentricity is 10%, but this increases to 35% in familial varieties. The inheritance pattern appears to be autosomal dominant with variable penetrance.

A classical clinical presentation would be of a painless, nontender mass located at the angle of the mandible. Although most tumors grow gradually, in one fifth of cases they may enlarge quickly, giving rise to pain and tenderness. Cases may also typically present with cranial nerve palsies that usually involve the vagus and hypoglossal nerves. These manifestations include hoarseness, pain, and deviation or atrophy of the tongue.

Carotid body tumors are composed of nests of epitheliod cells (Zellballen) with intervening vascular connective tissue. Carotid body tumors are generally classified as benign, locally invasive, or malignant (metastasizing). Locally invasive tumors constitute 3% to 13% of cases, with distant metastatic disease constituting 3%. However, histology appears to be a very poor guide for malignancy potential, since most carotid body tumors appear histologically benign.

Typical angiographic finding is a goblet-shaped splaying of the carotid bifurcation by a very vascular mass containing a cloud of fine tumor vessels. The tumor displaces the external carotid artery anteriorly and laterally and the internal carotid artery posterolaterally. On MR images, punctate flow voids are often seen within the tumor, and larger lesions have a typical salt-and-pepper pattern on T2-weighted images. Intense enhancement is seen after intravenous administration of gadolinium, which may be heterogeneous with areas of low signal intensity that may relate to fibrosis or flow dephasing.

Treatment is generally by surgery, since these tumors have a pattern of growth, local invasiveness, and malignant potential and since there is an absence of another treatment modality. Radiotherapy is occasionally used for palliative treatment.

## REFERENCES

Vogl T, Bruning R, Schedel H et al: Paragangliomas of the jugular bulb and carotid body: MR imaging with short sequences and Gd-DTPA, *AJR* 153:583-587, 1989.

Rippe DJ, Grist TM, Uglietta JP et al: Carotid body tumor: flow sensitive pulse sequences and MR angiography, *JCAT* 13(5):874-877, 1989.

Shamblin WR, Remine WH, Sheps SG, Harrison EG: Carotid body tumor (chemodectoma): clinicopathologic analysis of ninety cases, *Am J Surg* 122:732-739, 1971.

Lees GD, Levine HL, Beven EG, Tucker HM: Tumors of carotid body: experience with 41 operative cases, *Am J Surg* 142:362-365, 1981.

Idbohrn H. Angiographical diagnosis of carotid body tumors, *Acta Radiol* 35:115-123, 1951.

Berrett A: Value of angiography in the management of tumors of the head and neck, *Radiology* 84:1052-1058, 1965.

Barros D'Sa AAB: Management of carotid body tumors, *Curr Pract Surg* 4:36-48, 1992.

Pryse-Davis J, Dawson IMP, Westbury G: Some morphologic, histochemical, and chemical observations on chemodectomas and the normal carotid body, including a study of the chromaffin reaction and possible ganglion cell elements, *Cancer* 17:185-202, 1964.

Levit SA, Sheps SG, Espinosa RE et al: Catecholamine secreting paraganglioma of glomus-jugulare region resembling pheochromocytoma, *N Engl J Med* 281:805-811, 1969.

Meyer FB, Sundt TM, Pearson BW: Carotid body tumors: a subject review and suggested surgical approach, *J Neurosurg* 64:377-385, 1986.

# CASE 142
# GLOMUS VAGALE TUMOR

**History:** 56-year-old with a slowly increasing neck mass.

**Technique:** multiple axial volumes (multiple overlapping thin-slab acquisition), three-dimensional time-of-flight, 33/7/20, 256 × 128, one excitation, 1-mm thick, 64 slices, 20-cm field of view, 9:07.

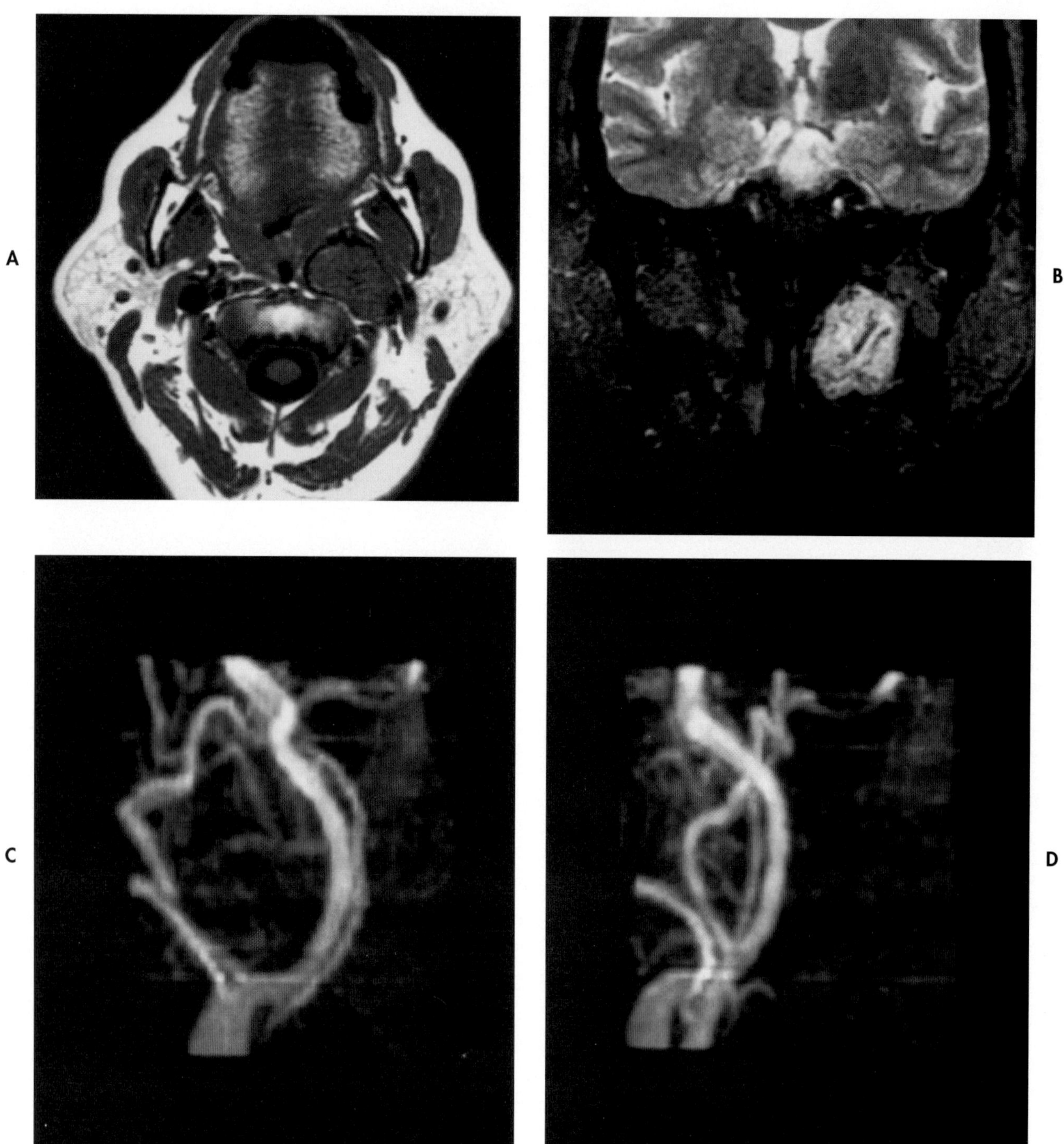

**Axial T1-weighted spin-echo image (A) shows a mass within the left carotid space, which has central punctate areas of low signal intensity. Heterogeneous signal intensity is present within the mass on the coronal T2-weighted image (B). Lateral maximum intensity projection view of the time-of-flight MRA (C) apparently shows the internal and external carotid arteries being splayed as with a carotid body tumor. However, the anteroposterior view (D) shows that the centering of the volume is slightly high and that the internal and external carotid arteries were overlapped on the lateral view, which made it look like the bifurcation. There is lateral displacement of the internal and external branches on the anteroposterior view. The mass is therefore above the carotid bifurcation within the carotid space and consistent with a glomus vagale tumor. (Courtesy Walter Kucharczyk, Toronto, Canada.)**

Chemoreceptor cells have been found in relation to the carotid body, aortic body, vagal ganglion, auricular branches of the ninth and tenth cranial nerves, superior and recurrent laryngeal nerves, iliac vessels, and pineal body. The vagal body is located in the perineurium of the vagus at the level of the nodose ganglion or within the ganglion itself. Glomus vagale tumors constitute approximately 10% of head and neck paragangliomas; women are more often affected than men. The incidence of multicentricity is 10%, with the most common combination being glomus vagale with glomus jugulare. Familial inheritance of glomus vagale tumors is quite rare in contrast to that for glomus jugulare and carotid body tumors. A glomus vagale tumor differs from a carotid body tumor in that it lies more cephalad in the neck, extending towards the skull base. Vagale tumors tend to invade the posterolateral pharyngeal wall and displace the carotid vessels anteriorly and medially without widening the carotid bifurcation. Some 50% of patients present with cranial neuropathies. Preoperative embolization with surgical excision is the treatment of choice. The vagus nerve is nearly always sacrificed during excision.

As in MR imaging of carotid body tumors, MR imaging of glomus vagale tumors demonstrates a characteristic appearance based on vasculature, including serpentine areas of flow void interspersed among high signal areas of tumor cells or slow flow. In larger lesions (greater than 2 cm) this salt-and-pepper pattern is consistently seen. This appearance is reported distinct from other tumors in this area, such as meningiomas, neuromas, and skull base tumors.

**REFERENCE**

Olsen WL, Dillon WP, Kelly W et al: MR imaging of paragangliomas, *AJR* 148:201-204, 1987.

# CASE 143
# GLOMUS JUGULARE

**History:** 40-year-old with pulsatile tinnitus.

**Technique:** axial volume; three-dimensional time-of-flight; 33/8/20 degrees; 192 × 512; 128 slices; 128-mm slab; tilted, optimized nonsaturating excitation pulse; 20-cm field of view; 13:34.

A

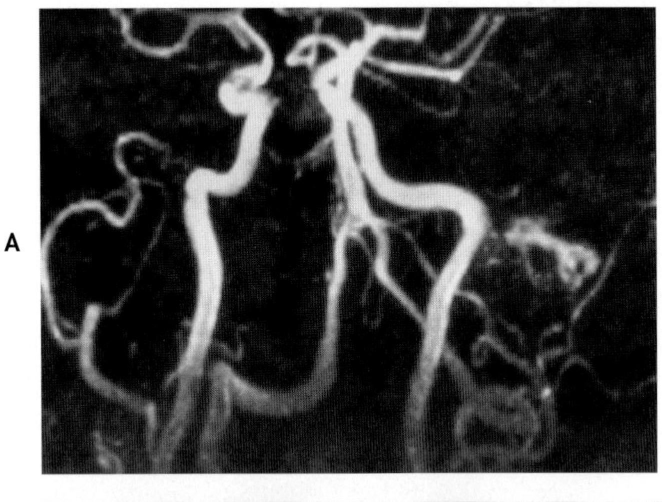

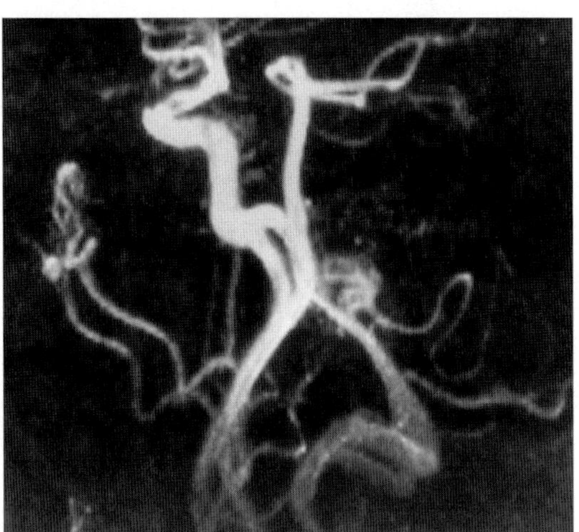

B

C

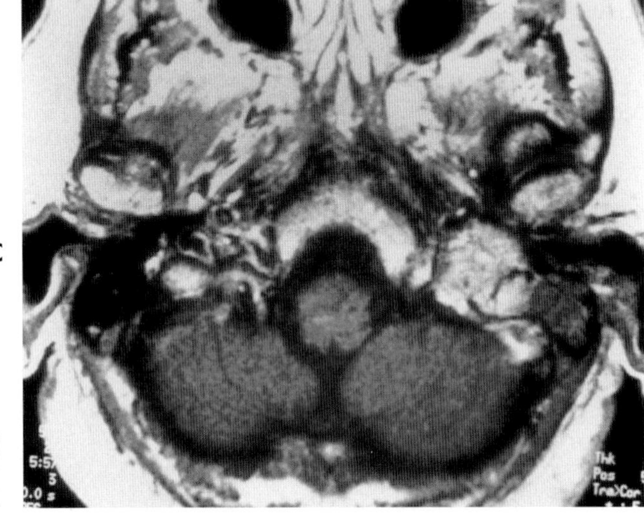

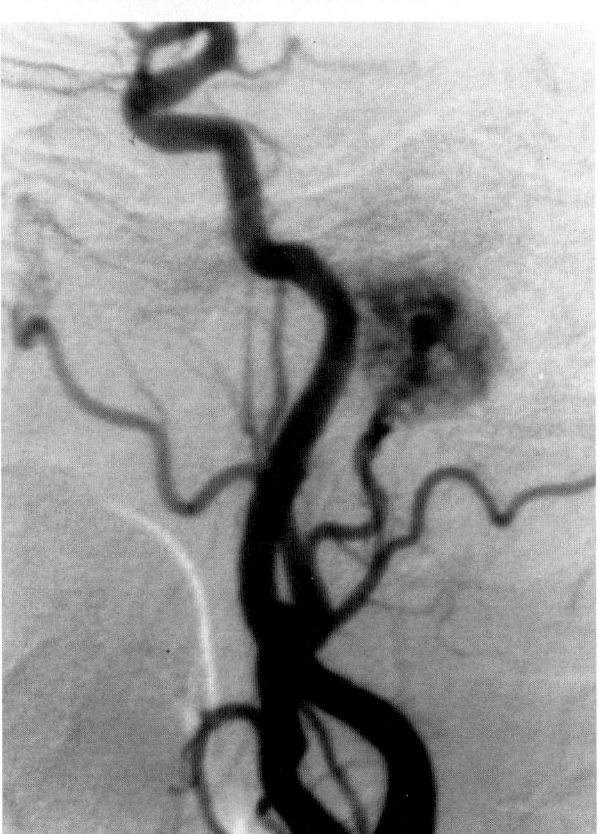

D

**Left anterior oblique (A) and lateral (B) maximum intensity projection views demonstrate an abnormal tangle of vessels in the region of the skull base on the left. The internal carotid arteries and vertebral arteries appear normal bilaterally. T1-weighted axial image of the skull base after contrast (C) demonstrates a large mass involving the left jugular foramen, with a spiculated appearance of low signal intensity within the central substance, which is consistent with a glomus jugulare. A lateral view from the left common carotid artery injection (D) demonstrates a large blush involving the left jugular foramen, which is supplied by an enlarged branch of the external carotid artery (posterior auricular artery). (Courtesy Alison S. Smith, Aultman Hospital, Canton, Ohio.)**

The region of the jugular foramen is the area of transition of the jugular bulb to the internal jugular vein, with the carotid artery positioned anteriorly. There is a thin, bony plate separating the vein from the artery. The ninth and tenth cranial nerves exit anteromedial to the jugular bulb. The inferior petrosal sinus drains in variable positions along the anterior margin of the jugular bulb and is separated from the exiting nerves by a small amount of connective tissue. The sigmoid sinus empties into the posterior part of the jugular bulb.

The main differential for such a skull base lesion involving the jugular foramen region would include glomus jugulare, metastasis, and meningioma. Glomus jugulare and meningiomas of the jugulare bulb have a propensity for slow, unremitting growth, with erosion of the skull base and neurologic involvement.

Meningiomas of the jugular foramen arise from the arachnoid lining cells in the arachnoid villi associated with the jugular bulb. As they grow, they envelope the cranial nerves and eventually spread to the temporal bone and posterior fossa. Unlike glomus jugulare tumors, meningiomas tend to spread along the neural sheaths. Thus ensuring that all the tumor is removed probably requires total removal of all cranial nerves surrounded by tumor. Meningioma recurrence is common, around 20%, in contrast to a 5% to 10% glomus recurrence rate.

**REFERENCE**

Molony TB, Brackmann DE, Lo W: Meningiomas of the jugular foramen, *Otolaryngol Head Neck Surg* 106:128-136, 1992.

## CASE 144
## GLOMUS TYMPANICUM

**History:** 55-year-old woman with left pulsatile tinnitus.

**Technique:** axial volume; three-dimensional time-of-flight; 45/7/20; 256 × 192; 64 slices; 60-mm slab; magnetization transfer saturation; tilted, optimized nonsaturating excitation radiofrequency pulse; 14-cm field of view; 9:15.

A

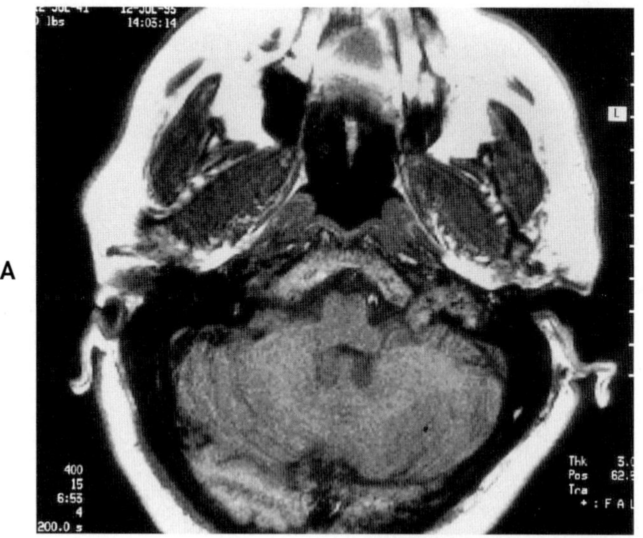


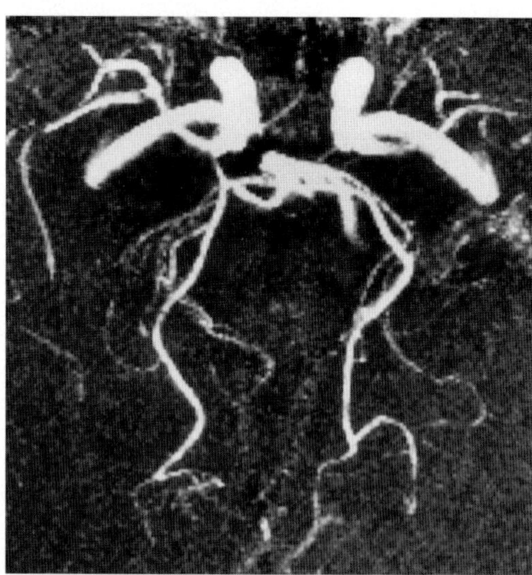

B

C

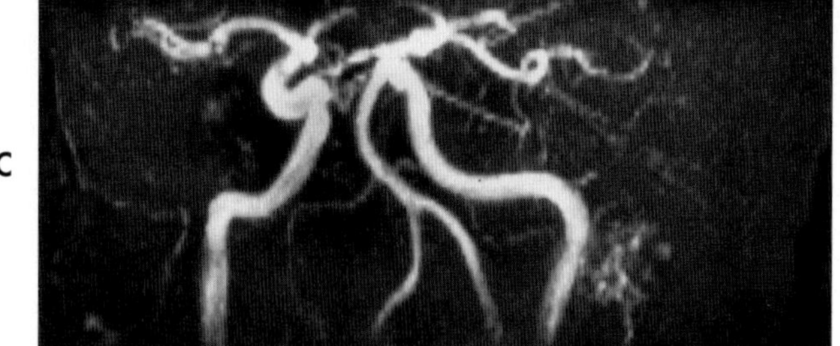

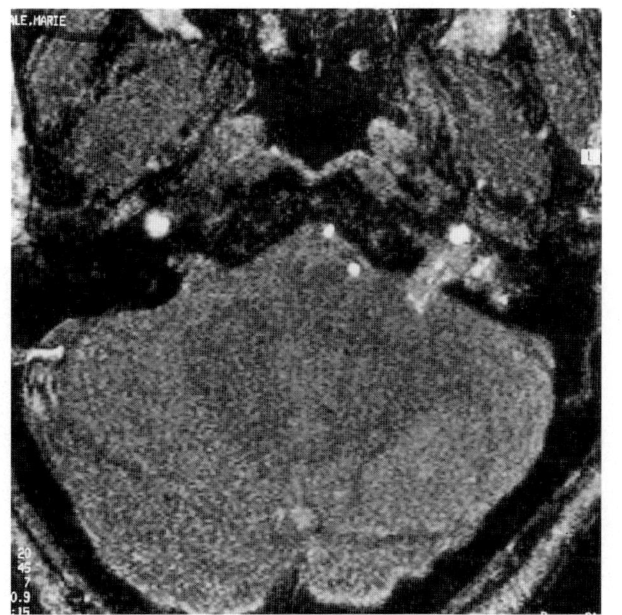

D

**Axial T1-weighted image shows a salt-and-pepper–appearing soft tissue mass in the petrous apex extending to the left middle ear (A). Base (B) and left anterior oblique (C) maximum intensity projection views of the MRA show a tangle of small vessels from the tumor, which is confirmed on the individual slice (D).**

Glomus tympanicum tumors are slow-growing chemodectomas similar to glomus jugulares and are the most common primary tumor of the middle ear. Glomus tympanicum tumors arise from glomus cells along the course of the tympanic branch of the ninth cranial nerve (Jacobson's nerve) within the middle ear. Clinical presentations include pulsatile tinnitus and hearing loss, and the majority of patients are women over the age of 40. The classic physical finding is a reddish-blue retrotympanic mass that blanches with pneumotoscopy. Typical findings include a markedly enhancing mass involving the middle ear and arising from the promontory without enlargement of the jugular fossa. Angiography shows a highly vascular mass within the middle ear that is most commonly fed by the ascending pharyngeal artery. These lesions do not seem to occur within families, and there does not seem to be a propensity toward bilaterality or multiplicity.

### REFERENCES

Larson TC III, Reese DF, Baker HL Jr, McDonald TJ: Glomus tympanicum chemodectomas: radiographic and clinical characteristics, *Radiology* 163:801-806, 1987.

O'Leary MJ, Shelton C, Giddings NA et al: Glomus tympanicum tumors: a clinical perspective, *Laryngoscope* 101:1038-1043, 1991.

## CASE 145
## BASILAR ARTERY LOOP COMPRESSING THE SEVENTH AND EIGHTH CRANIAL NERVES

**History:** 79-year-old with hemifacial spasm.

**Technique:** axial volume, three-dimensional time-of-flight, 40/7/15, 256 × 256, 64 slices, 60-mm slab, 25-cm field of view, 10:57.

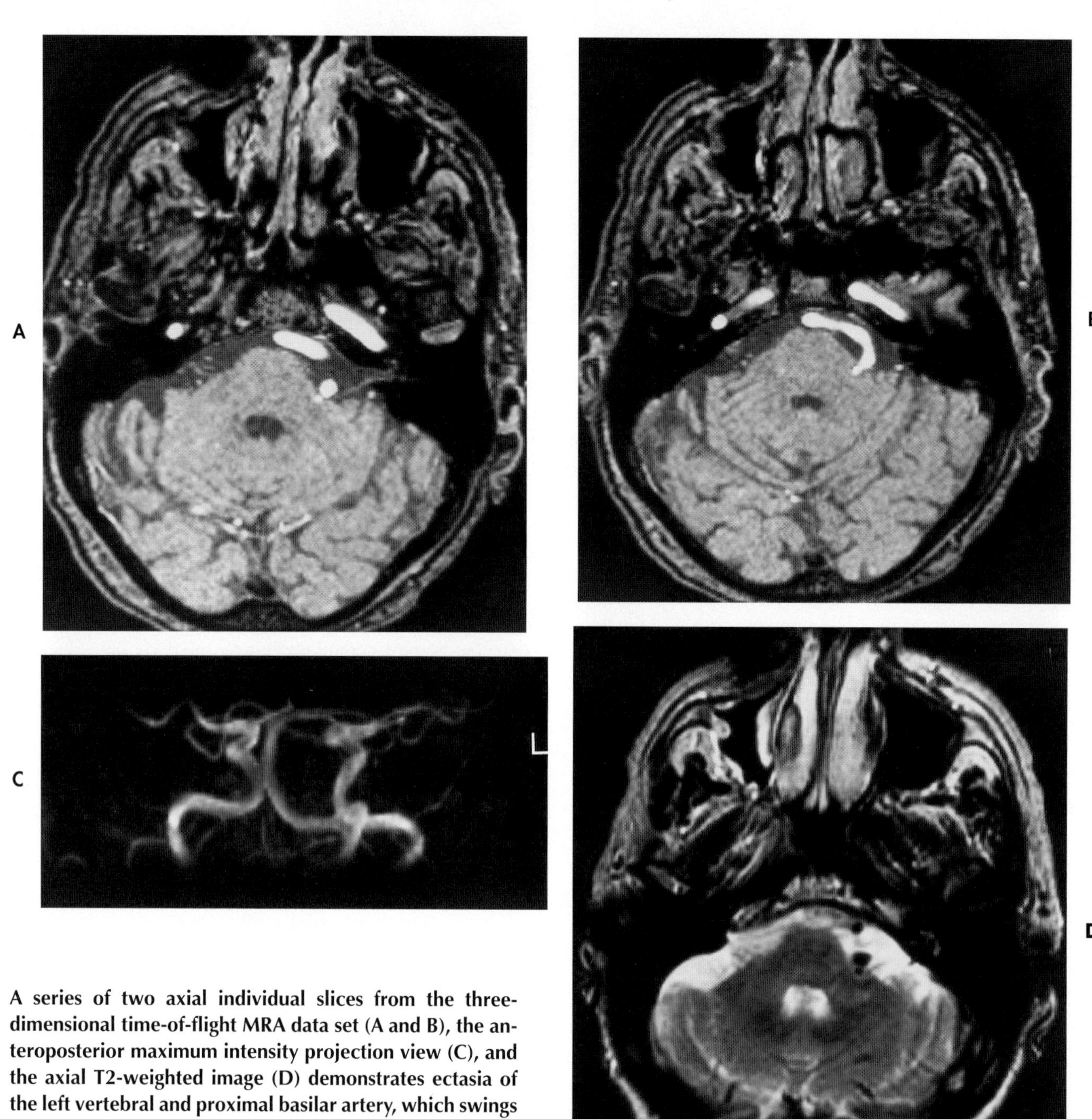


**A series of two axial individual slices from the three-dimensional time-of-flight MRA data set (A and B), the anteroposterior maximum intensity projection view (C), and the axial T2-weighted image (D) demonstrates ectasia of the left vertebral and proximal basilar artery, which swings into the left cerebellopontine angle and compresses the region of the exiting seventh and eighth nerve root complex.**

Hemifacial spasm is characterized by involuntary unilateral contractions of the muscles innervated by the seventh cranial nerve. Although most cases remain idiopathic, causes have been ascribed to extraaxial masses, intraparenchemal masses, multiple sclerosis, and vascular compression. Vascular compression is thought to occur at the root entry zone, which is the region of transition between central and peripheral myelin; this is proposed as a cause because of surgical visualization of compression and relief of symptoms after decompressive surgery. The causal mechanism of hemifacial spasm is thought to be continuous compression or pulsations that produce focal demyelination at the root entry zone, which would cause increased neuronal discharge in the facial nucleus. However, there is more than one mechanism, since supranuclear parenchymal lesions may also produce hemifacial spasm.

Adler et al evaluated 37 patients with hemifacial spasm and 16 age-matched controls with MRA and found that 65% of the patients with hemifacial spasm had ipsilateral vascular compression compared with 6% of the controls. Felber et al noted neurovascular contact in the root entry zone in 4 of 20 controls and 12 of 14 patients with hemifacial spasm; in the latter, MRA predicted the affected side. Venous disease has been described as causing root entry zone compression, so traditional time-of-flight techniques will not address this condition.

### REFERENCES

Adler CH, Zimmerman RA, Savino PJ et al: Hemifacial spasm: evaluation by magnetic resonance imaging and magnetic resonance tomographic angiography, *Ann Neurol* 32:502-506, 1992.

Felber S, Birbamer G, Aichner et al: Magnetic resonance imaging and angiography in hemifacial spasm, *Neuroradiolgy* 34:413-416, 1992.

Nielsen VK: Pathophysiology of hemifacial spasm. I. Ephaptic transmission and ectopic excitation, *Neurology* 34:418-426, 1984.

Tien RD, Wilkins RH: MRA deliniation of the vertebro-basilar system in patients with hemifacial spasm and trigeminal neuralgia, *AJNR* 14:34-36, 1993.

## CASE 146
## SECOND BRANCHIAL POUCH CYST

**History:** 34-year-old with a left nasopharyngeal pulsatile mass.

**Technique:** axial volume, three-dimensional time-of-flight, 40/7/15, 256 × 256, 64 slices, 60-mm slab, 25-cm field of view, 10:57.

A

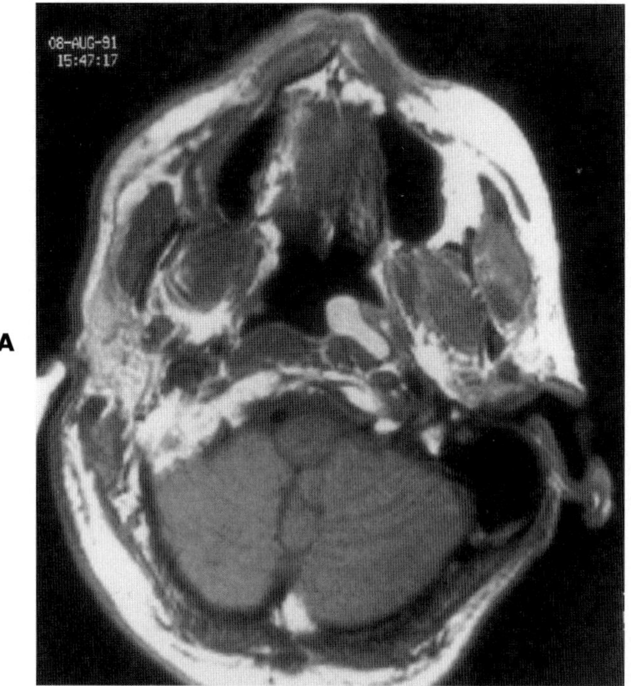


B

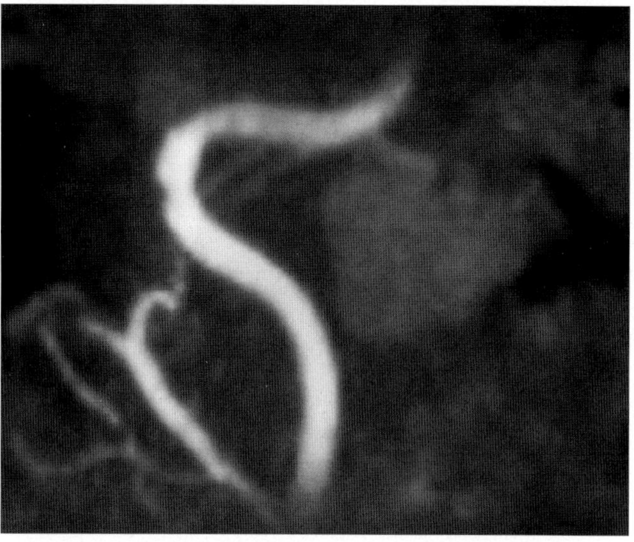

C

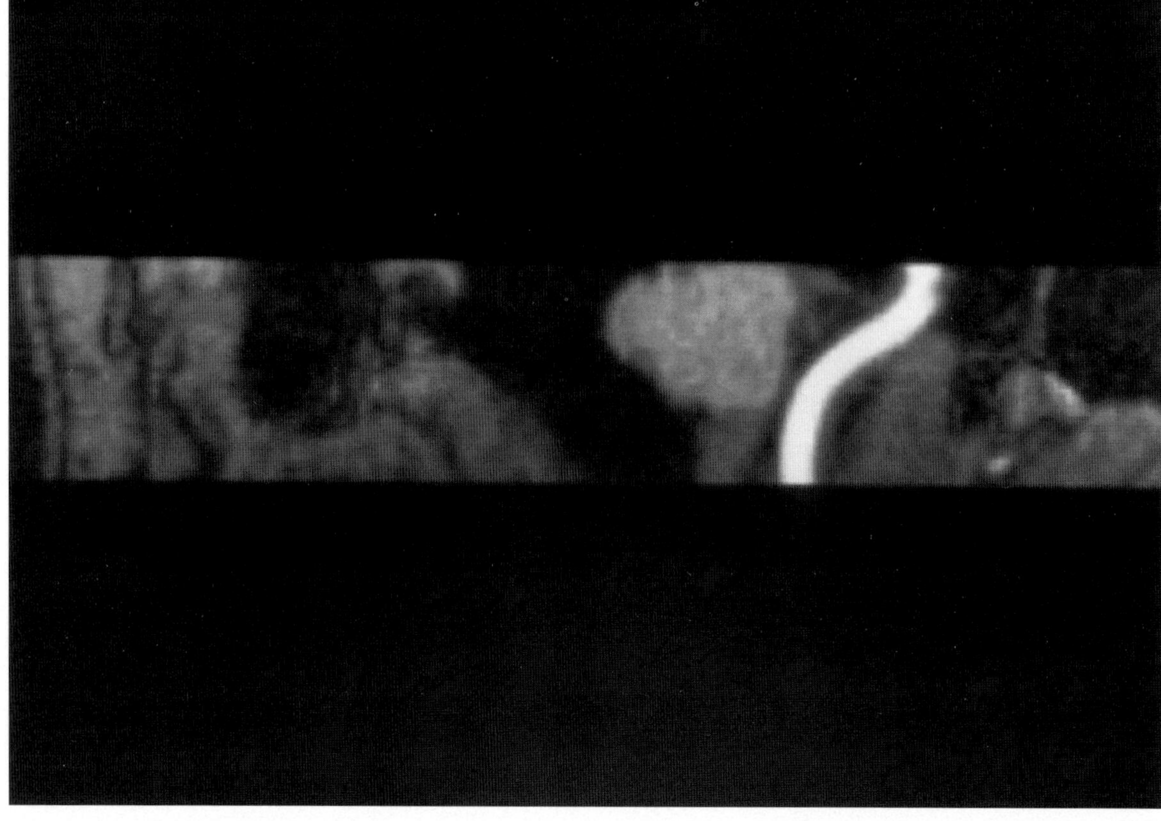

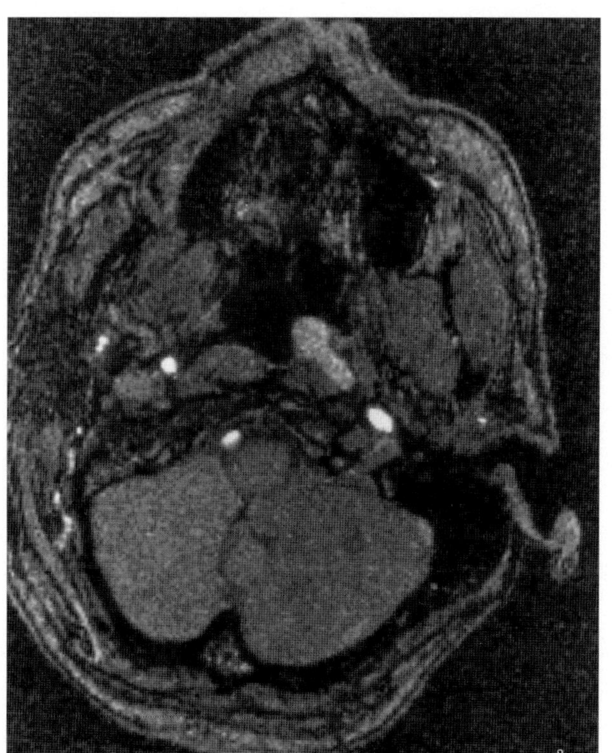


**Axial T1-weighted spin-echo study through the oral pharynx (A) demonstrates a well-defined mass of high signal intensity within the left fossa of Rosenmuller. Flow void of the carotid artery appears adjacent and lateral to the lesion. Right anterior oblique maximum intensity projection view of the MRA (B) demonstrates the normal-appearing cervical carotid artery lateral to the nasopharyngeal mass. The mass itself is vaguely seen as an area of increased signal intensity medial to the carotid. Sagittal reformatting from the MRA data (C) shows the separate nature of the cyst from the more laterally placed internal carotid artery. Individual slice from angiographic data set (D) confirms the separate nature of these lesions from the carotid. There is also quite different signal intensities from the flow within the carotid and from the cyst contents, which are causing T1 shortening. (From Ross JS: *Syllabus for the categorical course in neuroradiology,* pp. 21-29, 1992.)**

The location and signal intensity would be consistent with a second branchial pouch cyst with increased protein content, also called a *Bailey type IV cyst*. The T1-shortening effect is presumably similar to that possibly present within chronically obstructed sinonasal secretions. Anderson et al described a similar type of case, in which a thyroid cyst had increased signal intensity on T1-weighted images and mimicked a carotid pseudoaneurysm on carotid MRA.

The majority of branchial abnormalities arise from the second branchial apparatus, which is made up of ectoderm, mesoderm, and endoderm. The ectodermal component becomes part of the cervical sinus of His, the mesodermal component becomes the muscles of facial expression, and part of the hyoid and the endodermal component becomes the palatine tonsil. A persistent second branchial tract may extend from the anterior border of the sternocleidomastoid muscle, passing between the internal and external carotid arteries and above the hypoglossal and glossopharyngeal nerves toward the tonsillar fossae. The Bailey type IV cyst, as in this case, is a columnar, lined cyst believed to be a remnant of the pharyngeal pouch.

**REFERENCES**

Benson MT, Dalen K, Mancuso AA et al: Congenital anomalies of the branchial apparatus: embryology and pathologic anatomy, *Radiographics* 12:943-960, 1992.

Bailey H: *Branchial cysts and other essays on surgical subjects in the facio-cervical region,* London, 1929, Lewis.

Anderson CM, Gooding GAW, Lee RE: Thyroid cyst mistaken for carotid pseudoaneurysm by MR angiography, *Clinical imaging* 16:198-200, 1992.

Liston SL, Siegel LG: Branchial cysts, sinuses and fistulas, *Ear Nose Throat J* 58:9-17, 1979.

# CHAPTER 8

# Venous Disease (Excluding Vascular Malformations)

It is frequently necessary to evaluate the patency of dural venous sinuses in patients with contiguous mass lesions, meningeal inflammatory processes, or hypercoagulable states predisposing the patient to thrombosis. Until recently, venous disease was one of the few remaining indications for intravenouos digital subtraction angiography. MR imaging and MR venography are now the procedures of choice. Patients with dural sinus occlusion may have histories of otitis and mastoiditis, pregnancy, oral contraceptive use, malignancy or trauma, but the etiologies are many and varied (see box). Clinical symptomatology may be nonspecific but classically are manifestations of increased intracranial pressure (headache, nausea, and vomiting), focal neurologic deficit, and seizure. Less commonly associated clinical conditions include homocystinuria and collagen vascular diseases such as lupus and Behçet's syndrome. Blood disorders such as polycythemia and leukemia tend to produce thrombosis, as do deficiencies of certain vitamin K–dependent hepatically produced proteins (proteins C and S).

In the past, the diagnosis of venous occlusion was made directly with conventional angiography or with computed tomographic scanning by identification of thrombosed veins or the "empty delta," "sinus rectus," or "falx" signs.[1,2] However, these radiologic techniques are either invasive or limited in their ability to adequately visualize veins in the middle and posterior fossa because of artifact.

**CAUSES OF CEREBRAL VENOUS THROMBOSIS**

1. Infection: face, sinus, mastoid, systemic
2. Hematologic: polycythemia, sickle cell disease, leukemia, myeloproliferative disorders, protein C or S deficiency, antithrombin III deficiency
3. Collagen vascular disease
4. Dehydration
5. Pregnancy, oral contraceptive use, estrogen or androgen therapy
6. Trauma
7. Tumor: Local-venous sinus compression by meningioma, glomus, metastasis
8. Tumor: Systemic-carcinoid, carcinomatosis
9. Inflammation: sarcoid, Wegener's granulomatosis
10. Miscellaneous: L-asparaginase therapy, congestive heart failure

Spin-echo imaging can be useful in sinus thrombosis because it documents the lack of normal flow void within an occluded sinus. In a thrombosed sinus, spin-echo imaging demonstrates the signal intensity changes of the contained blood products, which are similar to those of a parenchymal hemorrhage.[3,4] In either case, it is also possible to demonstrate enlarged medullary or cortical veins and any adjacent parenchymal changes such as hemorrhage or infarction.[5]

The findings of occlusion or thrombosis are probably best appreciated on the coronal, long-echo-time, T2-weighted spin-echo studies, since the larger dural veins run predominantly perpendicular to this imaging plane. With through-plane flow, flowing blood normally demonstrates flow void because it is least apt to experience both the 90- and 180-degree pulses before leaving the imaging plane (because of the extended echo time) unless thrombosis is present. The spin-echo findings of dural sinus thrombosis can occasionally be confusing with slow flow or acute or early subacute thrombosis. The appearance varies, depending on the sequence parameters chosen (T1 vs. T2) and the imaging plane. In the case of slow flow, a hyperintense signal may simulate a thrombus. For example, high signal within the transverse sinus on T1-weighted spin-echo imaging is a common finding that is difficult to differentiate from thrombus with methemoglobin. Entry-slice flow-related enhancement must be distinguished from high signal intensity clot. In the case of acute or early subacute thrombus, the hypointense thrombus may simulate a flow void on T2-weighted images. In these situations, MR venograms can be most helpful in confirming or in excluding the presence of flow without having to do an invasive study such as an intravenous or an intraarterial digital subtraction angiography.

Three-dimensional time-of-flight techniques are not recommended for the evaluation of dural sinuses because of their normal slow flow. Slow flow causes artifactual signal loss within patent sinuses because of saturation effects that affect time-of-flight sequences and could mimic occlusion. A solution to this may be the concomitant use of gadolinium–DPTA.[6,7]

More appropriate for evaluation of the dural sinuses are two-dimensional time-of-flight techniques, which may be acquired several ways. Coronal images acquired posterior to anterior and against the direction of flow (countercurrent) make the best use of flow-related enhancement for the evaluation of the superior and inferior sagittal sinuses, transverse sinuses, and deep veins. However, the necessary distance for coverage of the superior sagittal sinus is greatest with the coronal acquisition, which increases the overall examination time. Likewise, the trade-off of axial images is the large distance that must be covered to visualize the superior sagittal sinus and transverse sinuses and the possibility of in-plane dephasing with signal loss for in-plane anatomy (such as the transverse sinuses). An oblique sagittal sequential two-dimensional sequence acquired from the posterior-to-anterior direction gives a good compromise between area of coverage and flow-related enhancement. Given the "normal" flow velocities of 20 to 46 cm/sec and the spatial resolution needed to demonstrate partial obstruction, the slice thickness for these two-dimensional slices should be as thin as possible to reduce the possibility of false-positive studies.[6] False-negative studies are also possible with this technique if the short T1 of methemoglobin within a thrombus is incorrectly interpreted as flow-related enhancement. The answer to this problem is simply to evaluate the T1- and T2-weighted spin-echo parenchymal examination for the high signal intensity methemoglobin or use a phase-contrast study.

Phase contrast techniques are particularly well suited to venous MRA applications, since stationary thrombus does not cause a phase shift over time and therefore appears as a filling defect in the dural sinus.[8,9] Although these images can be acquired with a three-dimensional phase-contrast technique that provides greater anatomic detail, the more time-efficient and clinically practical two-dimensional phase-contrast version is generally sufficient.[10] With imaging times around 2 to 3 minutes for single thick-slice versions, multiple velocity encodings may be acquired to maximize diagnostic confidence. Velocity-encoding settings at 10 to 20 cm/sec are usually sufficient for evaluation of venous anatomy. Artifacts also occur with the phase-contrast techniques. If the velocity encoding is set too low for the venous flow, there is signal loss that may mimic occlusion. Setting the velocity encoding to high causes aliasing, with central loss of signal in the sinus.

Other, less common techniques may be used to identify the diagnosis of sinus occlusion. Phase images could be reconstructed from a spin-echo study to confirm the presence of flow. These images have a sensitivity for velocities as low as 0.5 cm/sec in the slice-select direction or 2.5 cm/sec in the frequency direction if given the appropriate gradient construction.[11] A thin saturation pulse could be applied perpendicular to the direction of flow to perform bolus tagging. This can be used to quantitate flow velocity by simply measuring the distance that the saturation band moves within the imaging plane over time.[6,12] Phase information may also be obtained from paired gradient-recalled sequences, which can be used to quantitate the flow velocity and clearly distinguish slow flow from thrombus.[10,13]

## REFERENCES


1. Goldberg AL, Rosenbaum AE, Wang H et al: Computed tomography of dural sinus thrombosis, *JCAT* 10:16-20, 1986.
2. Virapongse C, Cazenave C, Quisling R et al: The empty delta sign: frequency and significance in 76 cases of dural sinus thrombosis, *Radiology* 162:779-785, 1978.
3. Macchi PJ, Grossman RI, Gomori JM et al: High field MR imaging of cerebral venous thrombosis, *JCAT* 10:10-15, 1986.
4. Sze G, Simmons B, Krol G et al: Dural sinus thrombosis: verification with spin-echo techniques, *AJNR* 9:679-686, 1988.
5. Anderson SC, Shah CP, Murtaugh FR: Congested deep subcortical veins as a sign of dural venous thrombosis: MR and CT correlations, *JCAT* 11:1050-1061, 1987.
6. Mattle H, Edelman RR, Reis MA, Atkinson DJ: Flow quantification in the superior sagittal sinus using magnetic resonance, *Neurology* 40:813-815, 1990.
7. Chakeres DW, Schmalbrock P, Brogan M et al: Normal venous anatomy of the brain: demonstration with gadopentetate dimeglumine in enhanced 3-D MRA, *AJNR* 11:1107-1118, 1990.
8. Rippe DJ, Boyko OB, Spritzer CE et al: Demonstration of dural sinus occlusion by the use of MRA, *AJNR* 11:199-201, 1990.
9. Dumoulin CL, Hart HR; Magnetic resonance angiography, *Radiology* 161:717-720, 1986.
10. Spritzer CE, Pelc NJ, Lee JN et al: Rapid MR imaging of blood flow with phase-sensitive, limited-flip angle gradient recalled pulse sequence: preliminary experience, *Radiology* 176:255-262, 1990.
11. Nadel L, Braun IF, Kraft KA et al: Intracranial vascular abnormalities: value of MR phase imaging to distinguish thrombus from flowing blood, *AJNR* 11:1133-1140, 1990.
12. Edelman RR, Mattle H, Kleenfield J, Silver MS: Quantification of blood flow with dynamic MR imaging and presaturation bolus tracking, *Radiology* 171:551-556, 1989.
13. Boyko O, Pelc NJ, Shimakawa A: *Application of velocity imaging and gradient recalled echo in neuro imaging.* In *Book of abstracts for RSNA 76th Annual Meeting,* Chicago, 1990, Radiological Society of North America.

## CASE 147
## PITFALL: MOTION ARTIFACT SIMULATING FOCAL OCCLUSION OF THE SAGITTAL SINUS

**History:** 40-year-old with pseudotumor cerebri.

**Technique:** oblique coronal, two-dimensional time-of-flight, 40/10/30, 256 × 256, 25-cm field of view, posterior-to-anterior direction, 9:23.

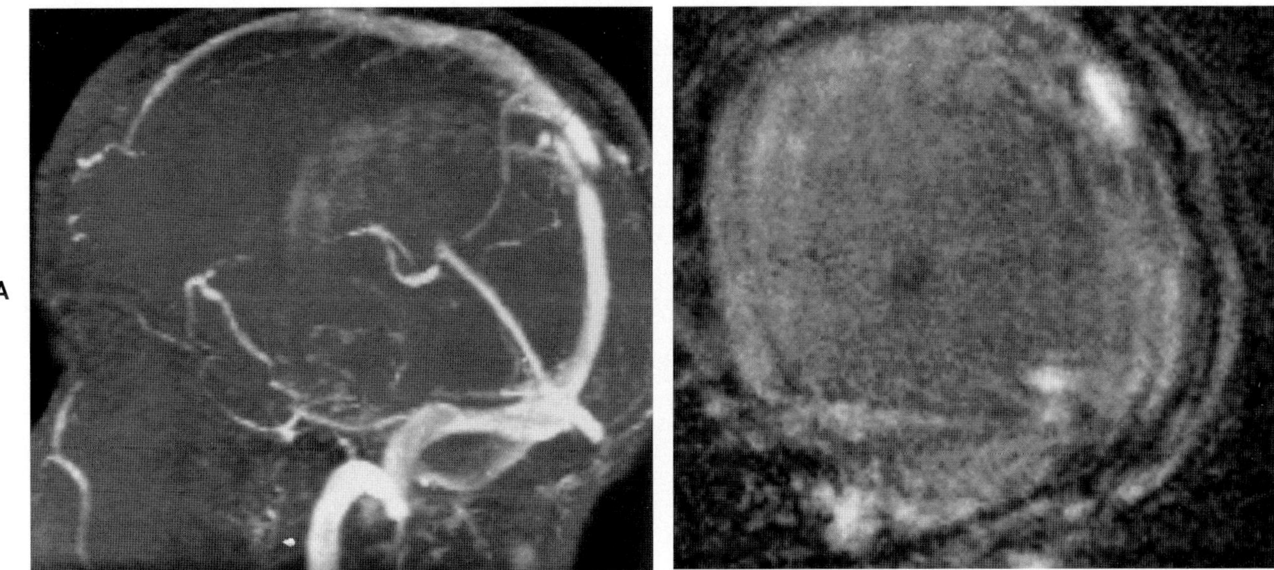


**Oblique maximum intensity projection view of the two-dimensional time-of-flight MRA (A) shows an apparent focal occlusion or stenosis of the posterior aspect of the superior sagittal sinus. There is an ill-defined curvilinear increased signal extending from right to left at the level of the sinus defect. Examination of the individual slice of this two-dimensional time-of-flight study shows gross motion artifact (B).**

The motion artifact in this case was present only on one slice, which was manifested on the maximum intensity projection view of all the acquired slices as a focal loss of signal intensity that mimicked stenosis or focal occlusion.

# CASE 148
# THROMBOSIS OF LEFT TRANSVERSE SINUS

**History:** 13-year-old boy with pseudotumor cerebri.

**Technique #1:** oblique sagittal, two-dimensional time-of-flight (head rotated 15 degrees), 45/9/60, 256 × 128, one excitation, 2.5-mm slices with 60 total slices, inferior saturation pulse, 20-cm field of view.

**Technique #2:** axial, two-dimensional phase-contrast, 30/8/20, 512 × 256, eight excitations, 60-mm thick section, 30 cm/sec velocity encoding, 20-cm field of view, 4 minutes.

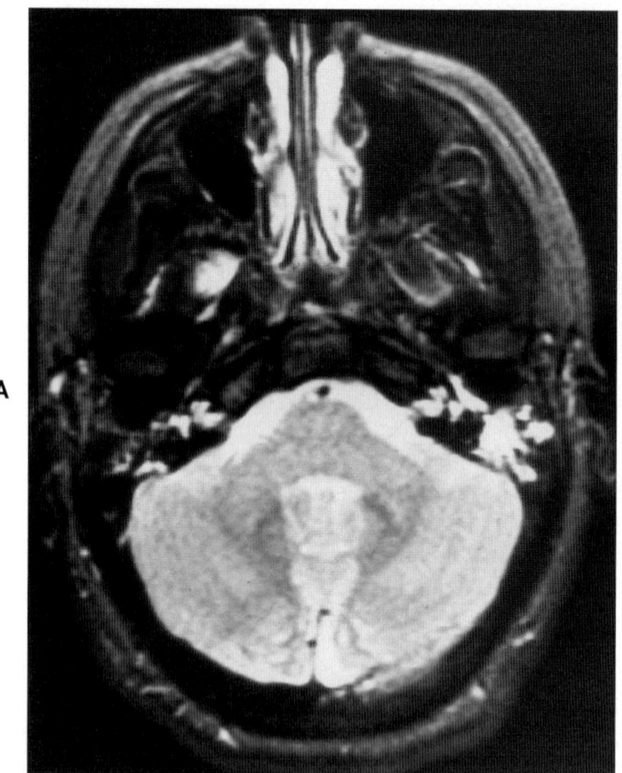

A

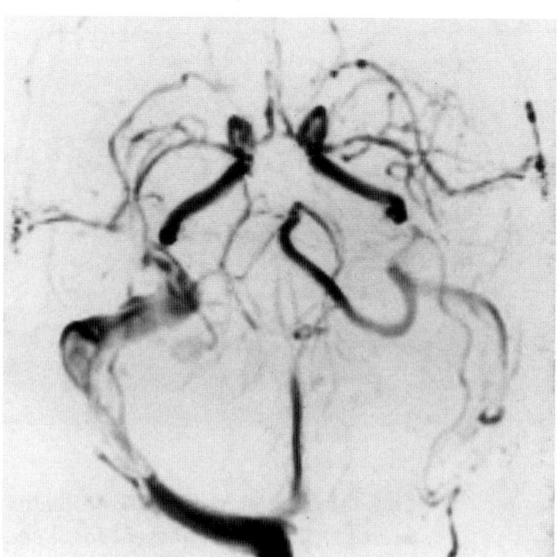

D

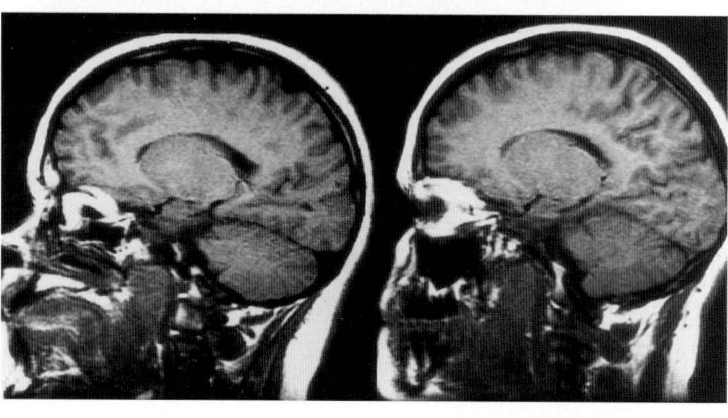

B C

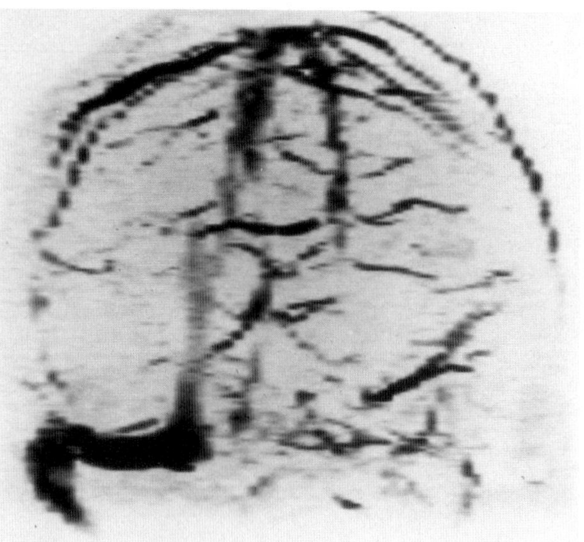

E

F

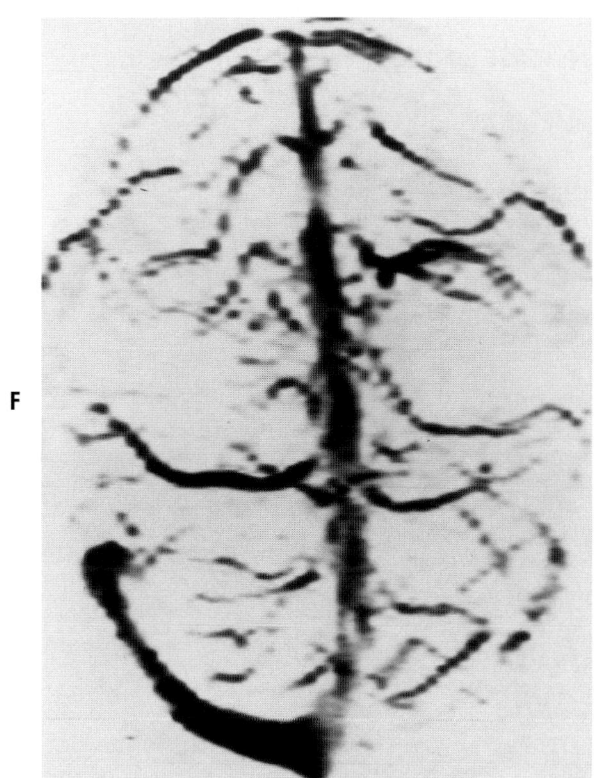

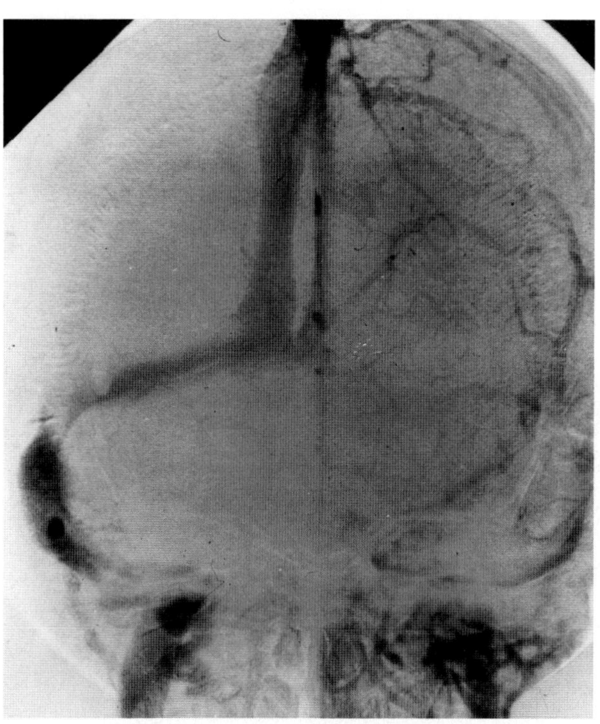

G

**A conventional T2-weighted axial MR (A) demonstrates high signal intensity bilateral otitis media and mastoiditis, more extensive on the left. Parasagittal T1-weighted spin-echo images on the right (B) and left sides (C) show asymmetry in the transverse sinus signals, with a normal flow void on the right and isointense signal within the transverse sinus on the left. Base view from a two-dimensional phase-contrast MRA demonstrates occlusion of the proximal left transverse and sigmoid sinuses, with reconstitution of the distal sigmoid sinus (D). A similar appearance is seen on the anteroposterior (E) and vertex (F) views of the two-dimensional time-of-flight MR venogram. There is also decreased signal from the lateral aspect of the right transverse sinus on the time-of-flight and phase-contrast MR venograms. (Courtesy John Huston, Mayo Clinic, Rochester, Minn.)**

The asymmetric appearance of the transverse sinuses on the sagittal T1-weighted images is suspicious for thrombosis. However, this must not be confused with increased signal within a sinus from entry-slice phenomenon, which is due to normal flow. In this case, the increased signal from the left transverse sinus on the T1-weighted image is due to thrombosis and is confirmed by the typical findings of sinus thrombosis on the phase-contrast and time-of-flight studies. In addition, the signal defect in the lateral aspect of the right transverse sinus suggests additional partial thrombosis of the right transverse sinus. The MRA findings of thrombosis of the left transverse sinus are confirmed on the anteroposterior venous phase of the conventional left carotid angiogram, as well as the partial filling defect in the right transverse sinus **(G).**

The finding of nonvisualization of the left transverse sinus on the phase-contrast study with a 30 cm/sec velocity encoding suggests occlusion. However, a small or hypoplastic transverse sinus with very slow flow may be seen only with a lower velocity encoding, such as 10 cm/sec. In this particular case, the question of a hypoplastic transverse sinus is excluded, since the T1-weighted spin-echo images show a normal-sized left sinus with abnormal signal intensity within it.

## CASE 149
## THROMBOSIS OF LEFT TRANSVERSE SINUS

**History:** 15-year-old girl with a congenital hematologic disorder.

**Technique #1:** axial, two-dimensional phase-contrast, 30/8/20, 512 × 256, eight excitations, 60-mm thick section, 30 cm/sec velocity encoding, 20-cm field of view, 4 minutes.

**Technique #2:** same as Technique #1 except with 15 cm/sec velocity encoding.

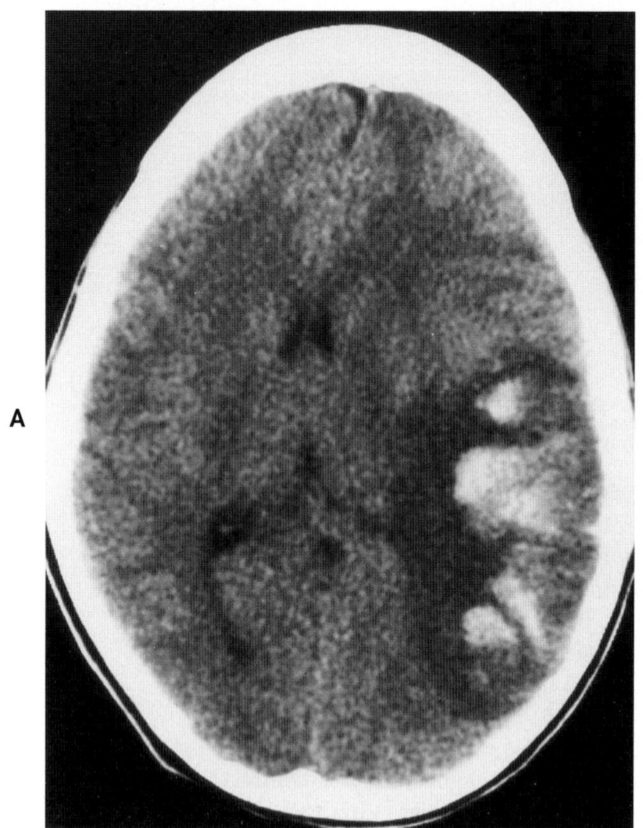

A

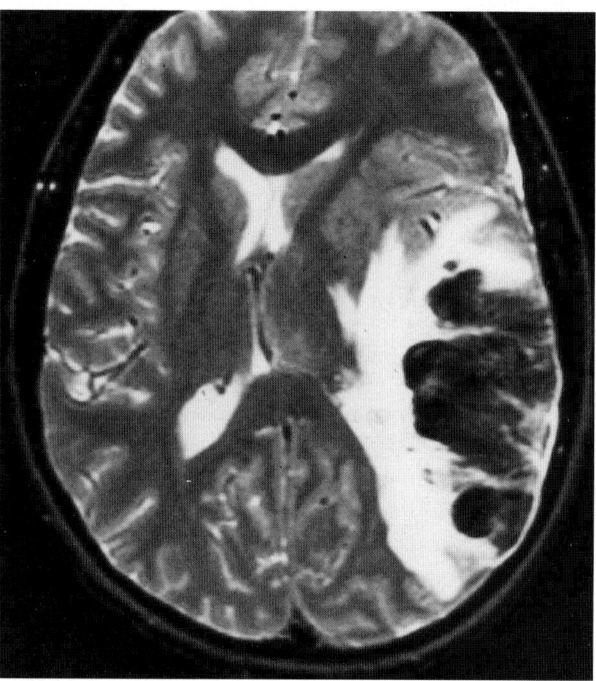

B

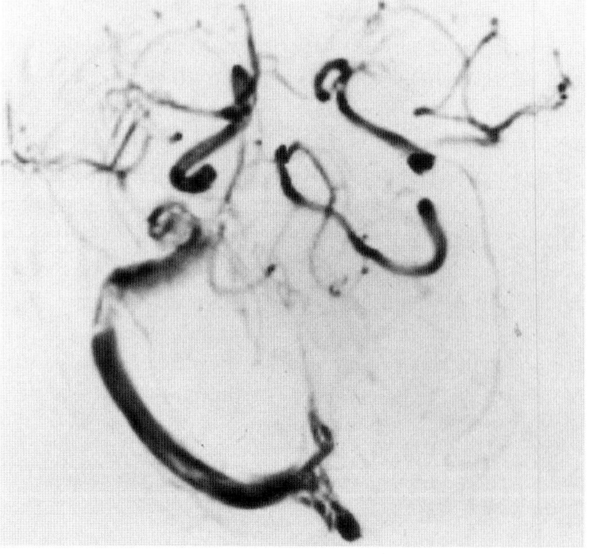

C

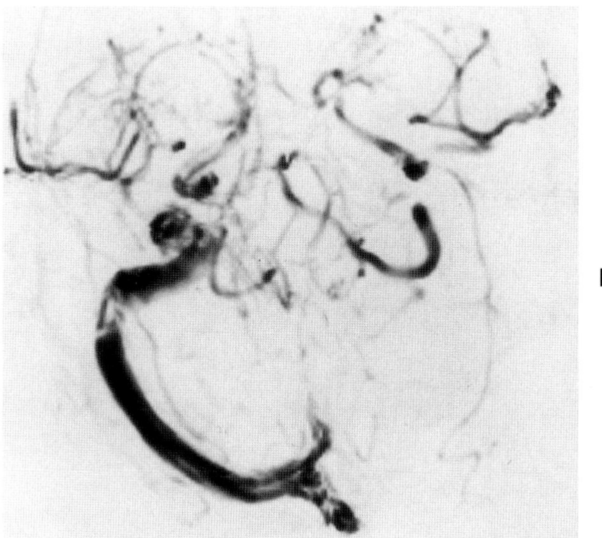

D

**Unenhanced axial computed tomographic examination demonstrates a well-defined area of decreased attenuation in the left parietal lobe with associated hemorrhage and subfacial herniation (A). T2-weighted axial MR image (B) shows the large hemorrhagic lesion with considerable mass effect and a small amount of vasogenic edema, which is consistent with a venous infarct. Base projections of two-dimensional phase-contrast MRAs with 30 cm/sec (C) and 15 cm/sec (D) velocity encodings show lack of signal from the left transverse sinus, which represents left transverse sinus thrombosis. (Courtesy John Huston, Mayo Clinic, Rochester, Minn.)**

The addition of the lower 15 cm/sec velocity encoding adds confidence to the diagnosis of left transverse sinus thrombosis by excluding very slow flow states.

## CASE 150
## SUPERIOR SAGITTAL SINUS THROMBOSIS

**History:** 14-day-old with decreased level of consciousness.

**Technique:** axial three-dimensional phase-contrast, 27/10/15, 256 × 128, one excitation, 1.5-mm slices with a total of 60 slices, velocity encoding of 15 cm/sec, 18-cm field of view, 14 minutes.

A

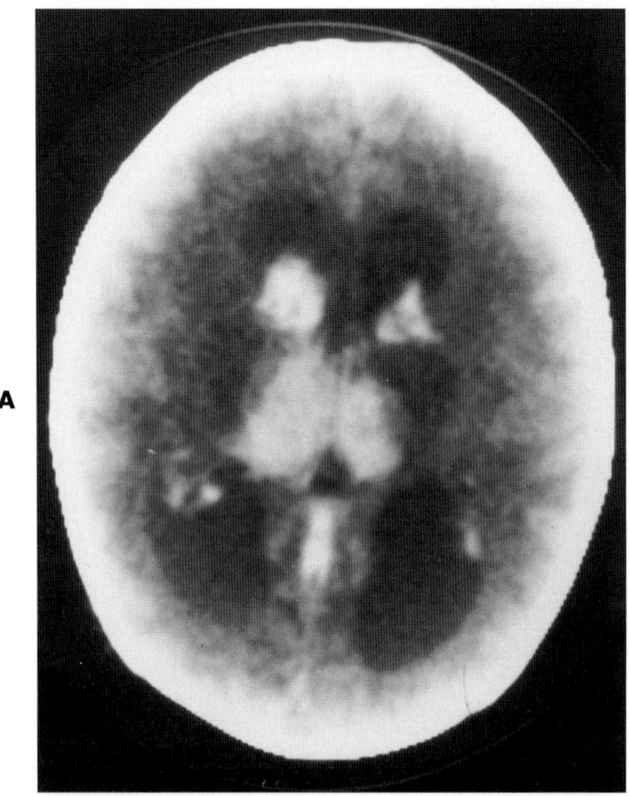

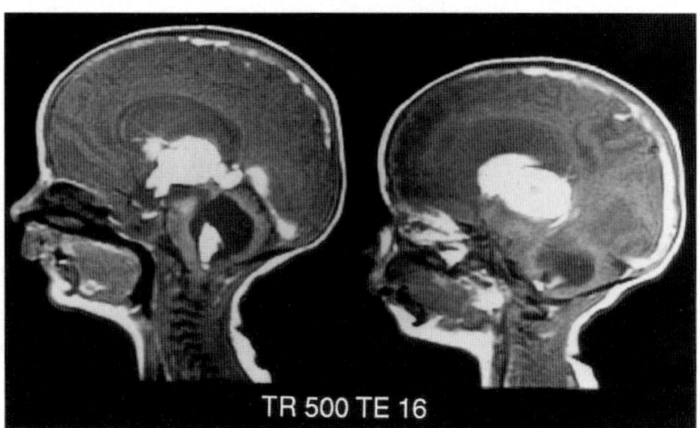


B

C

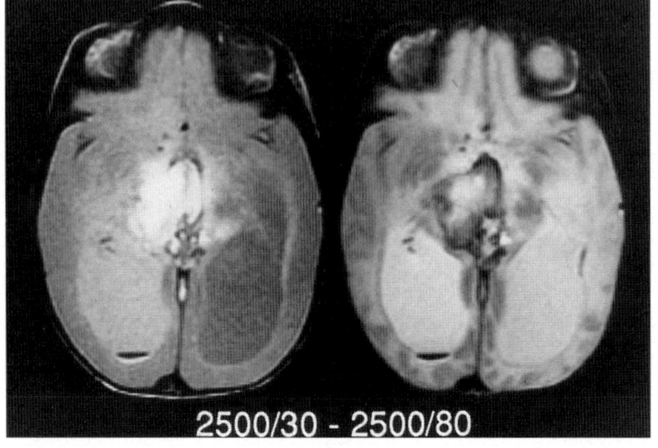


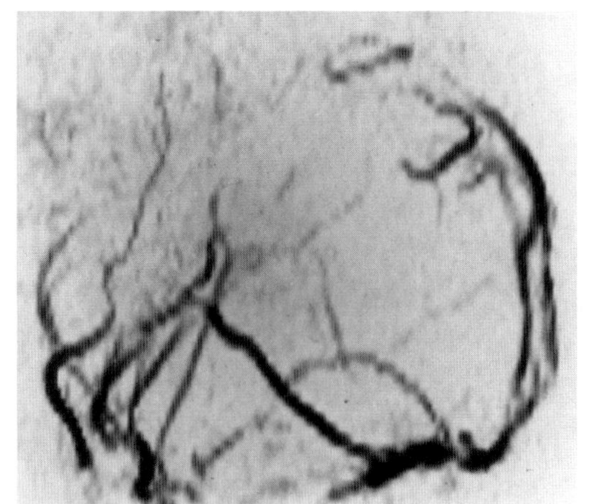

D

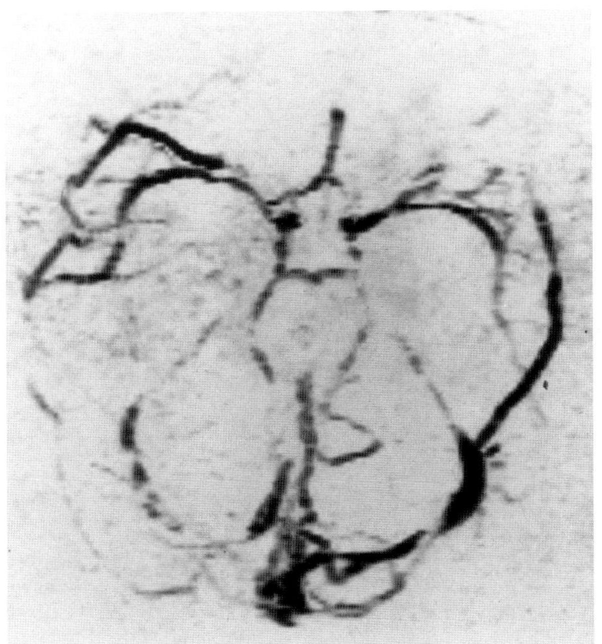


**A computed tomographic scan without contrast (A) demonstrates increased attenuation in both thalami and within the ventricles, which is consistent with thalamic and intraventricular hemorrhage. T1-weighted sagittal (B) and axial spin-density-weighted MR images (C) show the hemorrhage as increased signal (methemoglobin) within the lateral, third, and fourth ventricles and thalami. There is abnormal increased signal intensity from the superior sagittal and straight sinuses, which represents sinus thrombosis. The hemorrhage results in obstructive hydrocephalus and a trapped fourth ventricle. The lateral (D) and base (E) views of the three-dimensional phase-contrast angiogram show lack of signal from the superior sagittal and straight sinuses. (Courtesy John Huston, Mayo Clinic, Rochester, Minn.)**

There is excellent background suppression with the phase-contrast technique, with no interference from the high signal intensity methemoglobin. This amount of high signal intensity blood precludes the use of a time-of-flight technique to visualize the venous sinuses. The posterior aspect of the superior sagittal sinus demonstrates multiple patent channels resulting from reconstitution around the subacute thrombus.

## CASE 151
## SUPERIOR SAGITTAL SINUS THROMBOSIS

**History:** 32-year-old with a myeloproliferative disorder.

**Technique:** two-dimensional time-of-flight, 30/10/20, 256 × 192, 25-cm field of view, oblique coronal, posterior-to-anterior direction, 8:28.

A

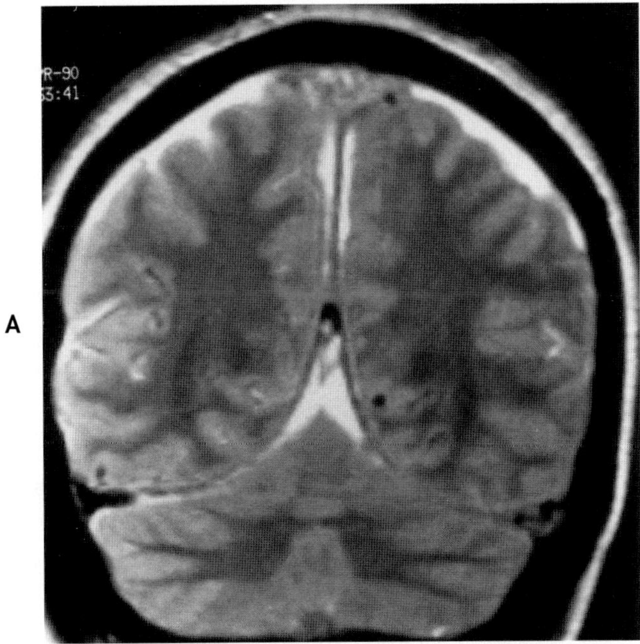

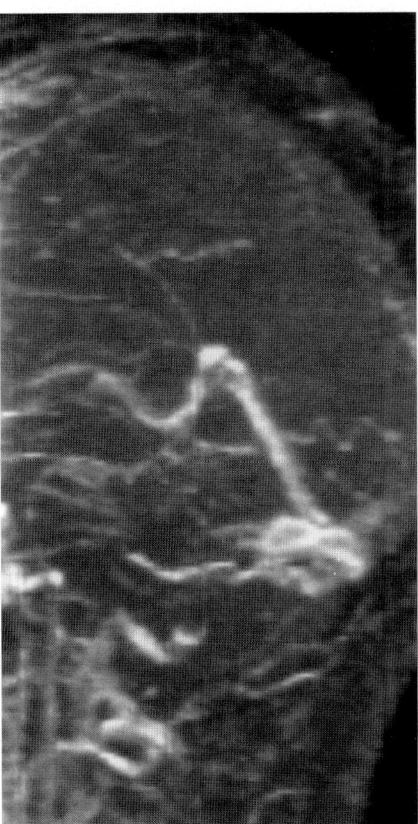

B

**Coronal spin-density-weighted image (A) shows small bilateral convexity and interhemispheric subdural hematomas. There is loss of the usual flow void from the superior sagittal sinus on this first echo and on the second echo (not shown). Lateral maximum intensity projection view of the MR venogram (B) of the posterior half of the head shows no flow within the superior sagittal sinus but patent internal cerebral veins, vein of Galen, and straight sinus.**

## CASE 152
## SUBACUTE SUPERIOR SAGITTAL SINUS THROMBOSIS

**History:** 66-year-old with transient visual obscuration for 2 weeks when bending over and a diagnosis of papilledema after physical examination.

**Technique #1:** oblique coronal, two-dimensional time-of-flight, 32/10/30, 256 × 192, 23-cm field of view, posterior-to-anterior direction, 5:58.

**Technique #2:** sagittal, two-dimensional phase-contrast, 33/8/20, 256 × 192, eight excitations, 60-mm thick section, 10 cm/sec velocity encoding, 20-cm field of view, 3:25.

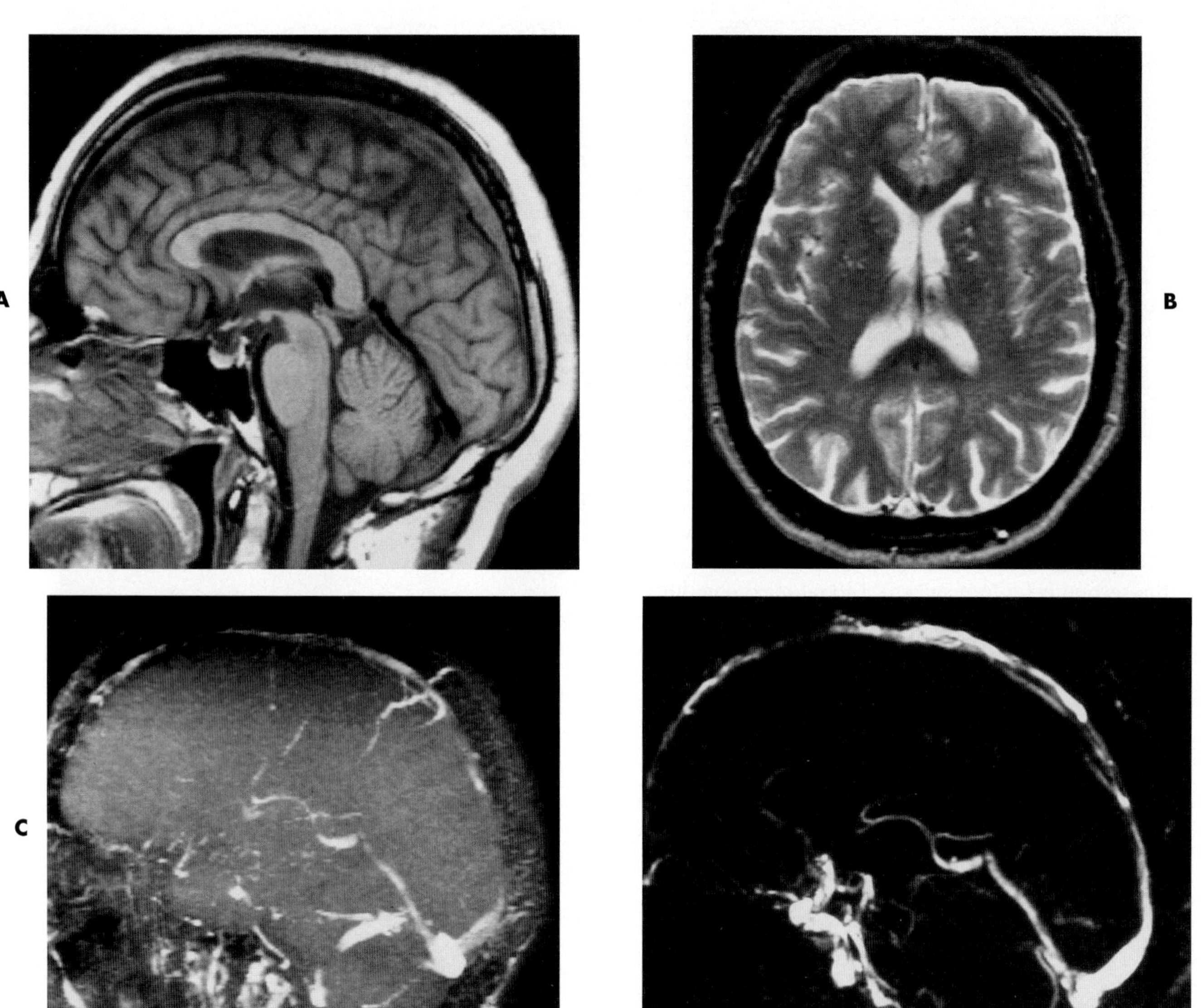

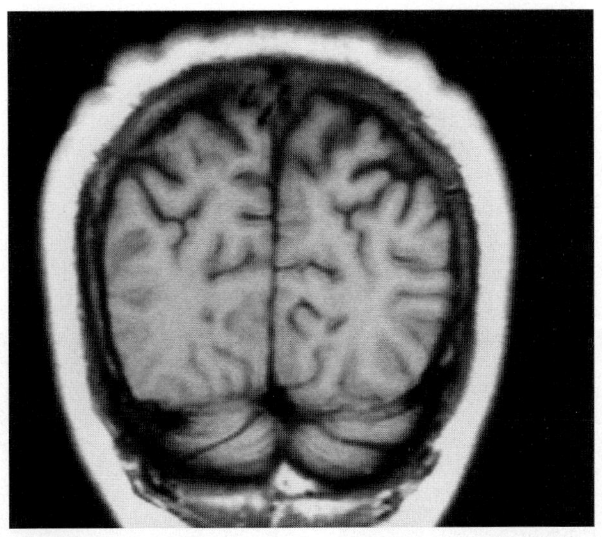

E

**Sagittal T1-weighted image (A) shows slightly increased signal from the superior sagittal sinus, which is suspicious for sinus thrombosis. Axial T2-weighted image (B) also shows abnormal signal from the posterior aspect of the superior sagittal sinus, with small areas of flow void around the sinus periphery. Sagittal maximum intensity projection view of the two-dimensional time-of-flight MRA (C) demonstrates lack of signal from the posterior portion of the superior sagittal sinus, with a patent torcula and deep veins. Sagittal view of the thick-slice two-dimensional phase-contrast study with a 10 cm/sec velocity encoding (D) shows only slight irregularity in the flow signal from the region of the superior sagittal sinus, which did not show flow on the two-dimensional time-of-flight study. A coronal T1-weighted image (E) shows isointense thrombus within the posterior sagittal sinus and small collateral vein flow void around the sinus periphery, as is seen on the axial T2-weighted study.**

The findings in this case relate to partial subacute thrombosis of the sagittal sinus. The signal from the sinus on the spin-echo images is abnormal but is not the classic high signal intensity from fresh methemoglobin. The discrepancy in appearance of the posterior portion of the superior sagittal sinus may be related to two factors: (1) partial thrombosis of the sinus, with a small peripheral rim of patent sinus with slow flow detected by the low velocity encoding of the two-dimensional phase-contrast study; and/or (2) slow flow signal from the small collateral veins demonstrated only on the phase-contrast study. The patient was placed on coumadin based on the clinical and MR findings.

## CASE 153
## DEEP VENOUS THROMBOSIS

**History:** 29-year-old with headaches and decreasing mental status, who was referred from outside the hospital with a possible diagnosis of herpes encephalitis.

**Technique:** oblique coronal, two-dimensional time-of-flight, 32/10/30, 256 × 192, 23-cm field of view, posterior-to-anterior direction, 5:58.

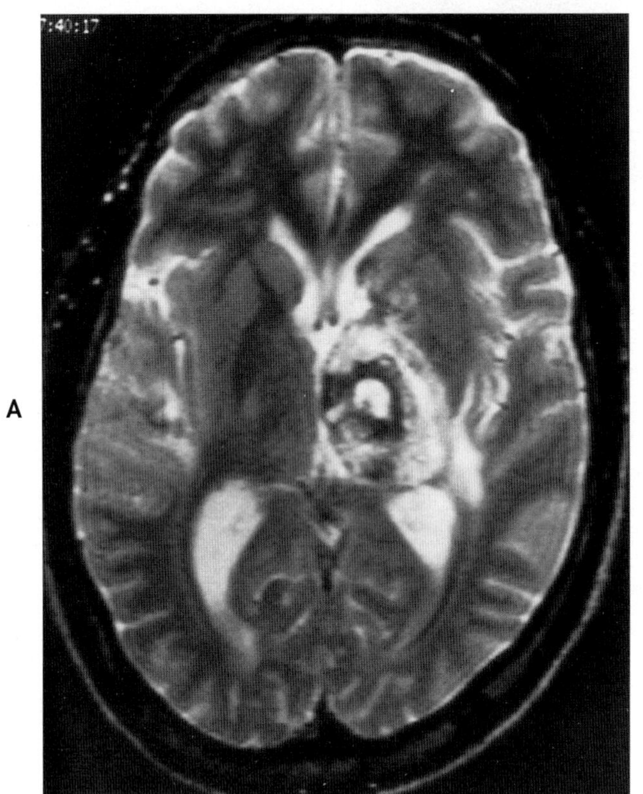


A

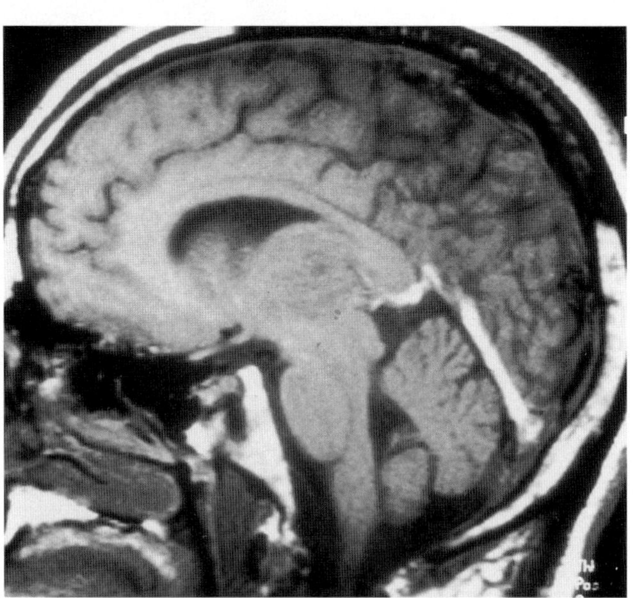

B

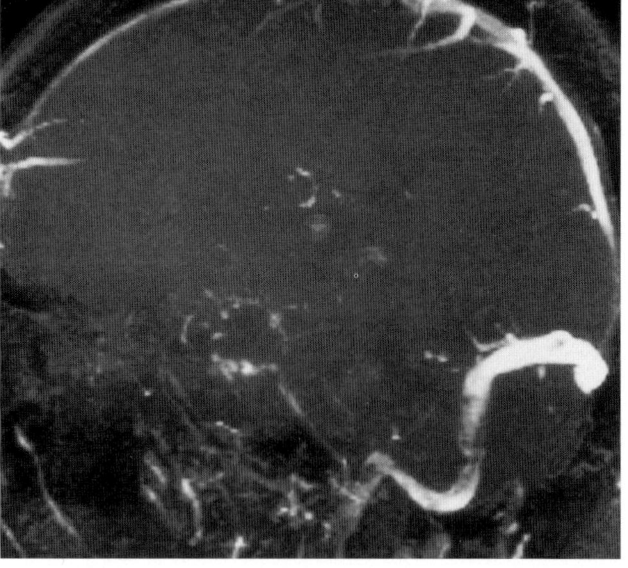

C

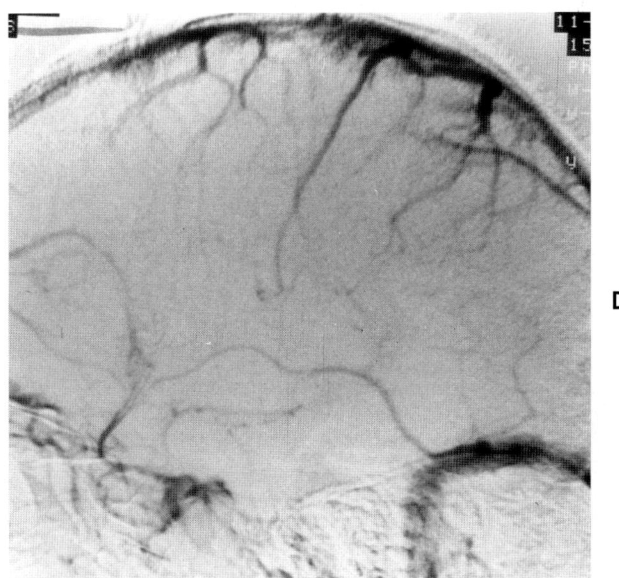

D

**T2-weighted axial image of the brain (A) shows rounded low signal intensity within the left thalamus, which is related to a hemorrhagic infarction with surrounding vasogenic edema, and a slight mass effect on the third ventricle. T1-weighted sagittal spin-echo image (B) shows abnormal increased signal from the straight sinus and vein of Galen. The lateral maximum intensity projection view of the MR venogram (C) shows lack of signal from the internal cerebral vein, vein of Galen, and straight sinus, with only slight "shine-through" from the methemoglobin within the thalamus. Lateral view of the conventional angiogram (D) shows no deep veins on the late venous image.**

The signs of deep venous thrombosis can be indirect or direct. Direct signs include thrombus visualized in the vein of Galen, straight sinus, internal cerebral vein, or thalamostriate veins by computed tomography or MR imaging. The indirct signs are infarctions in the thalamic and basal ganglia, enhancement of the venous infarcts, hemorrhagic infarction, hemorrhage into the velum interpositum, and ventricular dilatation. Ashforth et al described two patients with deep cerebral venous thrombosus diagnosed by computed tomography and MR imaging. Although they noted direct findings of hyperintense thrombus in the internal cerebral veins and vein of Galen on T1-weighted MR images, they were also struck by the marked amount of basal ganglia and thalamic edema, which extended into the internal and external capsules. In both cases, MR images showed basal ganglia and thalamic hemorrhage.

**REFERENCE**

Ashforth RA, Melanson D, Ethier R: MR of deep cerebral venous thrombosis, *Can J Neurol Sci* 16:417-421, 1989.

## CASE 154
## LEFT SIGMOID SINUS THROMBOSIS WITH SUBDURAL EMPYEMA AND CEREBITIS

**History:** 65-year-old with long-standing diabetes who now has fever and decreasing mental status.

**Technique:** axial volume, three-dimensional phase-contrast, 27/10.9/20, 256 × 128, velocity encoding of 10 cm/s, 60 slices, 72-mm slab, 20-cm field of view, 14:45.

A

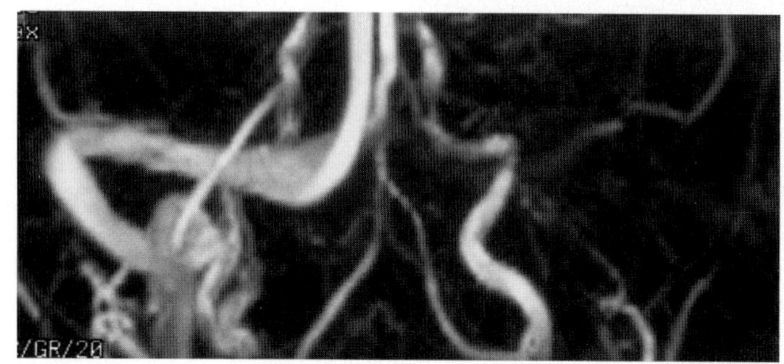


B

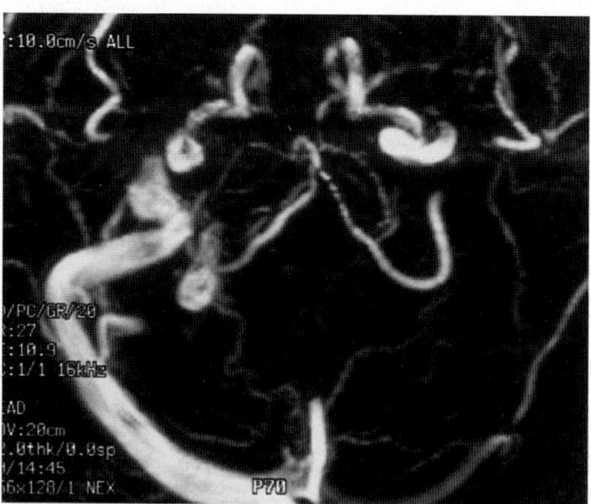


C

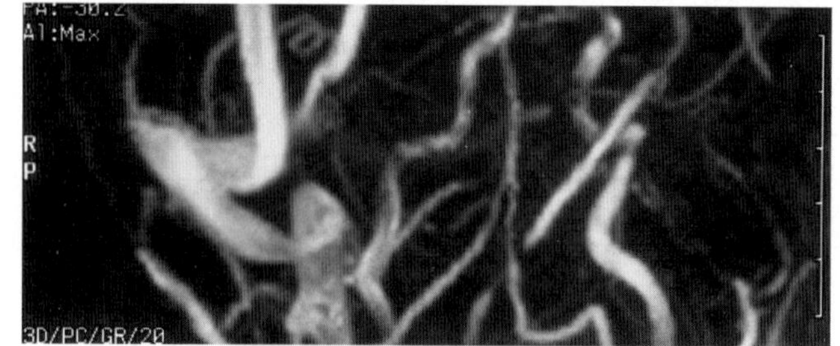


D

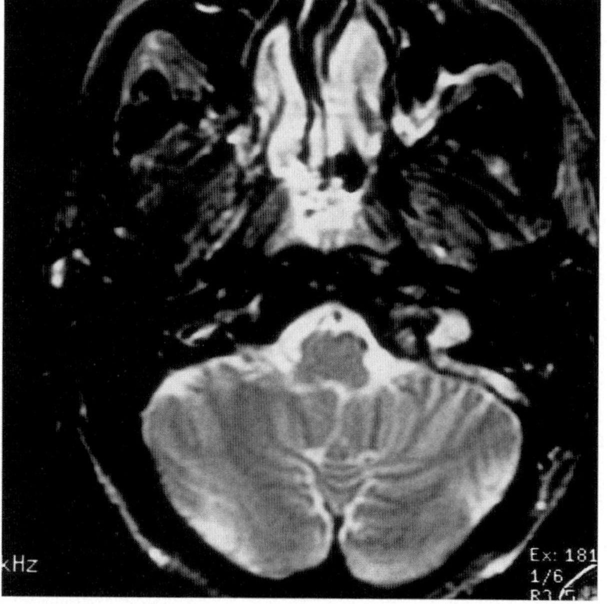

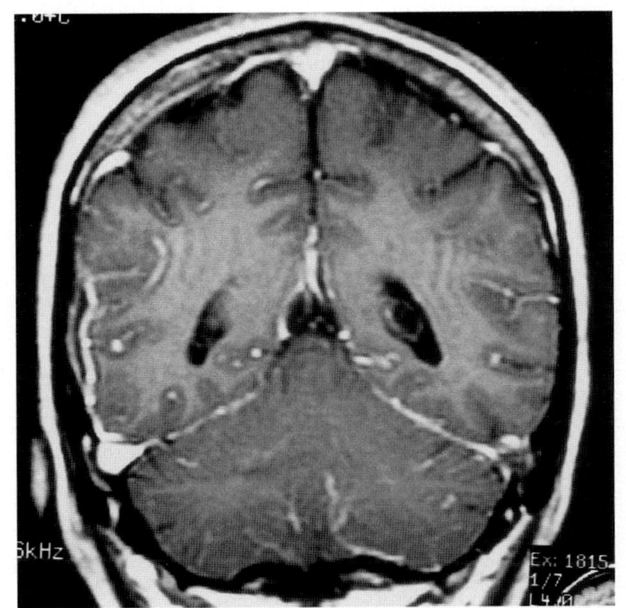


E

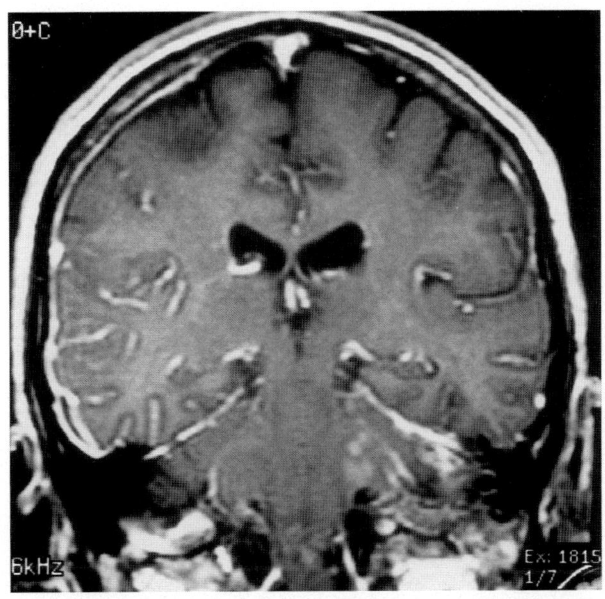


F

**Anteroposterior (A), base (B), and oblique (C) maximum intensity projection views of the three-dimensional phase-contrast study show attenuated flow signal from the left transverse sinus and no flow from the left sigmoid sinus or jugular vein. Thrombosis is further substantiated on the axial spin-density image (D) showing abnormal homogeneous increased signal from the left sigmoid sinus. The coronal T1-weighted image after contrast (E) shows a small amount of peripheral enhancement around the nonenhancing thrombus within the left transverse sinus (compared with the normal enhancement of the right transverse sinus). There is also abnormal enhancement on the T1-weighted image within the left cerebral peduncle (F) and around the right temporal lobe because of cerebritis and a right middle fossae subdural empyema.**

## CASE 155
## PARASAGITTAL MENINGIOMA WITH OCCLUSION OF THE SUPERIOR SAGITTAL SINUS

**History:** 44-year-old with headaches.

**Technique:** oblique sagittal, two-dimensional time-of-flight, 40/10/30, 256 × 256, posterior-to-anterior direction, 25-cm field of view, 9:23.

A

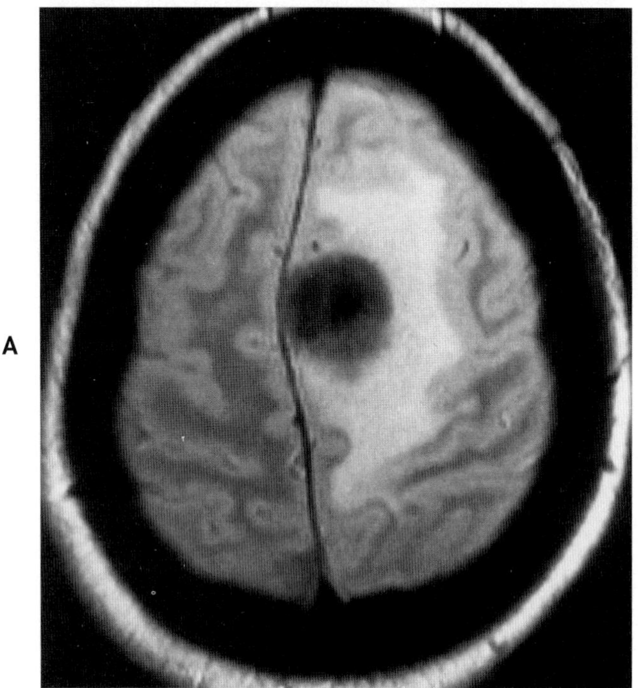

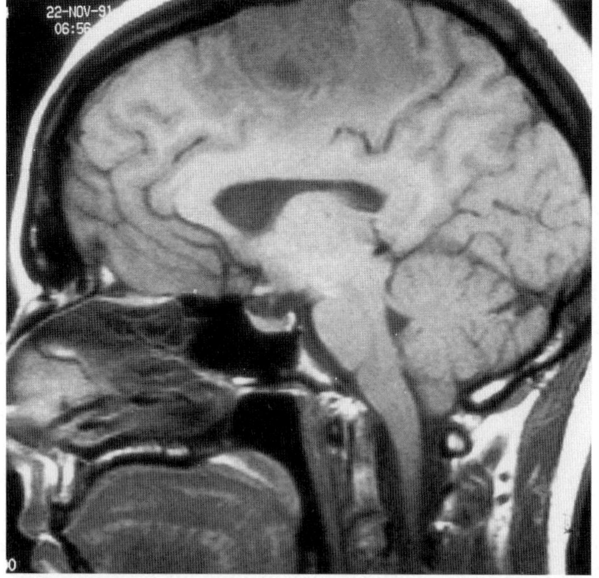


B

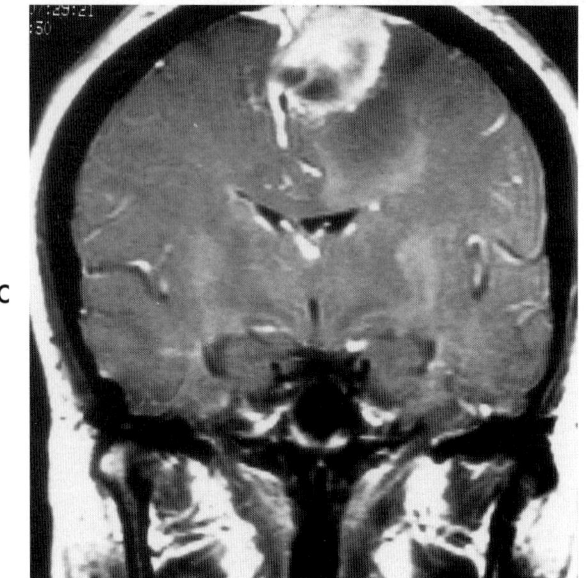

C

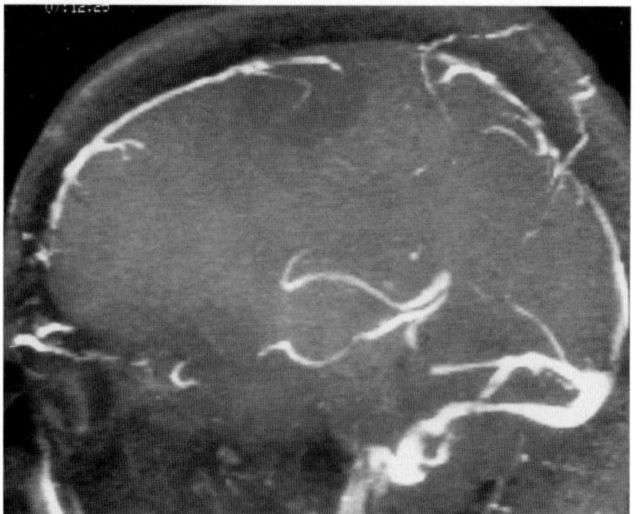

D

**Axial spin-density image (A) shows a well-defined left falcine meningioma with typical low signal intensity. The sagittal unenhanced T1-weighted (B) and coronal T1-weighted image (C) after contrast shows heterogeneous enhancement of the dural-based extraaxial lesion and the mass effect on the lateral ventricles. The lateral maximum intensity projection view of the MR venogram without contrast (D) shows lack of flow in the middle third of the superior sagittal sinus in the region of the meningioma, with prominent cortical collateral veins posteriorly.**


**REFERENCES**

Mattle HP, Wentz KU, Edelman RR et al: Cerebral venography with MR, *Radiology* 178(2):453-458, 1991.

Rippe DJ, Boyko OB, Spritzer CE et al: Demonstration of dural sinus occlusion by the use of MRA, *AJNR* 11(1):199-201, 1990.

## CASE 156
## RECURRENT MENINGIOMA WITH INVASION OF THE SUPERIOR SAGITTAL SINUS

**History:** 51-year-old after resection of meningioma.

**Technique:** oblique sagittal, two-dimensional time-of-flight, 40/10/30, 256 × 256, posterior-to-anterior direction, 25-cm field of view, 9:23.

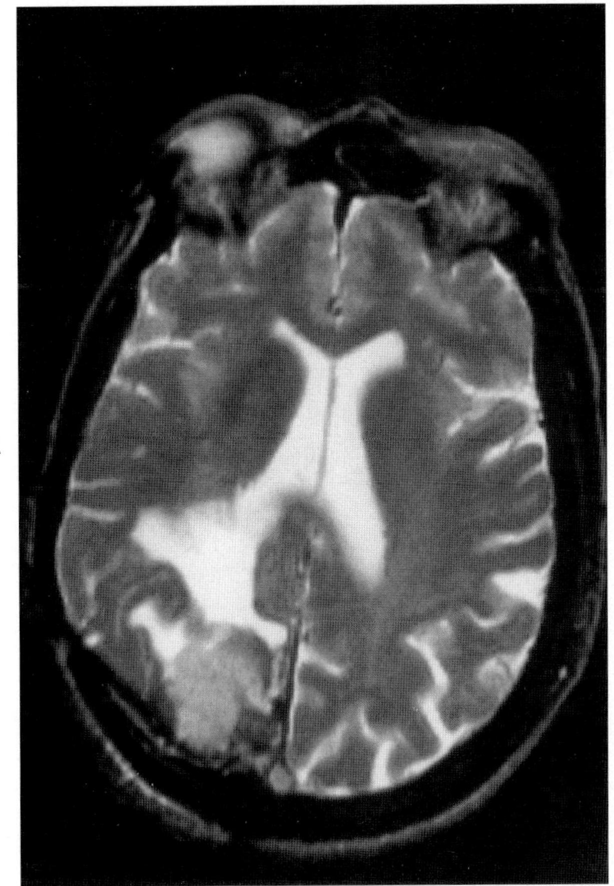

A

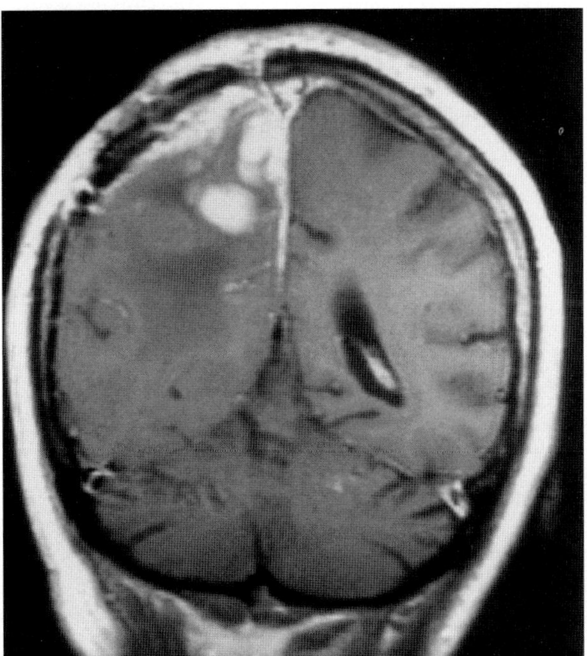

B

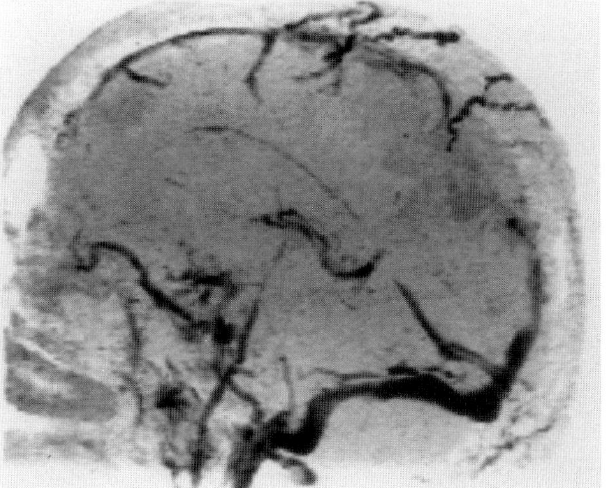

C

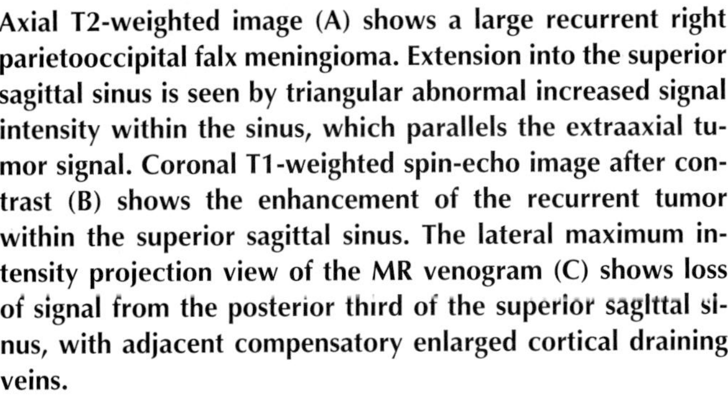

**Axial T2-weighted image (A) shows a large recurrent right parietooccipital falx meningioma. Extension into the superior sagittal sinus is seen by triangular abnormal increased signal intensity within the sinus, which parallels the extraaxial tumor signal. Coronal T1-weighted spin-echo image after contrast (B) shows the enhancement of the recurrent tumor within the superior sagittal sinus. The lateral maximum intensity projection view of the MR venogram (C) shows loss of signal from the posterior third of the superior sagittal sinus, with adjacent compensatory enlarged cortical draining veins.**

CHAPTER 9

# Carotid Bifurcation

The incidence of cerebrovascular disease and the prevalence of surgically accessible carotid stenoses have made the carotid bifurcation the most extensively studied arterial segment outside the coronary vessels.[1,2] In the 1950s, Fisher described the spectrum of pathologic changes in the carotid arteries in patients succumbing to cerebral ischemia.[3,4] Carotid bifurcation lesions produce cerebral ischemia by thrombotic or atheromatous embolization at sites of ulceration or by decreasing blood flow secondary to stenosis.[2,5-12] These ulcerations may be quite small, whereas the stenoses typically occur over a relatively confined region. The surgical and epidemiologic evidence incriminating atherosclerotic plaques as a cause of cerebrovascular disease has been paralleled by increasing demands for diagnostic studies that are less invasive and less expensive than conventional intraarterial arteriography.[5]

Controversy has surrounded the efficacy of carotid endarterectomy in stroke prevention. In the Joint Study of Extracranial Arterial Occlusion, there was no difference in total strokes and death between the medical and surgical groups when perioperative morbidity and mortality were included in the analysis.[13] Subsequent studies also failed to conclusively demonstrate any benefit to patients undergoing carotid endarterectomy, but controversy surrounding these reports related to study design.[14-17] The North American Symptomatic Carotid Endarterectomy Trial (NASCET) and the European Carotid Surgery Trial (ECST) results were published in 1991.[18-21] NASCET's objective was to determine whether carotid endarterectomy was superior to the best medical treatment in patients with carotid stenoses and transient cerebral ischemia or partial stroke.[7] The study was stopped when it was learned that patients with 70% to 99% stenosis who had undergone endarterectomy had an absolute 17% reduction in the risk of ipsilateral stroke at 2 years.[22] The study clearly defined the benefits of carotid endarterectomy in symptomatic patients without tandem lesions. If the surgeon has a low complication rate (perioperative major morbidity-mortality rate of 2.1% in NASCET) and the patient has a symptomatic 70% to 99% carotid stenosis, then endarterctomy is effective. The benefit of endarterectomy appears to be greater for patients with higher-grade stenoses.

From an imaging standpoint, important points to note in the NASCET imaging protocol were: (1) required selective carotid angiography in a minimum of two projections demonstrating the cervical and intracranial carotid territories, as well as a chest radiograph, duplex ultrasound of the carotid arteries, and computed tomography of the head; (2) percent stenosis of the carotid arteries determined in a reproducible fashion (stenosis / normal distal lumen × 100) and verified by an independent observer; and (3) exclusion of patients with tandem lesions of the carotid circulation from the study (approximately 2% of this population). These criteria must be taken into consideration if MRA is to have a significant impact on the clinical workup of carotid bifurcation atherosclerotic disease.

The value of endarterectomy for symptomatic patients with 30% to 70% stenosis and asymptomatic patients is under investigation. The number of endarterectomies performed in the United States dropped from an expected number of 127,000 to 83,000 in 1986 and to 67,000 in 1991 (the year of the NASCET report).[23]

## CURRENT EVALUATION

The workup of patients with cerebrovascular diseases proceeds along two separate lines: investigations of the underlying carotid lumenal morphology (accurate quantification of the degree of lumenal compromise at the bifurcation and demonstration of irregularities of the arterial wall) and studies of the brain parenchyma. Computed tomography and routine MR imaging are useful for showing the parenchymal changes of cerebrovascular disease. They are, however, unable to evaluate vessel morphology.

Intraarterial angiography continues to be the standard clinical test of vessel morphology by which other diagnostic studies are compared. However, conventional angiography cannot evaluate associated parenchymal changes; it is invasive and has a small risk of morbidity and mortality.

Several studies have shown duplex sonography to provide a useful, effective, and accurate for assessment of carotid atherosclerosis (sensitivities and specificities ranging from 84% to 95% for stenoses greater than 50%).[24-26] Color Doppler is at least as accurate as duplex and improves the confidence in diagnoses while reducing examination time.[26] Nevertheless, there continue to be reports of potential pitfalls such as operator dependence, machine variability, vessel tortuosity, high bifurcations and plaque calcification leading to nondiagnostic studies, overestimation of stenoses, and (although less commonly than with noncolor systems) misdiagnoses of complete occlusion at the bifurcation. Doppler ultrasound can provide flow information and morphologic data but is limited in terms of areas amenable to study and is insensitive to any concomitant parenchymal changes. Because of these limitations, there have been numerous reports describing MR techniques that exploit time-of-flight effects or spin-phase phenomena to image the carotid bifurcation.[27-44]

## TECHNIQUES

It is apparent from the number of methods discussed in Chapter 2 that no single MRA technique can answer all clinical questions and situations. Specific techniques and parameters will have to be tailored to individual patient needs. Although this makes the routine application of MRA more complex, it will also ensure that the maximum diagnostic yield is achieved.

In two-dimensional imaging, the carotid bifurcation is visualized by obtaining a series of thin two-dimensional axial gradient-echo images sequentially against the direction of flow. This stack of images with high signal intensity flowing blood may then be subjected to postprocessing to show just the vessel geometry, with the background stationary tissue suppressed.[40] If just the series of axial images were obtained, both in-flowing venous and arterial blood would be bright. The high signal from the adjacent venous structures, such as the jugular vein, would obscure the carotid bifurcation. To solve this problem, a saturation band is placed superior to each consecutive slice as it is obtained, which negates the signal from the caudally directed venous flow. Similarly, if venous anatomy is the goal, the slices are acquired in the reverse direction, and an inferiorly placed saturation pulse eliminates cranially directed arterial flow signal from the axial image stack.

Tissue contrast is affected in this technique by changing the signal of flowing blood or by altering the signal of the background tissue. The major parameters involved include (1) repetition time, (2) flip angle, and (3) slice orientation with respect to the vessel of interest. Ideally, the repetition time would be long enough to allow full replacement of the moving spins in the slice by fresh unsaturated spins to give high vascular signal. The trade-off is that a longer repetition time would also allow regrowth of the longitudinal magnetization from the background tissue. This would increase background signal and decrease vessel conspicuousness. A balance between these two factors is approximately 45 to 50 msec, allowing flow-related enhancement and an element of background suppression. A higher flip angle would provide a better signal-to-noise ratio and better suppression (saturation) of the background tissue. It would also cause increased saturation of the in-flowing blood. The ideal vessel orientation is perpendicular to the imaging slice, which maximizes flow-related enhancement and minimizes saturation of the blood. However, with this orientation it is difficult to cover large vessel lengths with axial two-dimensional slices.

A disadvantage of the two-dimensional technique includes patient motion manifested as vessel discontinuities or a stair-step configuration on the maximum intensity projection images. Motion artifacts are spread among all the slices in the three-dimensional time-of-flight technique, making them less obvious.[40] In addition, the necessity for thin slices in two-dimensional time-of-flight sequences requires higher gradient amplitudes, which limits the minimum echo time and field of view. The major advantages of two-dimensional techniques relate to the high signal intensity of blood related to excellent flow-related enhancement and the sensitivity of the technique to slow flow (as would occur with severe stenoses).

Three-dimensional time-of-flight techniques can also accurately depict the carotid bifurcation.[31,39] The optimal three-dimensional technique would combine factors that allow for the maximum flow-related enhancement and at the same time minimize motion-induced phase change. Flow-related enhancement may be maximized in three-dimensional time-of-flight MRA by using a transmit-receive head coil that localizes the region of excitation and saturation, allowing effective inflow of unsaturated spins. Optimization of the scan orientation relative to flow, the repetition time, and flip angle is as important in this technique as in two-dimensional time-of-flight angiography. To minimize motion-induced phase change, compensation gradients, echo times, and slice thicknesses must be optimized. Currently, flow-compensation gradients using correction for constant velocity (first order) in the read and slice-select directions with the shortest available opposed phase echo time appears to be the best compromise.[39,40] The extremely thin slices (and thus small voxels) available with three-dimensional Fourier transform imaging allow improved vascular signal by minimizing motion-induced phase change leading to signal loss.[39,45]

Advantages of the three-dimensional technique include a reduction of T2* effects in three-dimensional vs. two-dimensional[46] and a theoretical increase in the signal-to-noise ratio proportional to the square root of the number of slices (slice-select phase-encoding steps). Although the scan time is increased with three-dimensional imaging with the additional direction of phase encoding, overall imaging times are comparable for three-dimensional and sequential two-dimensional MRA techniques, with both being shorter than the three-dimensional phase-encoding technique.

A drawback to the three-dimensional Fourier transform time-of-flight method is the eventual saturation of moving spins as they reside longer (i.e., farther from the point of entry) within the region of excitation. Methods around this problem include multiple overlapping thin-slab acquisition and specialized radiofrequency pulses such as tilted, optimized nonsaturating excitation (see Chapter 2).

## COIL SELECTION

The orientation of the volume and the choice of coil can have a profound impact on image quality with three-dimensional time-of-flight imaging. For example, sagittal or coronal carotid acquisitions must be performed by a local transmit-receive head coil to produce the necessary contrast at the bifurcation.[39] If the same sequence is performed with a receive-only coil (i.e., the body coil acting as the transmitter), there is significant loss of signal intensity of spins inferior to the carotid bifurcation because of saturation. Similarly, sagittal acquisitions performed with a transmit-receive head coil require longer repetition times (in the 70- to 100-msec range) to provide adequate flow-related enhancement throughout the imaging volume relative to axial acquisitions, which have a more confined region of excitation. Axial acquisitions may be performed with both transmit-receive and receive-only coils because there is inflow of unsaturated spins from the edge of the volume rather than the edge of the coil. Alternatively, many more axial slices are needed to cover the region of interest adequately (with satisfactory spatial resolution in the slice-select direction), which may unduly prolong acquisition time.

Many techniques try to minimize problems of three-dimensional time-of-flight imaging, such as using a broad axial excitation pulse and then reading out the signal in the Z direction.[47] The current best three-dimensional technique is multiple overlaping thin three-dimensional slabs, which combines the advantages of the contiguous thin slices of three-dimensional imaging with the good flow-related enhancement of two-dimensional techniques.[48,49] One drawback of this technique is the "venetian blind" artifact, a striped appearance resulting from variations in the signal intensity of the vessels at the margins of the volume.[50] This artifact can be minimized by the proper amount of volume overlap and postprocessing.

Initial studies indicate that three-dimensional Fourier transform time-of-flight MRA has the capability to consistently approximate changes in arterial lumen relative to the gold standard, intraarterial angiography. The use of three-dimensional Fourier transform time-of-flight MRA as a screening tool for hemodynamically significant carotid stenoses does not appear to be limited by error in lumen definition secondary to artifacts inherent in the technique.[51] Recent studies have suggested that the combination of duplex ultrasound and MRA (two- and three-dimensional time-of-flight) may allow accurate assessment of the carotid bifurcation compared with conventional angiography in a noninvasive fashion.[52,53]

The ability of MRA techniques to accurately depict stenoses at the carotid bifurcation has dramatically improved in a short time.[36,39] The major limitation of MRA relates to loss of spin phase coherence which may result from higher-order motion (i.e., acceleration, jerk, or turbulent flow) with imaging gradients, magnetic susceptibility effects, and intravoxel variations in flow velocity. All of these causes may produce significant phase dispersion and vascular signal loss.[54,55] This signal loss may lead to the underestimation of vascular dimensions, overestimation of stenoses, and potentially, complete loss of lumen definition. These types of flow conditions are often present at and immediately distal to stenoses of the carotid bifurcation and may result in nonvisualization of the affected arterial segment.[54,55] Even the normal carotid bulb has very complex flow, with a zone of slowed or reversed flow along the outer wall of the carotid bulb[56] (see Case 157). These complicated spin-phase phenomena may in part be corrected by shorter echo-times, small voxels, and additional compensation gradients.

## RADIOFREQUENCY PULSE

An alternative type of radiofreqency pulse could compensate for the degree of spin saturation in a single large, axial three-dimensional volume. These ramp or tilted, optimized nonsaturating excitation pulses excite the spins with lower flip angles inferiorly and increasingly higher flip angles as the spins move superiorly in the imaging volume. The use of lower flip angles inferiorly limits the degree of saturation as the spins move through the volume. Exciting the spins at the superior aspect of the volume with higher flip angles partially compensates for the typical loss of signal in this portion of the volume (because of spin saturation) by giving a better signal-to-noise ratio.[57]

## BACKGROUND SUPPRESSION

The ability to accurately characterize a carotid stenosis by MRA is related not only to the problems of rapid complex flow, but also to the contrast-to-noise ratios of the MRA acquisitions. Phase-contrast techniques provide optimal contrast between the vessels and the adjacent stationary tissues, but these methods are limited by image degradation caused by prolonged acquisition times for three-dimensional methods (for resolutions similar to time-of-flight), susceptibility to a higher order of motion terms, and eddy currents.[58-60] Time-of-flight techniques are far less susceptible to these latter problems although the contrast-to-noise ratio is limiting. For this reason, various background suppression techniques have been implemented to suppress the stationary tissues for time-of-flight techniques.[61-64]

The time-of-flight techniques rely on the high signal intensity of inflowing unsaturated spins and a relative saturation of the stationary tissues to provide the necessary contrast. By necessity, the sequences are proton density and T1 weighted. Consequently, any tissue with a sufficiently short T1 or high proton density can also have a relatively high intensity in the MRA images. Because maximum intensity projections recognize only high intensity structures, these tissues can be confusing and can obscure the vessels of interest.[42] This problem is accentuated by patient motion, since the high intensity tissues account for the most prominent motion artifacts that further obscure the vessels. Routine two-dimensional and three-dimensional refocused sequences using fast imaging with steady-state free precession or gradient acquisition in steady state only suppress the short T1 tissues (such as fat) to a limited extent based on the intrinsic contrast behavior of these sequences at low-to-intermediate flip angles.

Tkach et al[64] compared the relative efficacy of a number of background-suppression techniques for improving carotid time-of-flight MRA images.[64] Conventional two- and three-dimensional fast imaging with steady-state free precession time-of-flight sequences with flow compensation were compared with the following suppression schemes: (1) a tracking saturation pulse (two-dimensional), (2) prolonged absolute echo times (two- and three-dimensional) for fat suppression based on T2* decay (Fig. 9-1), (3) frequency-selective saturation of fat (two- and three-dimensional), (4) in-plane spatial saturation (two-dimensional), and (5) magnetization transfer contrast (two- and three-dimensional).

Slight reductions in fat signal are appreciated with small variations in echo time for opposed-phase imaging. Larger variations in the absolute echo times yield greater reductions in the background tissues by taking advantage of the T2* phenomena to suppress the short T2* of fat as suggested by Laub et al.[62] With longer absolute echo times, fat is more effectively suppressed. However, there is a noticeable artifactual reduction in vessel caliber with longer absolute echo times. With any time-of-flight MRA technique incorporating gradient field echo sequences, tissue inhomogeneities set up local gradients through which the flowing blood passes. Similar, albeit smaller gradients exist at the edges of vessels. These local gradients cause more rapid dephasing of the spins, particularly for moving spins. Additional inhomogeneities related to factors such as coil construction and metallic foreign bodies can cause more rapid spin dephasing. The combination of these factors account for a reduction in vessel caliber and a variation of the vascular signal in the T2* suppression scheme (prolongation of the absolute echo times). This effect is more apparent in two-dimensional than in three-dimensional acquisitions because of the larger voxel size.[46]

The use of frequency-selective fat saturation radiofrequency pulses has two advantages; improving the vessel–soft tissue contrast and suppressing the tissue causing the greatest amount of motion artifact. The most important limitation of this strategy is the variability of suppression across the imaging volume caused by field nonuniformity related to tissue inhomogeneities, the coil choice, or the $B_0$ field. Incomplete suppression is often seen around the mouth and chin, where the local variations in the tissues (e.g., dental amalgam, air) are the most important factors. Any inhomogeneity can shift the precession frequencies of protons

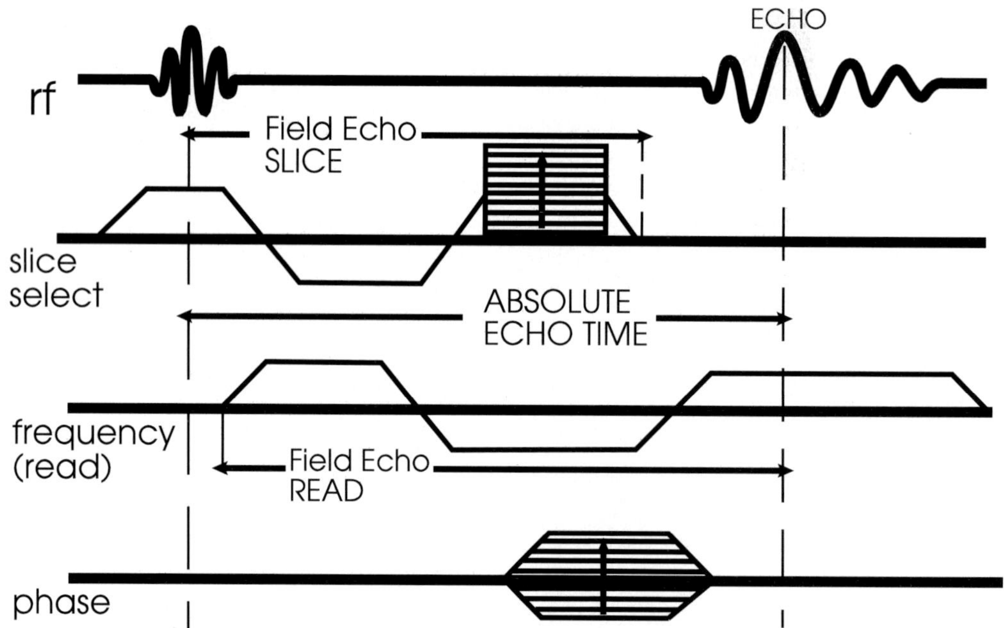


**Fig. 9-1** The "absolute echo time" represents the interval from the center of the radiofrequency pulse to the occurrence of the gradient-echo. The absolute echo time is important when considering the degree of signal loss associated with spin dephasing produced by motion of these spins through local field inhomogeneities as well as the normal signal loss from stationary tissues related to T2* dephasing. The "field echo time" in the slice-select direction is the interval from the center of the selective excitation pulse to the end of the last gradient pulse applied along this direction. Similarly, the field echo time in the frequency-encoding direction is the interval from the onset of the first gradient pulse applied along the read-out direction to the center of the gradient echo.

in an area so that the selected bandwidth and frequency offset of the radiofrequency pulse will not necessarily saturate the expected spins.

More complete suppression of the background is possible with a two-dimensional in-plane spatial saturation technique.[63] In this method, each slice is saturated and then excited by a second radiofrequency pulse after a sufficient time delay to allow arterial inflow but before significant relaxation of the stationary tissues. This technique produces base images in which the arteries are bright and the other tissues are reduced to the background noise level. However, the vessels often appear artifactually smaller with this technique. In this case, the vessel attenuation is most likely related to insufficient inflow of the slower-moving peripheral spins in the vessels. This artificial narrowing is eliminated by further offsetting the saturation slice away from the arterial inflow while maintaining only slight overlap of the saturation and excitation slices. This still produces a uniform and relatively effective suppression of the background.[64]

For three-dimensional time-of-flight carotid bifurcation MRA, of the various techniques for background suppression that have been described, incorporation of an additional frequency-selective spatial nonselective saturation pulse can be effective for improving the overall signal-to-noise ratio. However, routine application of this technique shows variation in image quality from patient to patient because of local field inhomogeneities disrupting the uniformity of the fat suppression. Some of the cases are beautiful, but many suffer in image quality. Because of this inconsistency, this type of fat suppression pulse is not recommended for routine carotid MRA. For the three-dimensional time-of-flight technique, a superior spatial-saturation slab to eliminate venous signal and the shortest possible opposed-phase echo time (7 msec at 1.5 Tesla) provide the most effective and consistent background suppression with excellent image quality. The shorter possible echo times and thinner slices would reduce the motion-induced phase dispersion expected in the region of a stenosis and would make three-dimensional imaging less vulnerable to the deleterious T2* effects. In addition, three-dimensional acquisition permits some degree of signal averaging to reduce motion artifact (i.e., ghosting) in mildly anxious patients. Finally, the radiofrequency power deposition associated with this three-dimensional strategy is typically lower than its two-dimensional counterpart by a factor of 2 or more.

A tracking saturation pulse that slightly overlaps the excitation slice, is the most efficacious two-dimensional time-of-flight technique. In practice, this technique provides not only effective venous suppression, but also a limited degree of background stationary tissue suppression because of the slight cross-talk between the excitation and saturation slices. This suppression is generally more uniform than a two-dimensional time-of-flight sequence with a frequency-selective saturation pulse, since the excitation produced by the higher bandwidth pulses (defining the tracking saturation pulses) is insensitive to the local field inhomogeneities. Compared with the three-dimensional sequences, this method is still limited by the longer echo times and thicker slices inherent to two-dimensional-techniques. These factors tend to increase the intravoxel phase dispersion, particularly in the region of a stenosis.

Investigators have incorporated very short echo times using a two-dimensional snapshot technique with an appropriate choice of preparatory pulses and pulse timing to suppress background tissues (e.g., two 180-degree pulses, appropriate inversion time to suppress the short T1 of fat),[65,66] Because of the gradient demands for these ultrashort echo times, these two-dimensional acquisitions must further compromise the through-plane and in-plane resolution. The development of stronger gradients capable of very rapid switching times would be very desirable in this setting. Although the technical constraints to designing a coil for the carotid arteries are considerable, prototype coils capable of 19 mT/m gradients in the Y direction and 38 mT/m peak gradient strength in the Z direction have been designed for the head and have shown promising results.[67,68]

## MAGNETIZATION TRANSFER CONTRAST

The degree of saturation with this technique is the greatest in the muscles of the neck, which are not a significant source of artifact for carotid bifurcation imaging. Fat, which is the source of greatest signal intensity competing with vascular signal in the neck, is not significantly affected by the off-resonance pulses used for magnetization transfer suppression.[69] Reducing the resonant offset or increasing the voltage and/or duration would enhance the muscle suppression but only at the expense of arterial signal intensity and examination time. Magnetization transfer contrast is very useful in intracranial MRA, since the background brain tissue is susceptible to the magnetization transfer suppression. This provides for higher vessel–soft tissue contrast, particularly in vessels with marginal flow-related enhancement such as small peripheral vessels.

## PHASE CONTRAST

Phase-contrast MRA may also be used to visualize the carotid bifurcation.[30,34,58,70] This technique uses bipolar flow-encoding gradients and subtraction to get signal from flowing blood, but stationary tissues does not contribute to the voxel signal.[71] The bipolar gradients cause a phase shift of spins proportional to their velocity. A second sequence is performed with inverted bipolar gradients. Both bipolar gradient sequences cause zero phase change of stationary spins and some net phase change of moving spins. The resultant subtracted image suppresses the background tissue and shows only the moving spins. The advantages of phase-encoding angiography compared with time-of-flight methods include direct and effective suppression of background (stationary) tissues and definition of slow-flow states. This method can also provide quantitative flow measurements. Because the signal of blood from this technique depends on flow-induced phase change, signal loss from more complex flow (as with carotid stenoses) that induces phase changes are more problematic with phase-encoding than with time-of-flight methods. These phase changes can more easily be corrected in time-of-flight methods because of the short echo times and the ability to use flow-compensation gradients.

## BLACK BLOOD

Although the previously discussed methods may be considered "bright blood" techniques in that they attempt to maximize signal from flowing blood, a "black blood" technique may also be useful in evaluation of the carotid bifurcation in which a uniform signal loss within the vessel lumen is desired.[72-75] This method uses a thin-slice (1.8 mm) sagittal two-dimensional spin-echo technique (1600/20/45) with flow presaturation by an axial slab inferior to the bifurcation to minimize signal from flowing blood. This technique has been suggested as an adjunct sequence that should be performed if the bright-blood technique has depicted a diseased carotid bifurcation, since the problem of overestimation of the severity of stenoses is not a problem with the black-blood technique.[73] Advantages of this technique include preservation of vessel contrast even with relatively slow flow and the fact that signal loss related to higher-order motion does not degrade image quality (since the purpose of the technique is to lose intravascular signal). Sagittal orientation was chosen to minimize imaging time, since fewer imaging sections are needed to encompass the bifurcation. There are several potential disadvantages. First, the method cannot be used in regions where vessels are in contact with bone, since there would be no contrast between the low signal vessel and the low signal bone; similarly, low signal intensity calcified plaque may cause an underestimation of stenosis, since it could have the same low signal intensity as blood. Second, the field of view is limited to the bifurcation and above, since a saturation pulse eliminates common carotid artery signal. Finally, there may be overlap of the jugular vein with the carotid artery.

### REFERENCES


1. Kurtzke JF: *Epidemiology of cerebrovascular disease.* In National Institutes of Health: *Cerebrovascular Survey Report 1985,* Bethesda, Md, 1985, The Institutes.
2. Joint Study of Extracranial Arterial Occlusion. I. Fields WS et al: Organization of study and survey of patient population, *JAMA* 203:955-960, 1968. II. Hass WK et al: Arteriography, techniques, sites, and complications, *JAMA* 203:961-968, 1968. III. Bauer BB et al: Progress report of controlled study of long term survival in patients with and without Operation, *JAMA* 208:509-518, 1969. IV. Blaisdell WF et al: A review of surgical considerations, *JAMA* 209:1889-1895, 1969. V. Fields WS et al: Progress report of prognosis following surgery or non-surgical treatment for transient ischemic attacks and cervical carotid artery lesions, *JAMA* 211:1993-2003, 1970. VI. Heyman A et al: Joint study of extracranial arterial occlusion: radical differences in ischemic stroke population, *JAMA* 222:285-289, 1972.
3. Fisher M: Occlusion of the internal carotid artery, *Arch Neurol Psychiat* 65:346-377, 1951.
4. Fisher M: Occlusion of the carotid arteries, *Arch Neurol Psychiat* 72:187-204, 1954.
5. Kricheff II: Arteriosclerotic ischemic cerebrovascular disease, *Radiology* 162:101-109, 1987.
6. Weinberger J, Robbins A: Neurologic symptoms associated with nonobstructive plaque at the carotid bifurcation, *Arch Neurol* 40:489-492, 1983.
7. Raichle ME: The pathophysiology of brain ischemia, *Ann Neurol* 13:2-10, 1983.
8. Busuttil RW, Baker JD, Davidson RK, Machleder HI: Carotid artery stenosis: hemodynamic significance and clinical course, *JAMA* 245:1438-1441. 1981.
9. Wood EH, Correll JW. Atheromatous ulceration in major neck vessels as a cause of cerebral embolism, *Acta Radiol* 9:520-536, 1969.
10. Robertson GH, Scott WR, Rosenbaum AE: Thrombi at the site of carotid stenosis, *Radiology* 109:353-356, 1973.
11. Kishore PRS, Chase NE, Kricheff II: Carotid stenosis and intracranial emboli, *Radiology* 100:351-356, 1971.
12. Howser OW, Sundt TM, Holman CB, Sandok BA, Burton RC. Atheromatous disease of the carotid artery, *J Neurosurg* 41:321-331, 1974.
13. Fields WS, Maslenikov V, Meyer JS et al: Joint Study of Extracranial Arterial Occlusion. V. Progress report of prognosis following surgery or nonsurgical treatment for transient cerebral ischemic attacks and cervical carotid artery lesions, *JAMA* 211(12):1993-2003, 1970.
14. Winslow CM, Solomon DH, Chassin MR et al: The appropriateness of carotid endarterectomy, *New Engl J Med* 318:721-727, 1988.
15. Pokras R, Kyken ML: Dramatic changes in the performance of endarterectomy for diseases of the extracranial arteries of the head, *Stroke* 19:1289-1290, 1988.
16. The Committee on Health Care Issues, American Neurological Association: Does carotid endarterectomy decrease stroke and death in patients with transient ischemic attacks? *Ann Neurol* 22(1):72-76, 1987.
17. The North American Symptomatic Carotid Endarterectomy Trial (NASCET) Steering Committee: North American Symptomatic Carotid Endarterectomy Trial: methods, patient characteristics, and progress, *Stroke* 22(6):711-720, 1991.
18. European Carotid Surgery Trialists' Collaborative Group: MRC European carotid surgery trial: interim results for symptomatic patients with severe (70-99%) or with mild (0-29%) carotid stenosis, *Lancet* 337:1235-1243, 1991.
19. Editorial: Operating to prevent stroke, *Lancet* 337:1255-1256, 1991.
20. North American Symptomatic Carotid Endarterectomy Trial Investigators: Clinical alert: benefit of carotid endarterectomy for patients with high-grade stenosis of the internal carotid artery, *Stroke* 22:816-817, 1991.
21. Reinmuth OM, Dyken ML: Carotid endarterectomy: bright light at the end of the tunnel, *Stroke* 22:835-836, 1991.
22. North American Symptomatic Carotid Endarterectomy Trial Collaborators: Beneficial effect of carotid endarterectomy in symptomatic patients with high-grade carotid stenosis, *New Engl J Med* 325(7):445-453, 1991.
23. Dyken ML: Controversies in stroke: past and present: The Willis Lecture, *Stroke* 24(8):1251-1258, 1993.
24. Robinson ML, Sacks D, Perlmutter GS, Marinelli DL: Diagnostic criteria for carotid duplex sonography, *AJR* 151:1045-1049, 1988.

25. Jacobs NM, Grant EG, Schellinger D et al: Duplex carotid sonography: criteria for stenosis, accuracy and pitfalls, *Radiology* 154:385-391, 1985.
26. Carroll BA: Carotid sonography, *Radiology* 178:303-313, 1991.
27. Axel L, Morton D: A method for imaging blood vessels by phase compensated/uncompensated difference images, *Magn Reson Imag* 4:153, 1986.
28. Pattany PM, Marino R, McNally JM: Velocity and acceleration desensitization in 2DFT MR imaging, *Magn Reson Imag* 4:154-155, 1986.
29. Naylor W, Firmin DN: Multislice MR angiography, *Magn Reson Imag* 4:156, 1986.
30. Dumoulin CL, Hart HR: Magnetic resonance angiography, *Radiology* 161:717-720, 1986.
31. Masaryk TJ, Ross JS, Modic MT et al: Carotid bifurcation: MR imaging, *Radiology* 166:461-466, 1988.
32. Lenz GW, Haacke EM, Masaryk TJ et al: In-plane vascular imaging: pulse sequence design and strategy, *Radiology* 166:875-882, 1988.
33. Laub G, Kaiser W: MR angiography with gradient motion refocussing, *JCAT* 12(3):377-382, 1988.
34. Dumoulin CL, Souza SP, Walker MF, Wagle W: Three-dimensional phase contrast angiography, *Magn Reson Med* 9:139-149, 1989.
35. Dixon WT, Du LN, Gado M, Rossnick S: Projection angiograms of blood labeled by adiabatic fast passage, *Magn Reson Med* 3:454-462, 1986.
36. Nishimura DG, Macovski A, Pauly JM, Conolly SM: MR angiography by selective inversion recovery, *Magn Reson Med* 4:193-202, 1987.
37. Wehrli FW, Shimakawa A, Gullberg GT, MacFall JR: Time-of-Flight MR flow imaging: selective saturation recovery with gradient refocussing, *Radiology* 160:781-785, 1986.
38. Gullberg GT, Wehrli FW, Shimakawa A, Simmons MA: MR vascular imaging with fast gradient refocussing pulse sequence and reformatted images from transaxial sections, *Radiology* 165:241-246, 1987.
39. Masaryk TJ, Modic MT, Ruggieri PM et al: Three-dimensional (volume) gradient-echo imaging of the carotid bifurcation: preliminary clinical experience, *Radiology* 171:801-806, 1989.
40. Keller PJ, Drayer BP, Fram EK et al: MR angiography with two-dimensional acquisition and three-dimensional display, *Radiology* 173:527-532, 1989.
41. Sardashti M, Schwartzberg DG, Stomp GP et al: *Spin labeling angiography of the carotids by presaturation and adiabatic inversion.* Paper presented at the Eighth Annual Meeting of the Society of Magnetic Resonance in Medicine, Amsterdam, The Netherlands, Aug 12-18, 1989.
42. Anderson CM, Saloner D, Tsuruda J et al: Artifacts in maximum-intensity-projection display of MR angiograms, *AJR* 154:623-629, 1990.
43. Daniels DL, Kneeland JB, Foley WD et al: Cardiac-gated local coil MR imaging of the carotid neck bifurcation, *AJNR* 7:1036-1037, 1986.
44. Ruskowski JT, Damadian R, Giambalvo A et al: MRI angiography of the carotid artery, *Magn Reson Imag* 4:497-502, 1986.
45. Ruggieri PM, Laub GA, Masaryk TJ, Modic MT: Intracranial circulation: pulse sequence considerations in three-dimensional (volume) MR angiography, *Radiology* 171:785-791, 1989.
46. Haacke EM, Tkach JA, Parrish TB: Reduction of T2* dephasing in gradient field-echo imaging, *Radiology* 170:457-462, 1989.
47. Masaryk TJ, Laub G, Modic MT et al: *3DFT MR angiography: a comparison of time-of-flight techniques.* Paper presented at the Eighth Annual Meeting of the Society of Magnetic Resonance in Medicine, Amsterdam, The Netherlands, Aug 12-18, 1989.
48. Parker DL, Blatter DD: Multiple thin slab magnetic resonance angiography, *Neuroimag Clin North Am* 2(4):677-692, 1992.
49. Parker DL, Yuan C, Blatter DD: MR angiography by multiple thin slab 3D acquisition, *Magn Reson Med* 17:434-451, 1991.
50. Blatter DD, Parker DI, Schwartz R, Robinson RO: Intracranial MR angiography with multiple thin-slab three-dimensional acquisition: preliminary clinical experience in 80 patients, *Radiology* 177(P):89, 1990 (abstract).
51. Masaryk AM, Ross JS, DiCello M et al: 3DFT magnetic resonance angiography of the carotid bifurcation: potential and limitations as a screening examination, *Radiology* 179:797-804, 1991.
52. Porges R, Grist TM, Boyko OB et al: Potential role of MR angiography as a screening modality for carotid artery disease, *Radiology* 177(P):89, 1990 (abstract).
53. Riles TS, Eidelman EM, Litt AW et al: Comparison of MR angiography, conventional angiography and duplex scanning, *Stroke* 23(3):341-346, 1992.
54. Evans AJ, Blinder RA, Herfkins RJ et al: Effects of turbulence on signal intensity in gradient echo images, *Invest Radiol* 23(7):512-518, 1988.
55. Podolak MJ, Hedlund LW, Evans AJ, Herfkins RJ: Evaluation of flow through simulated vascular stenoses with gradient echo magnetic resonance imaging, *Invest Radiol* 24(3):184-189, 1989.
56. Karino T, Goldsmith HL, Motomiya M et al: Flow patterns in vessels of simple and complex geometries, *Ann N Y Acad Sci* 516:422-441, 1987.
57. Laub G, Purdy DE: *Variable tip angle slab selection for improved three dimensional MR angiography.* In *Book of abstracts: Society of Magnetic Resonance in Medicine, 1992,* Berkeley, Calif, 1992, Society of Magnetic Resonance in Medicine.
58. Dumoulin CL, Cline HE, Souza SP et al: Three-dimensional time-of-flight magnetic resonance angiography using spin saturation, *Magn Reson Med* 11:35-46, 1989.
59. Edelman RR, Wentz KU, Mattle H et al: Projection arteriography and venography: initial clinical results with MR, *Radiology* 172:351-357, 1989.
60. Pernicone JR, Siebert JE, Potchen EJ et al: Three-dimensional phase contrast MR angiography in the head and neck: preliminary report, *AJNR* 11:457-466, 1990.
61. Keller PJ, Hunter WW, Schmalbrock P: Multisection fat-water imaging with chemical shift selective presaturation, *Radiology* 164:539-541, 1987.
62. Laub G, Lewin J: *T2-enhanced time-of-flight magnetic resonance angiography.* Paper presented at the Eighth Annual Meeting of the Society of Magnetic Resonance Imaging, Boston, 1990 (abstract).
63. Hu X, Yuan C: *Techniques for elimination of stationary tissue signal in 2DFT MR angiography.* Paper presented at the Ninth Annual Meeting of the Society of Magnetic Resonance in Medicine, New York, 1990.
64. Tkach J, Ruggieri P, Ross JS et al: Pulse sequence strategies for vascular contrast in time-of-flight MR angiography, *JMRI* 3:811-820, 1993.
65. Riederer SJ: *Rapid scan angiography.* Paper presented at the Second Annual Workshop in Magnetic Resonance Angiography, East Lansing, Mich, 1990.
66. Lewin JS: *Ultra-fast time-of-flight MRA and spin saturation.* Paper presented at the Second Annual Workshop in Magnetic Resonance Angiography, East Lansing, Mich, 1990.
67. Masaryk TJ: MR angiography in cerebrovascular disease (course), *Radiology* 177(P):course 202, 1990.
68. Chew W, Tsuruda JS: Advantages of high resolution MR angiographic imaging, *Radiology* 177(P):1025, 1990.
69. Wolff SD, Balaban RS: Magnetization transfer contrast (MTC) and tissue water proton relaxation in vivo, *Magn Res Med* 10:135-144, 1989.

70. Wagle WA, Dumoulin CL, Souza SP, Cline HE: 3DFT MR angiography of carotid and basilar arteries, *AJNR* 10:911-919, 1989.
71. Dumoulin CL, Souza SP, Hart HR: Rapid scan magnetic resonance angiography, *Magn Reson Med* 5:238-245, 1987.
72. Edelman RR, Mattle H, Wallner B et al: Extracranial carotid arteries: evaluation with "black blood" MR angiography, *Radiology* 177:45-50, 1990.
73. Edelman RR, Mattle HP, Wallner B et al: MR angiography of the extracranial carotid arteries: evaluation of bright and black blood techniques, *Radiology* 177(P):89, 1990 (abstract).
74. Edelman RR, Chien D, Kim D: Fast selective black blood MR imaging, *Radiology* 181(3):655-660, 1991.
75. Mattle HP, Kent KC, Edelman RR et al: Evaluation of the extracranial carotid arteries: correlation of magnetic resonance angiography, duplex ultrasonography, and conventional angiography, *J Vasc Surg* 13(6):838-845, 1991.

## CASE 157
## PITFALL: NORMAL CAROTID BULB SIGNAL LOSS

**History:** 25-year-old being evaluated for seizures.

**Technique:** axial volume, three-dimensional time-of-flight, 39/7/25, 160 × 256, 64 slices, 80-mm slab, 25-cm field of view (rectangular), 6:42.

A

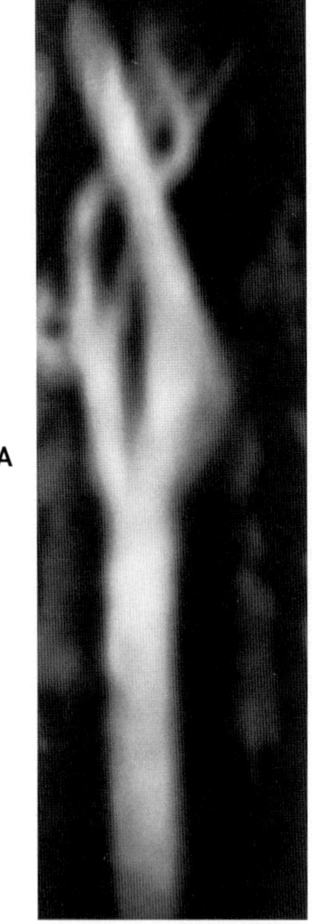

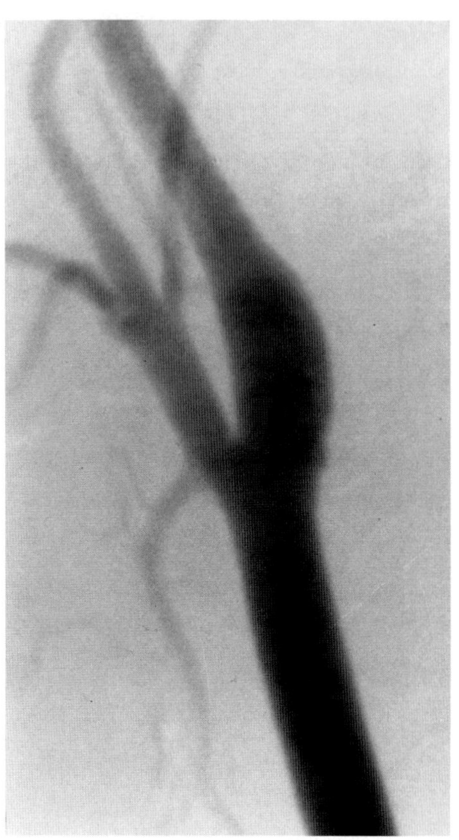

B

**A is a lateral maximum intensity projection view that shows slight loss of signal involving the proximal internal carotid artery along the posterior wall. Signal loss is invariably seen along the posterior aspect of the normal proximal carotid bulb. The flow reversal causes saturation and turbulent dephasing of that arterial segment. The conventional intraarterial angiogram is entirely normal (B). This gradual signal loss of the posterior margin of the vessel by MRA should not be misconstrued as mild narrowing.**

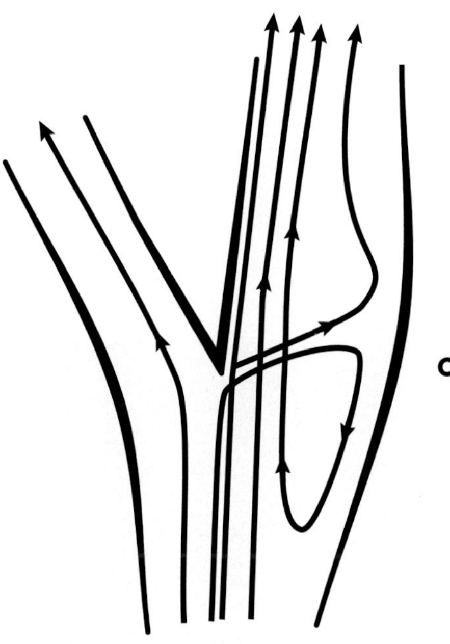


FLOW SEPARATION AT CAROTID BULB

**C shows the type of flow present in the normal carotid bifurcation. Flow streamlines along the anterior wall are straight, whereas the posterior wall streamlines show nonlaminar flow and areas of flow reversal. This nonlaminar and even turbulent flow gives rise to a wide variety of phases on the MRA, which is seen as loss of signal (phase dispersion). (Modified from Karino T, Goldsmith H, Motomiya M: *Ann N Y Acad Sci* 516:422-441, 1987.)**

## REFERENCE

Karino T, Goldsmith H, Motomiya M: Flow patterns in vessels of simple and complex geometries, *Ann N Y Acad Sci* 516:422-441, 1987.

## CASE 158
## PITFALL: MOTION ARTIFACT ON TWO-DIMENSIONAL TIME-OF-FLIGHT STUDY WITH SEVERE RIGHT INTERNAL CAROTID STENOSIS

**History:** 63-year-old with right hemispheric transient ischemic attacks.

**Technique:** axial two-dimensional time-of-flight, spoiled gradient acquisition in steady state 45/8.7/60, 256 × 128, 64 slices, 1.5-mm thickness, 20-cm field of view, 6:27.

A

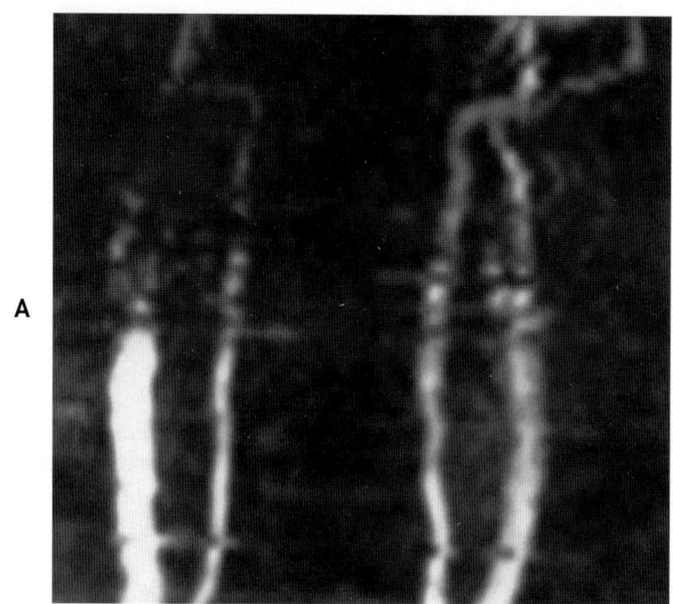

**Single anteroposterior projection from an axial two-dimensional time-of-flight MRA (A) shows multiple areas of horizontal motion artifact demonstrated by the misregistration effects throughout the vessels. There is significant degradation of the appearance of the bifurcations, but there is still evidence of flow through the left internal carotid artery. Given that this is a two-dimensional technique, severe stenosis (greater than 70%) will be manifested as a segment of signal loss. Therefore it is unlikely that there is more than a moderate stenosis at the origin of the left internal carotid artery, since the proximal internal carotid is visible, albeit severely degraded, in quality. However, on the right, there is a considerable area of signal loss involving the proximal internal carotid artery with faint reconstitution distally, which suggests a greater than 70% stenosis.**

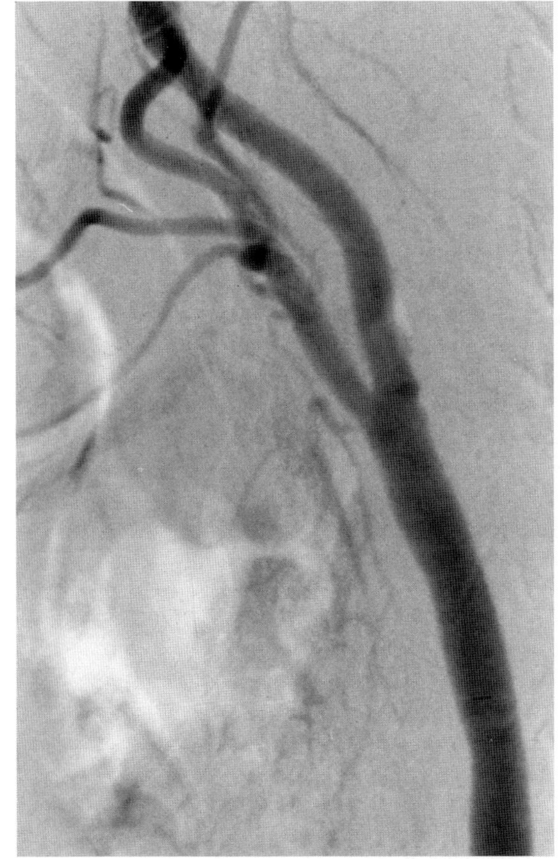

B

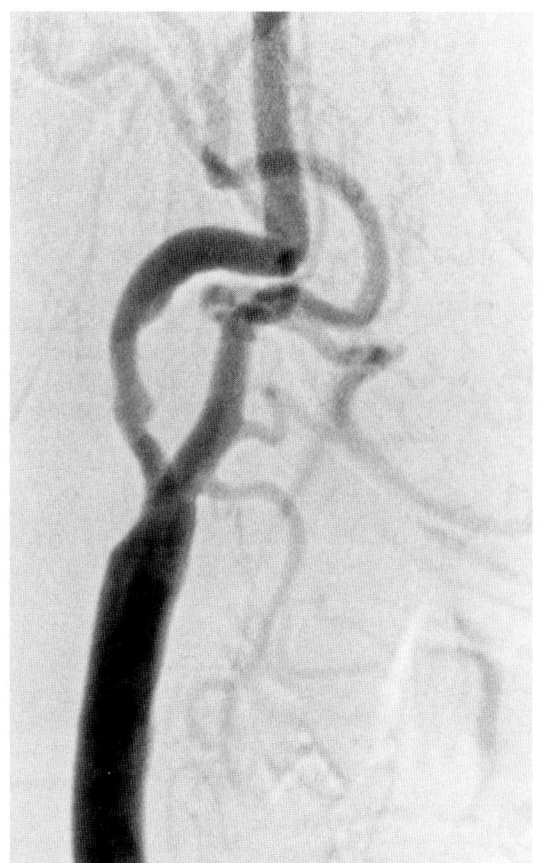

C

**A common carotid artery injection on the left (B) demonstrates a mild stenosis involving the proximal internal carotid artery. On the right common carotid injection (C), there is a severe stenosis involving the proximal internal carotid artery, as suggested by the area of signal loss on the two-dimensional time-of-flight study.**

## REFERENCES

Polak JE, Kalina P, Donaldson M et al: Carotid endarterectomy: preoperative evaluation of candidates with combined Doppler sonography and MR angiography, *Radiology*, 186:333-338, 1993.

Huston J, Lewis BD, Wiebers DO et al: Carotid artery: prospective blinded comparison of two dimensional time of flight MR angiography with conventional angiography and duplex US, *Radiology* 186(3)339-344, 1993.

## CASE 159
## PITFALL: FLOW SATURATION RESULTING FROM A VASCULAR LOOP

**History:** 70-year-old with left hemispheric infarct.

**Technique:** axial two-dimensional time-of-flight, spoiled gradient acquisition in steady-state, 45/8.7/60, 256 × 128, 64 slices, 1.5-mm thickness, 20-cm field of view, 6:27.

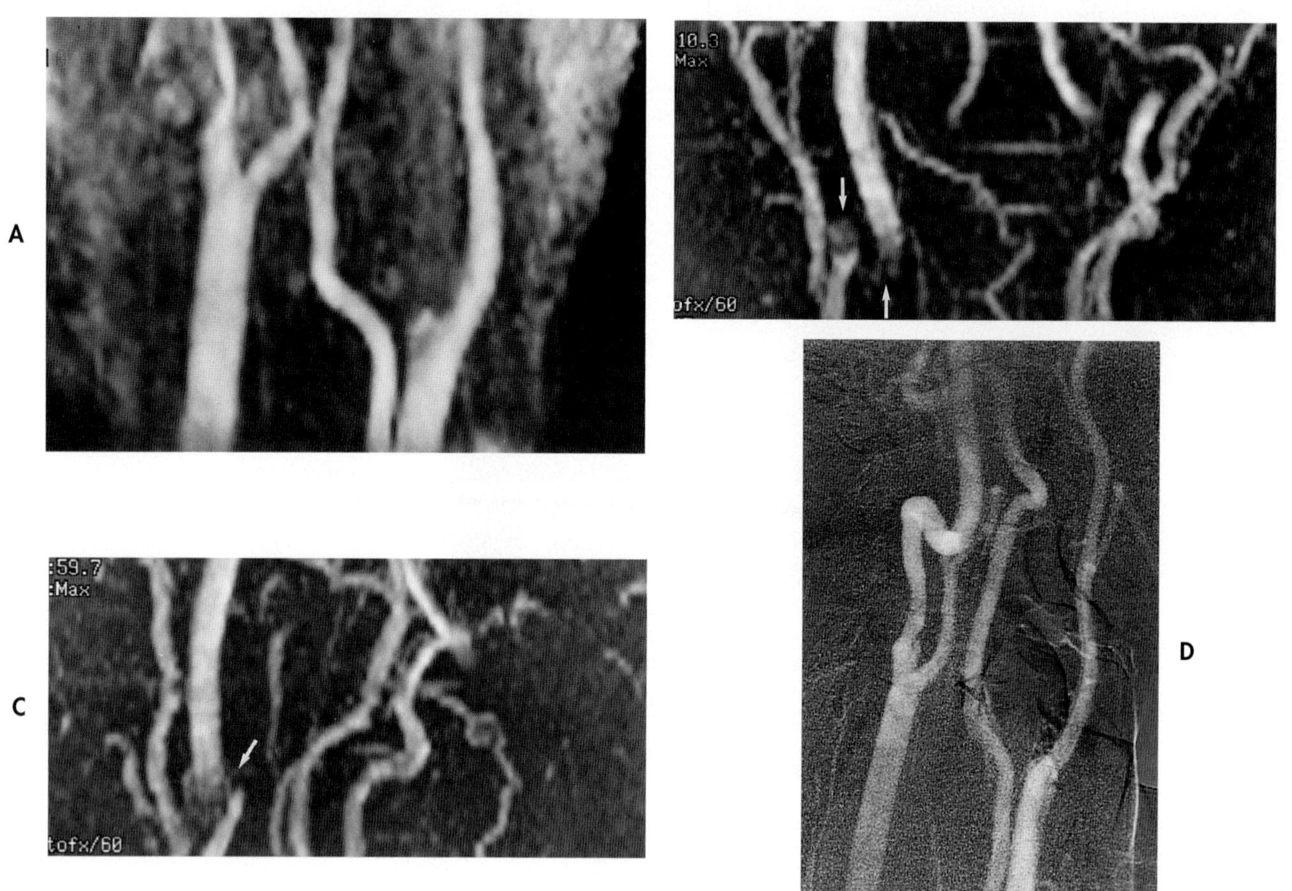

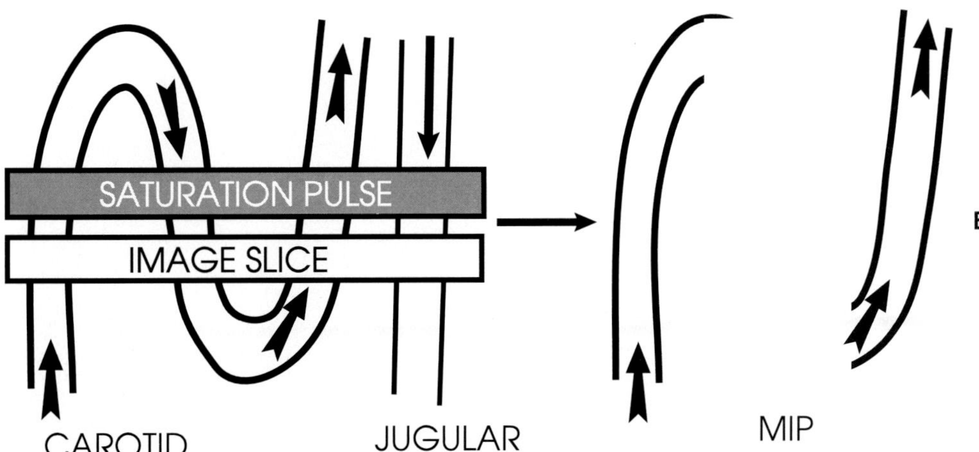


**A right anterior oblique maximum intensity projection of the two-dimensional time-of-flight study of the carotid bifurcations (A) shows a moderate stenosis of the right proximal internal carotid artery just distal to the bifurcation. The left internal carotid artery is occluded at its origin. An additional two-dimensional time-of-flight study of the upper cervical carotid artery above the bifurcation (B is an anteroposterior maximum intensity projection view, and C is a left anterior oblique maximum intensity projection view) shows an offset in the location of vascular signal of the proximal portion of the right internal carotid artery with intervening marked signal loss *(arrows),* which could result from a severe stenosis. However, the offset suggests the possibility of a vascular loop in this region, which could also give signal loss and a false-positive appearance of stenosis on the two-dimensional time-of-flight study. Conventional intraarterial angiography (D) shows the moderate stenosis at the origin of the right internal carotid artery, as well as the vascular loop more superiorly, without significant stenosis. The left internal carotid artery is occluded at its origin.**

The cause of this artifact is related to the presence of the "tracking" saturation pulses used in two-dimensional time-of-flight studies to "saturate out" unwanted venous blood flow signal. As the diagram illustrates, this saturation pulse causes signal loss and a false appearance of a "severe" stenosis when there is a vascular loop causing the vessel orientation to be reversed into a "venous" flow direction.

**E,** Axial two-dimensional time-of-flight images are acquired with a saturation pulse superior to the image slice to purposely eliminate venous signal. In cases with vascular loops, the saturation pulse may be oriented upstream to sections of the artery, which causes unwanted signal loss. The left side shows the positions of an imaging slice and tracking saturation pulse relative to a vascular arterial loop and the jugular vein and the resultant MRA image on the right. The MRA shows only the arterial segments where the saturation pulse is downstream to the image slice and the jugular vein signal is eliminated.

## CASE 160
## PITFALL: ENDARTERECTOMY CLIP MIMICKING STENOSIS

**History:** 62-year-old with a new onset of left hemispheric transient ischemic attacks and a history of endarterctomy 5 years before.

**Technique:** axial volume, three-dimensional time-of-flight, 39/7/25, 256 × 160, 64 slices, 80-mm slab, 25-cm field of view (rectangular), 6:42.

A

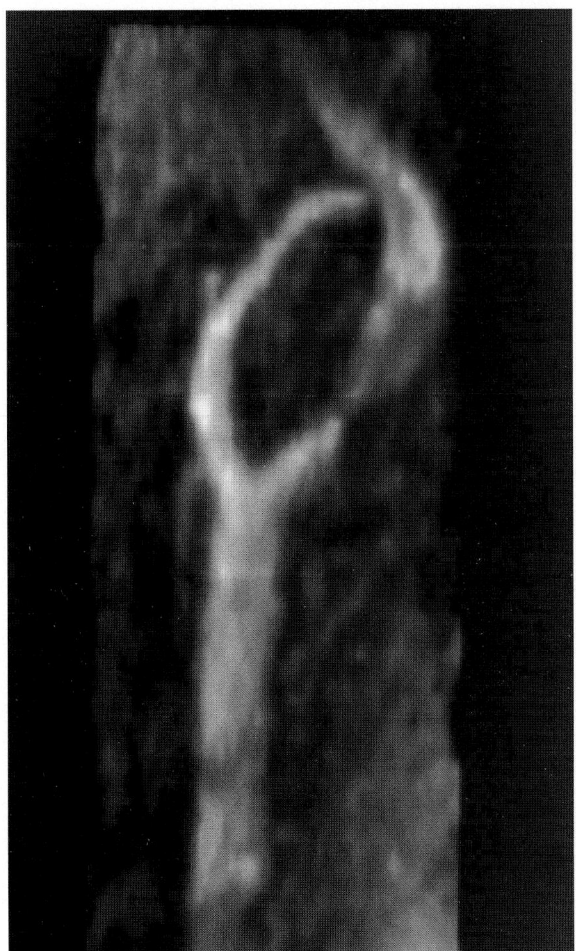

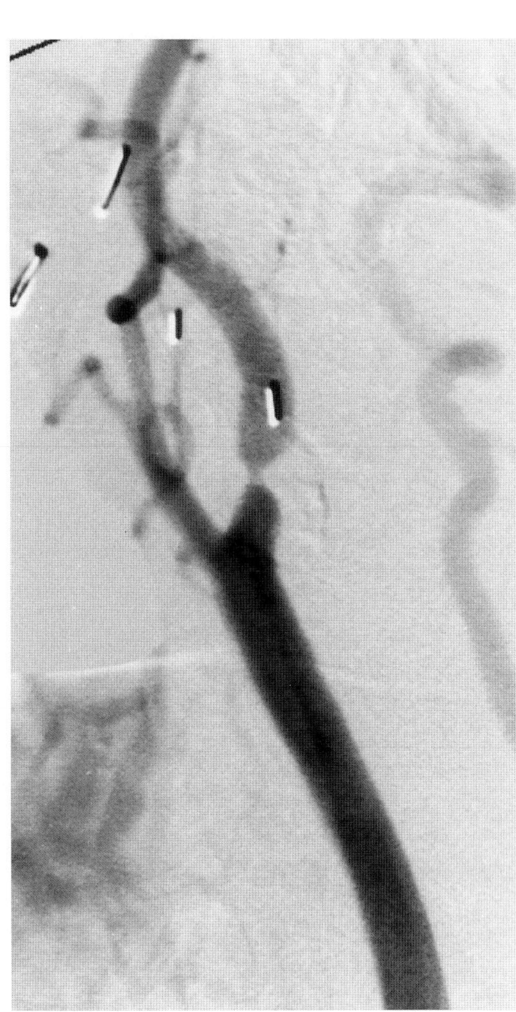

B

**MRA (A) shows an apparent long segment of severe stenosis involving the internal carotid artery, approximately 1 cm beyond the bifurcation. Conventional common carotid angiogram (B) shows that there is indeed a severe stenosis just distal to the internal carotid origin, but the length is overestimated on the MRA because of the presence of a surgical clip from prior endarterectomy. The metal introduces a local field inhomogeneity, spin dephasing, and signal loss.**

## CASE 161
## PITFALL: INTERNAL CAROTID OCCLUSION WITH OVERLAP ON MAXIMUM INTENSITY PROJECTION MIMICKING A PATENT VESSEL

**History:** 70-year-old with left hemispheric transient ischemic attacks.

**Technique:** axial volume, three-dimensional time-of-flight, 50/7/20, 256 × 192, 64 slices, 80-mm slab, 23-cm field of view, 10:17.

A

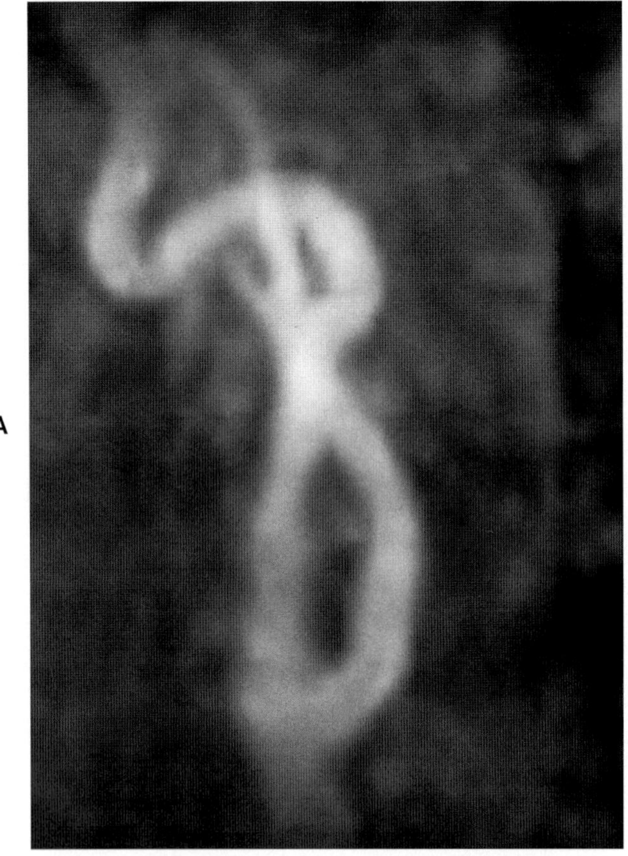

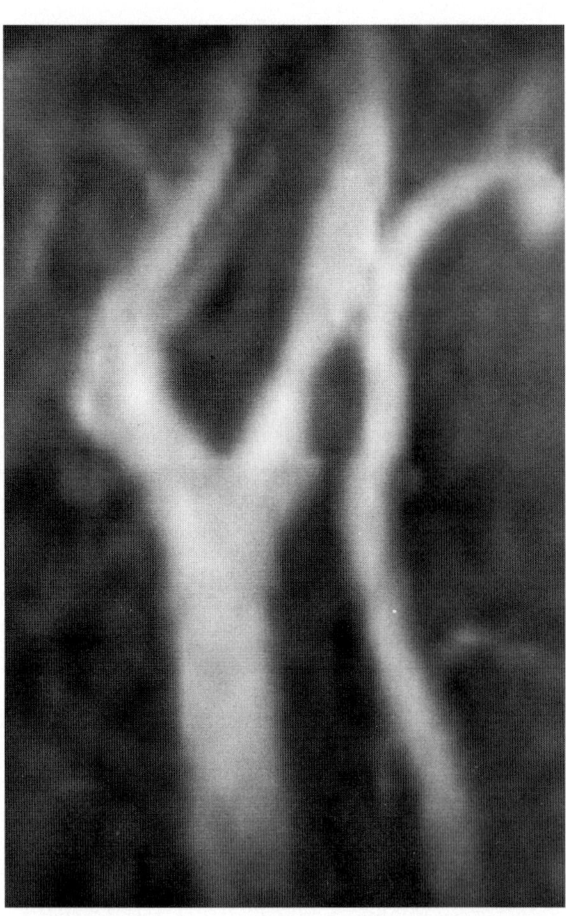

B

C

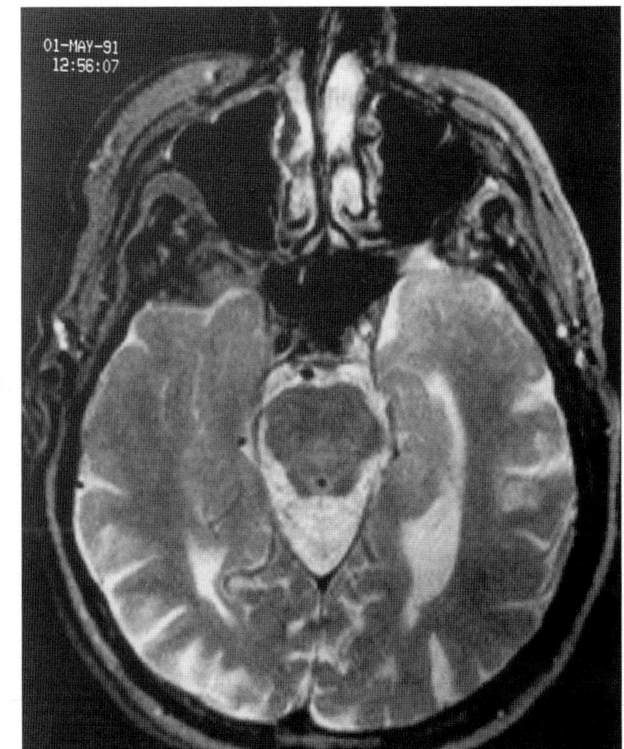


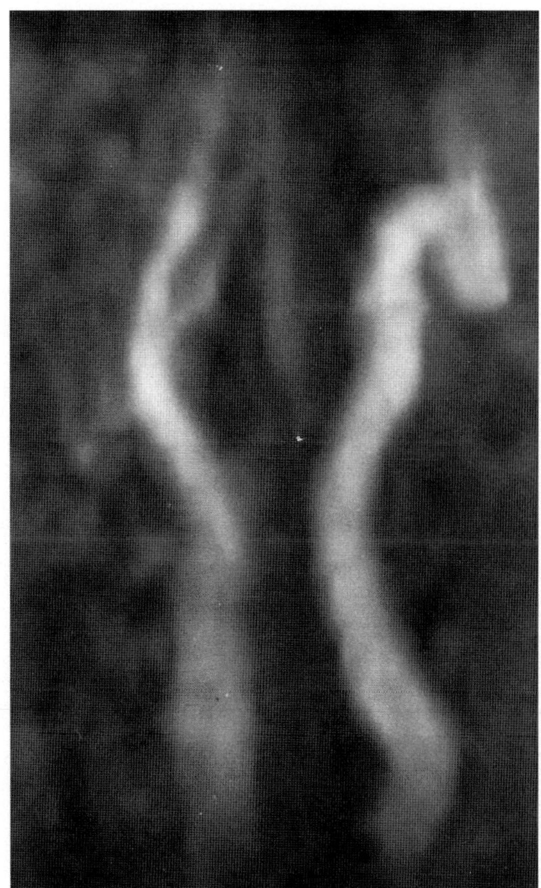

D

**Lateral views of the right and left carotid bifurcations show an apparently patent left bifurcation (A) and moderate smooth stenosis of the right bifurcation (B). However, the T2-weighted image (C) shows abnormal signal from the left carotid siphon, which represents abnormally slowed flow or occlusion, the cause of which is not apparent from the single view of the left carotid bifurcation. An oblique view of the left common carotid bifurcation (D) demonstrates two serpentine vessels extending through the course of the volume, without a bifurcation. The posterior vessel (at the right) has the characteristic turn of the vertebral artery at the craniovertebral junction. The anterior vessel branches, so it is the external carotid artery. In A, overlap of the external carotid and vertebral arteries falsely mimics a common carotid bifurcation. The oblique view allows a correct interpretation, differentiating the vessels into the posterior vertebral artery, the anterior external carotid artery, and an occluded internal carotid artery. This occlusion is also suggested by the axial T2-weighted spin-echo study showing abnormal increased signal intensity within the left carotid siphon.**

## CASE 162
## PITFALL: ARTIFACT MIMICKING STENOSIS AND STRING SIGN

**History:** 65-year-old with remote right hemispheric infarct.

**Technique:** axial two-dimensional time-of-flight, spoiled gradient acquisition in steady-state, 45/8.7/60, 256 × 128, 64 slices, 1.5-mm thickness, 18-cm field of view, 6:27.

A

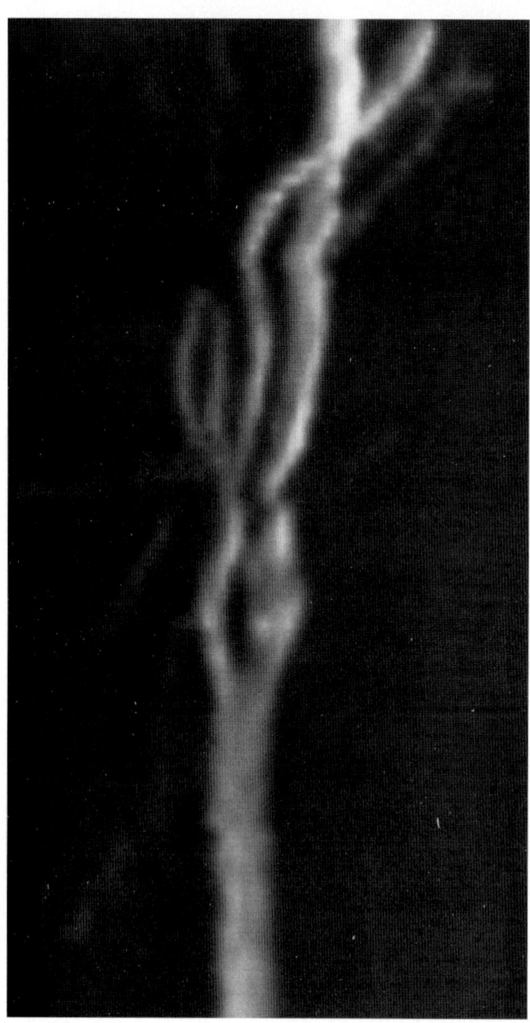

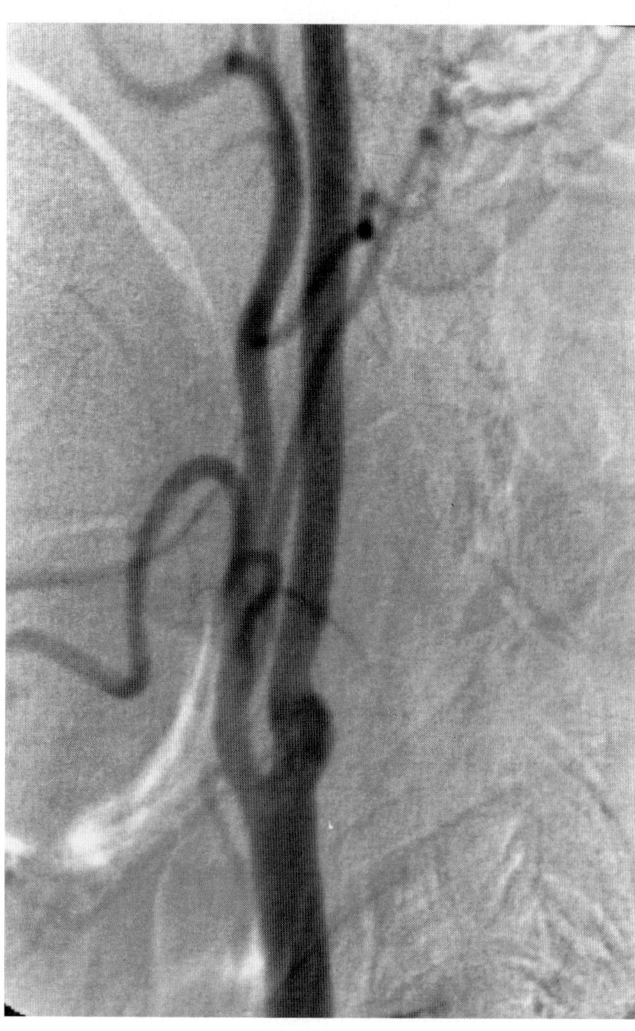

B

C 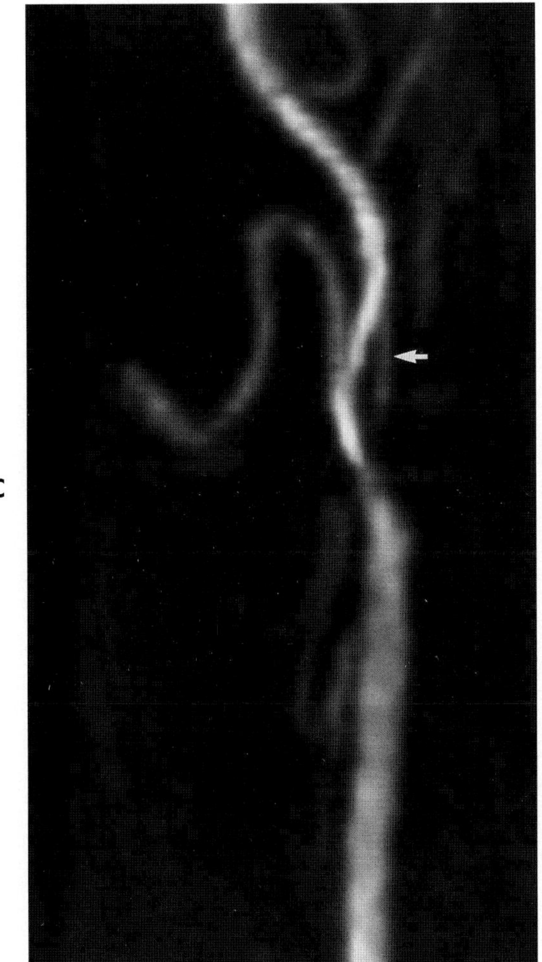

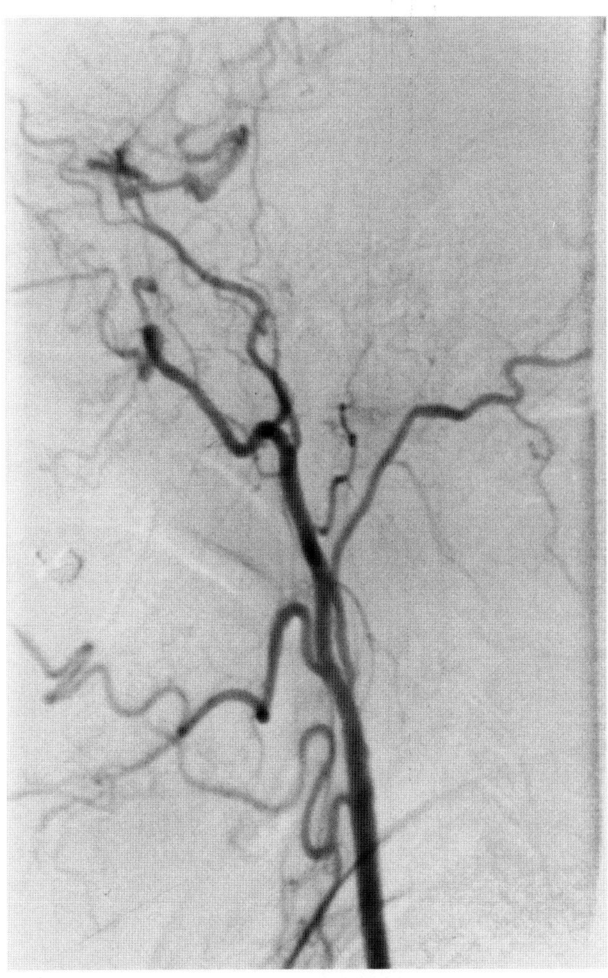 D

**Targeted lateral maximum intensity projection of the left carotid bifurcation (A) shows an apparent focal severe stenosis of the proximal internal carotid artery. Conventional angiography of the left bifurcation (B) fails to show any stenosis, which was produced on the MRA by patient motion during only one slice of the two-dimensional acquisition. Targeted lateral maximum intensity projection of the right bifurcation (C) shows an apparently high-grade stenosis of the proximal internal carotid artery, with only faint signal from the internal carotid (a string sign *[arrow]*). Again, conventional angiography (D) fails to confirm the MRA findings and instead shows an occlusion of the internal carotid artery. The linear signal intensity thought to be the internal carotid artery is probably the occipital branch of the external carotid artery.**

# CASE 163
## PITFALL: RECANALIZED INTERNAL CAROTID MIMICKING STRING SIGN

**History:** 74-year-old with transient ischemic attacks.

**Technique:** axial two-dimensional time-of-flight, spoiled gradient acquisition in steady-state, 45/8.7/60, 256 × 128, 64 slices, 1.5-mm thickness, 18-cm field of view, 6:27.

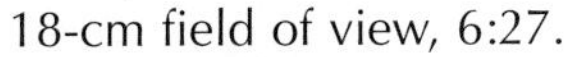

A

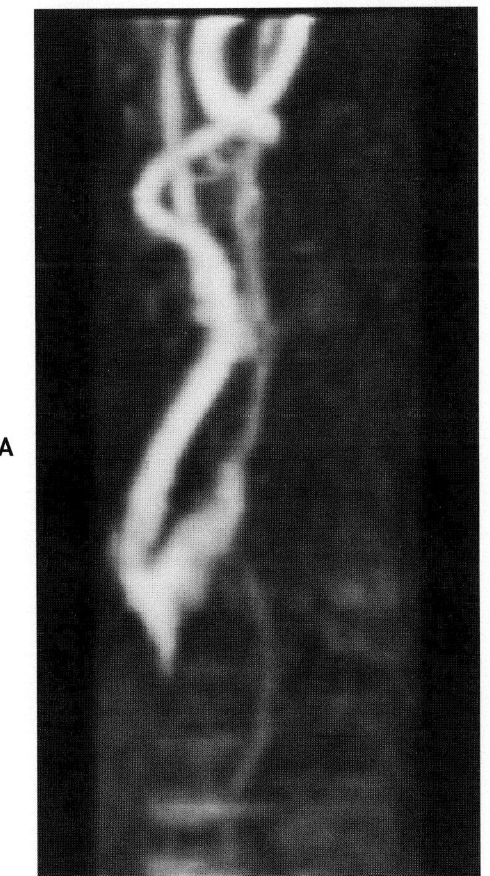

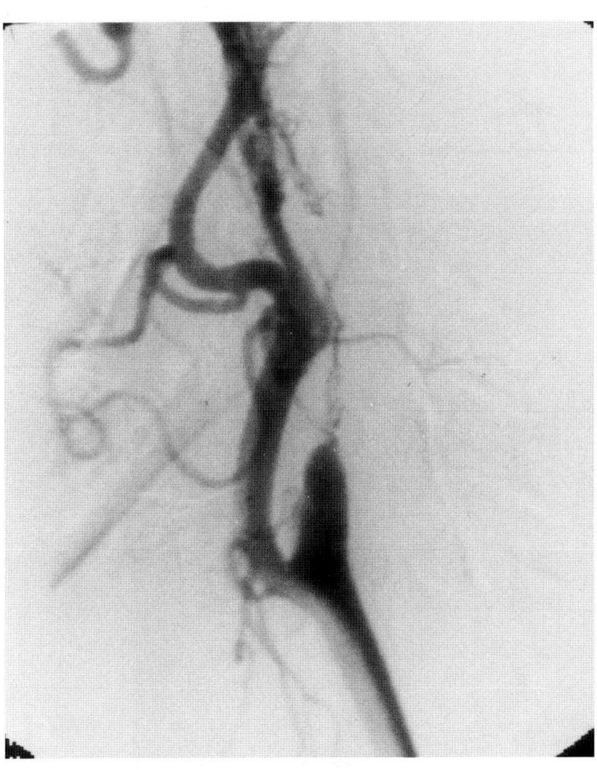

B

**Targeted lateral view of the maximum intensity projection (A) demonstrates a normal external carotid artery but a markedly narrowed, long, irregular segment of the internal carotid artery. This would be consistent with a string sign by MRA in atherosclerotic stenosis or carotid dissection. There is abrupt loss of signal within the distal common carotid artery resulting from artifactual cutoff of that portion by the margin of the targeted maximum intensity projection. Lateral view from the conventional angiogram (B) demonstrates the typical appearance of a chronic occlusion of the left internal carotid artery, with small irregular vessels extending up the path of the internal carotid artery related to recanalization.**

In this instance, the resolution of the two-dimensional time-of-flight MRA could not differentiate the appearance of a small tortuous recanalized internal carotid artery from a severe stenosis with a string sign.

## CASE 164
## PITFALL: HEMORRHAGIC PLAQUE

**History:** 68-year-old with left hemispheric transient ischemic attacks.

**Technique:** axial volume, three-dimensional time-of-flight, 39/7/25, 256 × 160, 64 slices, 80-mm slab, 25-cm field of view (rectangular), 6:42.

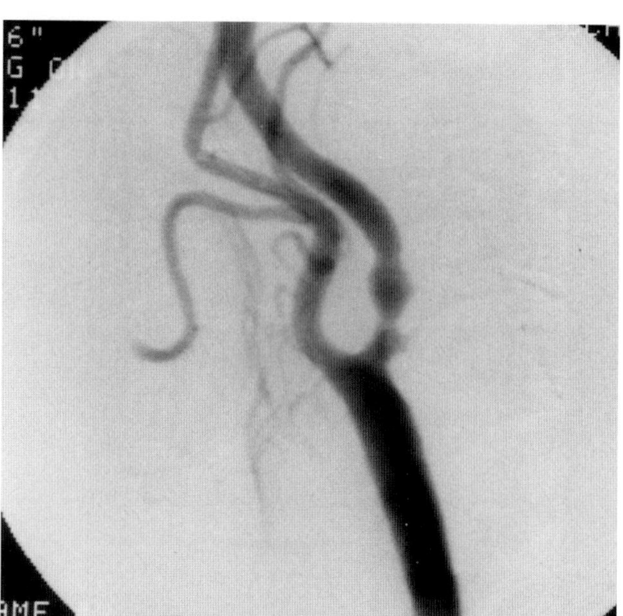

B

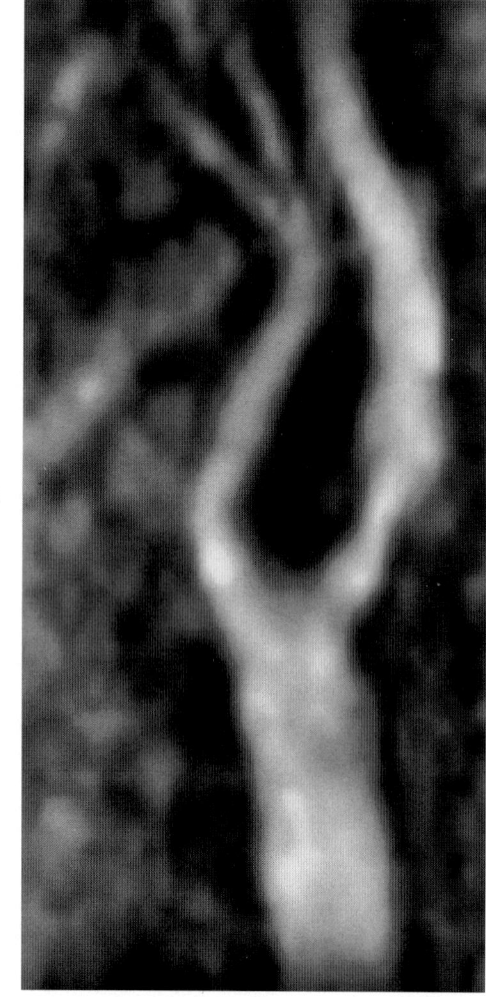

A

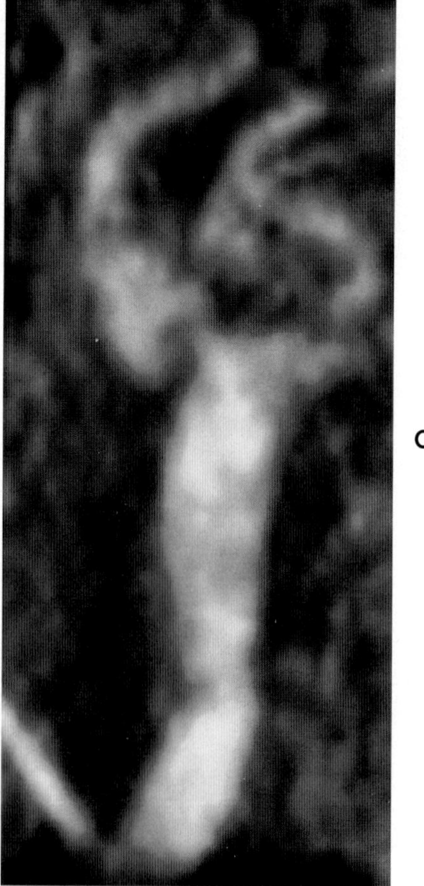

C

D

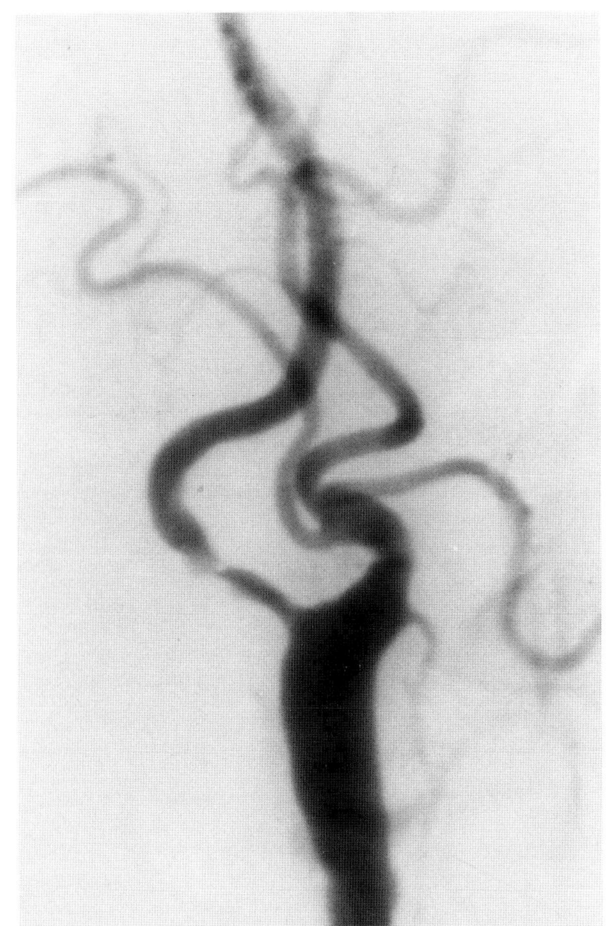

**Lateral maximum intensity projection view of the left carotid bifurcation (A) shows a severe stenosis at the origin of the internal carotid artery. Conventional common carotid angiogram (B) confirms the presence of a severe internal carotid stenosis. Lateral maximum intensity projection view of the right carotid bifurcation (C) shows a severe stenosis at the origin of the internal carotid artery, with a more normal-sized carotid artery seen distal to the focal stenosis. The conventional angiogram (D) shows that the stenosis is considerably longer than appreciated on the MRA and that it does not have the poststenotic dilated segment.**

E

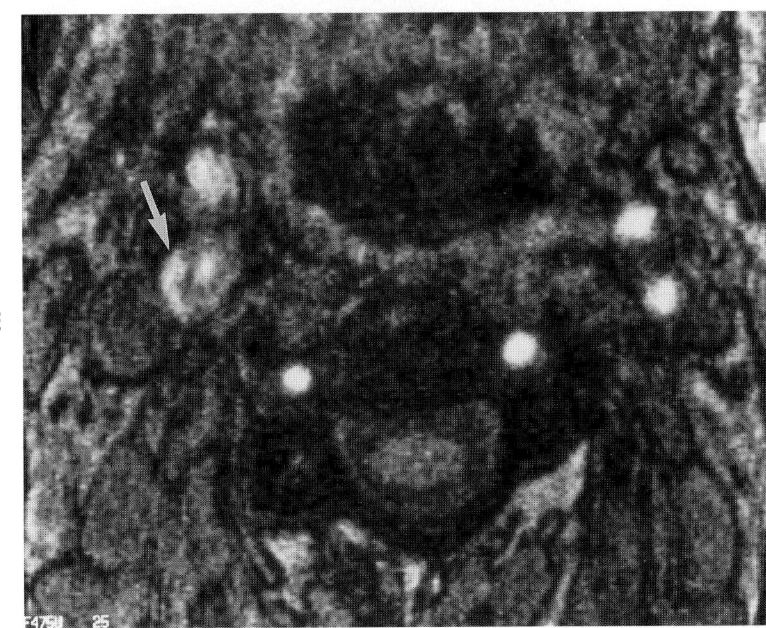

The discrepancy relates to high signal intensity hemorrhagic plaque (methemoglobin) falsely appearing as flow on the time-of-flight MRA maximum intensity projection view. The intraplaque hemorrhage is better appreciated on the individual slice as a cresent region of increased signal lateral to the more punctate lumen of the right internal carotid artery **(E)** ***(arrow)***.

## CASE 165
## PITFALL: OVERESTIMATION OF CAROTID STENOSIS

**History:** 64-year-old with left hemispheric transient ischemic attacks.

**Technique:** axial volume, three-dimensional time-of-flight, 39/7/25, 256 × 160, 64 slices, 80-mm slab, 25-cm field of view (rectangular), 6:42.

A

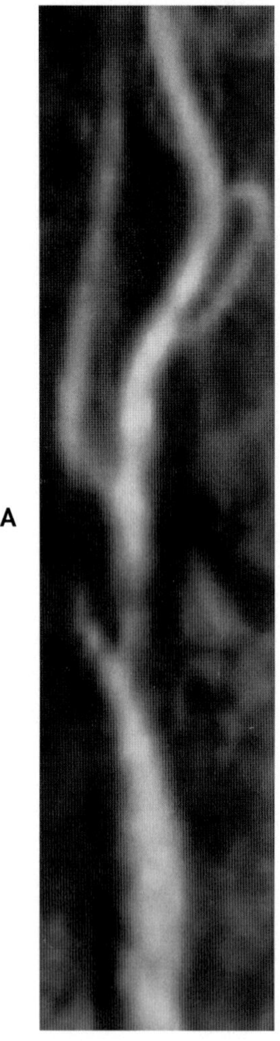

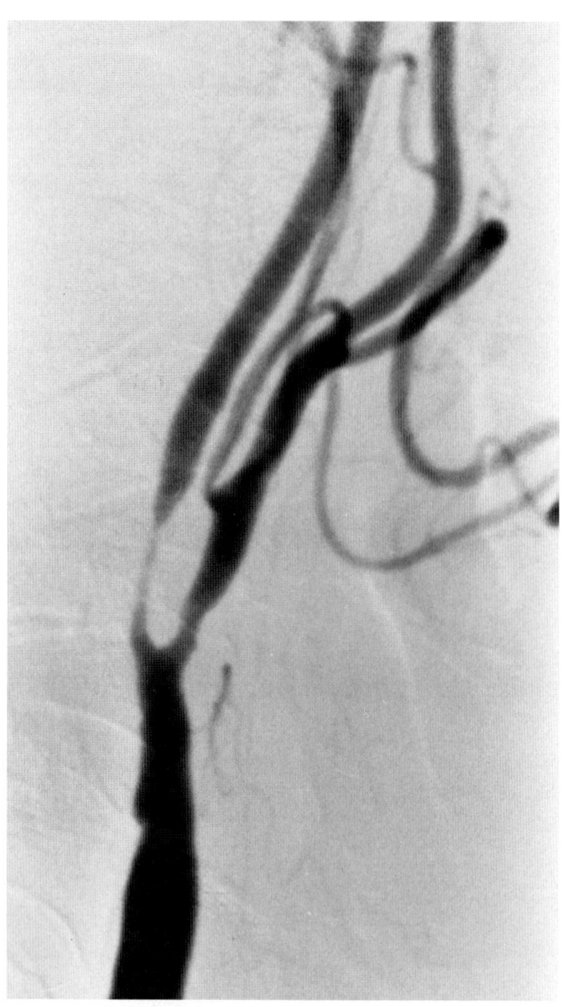

B

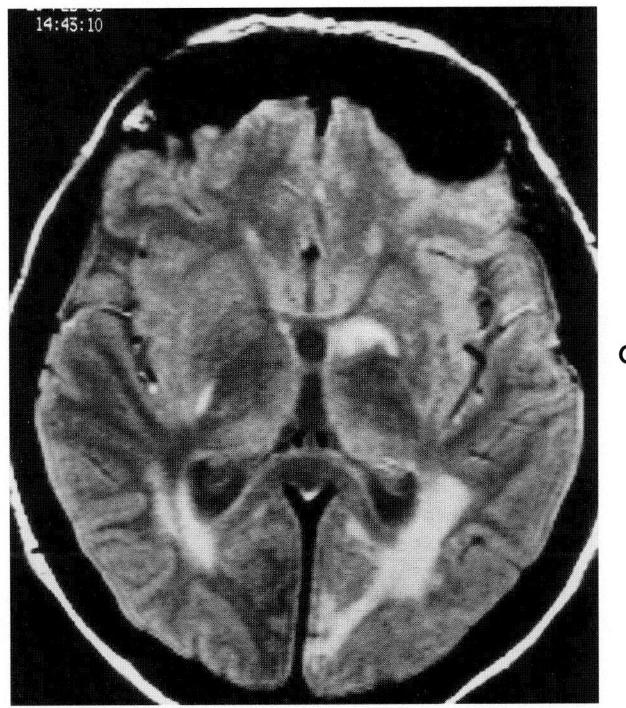


C

**Lateral maximum intensity projection view (A) shows a severe stenosis at the origin of the left internal carotid artery, which is manifested as a long segment of signal loss on this three-dimensional time-of-flight MRA. The more distal cervical internal carotid shows attenuated caliber and decreased signal, which represents slowed flow with an element of flow saturation. There is also a severe stenosis at the origin of the external carotid artery and moderate narrowing involving the distal common carotid artery. The findings are confirmed on the conventional common carotid angiographic injection (B) showing the severe internal carotid stenosis. Spin-density brain image (C) shows infarcts in the left basal ganglia, left occipital lobe, right periatrial white matter, and right posterior limb of the internal capsule.**

This is the typical pattern of signal loss at the carotid bifurcation with a severe stenosis (less than 90%) using a three-dimensional time-of-flight technique. Accelerated flow at the stenosis and complex flow immediately downstream from the stenosis causes signal loss and overestimation of stenosis. However, such signal loss is a reliable guide of severe stenosis.

## CASE 166
## PITFALL: OVERESTIMATION OF STENOSIS WITH TWO- VS. THREE-DIMENSIONAL TIME-OF-FLIGHT TECHNIQUES

**History:** 69-year-old with carotid bruit.

**Technique #1:** axial volume, three-dimensional time-of-flight, 40/6.9/20, 256 × 256, 60 slices, 72-mm slab, 10:56.

**Technique #2:** axial two-dimensional time-of-flight, spoiled gradient acquisition in steady-state, 45/8.8/60, 256 × 128, 52 slices, 1.5-mm thickness, 18-cm field of view, 5:11.

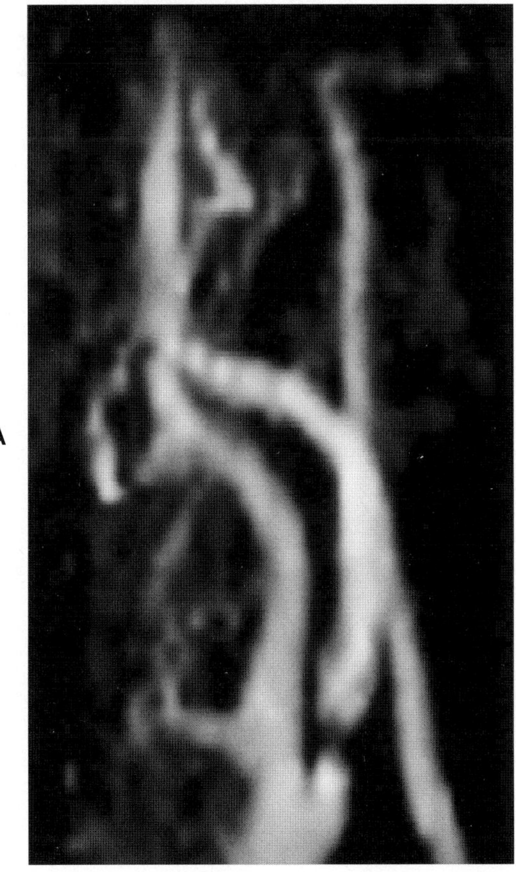

A

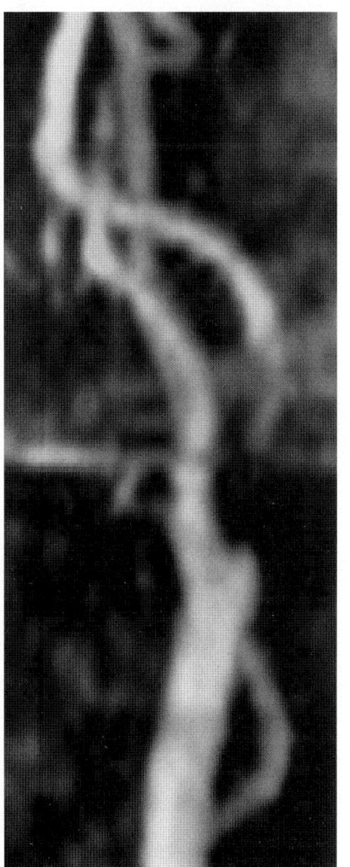

B

**Severe stenosis of the proximal internal carotid artery is present on the three-dimensional time-of-flight MRA (A), with loss of signal just at the stenosis and maintenance of signal distal to the stenosis. On the two-dimensional time-of-flight study (B), the severe stenosis is seen as a segment of signal loss at and distal to the stenosis compared with the three-dimensional time-of-flight study.**

The improved appearance of the stenosis on the three-dimensional study relates to (1) thinner slice thickness and increased inplane matrix, giving a smaller voxel that decreases intravoxel dephasing, and (2) a shorter echo time that minimizes phase dispersion.

Rough guidelines for the presence of signal loss on time-of-flight MRA is that signal loss resulting from stenosis with acceleration of flow and turbulent flow occurs with 70% or greater stenosis for two-dimensional time-of-flight techniques and around 90% stenosis for three-dimensional time-of-flight techniques.

### REFERENCE

Huston J, Lewis BD, Wiebers DO et al: Carotid artery: prospective blinded comparison of two dimensional time of flight MR angiography with conventional angiography and duplex US, *Radiology* 186(3):339-344, 1993.

## CASE 167
## PITFALL: CAROTID STENOSIS WITH OUTPOUCHING

**History:** left hemispheric transient ischemic attacks.

**Technique:** dual sagittal volumes, three-dimensional time-of-flight, 80/7/40, 256 × 256, two 16-slice volumes (32 slices total), 32-mm thick slab, 23-cm field of view, 10:56.

A

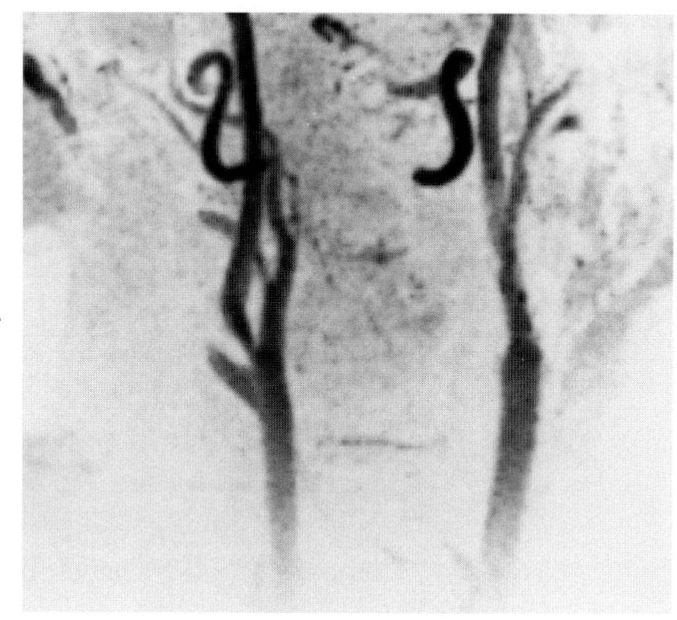

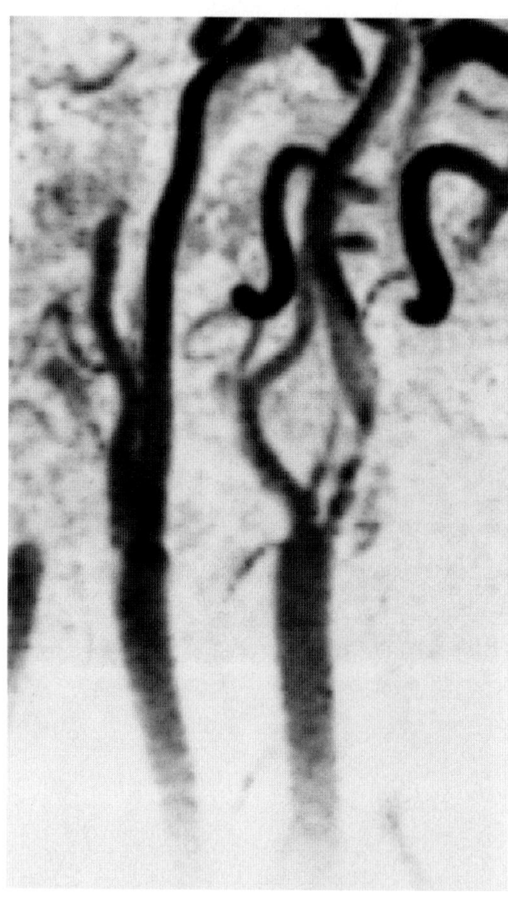

B

C

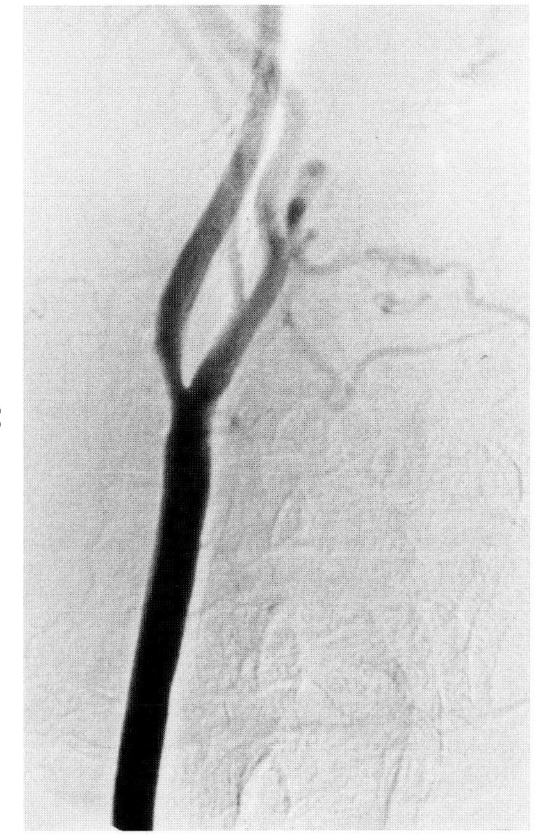

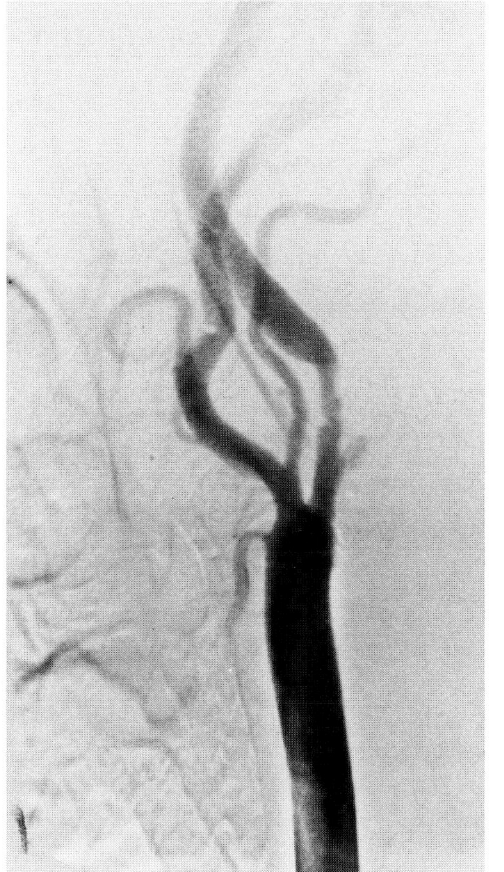

D

**Right (A) and left (B) anterior oblique maximum intensity projection views of the carotid bifurcations show a severe irregular stenosis involving the proximal portion of the left internal carotid artery and a moderate smooth stenosis involving the right internal carotid artery. Selective injection of the right common carotid artery confirms the moderate smooth stenosis (C). Selective injection of the left common carotid artery (D) demonstrates the severe stenosis involving the proximal internal carotid artery and an outpouching off the posterior wall of the proximal internal carotid artery, which was not seen on the MRA. (From Masaryk T, Ross JS: *MR angiography: clinical applications.* In Atlas S, ed: *Magnetic resonance imaging of the brain and spine,* New York, 1991, Raven.)**

Slow, stagnant, or complex flow within the outpouching leads to flow saturation and dephasing that is not visualized on the three-dimensional time-of-flight MRA. This has a considerable clinical significance, since this can be a site of embolus formation. In such cases, two-dimensional time-of-flight or phase-contrast techniques have an advantage because of their ability to define slower flow components.

## REFERENCE

Masaryk TJ, Modic MT, Ruggieri PM et al: Three-dimensional (volume) gradient-echo imaging of the carotid bifurcation: preliminary clinical experience, *Radiology* 171:801-806, 1989.

## CASE 168
## RIGHT INTERNAL CAROTID ARTERY OCCLUSION

**History:** 71-year-old with left hemiplegia.

**Technique:** axial two-dimensional time-of-flight, spoiled gradient acquisition in steady-state, 45/8.7/60, 256 × 128, 64 slices, 1.5-mm thickness, 18-cm field of view, 6:27.

A

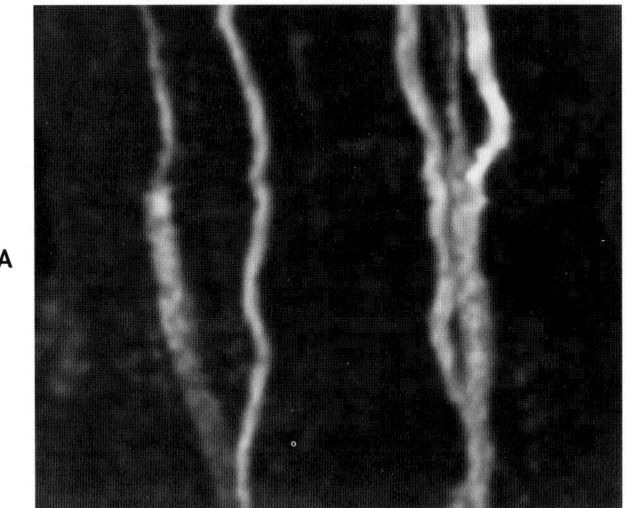

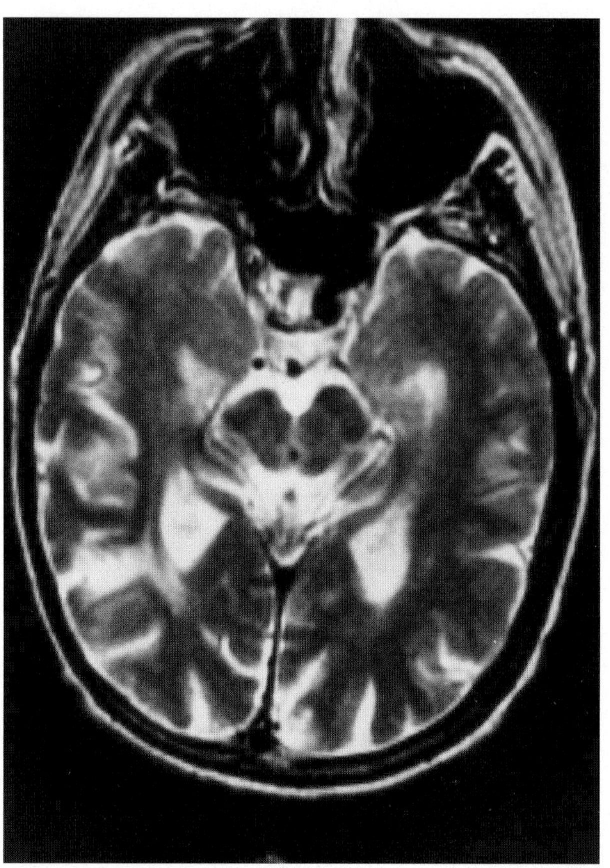

B

C

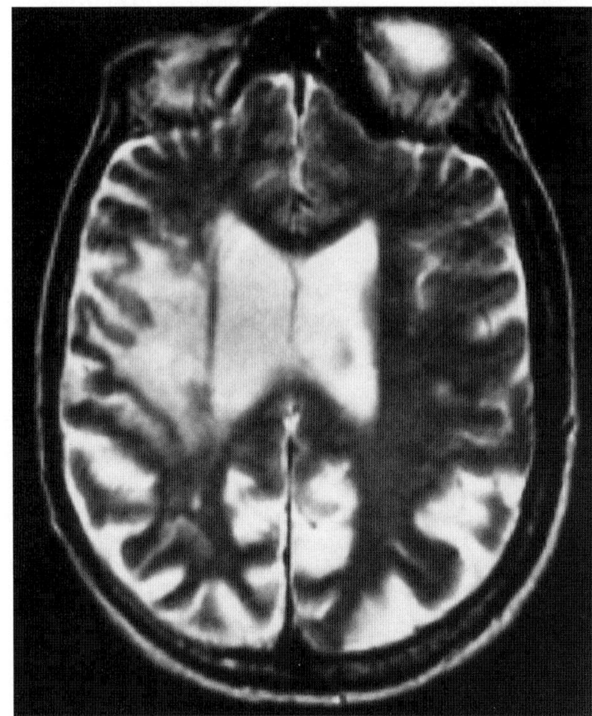

**A two-dimensional time-of-flight MRA of the carotid bifurcation (A) demonstrates a mild stenosis at the origin of the left internal carotid artery but otherwise patent common carotid and vertebral arteries bilaterally. On the right, the common carotid artery ends in a single vessel, most likely the external carotid artery. However, no significant branching is seen on the MRA to provide a definitive diagnosis. Confirmation is provided by the conventional spin-echo imaging of the brain (B), which at the level of the carotid siphon shows absent flow within the right carotid siphon compared with a normal flow void on the left. There is also an infarct involving the right middle cerebral artery distribution, which is seen as abnormally increased signal intensity within the right corona radiata (C).**

Laster et al compared two-dimensional time-of-flight MRA with conventional angiography in 101 patients and found that MRA showed a high rate of agreement with conventional angiography. They graded the MRA studies into the following categories: (1) "normal or mildly narrowed" (0% to 29%) if the vessel contour was normal or very minimally narrowed, (2) "moderately narrowed" (30% to 69%) if significant vessel narrowing but no focal signal loss was seen with the narrowing, and (3) "severely narrowed" (70% to 99%) if there was signal void with signal present proximally and distally (i.e., no occlusion present). Advantages of such a technique for the carotid bifurcation include good assessment of slow flow compared with that on three-dimensional time-of-flight techniques (no flow saturation), good length of coverage (10 cm), and minimal motion artifacts. The authors make the point that, with the two-dimensional technique, motion artifact affects only one or a few slices, not the whole imaging volume, as occurs with three-dimensional studies.

## REFERENCES

Laster RE, Acker JD, Halford HH et al: Assessment of MR angiography versus arteriography for evaluation of cervical carotid bifurcation disease, *AJNR* 14:681-688, 1993.

Heiserman JE, Drayer BP, Fram EK et al: Carotid artery stenosis: clinical efficacy of 2D time-of-flight MR angiography, *Radiology* 182(3):761-768, 1992.

Litt AW, Edelman EM, Pinto RS et al: Diagnosis of carotid artery stenosis: comparison of 2DFT time-of-flight MR angiography with contrast angiography in 50 patients, *AJNR* 12:611-616, 1991.

## CASE 169
## RIGHT INTERNAL CAROTID ARTERY OCCLUSION

**History:** 77-year-old with right hemispheric transient ischemic attacks.

**Technique:** coronal volume, three-dimensional time-of-flight, 50/6/15, 256 × 128, 64 slices, 84-mm thick, 23-cm field of view, 6:53. The repetition time is slightly prolonged with use of the coronal volume compared with the axial volumes, since time-of-flight geometry is not optimal. Prolonging the repetition time allows more time for inflow of fresh unsaturated spins into the volume to improve vascular signal.

A

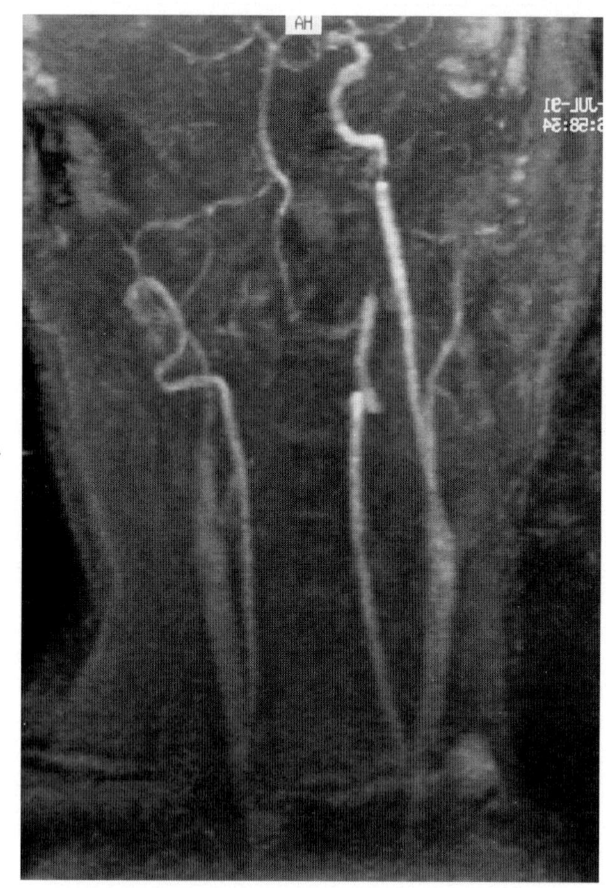

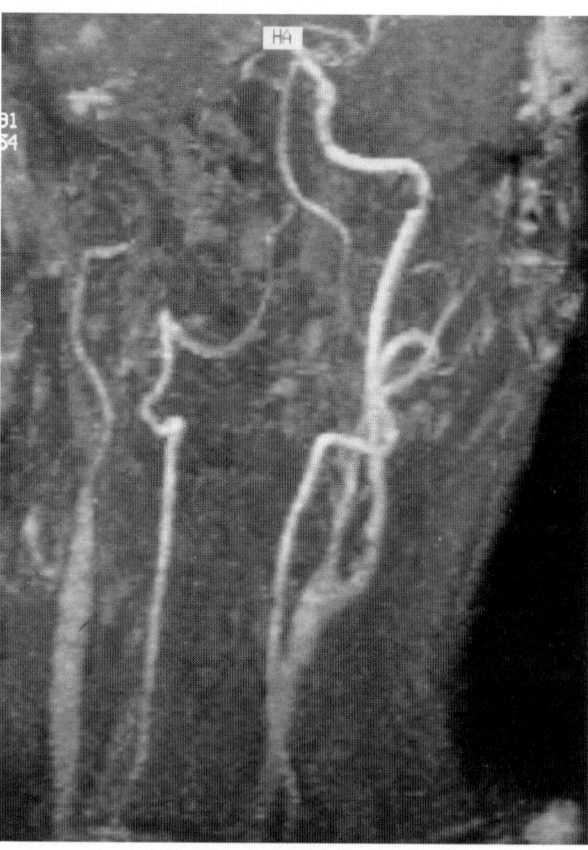

B

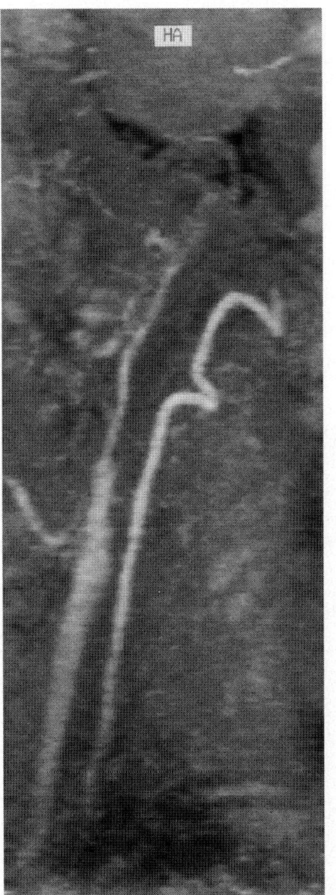


C

Anteroposterior (A) and left anterior oblique (B) whole volume maximum intensity projection views of the coronally acquired volume and targeted maximum intensity projection view of the right carotid bifurcation (C) demonstrate an occlusion of the right internal carotid artery. The right external carotid origin appears widely patent. On the left, there is a mild stenosis involving the origin of the internal carotid artery, but good flow is maintained distally. The distal left common carotid and external carotid are widely patent. Note the artifactual narrowing of the distal left internal carotid artery resulting from the susceptibility effects at the junction with the skull base.

## CASE 170
## LEFT INTERNAL CAROTID ARTERY OCCLUSION WITH INFARCT

**History:** 66-year-old with sudden onset right-sided weakness.

**Technique:** coronal volume, three-dimensional time-of-flight, 50/6/15, 256 × 128, 64 slices, 84-mm thick, 23-cm field of view, 6:53. Repetition time is slightly prolonged with use of the coronal volume compared with the axial volumes, since time-of-flight geometry is not optimal. Prolonging the repetition time allows more time for inflow of fresh unsaturated spins into the volume to improve vascular signal.

A

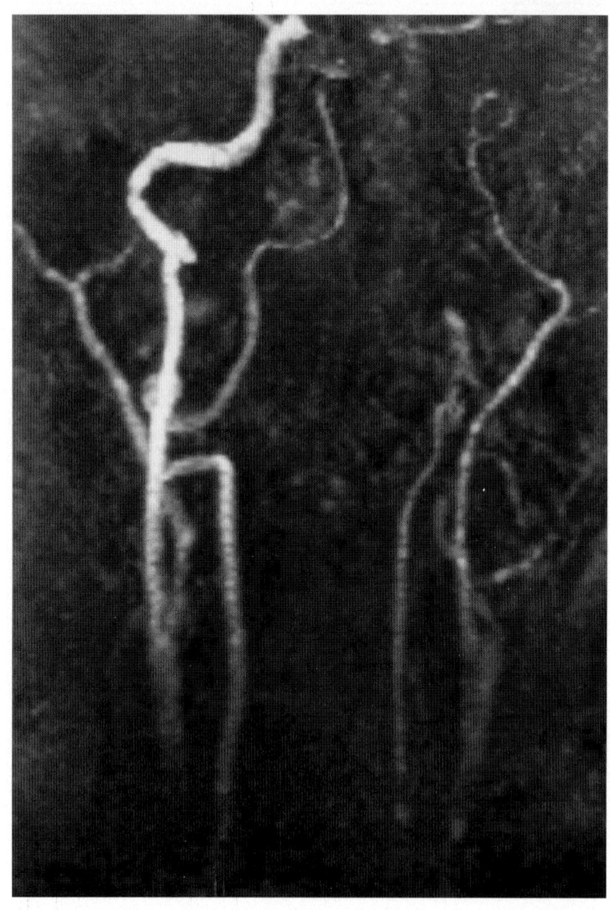

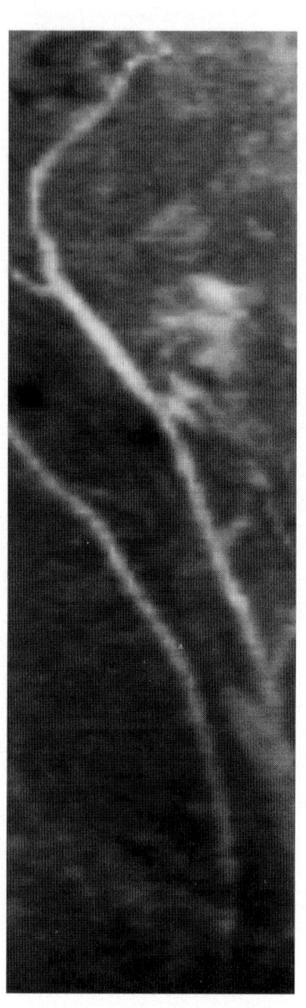

B

C

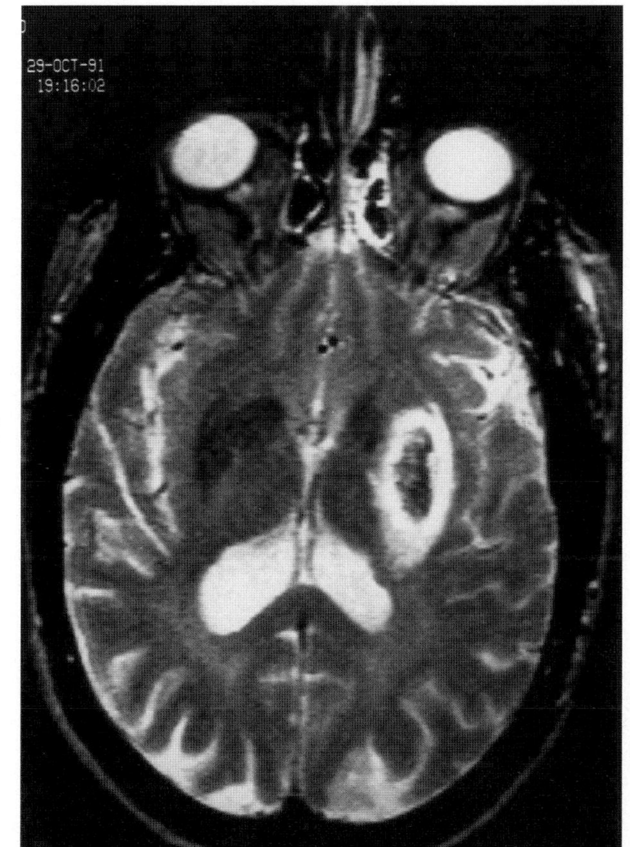


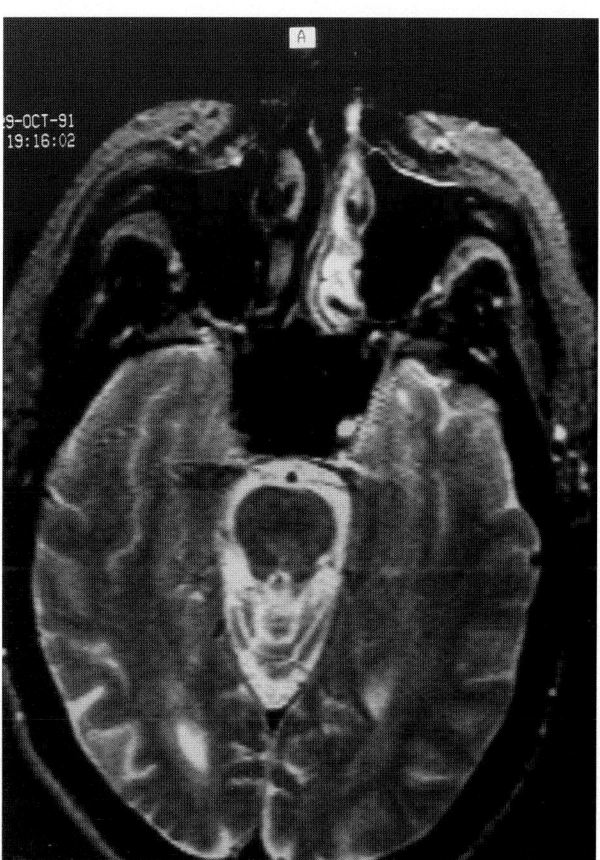


D

**Anteroposterior whole volume maximum intensity projection (A) and targeted lateral maximum intensity projection (B) of the left bifurcation demonstrate occlusion of the left internal carotid artery. Note the branching of the distal portions of the left external carotid artery, which confirms the vessel's identity. On the right, there is moderate stenosis of the external origin, but the internal carotid is widely patent. Artifactual narrowing of the distal internal carotid artery is noted at the skull base. T2-weighted spin-echo MR image of the head demonstrates an infarct involving the left basal ganglia (C). There is also abnormal increased signal and absence of the flow void within the left internal carotid artery related to the occlusion (D).**

## CASE 171
## LEFT INTERNAL CAROTID OCCLUSION AND RIGHT CAROTID STENOSIS

**History:** 54-year-old with right carotid bruit.

**Technique:** coronal volume, three-dimensional time-of-flight, 50/6/15, 256 × 128, 64 slices, 84-mm thick, 23-cm field of view, 6:53. Repetition time is slightly prolonged with use of the coronal volume compared with the axial volumes, since time-of-flight geometry is not optimal. Prolonging the repetition time allows more time for inflow of fresh unsaturated spins into the volume to improve vascular signal.

A

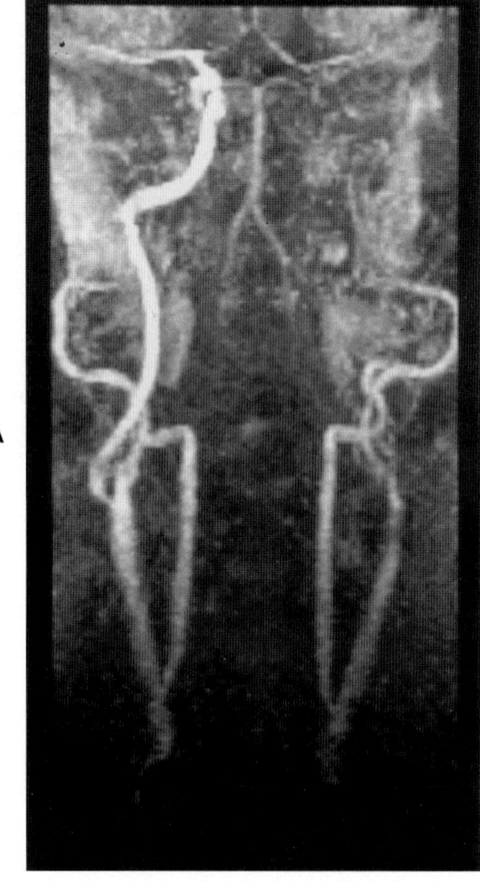

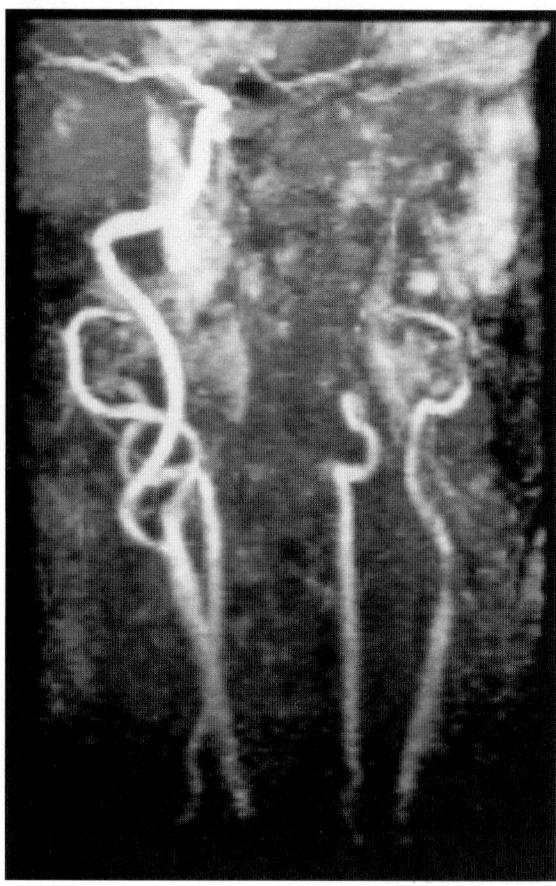

B

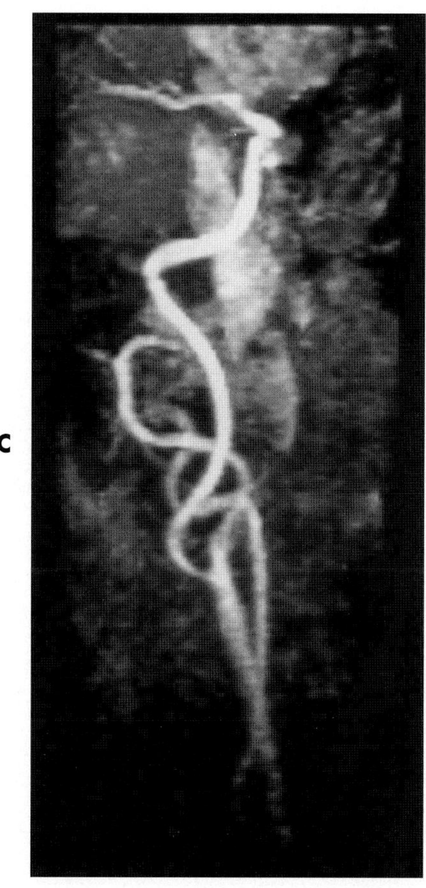

C

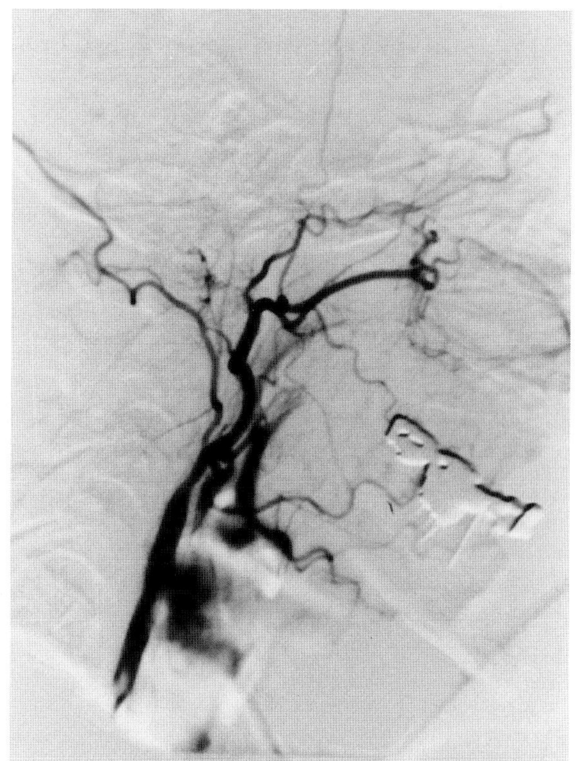

D

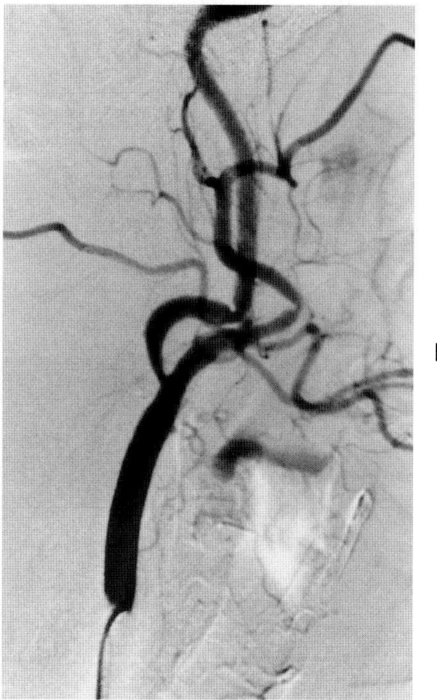

E

**Anteroposterior (A) and right anterior oblique (B) whole volume maximum intensity projection and targeted lateral maximum intensity projection (C) of the right bifurcation of the coronal three-dimensional volume demonstrate a severe stenosis involving the origin of the right internal carotid artery. There is occlusion of the left internal carotid artery, with only the branching visualized of the left external carotid artery.**

The advantage of obtaining a coronal volume is its increased superior-to-inferior coverage of the neck vessels. However, overall resolution for any one area is decreased because of the enlarged field of view. There is also cutoff of a portion of the superior vertebral arteries, which is related to the positioning of the volume. An additional, potentially more serious disadvantage with the coronal volume is the increased in-plane dephasing that occurs because the carotids are oriented parallel to the slices. This can accentuate signal loss at sites of stenosis and cause worse overestimation of stenoses compared with an axially acquired volume. Conventional angiogram confirms the occlusion of the left internal carotid artery **(D)** and the smooth severe stenosis at the origin of the right internal carotid artery **(E).**

## CASE 172
## SEVERE CAROTID BIFURCATION STENOSIS WITH DECREASED INTRACRANIAL SIGNAL

**History:** 55-year-old with episodic right extremity weakness.

**Technique:** axial volume, three-dimensional time-of-flight, 34/6/20, 256 × 128, 64 slices, 80-mm slab, 23-cm field of view (rectangular), 9:19.

A

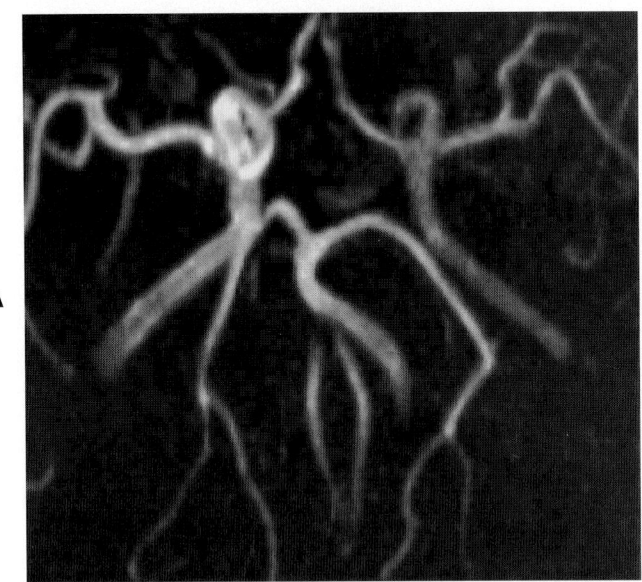

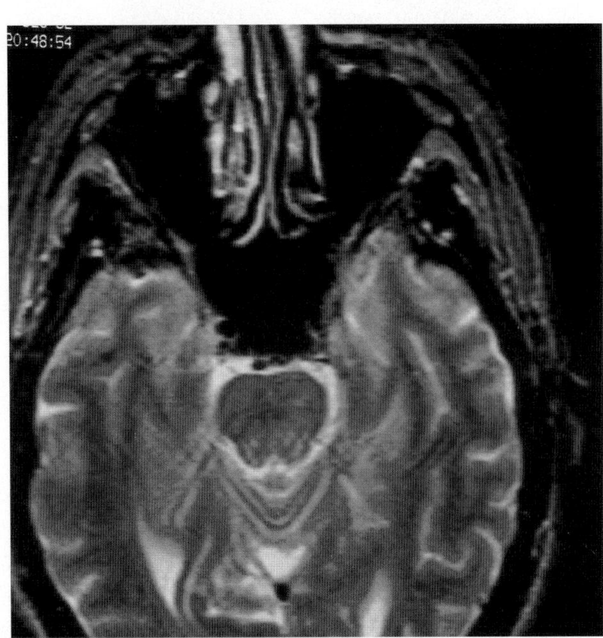


B

C

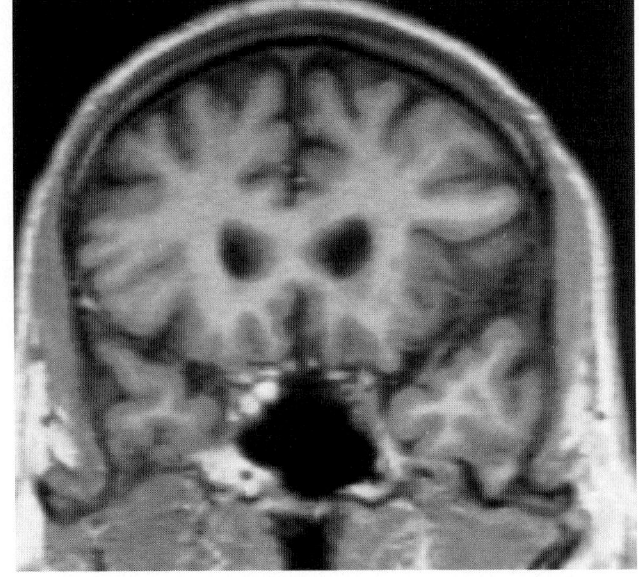

D

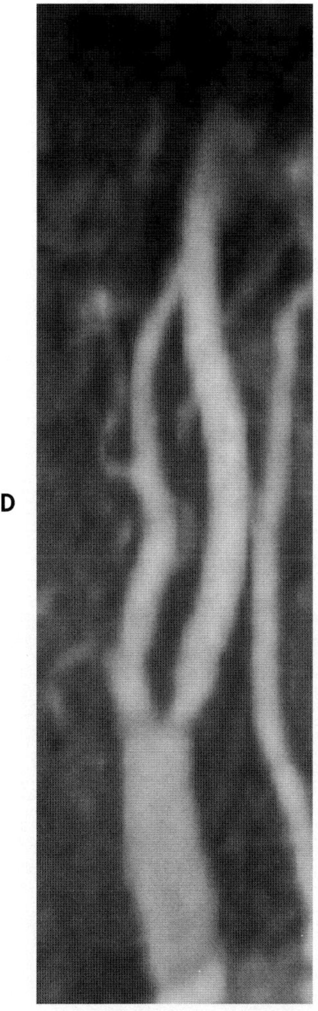

E

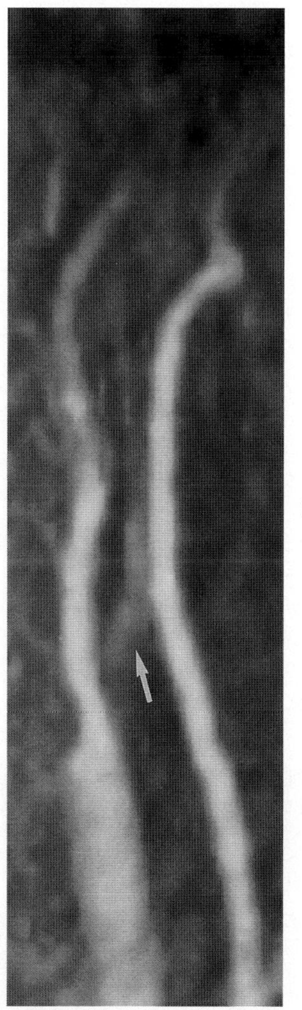

**Base view maximum intensity projection of the intracranial circulation (A) shows abnormally decreased signal intensity involving the distal left internal carotid artery and the middle cerebral artery branches compared with the normal signal intensity of the right internal carotid and basilar distributions. Abnormality of flow is further identified on the axial T2-weighted study of the head, which shows lack of the usual flow void within the left carotid siphon (B). The presence of this signal intensity on the head MRA indicates at least slow flow and not an occlusion. The coronal T1-weighted gradient-echo study (C) shows normal-appearing flow-related enhancement within the right carotid siphon and no evidence of acute methemoglobin within the carotid siphon to mimic a patent vessel on the MRA maximum intensity projection view. Because of the questionable slow flow within the distal internal carotid artery, MRA of the carotid bifurcation was performed. The right carotid bifurcation shows moderate stenosis involving the origin of the internal carotid artery (D). On the left (E), there is a severe stenosis at the origin of the internal carotid artery, with a small threadlike amount of signal intensity within the cervical internal carotid (the MR equivalent of the angiographic string sign) *(arrow).***

This finding on the intracranial MRA (decreased signal intensity within the internal carotid distribution) is a typical time-of-flight finding for severe stenosis that is more proximal; this finding requires that additional imaging of the carotid bifurcation or aortic arch be performed. The slowed flow resulting from the proximal stenosis allows increased flow saturation effects, thus decreasing the signal intensity.

## CASE 173
## SEVERE CAROTID BIFURCATION STENOSIS WITH DECREASED INTRACRANIAL SIGNAL

**History:** 59-year-old with left carotid bruit.

**Technique #1:** carotid (1.0-Tesla magnet), axial volume, three-dimensional time-of-flight, 40/11/25, 256 × 256, 64 slices, 80-mm slab, 20-cm field of view, 10:57. Echo time is prolonged relative to the usual 7-msec echo time at 1.5 Tesla, since fat and water cycle inphase at 1.0 Tesla with 7-msec echo time and opposed phase at echo time 11. Prolonging the echo time to the opposed phase improves the background enough to outweigh the increased dephasing that might occur.

**Technique #2:** intracranial, axial volume, three-dimensional time-of-flight, 40/7/15, 256 × 256, 64 slices, 80-mm slab, 20-cm field of view, 10:57. Since the background signal of fat is not a problem in intracranial imaging, the echo time can be safely reduced to 7 msec.

A

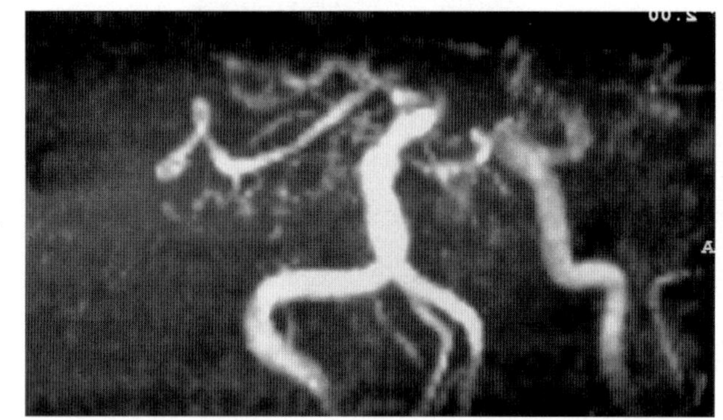

B

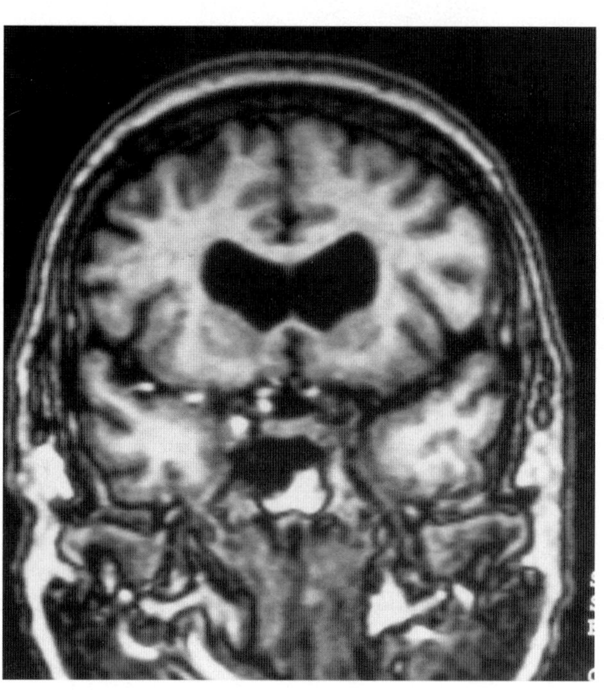

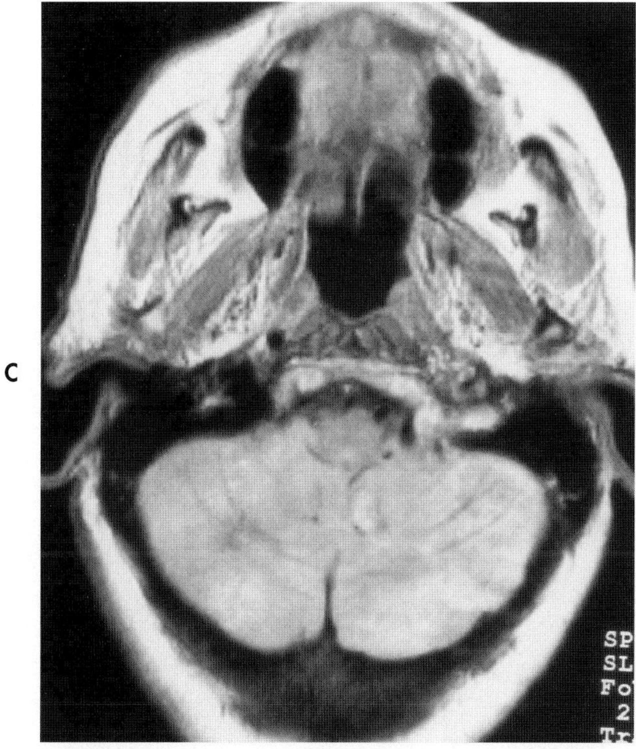


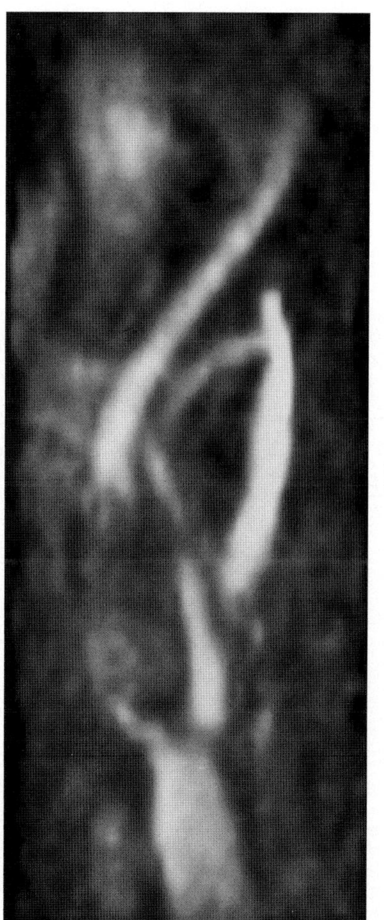


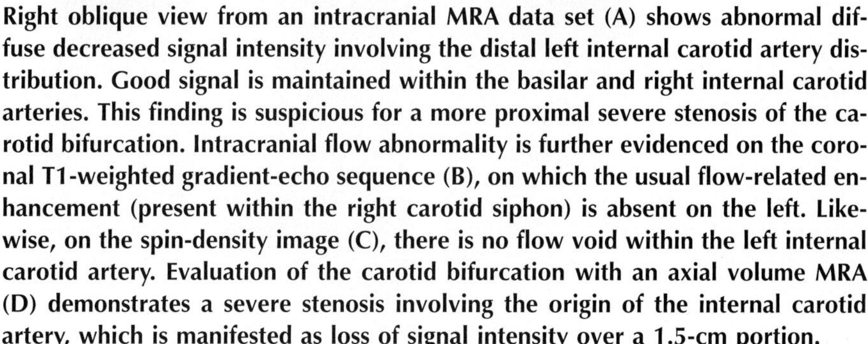
**Right oblique view from an intracranial MRA data set (A) shows abnormal diffuse decreased signal intensity involving the distal left internal carotid artery distribution. Good signal is maintained within the basilar and right internal carotid arteries. This finding is suspicious for a more proximal severe stenosis of the carotid bifurcation. Intracranial flow abnormality is further evidenced on the coronal T1-weighted gradient-echo sequence (B), on which the usual flow-related enhancement (present within the right carotid siphon) is absent on the left. Likewise, on the spin-density image (C), there is no flow void within the left internal carotid artery. Evaluation of the carotid bifurcation with an axial volume MRA (D) demonstrates a severe stenosis involving the origin of the internal carotid artery, which is manifested as loss of signal intensity over a 1.5-cm portion.**

There is maintenance of signal intensity within the more distal aspect of the internal carotid artery, which excludes the presence of total vessel occlusion. The loss of signal intensity in the intracranial MRA relates to flow saturation effects resulting from the slowed flow occurring because of the proximal bifurcation stenosis.

## CASE 174
## SEVERE CAROTID STENOSIS ON MRA THAT DIRECTED THE CONVENTIONAL ANGIOGRAPHIC VIEWS

**History:** 55-year-old with carotid bruit.

**Technique:** axial volume, three-dimensional time-of-flight, 50/7/20, 256 × 192, 64 slices, 80-mm slab, 23-cm field of view, 10:16.

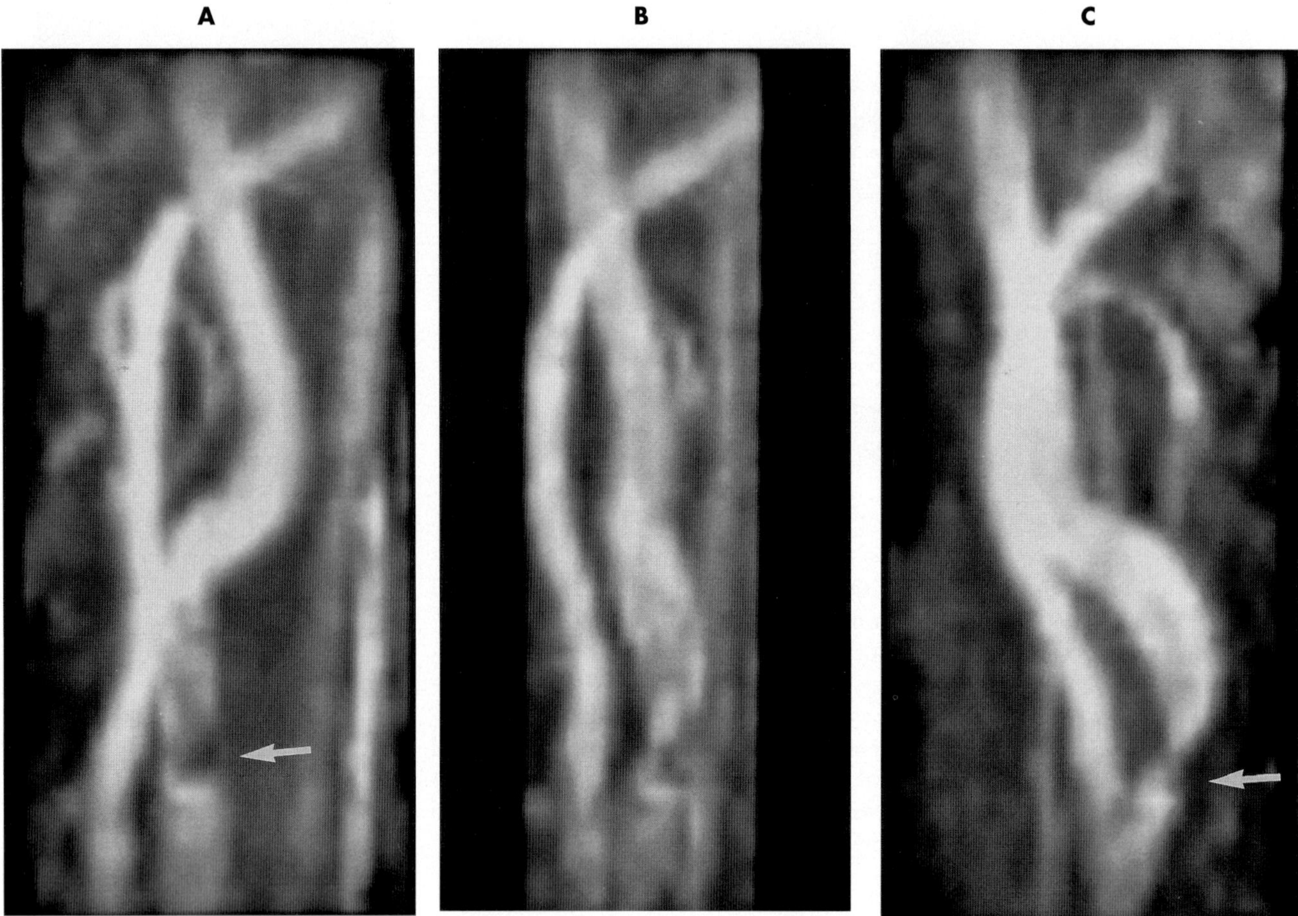


**Three oblique maximum intensity projection views (A to C) of the region of the right carotid bifurcation show two vessels. The smaller vessel is without evidence of stenosis, has branches, and is the external carotid artery. The other, larger vessel is the internal carotid artery and shows a severe shelf stenosis *(arrow)*. The carotid bifurcation proper was missed by an incorrect cephalad placement of the imaging volume.**

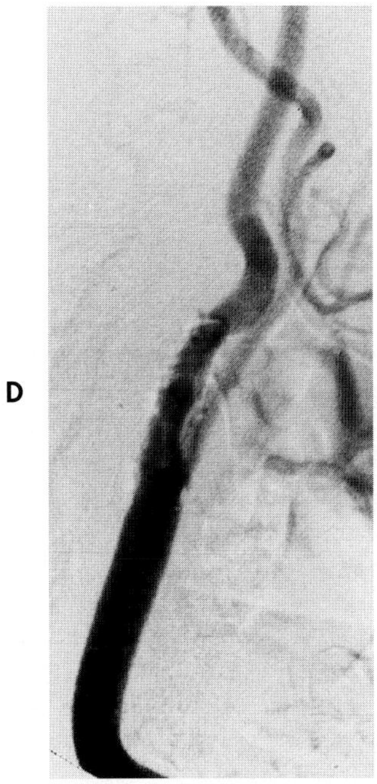
D

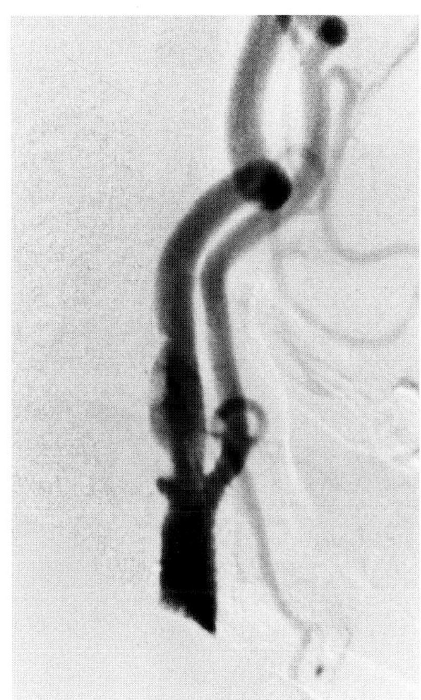
E

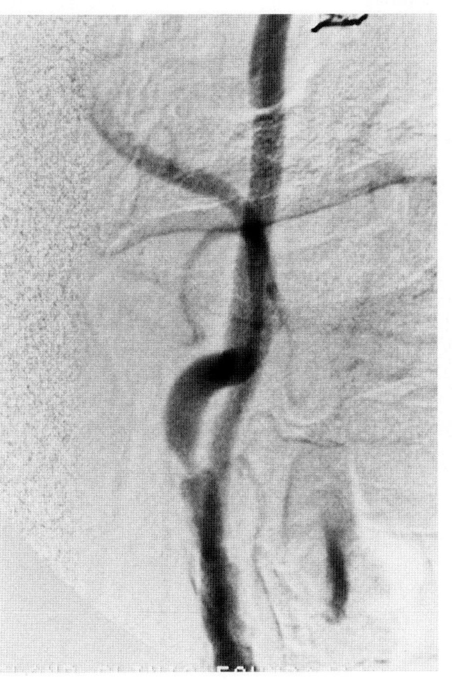
F

**Right anterior oblique (D) view and lateral view (E) from the conventional angiogram shows a large, calcified plaque around the bifurcation but no severe stenosis. Because of the information gained by MRA, additional conventional angiographic views were performed before the severe ribbon stenosis of the internal carotid artery was defined on an anteroposterior view with cephalocaudad angulation (F).**

In this instance, the information from the MRA (even though incorrectly positioned) altered the course of the conventional angiogram to more fully characterize the stenosis by obtaining additional views when the initial conventional angiogram images did not match the MRA information.

## CASE 175
## BILATERAL CAROTID STENOSES

**History:** 70-year-old being evaluated for carotid disease before cardiac bypass.

**Technique:** axial volume, three-dimensional time-of-flight, 39/7/25, 256 × 160 (rectangular field of view), 64 slices, 80-mm slab, 25-cm field of view, 6:42.

A

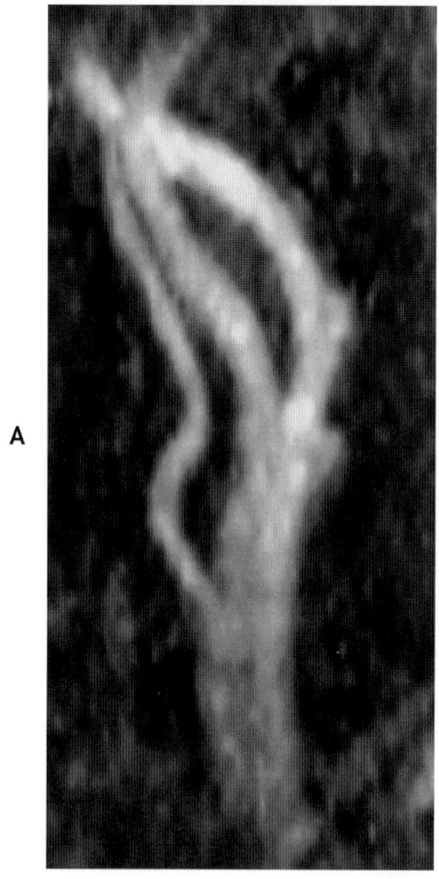

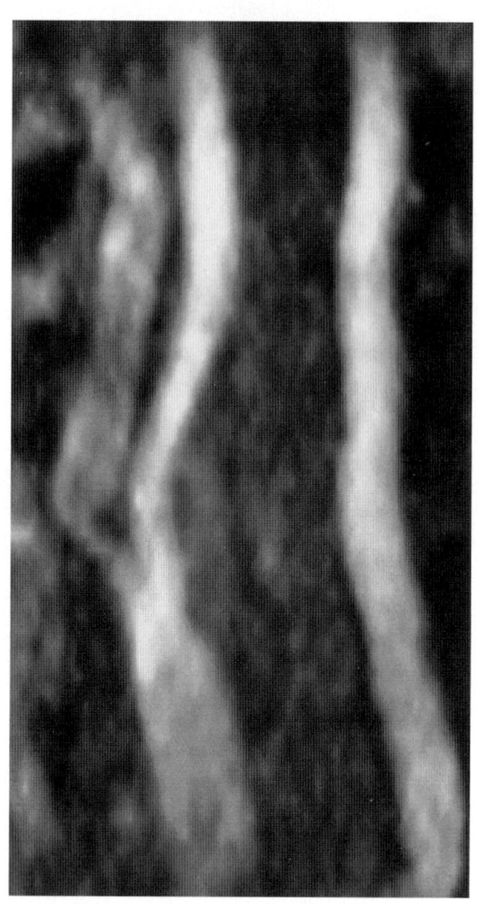

B

C

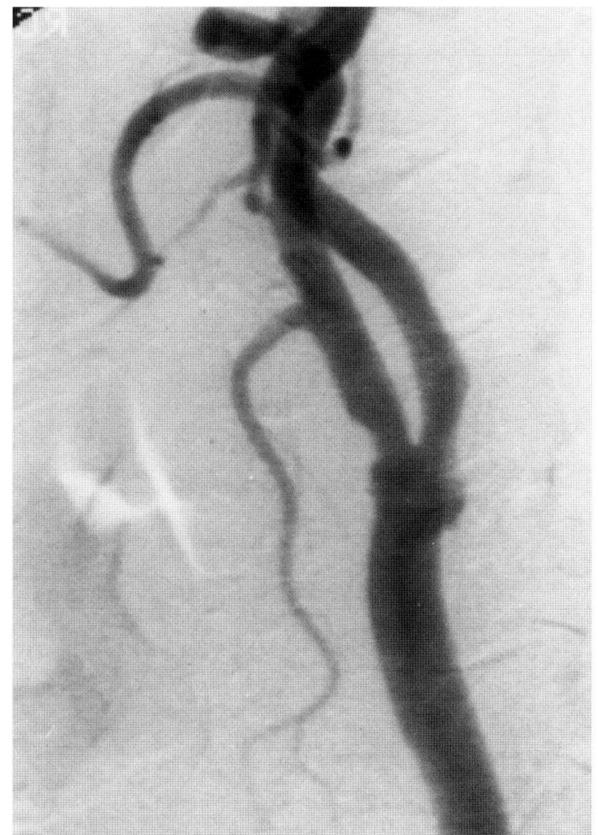

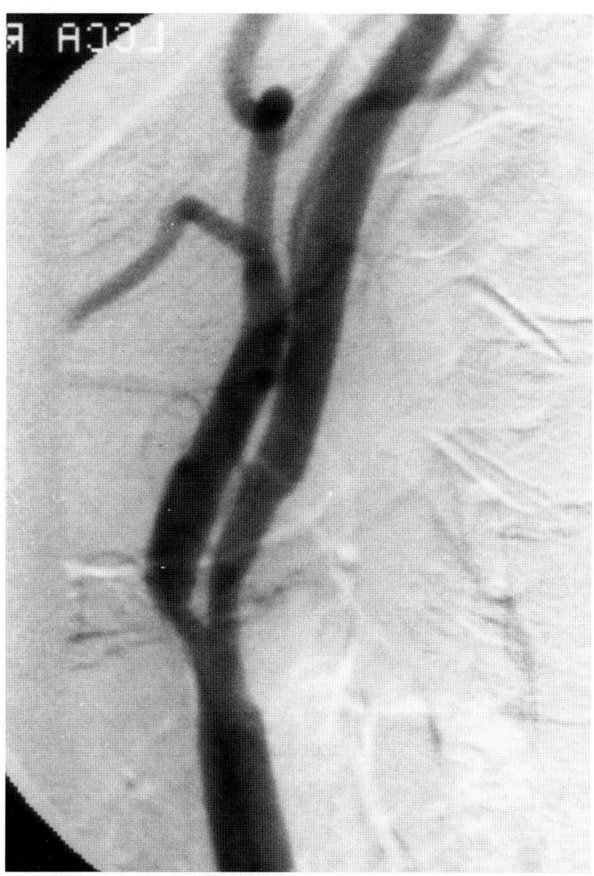

D

**Lateral views of the right and left carotid bifurcation maximum intensity projection (A and B) demonstrate moderate stenosis involving the origin of the left and right internal carotid arteries. There is good reproduction of the irregularity of the posterior wall of the left internal carotid artery. There are mild stenoses of the external carotid arteries bilaterally. The findings are confirmed on the conventional angiographic views (C and D) of the carotid bifurcations, again demonstrating the moderate internal carotid stenoses.**

# CASE 176
# CAROTID STENOSES

**History:** right hemispheric transient ischemic attacks.

**Technique:** axial volume, three-dimensional time-of-flight, 40/7/25, 256 × 256, 64 slices, 80-mm slab, 23-cm field of view, 10:57.

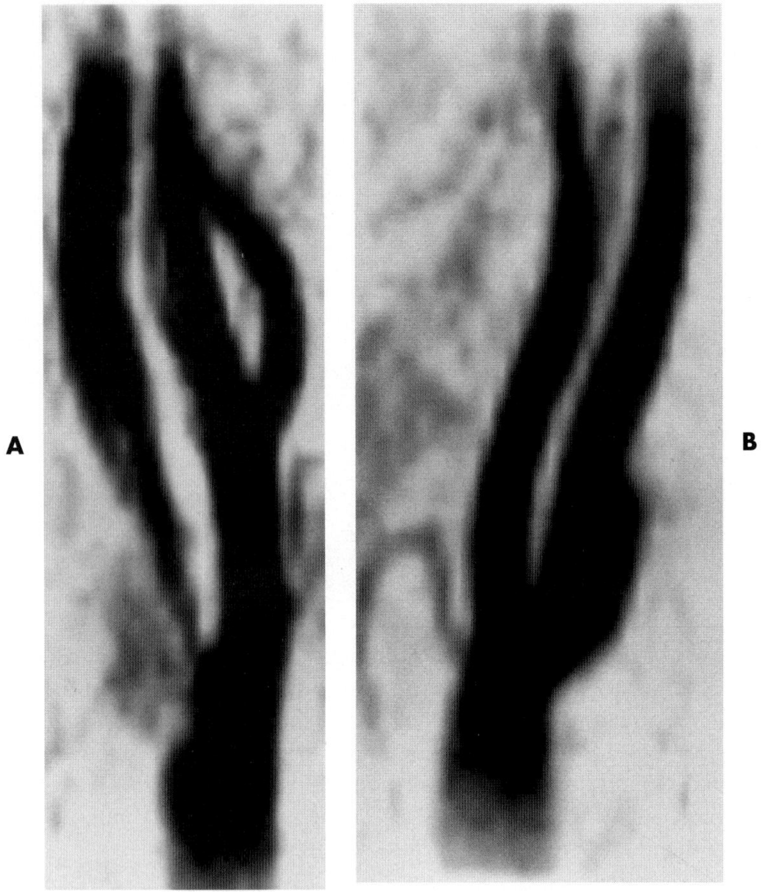

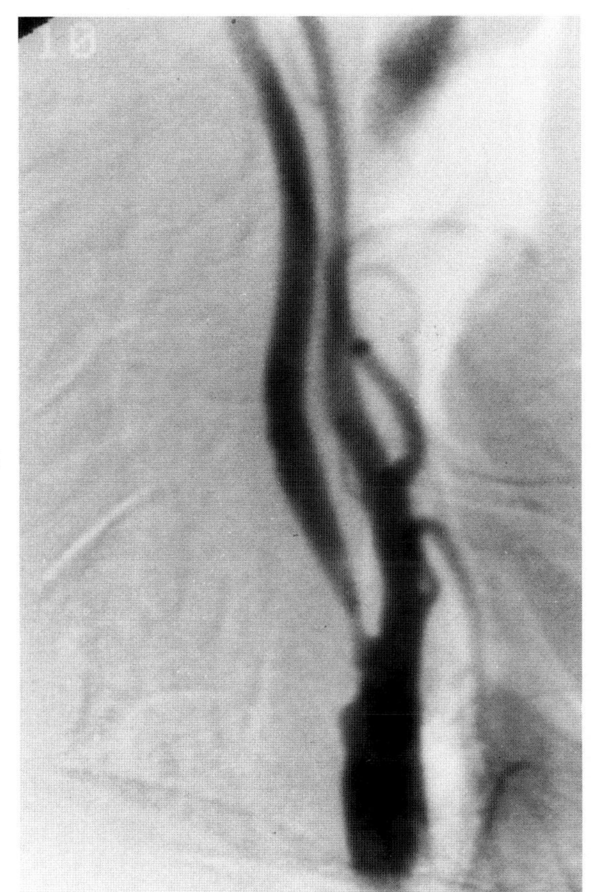
C

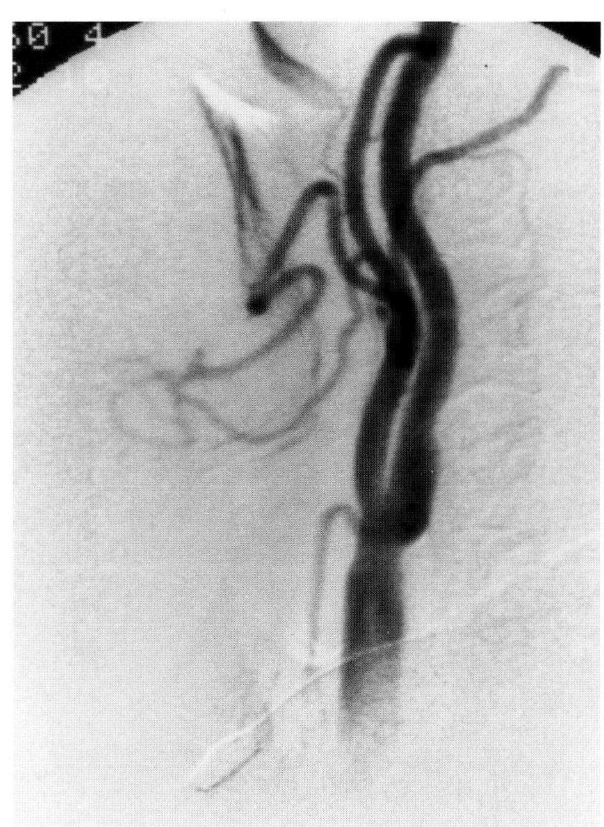
D

**Lateral maximum intensity projection view of the left carotid bifurcation (A) demonstrates a mild stenosis involving the origin of the left internal carotid artery, with widely patent distal common carotid and external carotid arteries. The MRA of the right bifurcation (B) shows a severe stenosis involving the origin of the internal carotid artery. There is a widely patent external carotid artery. The findings are confirmed on the conventional angiographic views of the left (C) and right (D) carotid bifurcations, again demonstrating the mild and severe stenoses.**

In this example, despite the severe stenosis at the origin, which would produce acceleration of blood flow and higher-order motion through it, there continues to be good correlation in the depiction of the stenosis with the conventional angiogram.

Masaryk et al reviewed and quantitatively compared three dimensional time of flight MRAs (three dimensional Fourier transform time-of-flight MRAs) in 38 patients initially studied by intraarterial digital subtraction angiography for suspected arteriosclerotic disease of the carotid bifurcation. A total of 75 vessels were studied by intraarterial angiography; MRAs were successfully obtained in 65 (87%). Intraarterial digital subtraction angiography and MRA studies were assessed for percent area stenosis by two independent observers on two separate occasions. Spearman-correlation and Wilcoxon-signed rank tests indicate consistency in interpretation for each observer as well as between observers. In addition, no significant difference was found between the two modalities in their ability to depict changes in percent area stenosis. Analysis of receiver operating characteristics indicated that technically adequate MRAs may act as a sensitive screening test for hemodynamically significant carotid stenoses. The authors conclude that motion-induced spin dephasing artifacts may not be a significant impediment to the clinical use of three-dimensional Fourier transform time-of-flight MRA for the evaluation of carotid arteriosclerotic disease.

## REFERENCES

Masaryk TJ, Modic MT, Ruggieri PM et al: Three-dimensional (volume) gradient-echo imaging of the carotid bifurcation: preliminary clinical experience, *Radiology* 171:801-806, 1989.

Masaryk AM, Ross JS, DiCello M et al: 3DFT magnetic resonance angiography of the carotid bifurcation: potential and limitations as a screening examination, *Radiology* 179:797-804, 1991.

# CASE 177
# BILATERAL SEVERE CAROTID STENOSIS

**History:** 71-year-old with right hemispheric transient ischemic attacks.

**Technique:** coronal and sagittal volumes, 80/8/40, 256 × 128, 32 slices (sagittal) and 64 slices (coronal), 2-mm thick slices, 23-cm field of view, 5:28 and 11:00.

A

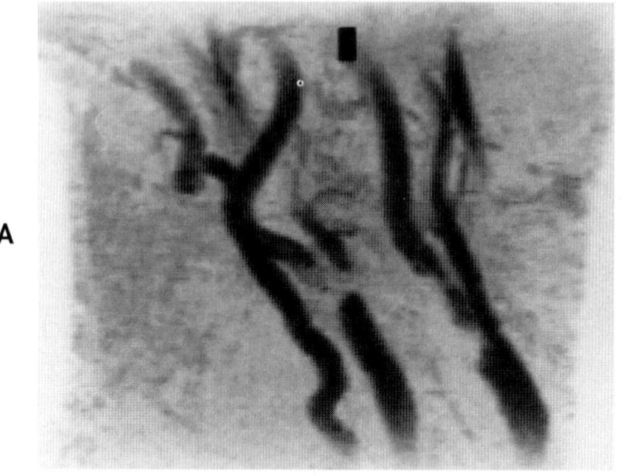

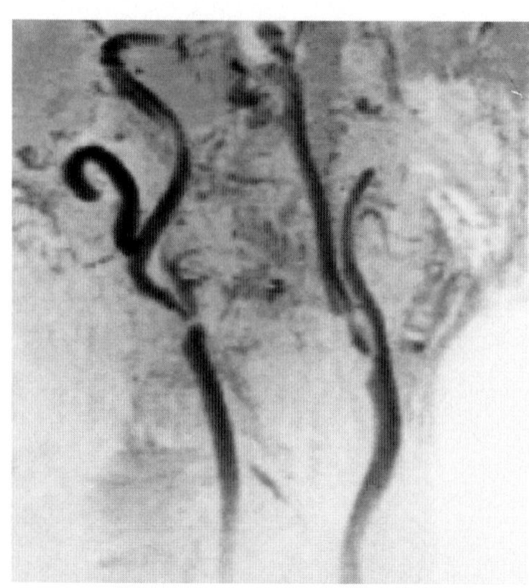

B

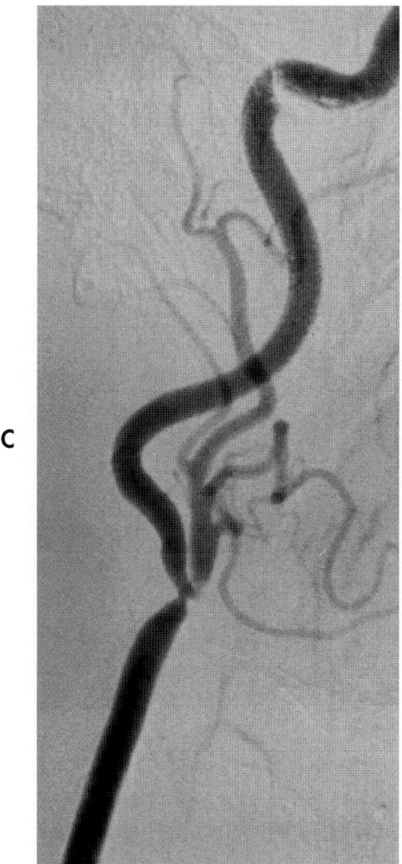


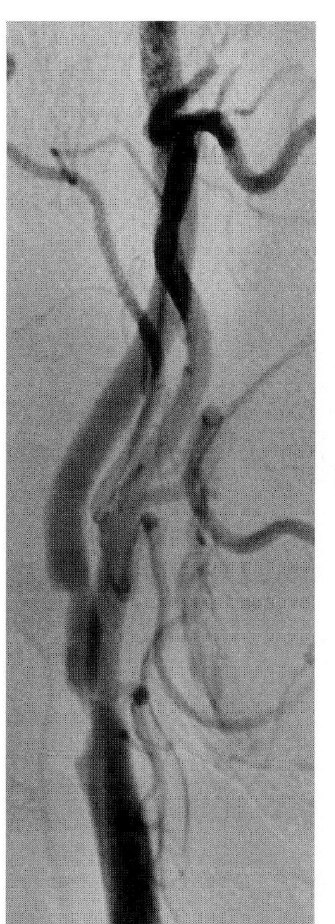


**Right anterior oblique views from a coronal volume acquisition (A) and dual sagittal slab three-dimensional acquisition (B) show a severe stenosis involving the right carotid bifurcation, which is manifested as a signal loss involving the distal common carotid as well as the proximal internal and external carotid arteries. On the left, there is a longer segment of irregular severe stenosis involving the internal carotid artery. These findings are confirmed on the lateral views from the conventional intraarterial angiograms, with the severe stenosis involving the bifurcation on the right (C) and the moderate, complex stenosis involving the bifurcation on the left (D).**

There is slightly improved signal involving the left bifurcation on the coronal acquisition, which may relate to slightly improved time-of-flight effects resulting from the tilt of the carotid bifurcations in regard to the coronal volume. That is, with the coronal acquisition, the carotid bifurcations are angled in a slightly more anterior-to-posterior direction and are thus more perpendicular to the direction of flow (better flow-related enhancement) than is achieved with a sagittally oriented volume.

## CASE 178
## SEVERE CAROTID STENOSIS WITH STRING SIGN

**History:** 69-year-old with left hemispheric transient ischemic attacks.

**Technique:** axial volume, three-dimensional time-of-flight, 41/6/20, 128 × 256 (rectangular field of view), 64 slices, 64-mm slab, 25-cm field of view, 11:14.

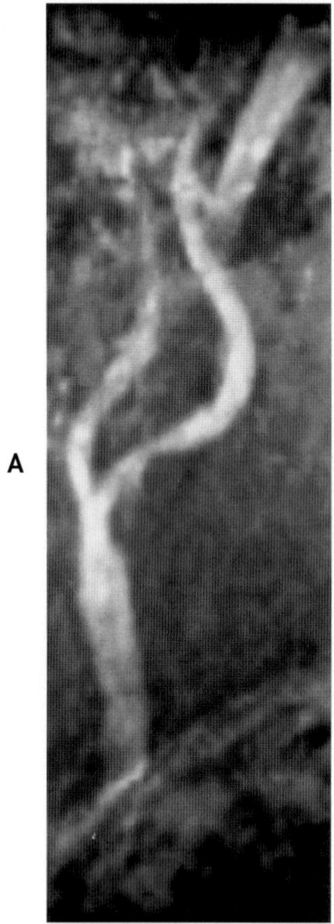

A

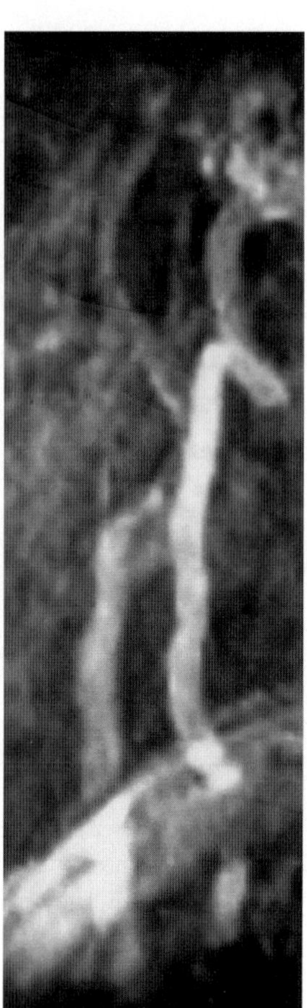

B

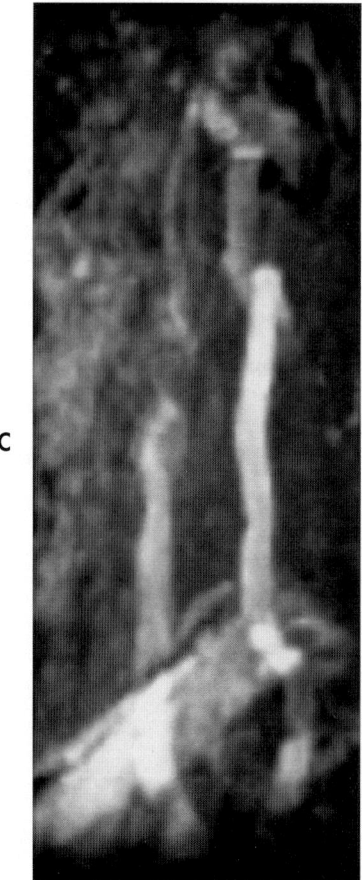

C

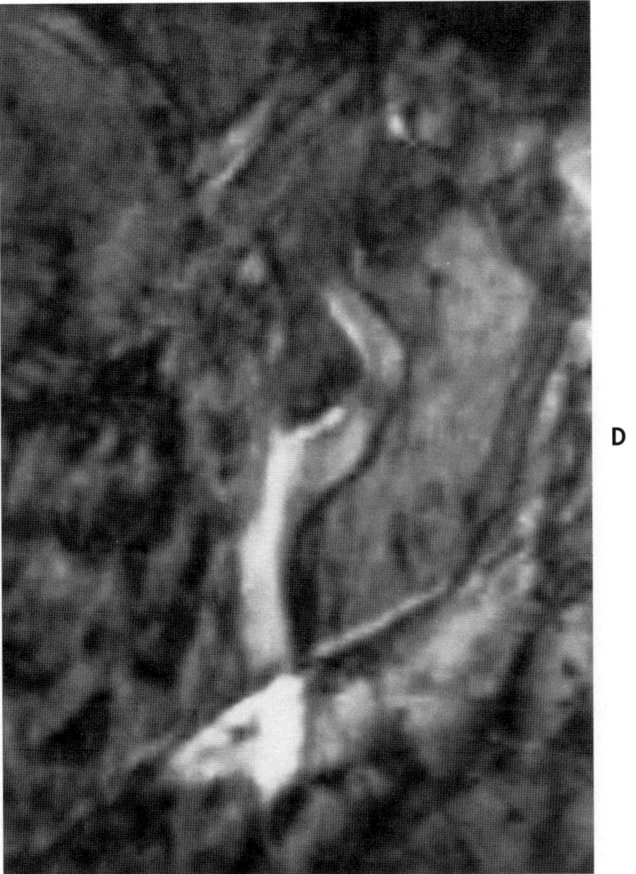


**Lateral maximum intensity projection view of the right carotid bifurcation (A) demonstrates a moderate long-segment stenosis involving the distal common carotid and right internal carotid arteries. Lateral (B) and oblique (C) maximum intensity projection views of the left bifurcation shows a long segment of severe stenosis, with loss of signal intensity involving the distal portion of the internal carotid artery. Sagittal multiplanar reformat of the angiographic data (D) demonstrates a stringlike region of high signal intensity along the anterior wall of the internal carotid artery, which represents patent lumenal flow (a string sign). The remainder of the posterior margin of the carotid relates to the thickened arterial wall or thrombus.**

The loss of signal intensity involving the distal portion of the carotid relates to very slow flow, with flow saturation on the three-dimensional time-of-flight study. This patient had ultrasound correlation, which also demonstrated a severe stenosis on the left (greater than 95%). The patient then underwent left carotid endarterectomy, during which confirmation of the severe left carotid stenosis occurred. Conventional angiography was not performed because of poor renal function.

Evaluation of the individual slices and reformatting the data for coronal or sagittal images can be as essential for evaluation of the carotid bifurcation as it is with evaluation of intracranial pathology.

## CASE 179
## BILATERAL SEVERE STENOSES WITH MULTIPLANAR REFORMATS

**History:** 70-year-old with multiple infarcts.

**Technique:** axial volume; three-dimensional time-of-flight; 30/6/25; 96 × 256 (rectangular field of view); 128 slices; 128-mm slab; 25-cm field of view; tilted, optimized nonsaturating excitation pulse; 6:11.

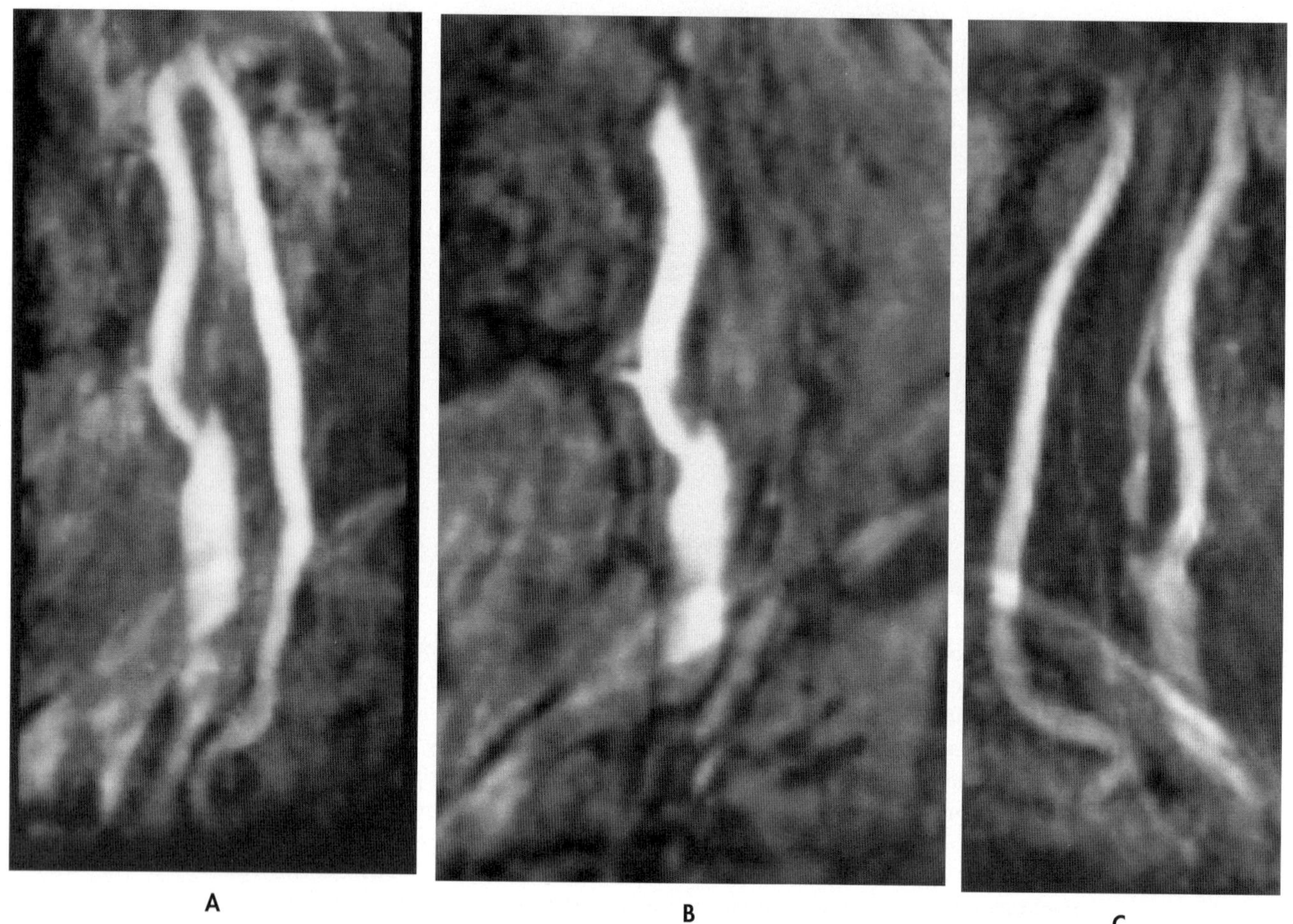

A B C

D

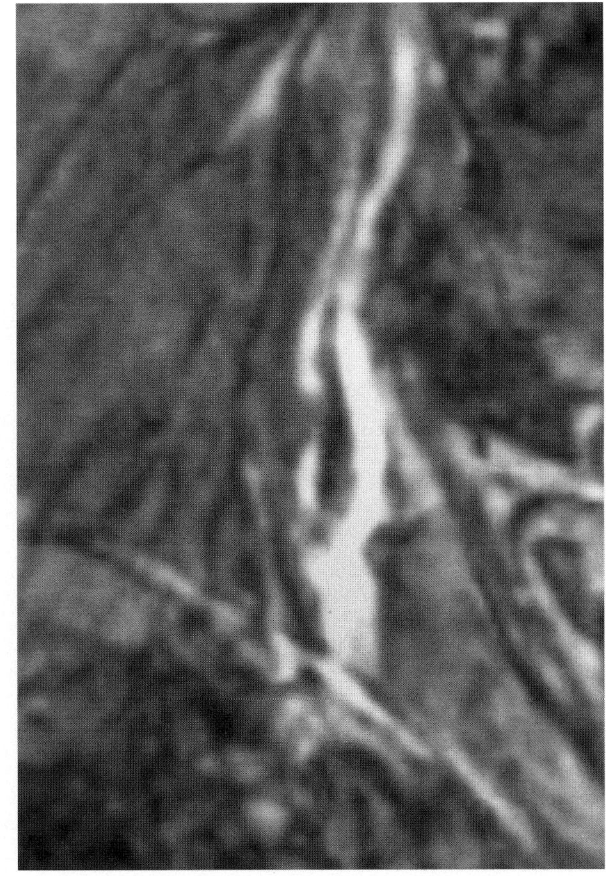

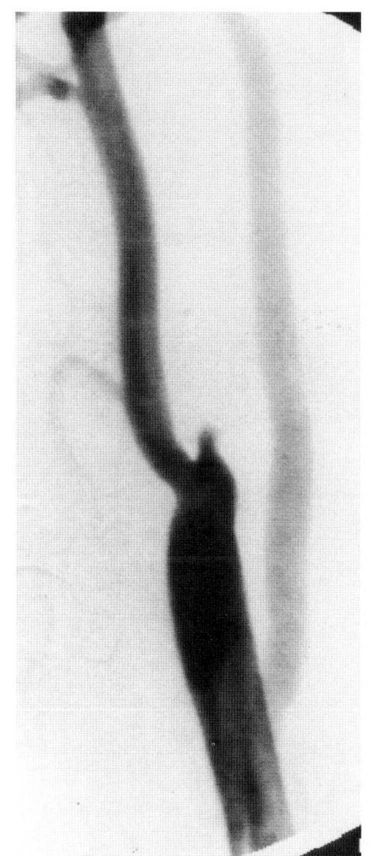

E

Lateral maximum intensity projection view of the right carotid bifurcation (A) demonstrates occlusion of the right internal carotid artery, with mild narrowing involving the external carotid artery. The visualized portion of the vertebral artery is patent. Multiplanar reformat in the sagittal plane off the axial angiographic volume (B) confirms the occlusion of the internal carotid artery. Lateral maximum intensity projection view of the left bifurcation (C) shows a focal area of very severe stenosis at the origin of the internal carotid artery and a small irregular internal carotid artery distal to this region. These findings indicate either a very severe focal stenosis involving the origin, with subsequent flow saturation distally of a more normal-appearing lumen, or irregularity involving the distal internal carotid, which is not easily identified on the MRA. Sagittal reformatting of the angiographic data on the left (D) also shows this severe focal stenosis at the origin and a very small string sign of the distal portion of the internal carotid artery. Conventional angiography confirms the findings on the MRA, with an occluded internal carotid artery on the right (E) and a severely stenotic left internal carotid artery (F).

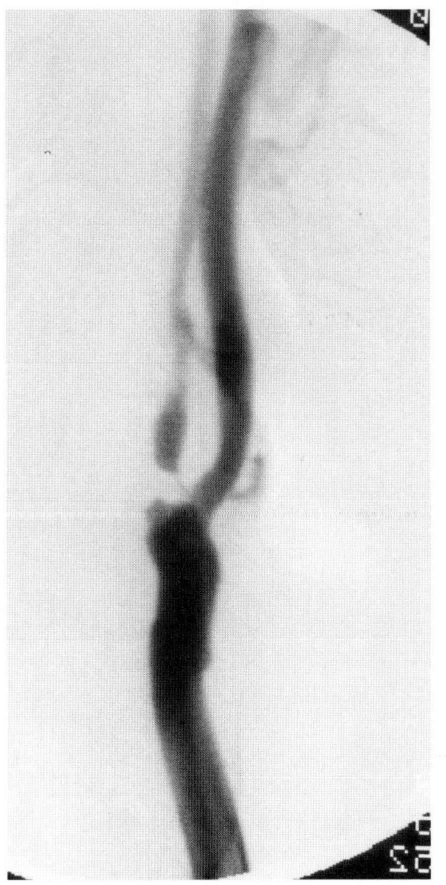

F

## CASE 180
## SEVERE RIGHT CAROTID BIFURCATION STENOSIS AND MODERATE LEFT STENOSIS

**History:** 76-year-old with carotid bruit.

**Technique:** axial two-dimensional time-of-flight, spoiled gradient acquisition in steady-state, 45/8.7/60, 256 × 128, 64 slices, 1.5-mm thickness, 18-cm field of view, 6:27.

A

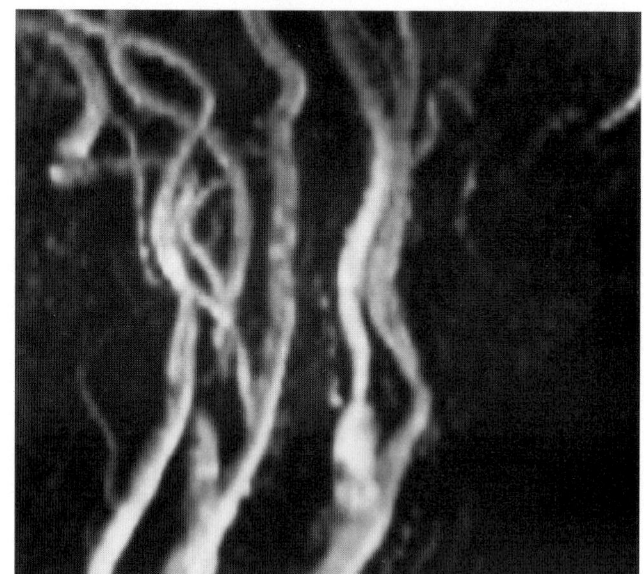

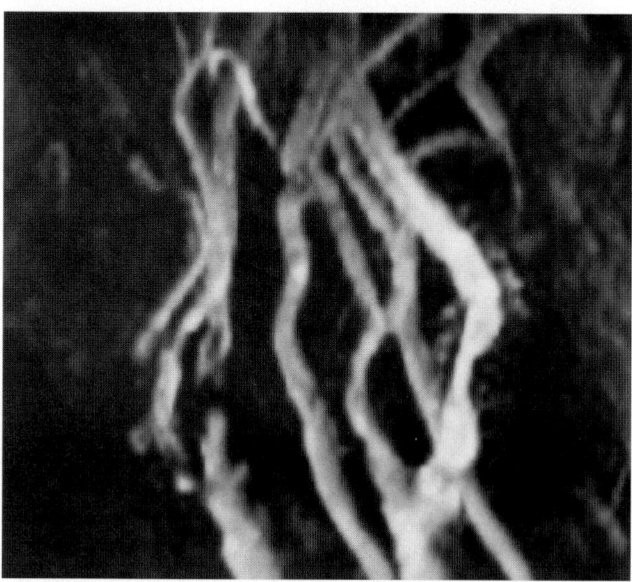

B

C

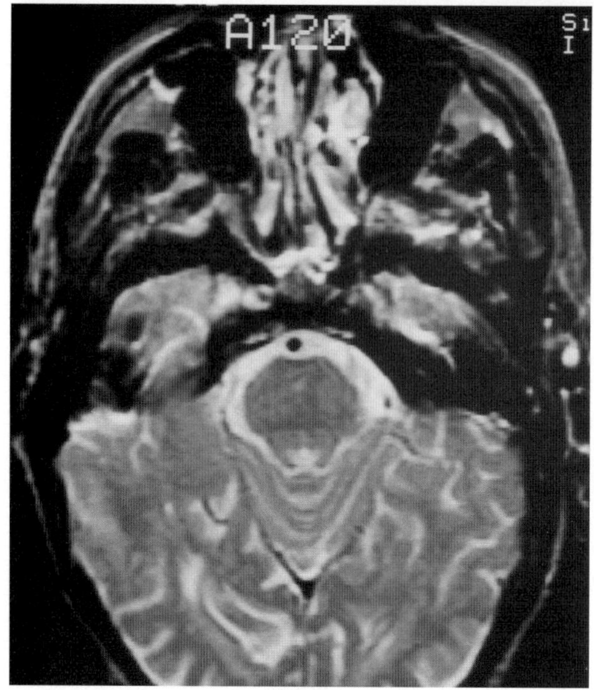


**Right (A) and left (B) anterior oblique views from a two-dimensional time-of-flight sequence show a severe stenosis involving the proximal right internal carotid artery, which is demonstrated as a signal loss in this region. However, good signal intensity is maintained throughout the remainder of the left internal carotid artery. This finding would be consistent with a greater than 70% stenosis of the right internal carotid artery on the two-dimensional time-of-flight study. On the left, there is a moderate complex stenosis involving the proximal internal carotid artery. The nonspecificity of the signal intensity changes within the carotid siphon are evidenced in this case, since the T2-weighted study of the head shows abnormal increased signal intensity on the right (C). This is occurring with slow flow, and does not necessarily indicate occlusion, since the carotid artery is patent on the two-dimensional time-of-flight study.**

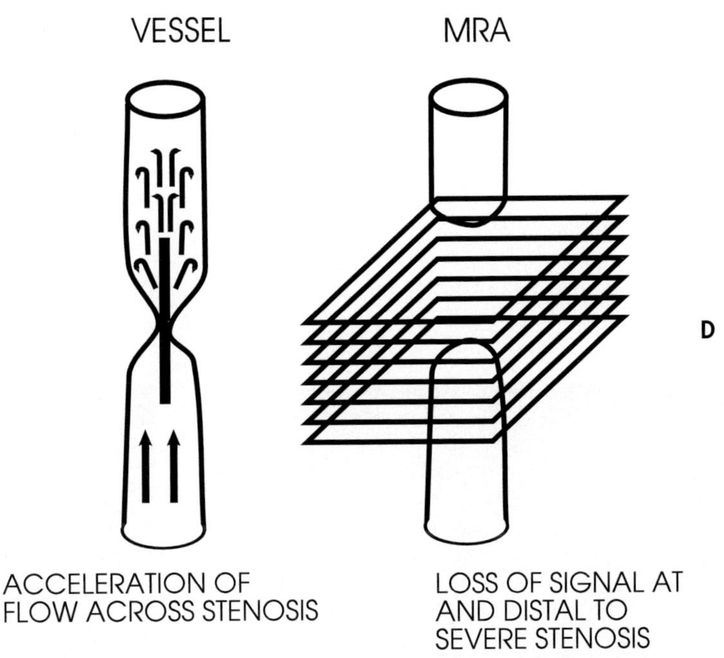


**D, With a stenoses, there must be acceleration of blood flow at the stenosis to maintain overall blood flow. Distal to the stenosis, chaotic flow can occur with vortices and reversed flow. The acceleration of flow and complex flow seen distal to the stenosis may be manifested as signal loss on MRA. Two-dimensional time-of-flight MRA is, in general, more sensitive to this type of signal loss than three-dimensional time-of-flight MRA.**

Huston et al evaluated two-dimensional time-of-flight MRA of the carotid bifurcation to color duplex flow ultrasound in 50 patients, using the guidelines of NASCET for measuring the stenosis. They noted that a signal void on the maximum intensity projection images corresponded to a 70% or greater stenosis (see diagram). They found that the accuracy of two-dimensional time-of-flight MRA was equal to that of ultrasound in characterizing the degree of stenosis (similar receiver operating characteristic curves).

Anson et al evaluated two-dimensional time-of-flight MRA in 20 patients and compared it with conventional angiography and surgery. Conventional angiography and MRA were highly correlated, particularly with respect to severe stenosis and occlusion. Significantly, there were no false-negative studies that missed surgical lesions. They came to conclusions similar to those of Huston et al, in that surgically significant stenoses (70%) appear as areas of signal void at the stenosis, with reappearance of signal more distally in the internal carotid artery. Failure to visualize the distal internal carotid artery indicates vessel occlusion.

#### REFERENCES

Polak JR, Bajakian RL, O'Leary KD et al: Detection of internal carotid artery stenosis: comparison of MR angiography, color Doppler sonography, and arteriography, *Radiology* 182:35-40, 1992.

Huston J, Lewis BD, Wiebers DO et al: Carotid artery: prospective blinded comparison of two dimensional time of flight MR angiography with conventional angiography and duplex US, *Radiology* 186(3):339-344, 1993.

Anson JA, Heiserman JE, Drayer BP, Spetzler RF: Surgical decisions on the basis of magnetic resonance angiography of the carotid arteries, *Neurosurgery* 32(3):335-343, 1993.

## CASE 181
## SEVERE LEFT CAROTID BIFURCATION STENOSIS WITH DECREASED INTRACRANIAL SIGNAL AND INTRALUMINAL THROMBUS

**History:** 77-year-old with left hemispheric transient ischemic attacks.

**Technique #1:** carotid, 34/6/20, 256 × 128, 128 slices, 25-cm field of view (rectangular), 9:19.

**Technique #2:** intracranial, 45/7/20, 256 × 256, 64 slices, 60-mm slab, magnetization transfer background suppression, 14-cm field of view, 12:20.

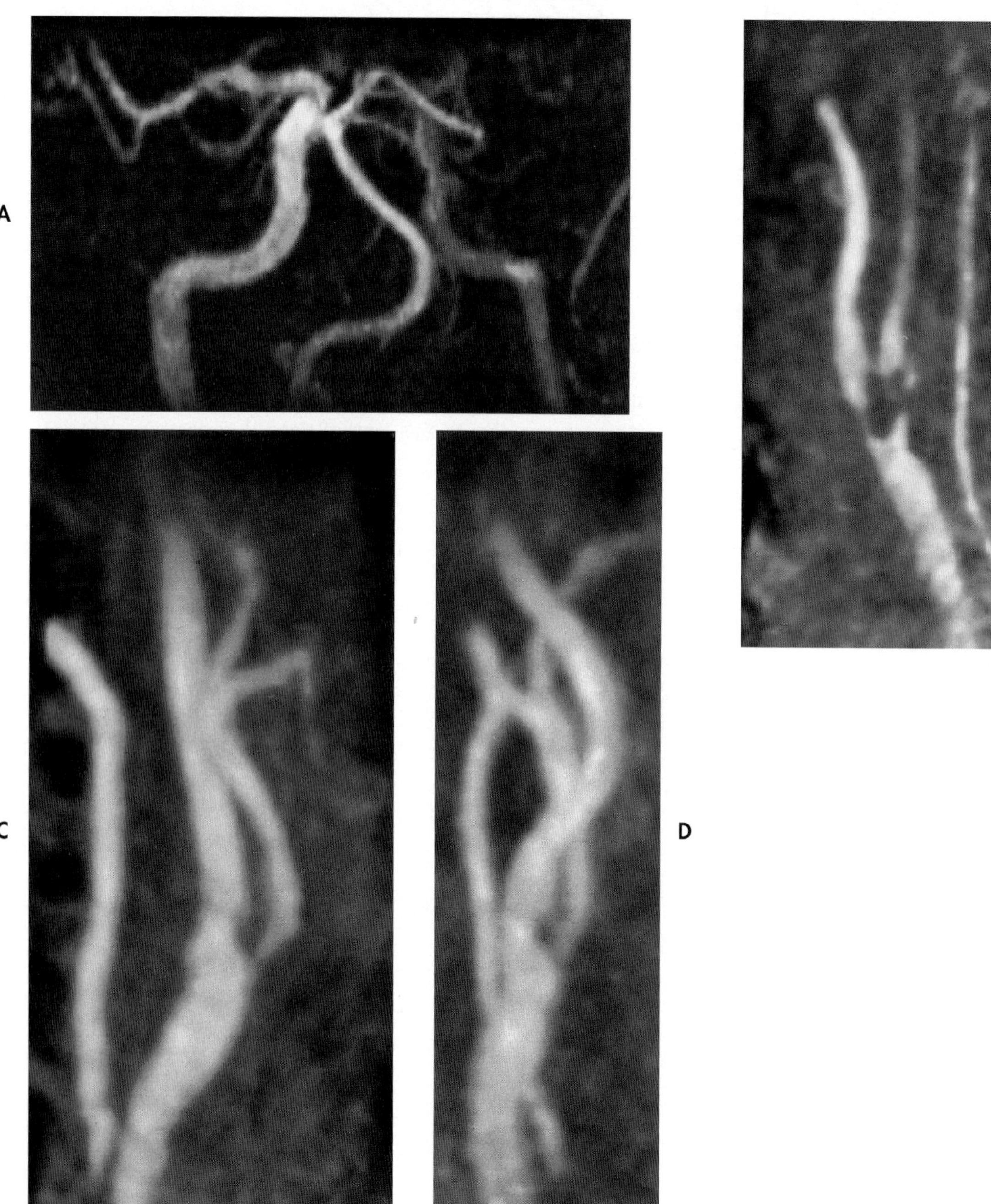

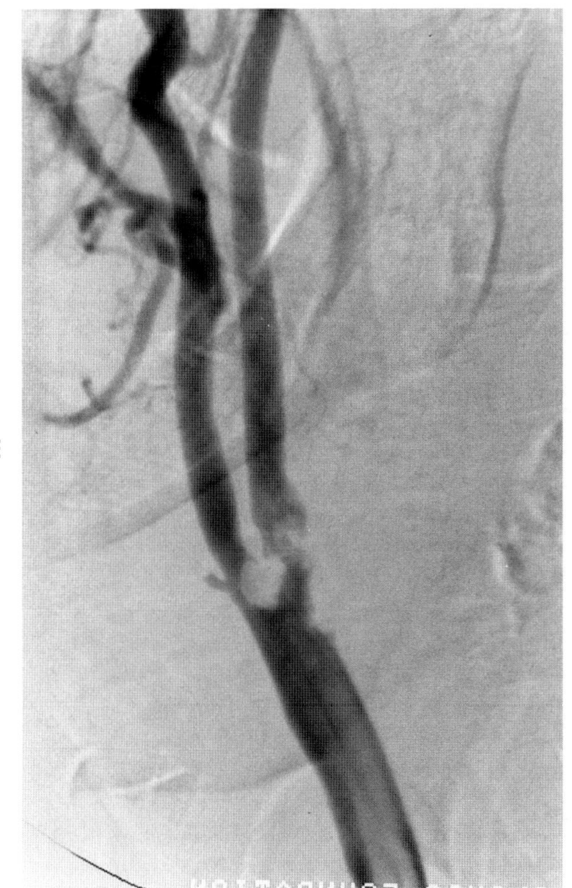

E

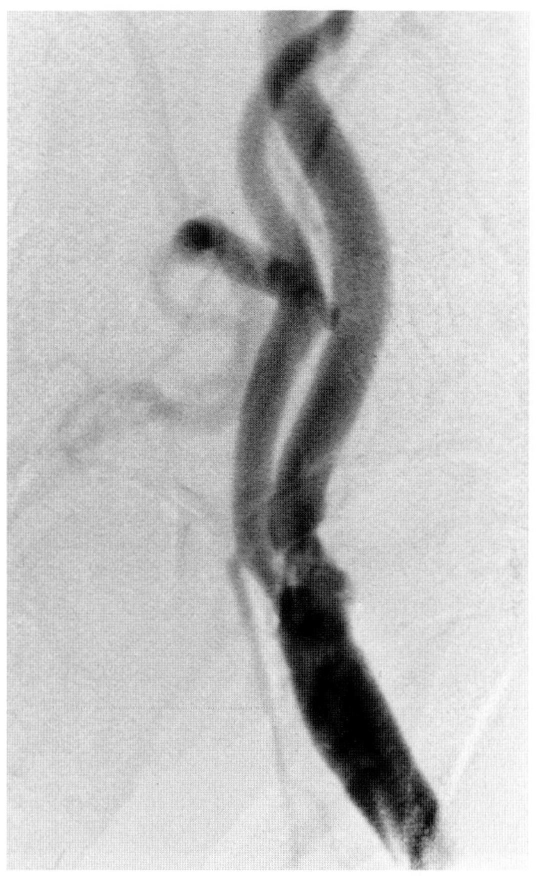

F

**Anteroposterior view of the intracranial circulation (A) demonstrates a marked decrease in diffuse signal throughout the left internal carotid distribution, which would be highly suspicious for a severe stenosis at the carotid bifurcation. Lateral view from a maximum intensity projection of the left carotid bifurcation (B) demonstrates a very severe stenosis involving the origin of the internal carotid artery, with loss of signal within the internal carotid artery distally because of slow flow. There is also a severe stenosis involving the origin of the external carotid artery. Lateral maximum intensity projection view of the right (C) shows a mild stenosis involving the origin of the internal carotid artery, with a line of low signal intensity extending throughout the carotid, which may reflect a shelflike plaque. This stenosis is confirmed on the additional oblique projection (D) showing a moderate stenosis.**

Comparison with conventional angiography of the left **(E)** and right bifurcations **(F)** confirms the severe stenosis involving the origin of the left internal and external carotid arteries. However, the conventional angiogram gives more convincing evidence of the complex irregularity of the stenosis, which the MRA does not convey. The smooth filling defect extending inferiorly from the crotch of the bifurcation is highly suspicious for intraluminal thrombus, which was not conveyed on the MRA images. This finding has an obvious dramatic clinical impact on the workup, since the patient's blood will be anticoagulated and the patient will be taken rapidly to surgery to prevent distal embolization of the thrombus. On the right side, there is confirmation of this moderate stenosis with a shelflike plaque involving the origin of the internal carotid.

## CASE 182
## ANEURYSMALLY DILATED ENDARTERECTOMY PATCH GRAFT

**History:** 77-year-old after endarterectomy.

**Technique:** axial two-dimensional time-of-flight, spoiled gradient acquisition in steady-state, 45/8.7/60, 256 × 128, 64 slices, 1.5-mm thickness, 18-cm field of view, 6:27.

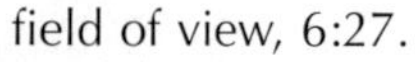

A 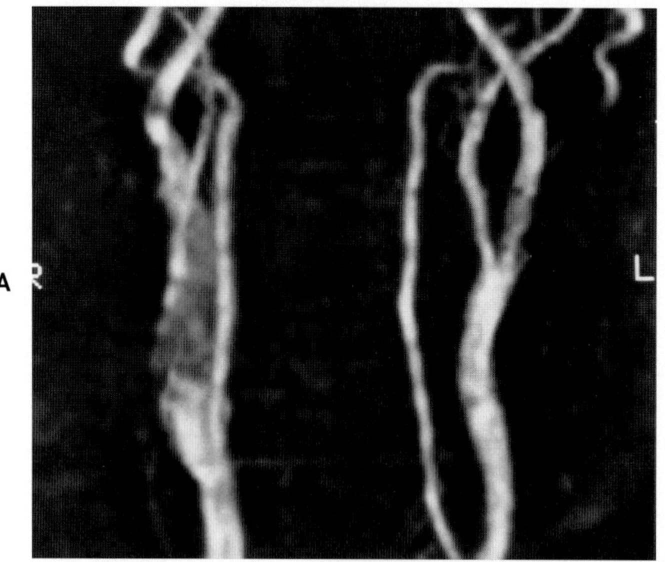


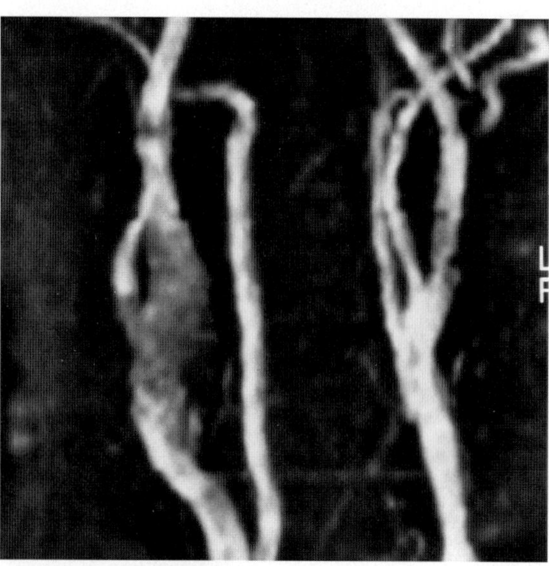 B


C 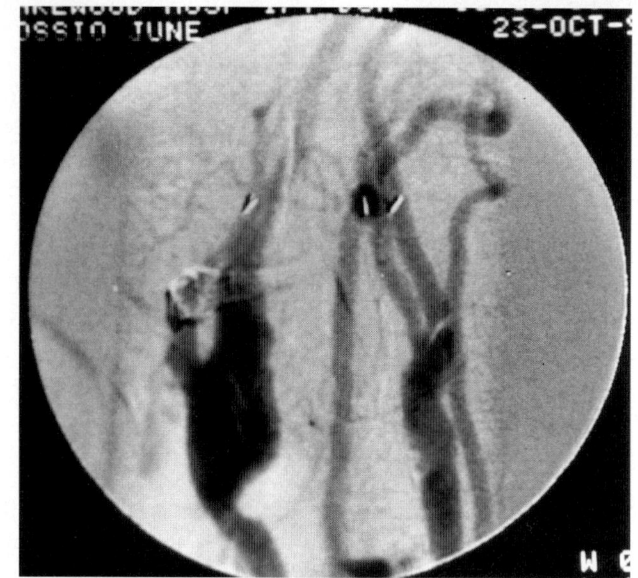

**Anteroposterior (A) and left anterior oblique (B) maximum intensity projection views of the two-dimensional time-of-flight MRA show a mild stenosis of the origin of the left internal carotid artery. The distal right common carotid artery and the proximal internal carotid artery appear dilated and have decreased signal intensity. There is a relatively narrowed portion along the posterior wall of the internal carotid artery. Oblique view of an intravenous digital subtraction angiographic study (C) shows marked dilatation of the right carotid bifurcation at the patch graft site. The area of narrowing on the MRA is not present on the intravenous digital subtraction angiographic study and represents a false-positive area of narrowing because of dephasing related to slowed and/or complex flow.**

# CHAPTER 10

# Dissection

Spontaneous hemorrhagic dissection of the internal carotid artery is a cause of transient ischemic attack or stroke in relatively young patients and may be the cause for up to 2% of all strokes. The diagnosis of dissection has been based on conventional intraarterial angiography, which demonstrates a long, tapered, and eccentric narrowing of the cervical internal carotid artery (the string sign or "rat-tail"), often beginning 3 to 4 cm beyond the origin and extending to the base of the skull.[1-6] The petrous bone tends to limit further extension of the dissection cephalad. An additional type of angiographic finding is a short, irregular arterial segment with a variable degree of narrowing in the upper cervical region. Both of these findings are characteristic but not completely specific.

The cause of hemorrhagic dissection is unknown. Associations with dissection include hypertension, fibromuscular dysplasia, oral contraceptive use, trauma, atherosclerosis, previous viral illness, and neck manipulation. Patients are typically in the second through fifth decades of life and have ischemic neurologic deficits, either transient ischemic attack or complete embolic stroke. This may be also associated with face, head, or neck pain or an incomplete Horner's syndrome or with a cervical bruit. Saccular pseudoaneurysms occurring as sequelae of the arterial dissection have been described and have a variable course. These pseudoaneurysms may remain unchanged, decrease in size, or even resolve over time. Rarely, these aneurysms enlarge, and there may be a delayed appearance of pseudoaneurysm formation in approximately 5% of cases. Petro et al[5] noted that the pseudoaneurysms in their series occurred with marked tortuosity or coiling of the cervical internal carotid artery, which is associated with the dissected vessels. They concluded that demonstration of an aneurysm-like outpouching of the arterial lumen on a coiled cervical carotid artery makes dissection highly likely. Treatment is generally by anticoagulation, the object of which is to minimize embolic events while the wall is healing.

MR imaging can demonstrate the patent vascular lumen and arterial wall noninvasively. Saturation pulses placed below the imaging area are useful in the spin-echo images to completely dephase the signal intensity in the patent arterial lumen to maximize the contrast of the hematoma within the arterial wall. If the examination is performed in the subacute phase, the clot will be methemoglobin and will show high signal intensity on T1-weighted images. The hyperintensity of fat surrounding the internal carotid artery can create difficulty in recognition of these high signal intensity hematomas. Therefore frequency-selective fat-saturated T1-weighted images are also useful. The typical appearance of dissection on conventional spin-echo imaging is a peripheral high signal intensity collar of intramural blood with a central flow void, which represents the patent lumen (which is generally smaller than on the opposite, normal side). Findings on MRA include segmental vessel narrowing, definition of the intimal flap, and outpouchings of pseudoaneurysms. Intramural blood can be seen on the maximum intensity projection views as a hazy collar surrounding the residual patent lumen signal. The combination of MR imaging and MRA is ideal for the evaluation of cervical dissections.[7-10] The intramural clot is best identified on the fat-saturated or regular T1-weighted axial views, which may also show the patent lumen. The MRA allows for better definition of the length of involvement, vessel narrowing, and pseudoaneurysms (Fig. 10-1). MR imaging and MRA also allow noninvasive follow-up after anticoagulant therapy has begun.

Pitfalls are mainly technique related. This would include poor or variable fat saturation on the T1-weighted spin-echo images resulting from susceptibility effects from the neck/air or chin/air interface or from dental amalgam or braces. In these cases, use of the routine axial T1-weighted images suffices. Use of an inferior saturation pulse is a must if all signal from flowing arterial blood is to be eliminated. This is necessary so that there is no confusion of entry-slice signal with that of intramural hematoma. A superior saturation pulse for venous saturation helps the image aesthetics but is not critical for diagnosis of dissection. If a time-of-flight technique is used, care must be taken where there is apparent occlusion of the vessel associated with dissection. Just as with atherosclerotic narrowing with slowed distal flow, there may be saturation of flow distal to a critical stenosis or distal turbulence with dephasing and a false-positive result for occlusion. In this case, referring to the

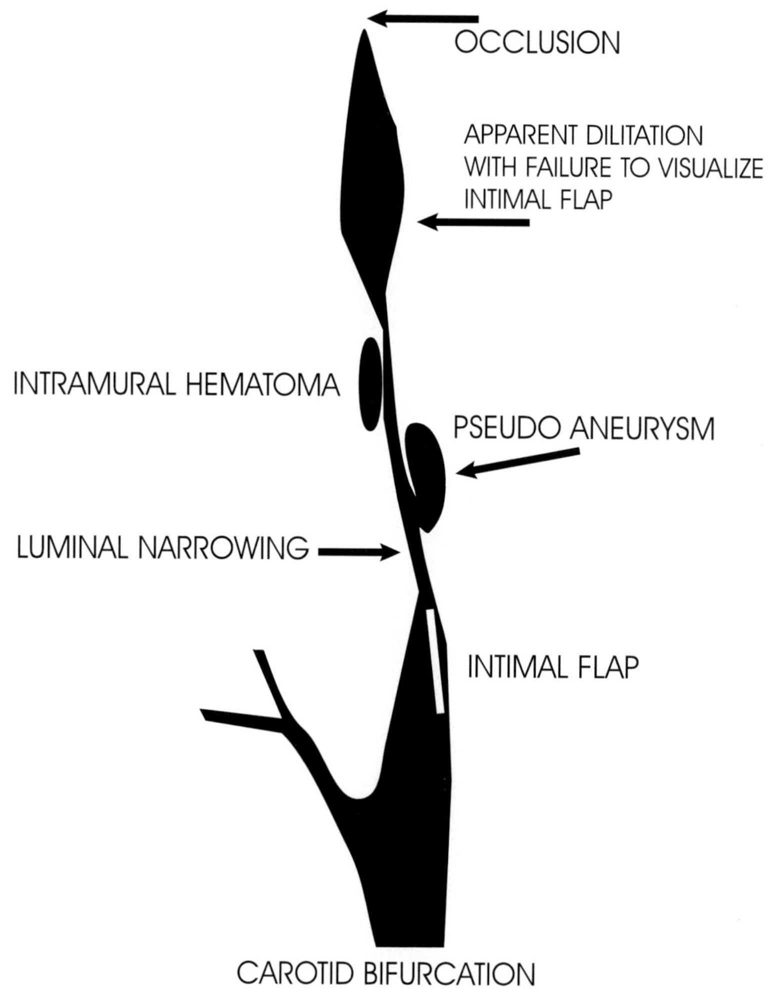


**Fig. 10-1** Schematic of different appearances of carotid dissection. Findings can vary from a classic rattail type of narrowing with occlusion to a very subtle intimal flap.

conventional T1-weighted images and looking for the central flow or using a phase-contrast technique with a low velocity encoding void may help confirm or refute the presence of occlusion. Susceptibility effects presumably related to the mastoid air cells and skull base may also cause a false lumenal narrowing at the junction of the cervical and petrous carotids, which must be distinguished from dissection.

## REFERENCES

1. Luken MG, Ascherl GF, Correll JW, Hilal SK: Spontaneous dissecting aneurysms of the extracranial internal carotid artery, *Clin Neurosurg* 26:353-375, 1979.
2. Houser OW, Mokri B, Sundt TM Jr et al: Spontaneous cervical cephalic arterial dissection and its residuum: angiographic spectrum, *AJNR* 5:27-34, 1984.
3. Mokri B, Sundt TM Jr, Houser OW: Spontaneous internal carotid dissection, hemicrania and Horner's syndrome, *Arch Neurol* 36:677-680, 1979.
4. Quisling RG, Friedman WA, Rhoton AL: High cervical carotid artery dissection: spontaneous resolution, *AJNR* 1:463-468, 1980.
5. Petro GR, Witwer GA, Cacayorin ED et al: Spontaneous dissection of the cervical intenal carotid artery: correlation of arteriography, CT, and pathology, *AJR* 148:393-398, 1987.
6. Biller J, Hingtgen W, Adams H et al: Cervicocephalic arterial dissections: a ten year experience, *Arch Neurol* 43:1234-1238, 1986.
7. Bui LN, Brant-Zawadzki M, Verghese P, Gillan G: Magnetic resonance angiography of cervicocranial dissection, *Stroke* 24(1):126-131, 1993.
8. Goldberg H, Grossman R, Gomori J et al: Cervical internal carotid artery dissecting hemorrhage: diagnosis using MRI, *Radiology* 158:157-161, 1986.
9. Gelbert F, Assouline E, Hodes J et al: MRI in spontaneous dissection of vertebral and carotid arteries, *Neuroradiology* 33:111-113, 1991.
10. Mann CI, Dietrich RB, Schrader MT et al: Posttraumatic carotid artery dissection in children: evaluation with MR angiography, *AJR* 160:134-136, 1993.

## CASE 183
## PITFALL: CAROTID OCCLUSION RELATED TO TUMOR EMBOLUS

**History:** 25-year-old with acute onset of right-sided hemiplegia with a clinical concern of carotid dissection.

**Technique #1:** carotid, axial two-dimensional time-of-flight, spoiled gradient acquisition in steady state, 45/8.7/60, 256 × 128, 64 slices, 1.5-mm thickness, 18-cm field-of-view, 6:27.

**Technique #2:** intracranial, axial volume, three-dimensional time-of-flight, 45/7/20, 256 × 128, 60 slices, 72-mm slab, 18-cm field-of-view, 6:09.

A

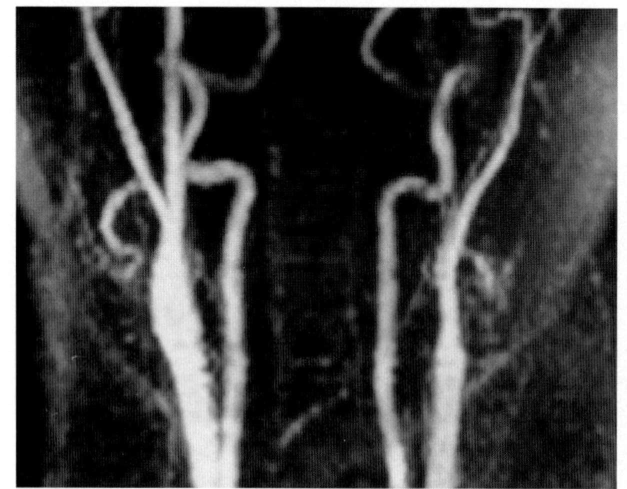

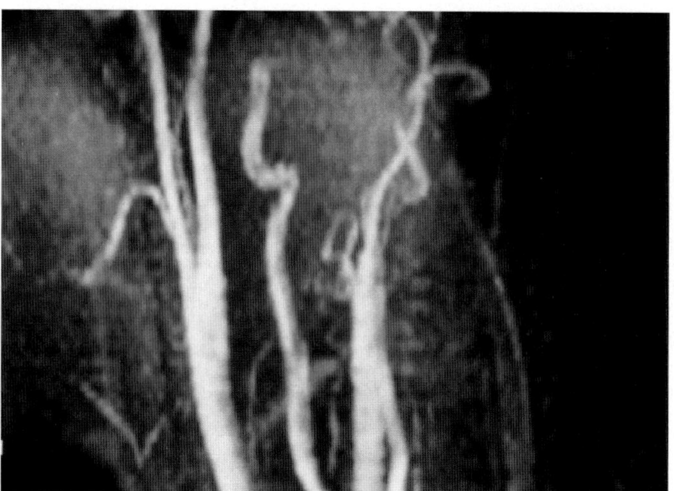

B

C

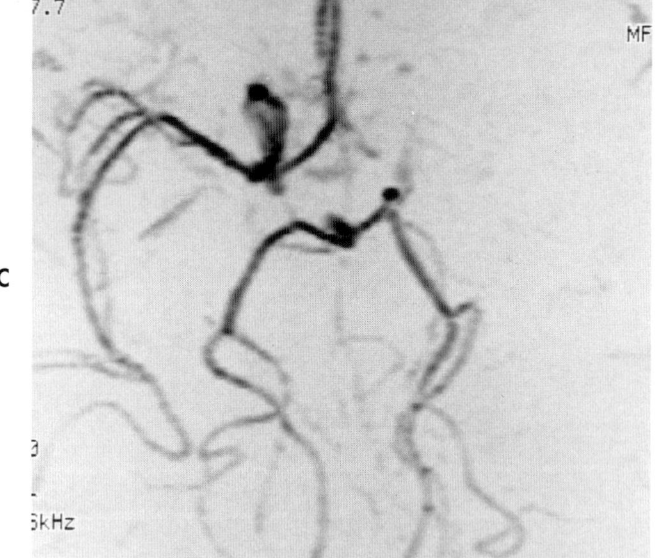

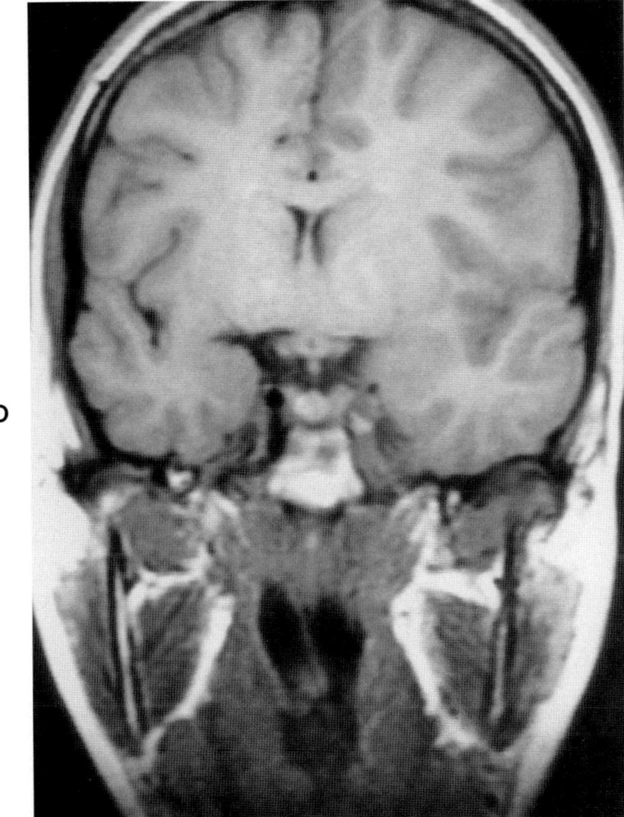


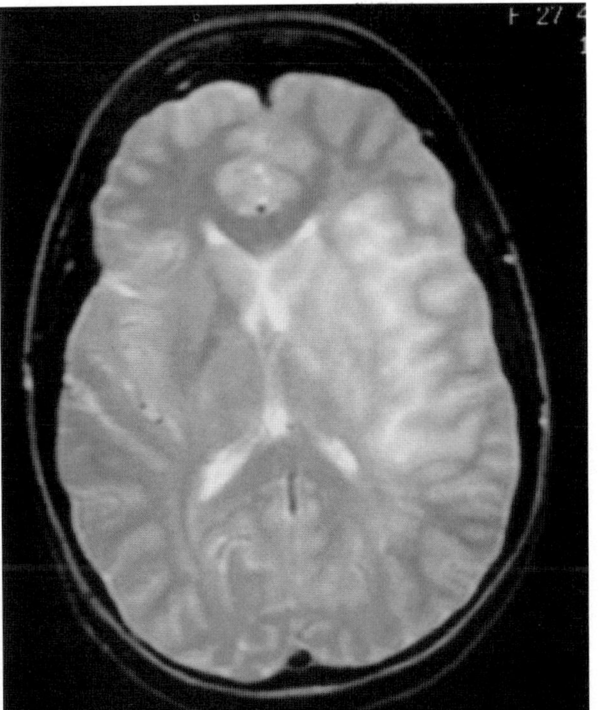


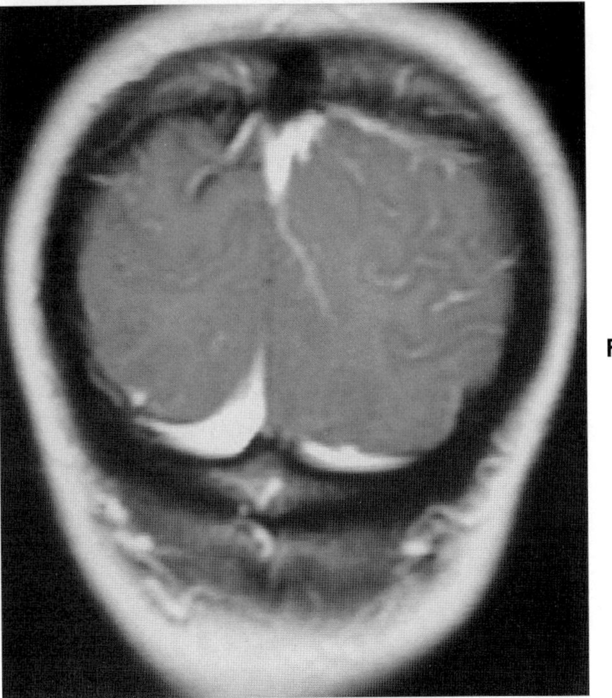


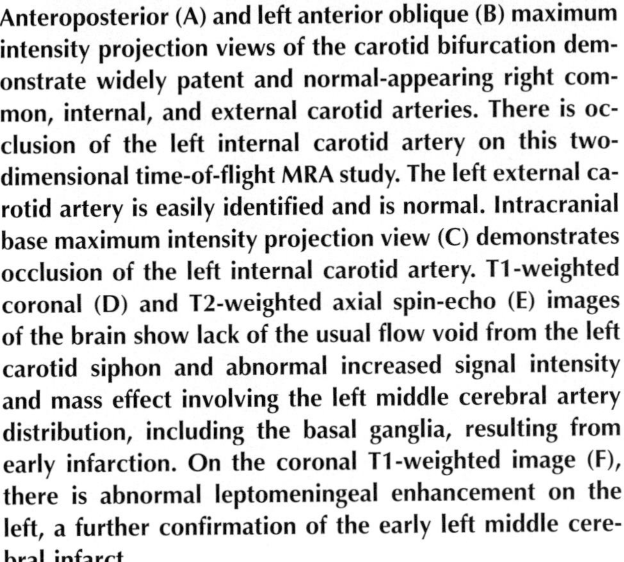
**Anteroposterior (A) and left anterior oblique (B) maximum intensity projection views of the carotid bifurcation demonstrate widely patent and normal-appearing right common, internal, and external carotid arteries. There is occlusion of the left internal carotid artery on this two-dimensional time-of-flight MRA study. The left external carotid artery is easily identified and is normal. Intracranial base maximum intensity projection view (C) demonstrates occlusion of the left internal carotid artery. T1-weighted coronal (D) and T2-weighted axial spin-echo (E) images of the brain show lack of the usual flow void from the left carotid siphon and abnormal increased signal intensity and mass effect involving the left middle cerebral artery distribution, including the basal ganglia, resulting from early infarction. On the coronal T1-weighted image (F), there is abnormal leptomeningeal enhancement on the left, a further confirmation of the early left middle cerebral infarct.**

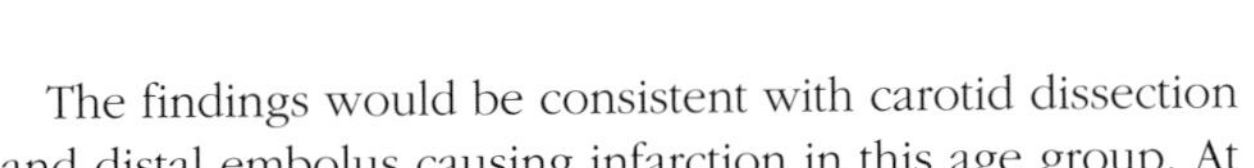

The findings would be consistent with carotid dissection and distal embolus causing infarction in this age group. At surgery, the carotid artery was occluded because of an embolus from a left atrial myxoma.

## CASE 184
## LEFT CAROTID DISSECTION

**History:** 57-year-old with new onset of Horner's syndrome and neck pain.

**Technique:** sagittal volume, three-dimensional time-of-flight, 50/7/20, 256 × 256, 64 slices, 60-mm slab, 20-cm field of view, 13:41.

A

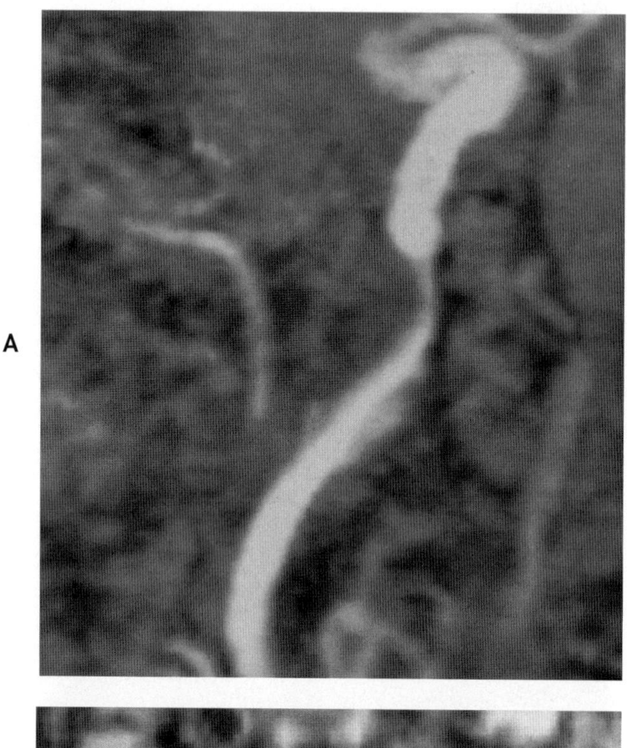

C

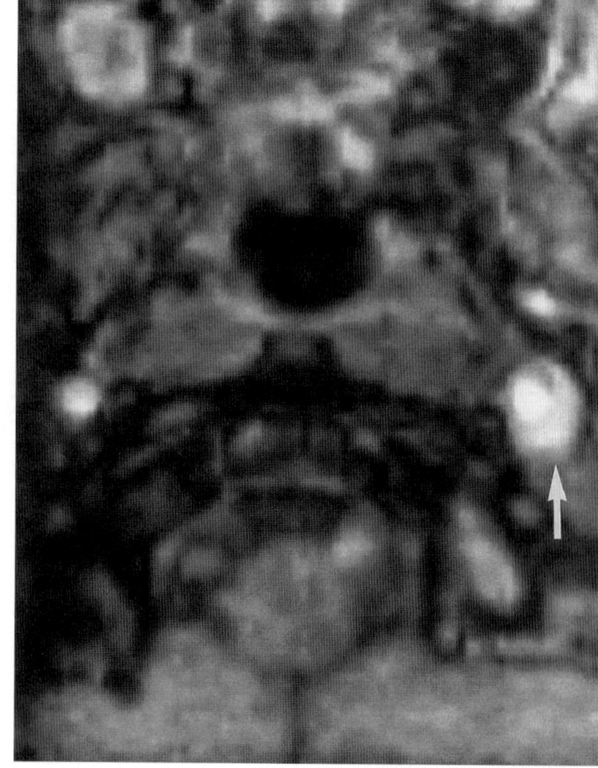

B

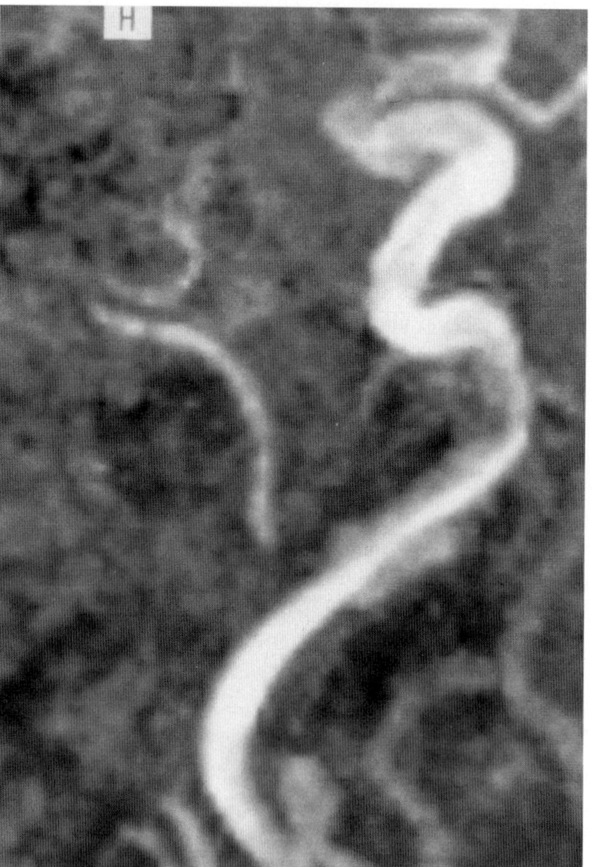

D

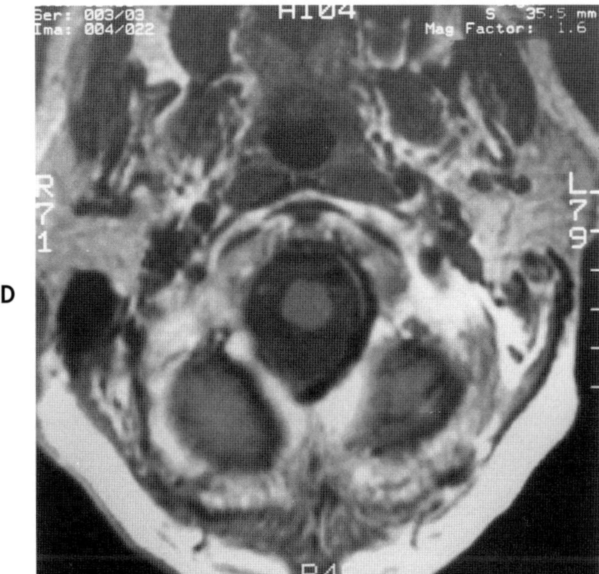

E

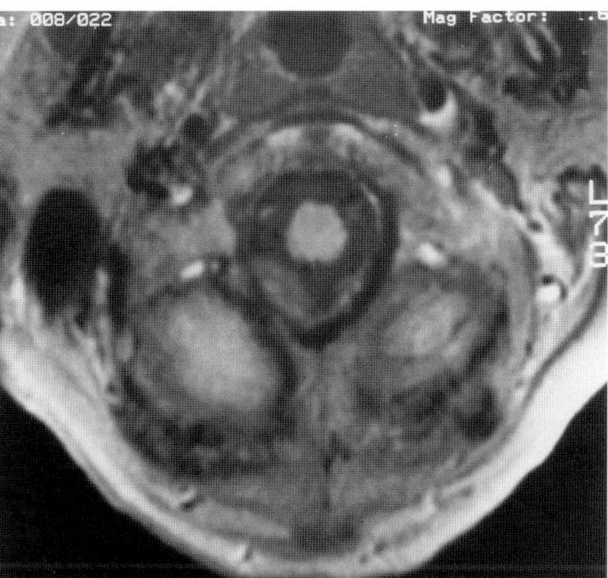

**Lateral (A) and oblique (B) targeted maximum intensity projection views of the left internal carotid artery demonstrate a smooth narrowing involving the mid-portion of the cervical internal carotid artery. There is also the slightly ill-defined increased signal intensity from the subintimal methemoglobin surrounding the midportion of the internal carotid artery. Axial reformat of the MRA data (C) shows to better advantage the intramural high signal hemorrhage peripherally *(arrow)*, which surrounds the central high signal from the patent lumen. Axial T1-weighted spin-echo image (D) through the neck demonstrates a concentric area of abnormally increased signal intensity along the posterior margin of the left internal carotid artery, which represents the false lumen containing methemoglobin. Confirmation is also present on the axial T1-weighted image with fat saturation (E), which improves the delineation of the abnormal high signal intensity along the posterior margin of the carotid artery.**

Small subintimal and subadventitial dissections may have very mild findings or no findings on conventional angiography. The findings are more obvious on the conventional spin-echo images and MRA because of the presence of the methemoglobin, which gives the high signal intensity on the T1-weighted images.

## REFERENCE

Sue DE, Brant-Zawadzki MN, Chance J: Dissection of cranial arteries in the neck: correlation of MRI and arteriography, *Neuroradiology* 34:273-278, 1992.

## CASE 185
## LEFT VERTEBRAL OCCLUSION RESULTING FROM DISSECTION

**History:** 46-year-old with sudden onset of vertigo while playing racketball.

**Technique:** axial volume, three-dimensional phase-contrast, 24/8.8/20, 256 × 128, 60 slices, 80-mm slab, velocity encoding of 60 cm/sec, 18-cm field of view, 13:08.

A

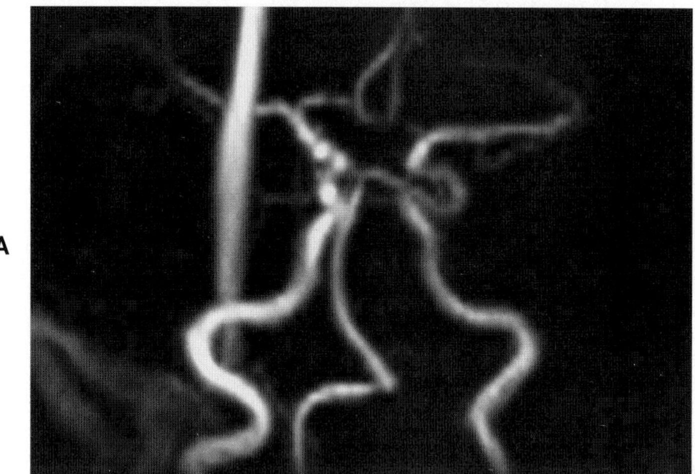

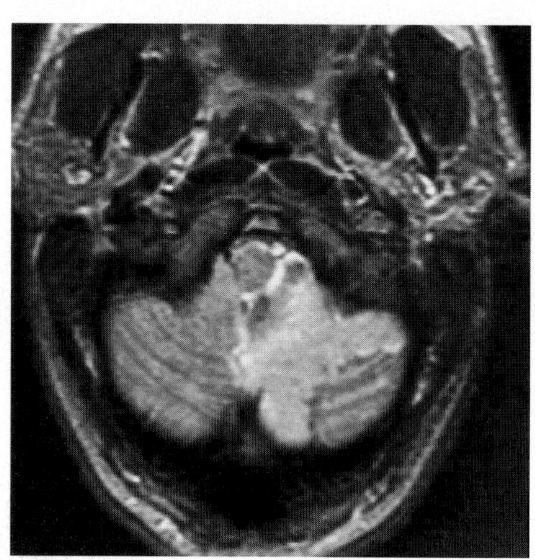

B

C

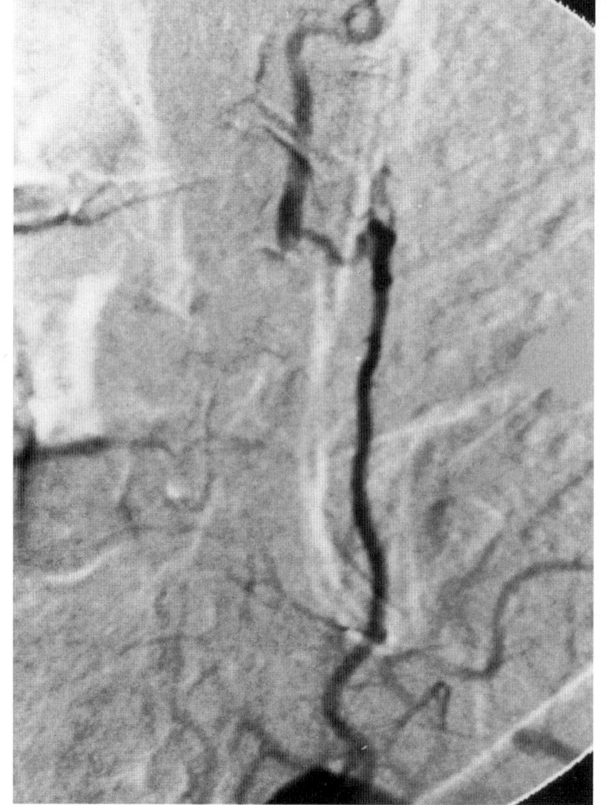

**Anteroposterior maximum intensity projection view of the phase-contrast angiogram (A) of the intracranial circulation demonstrates absent flow within the left vertebral artery. The right vertebral and basilar arteries appear widely patent, as do the anterior circulation vessels. From this clinical history, findings are to be highly suspicious for vertebral artery occlusion related to dissection. Spin-echo T2-weighted image through the posterior fossa demonstrates a large infarct involving the distribution of the left posterior inferior cerebellar artery (B). Note the normal flow void within the right vertebral artery and abnormal increased signal intensity within the left vertebral artery, which could relate to slow flow or occlusion. Conventional angiographic view from a left subclavian artery injection demonstrates occlusion of the left vertebral artery at its origin, with a large lateral supply through the costocervical trunk and cervical muscular branches (C). There was very slow flow in the reconstituted distal left vertebral artery. The very slow flow within the distal left vertebral artery was not imaged on the phase-contrast study because of the velocity-encoding setting of 60 cm/sec.**

The list of apparently benign activities linked to vertebral artery dissection is amazing. The reported causes of vertebral dissection include yoga, calisthenics, aerobic exercise, ceiling painting, trampoline exercise, and chiropractic manipulation. Vertebral artery dissection most commonly affects young adults and has an overall good prognosis, with resolution of vessel abnormalities from 63% to 88% after 2 to 3 months. Neurologic deficits from vertebral artery dissection are quite variable, extending from none to partial brainstem syndromes and Wallenberg's lateral medullary syndome to "locked-in" syndrome. The preferred treatment is with antiplatelet drugs and anticoagulation.

## REFERENCES

Hart RG: Vertebral artery dissection, *Neurology* 38:987-989, 1988.

Robertson JT: Neck manipulation as a cause of stroke, *Stroke* 12:1, 1981 (editorial).

Aston JD, Sherman DG: Cervical manipulation and stroke, *Stroke* 8:594-597, 1977.

Rae-Grant AD, Lin F, Yaeger BA et al: Post traumatic extracranial vertebral artery dissection with locked-in syndrome: a case with MRI documentation and unusually favorable outcome, *J Neurol Neurosurg Psychiatr* 52:1191-1193, 1989.

## CASE 186
## CAROTID DISSECTIONS WITH PSUEDOANEURYSMS

**History:** 38-year-old with new onset of mild weakness on the left side after a motor vehicle accident.

**Technique:** axial volume, three-dimensional time-of-flight, 30/6/25, 256 × 128, 128 slices, 128-mm slab, 25-cm field of view (1/2 rectangular), 8:14.

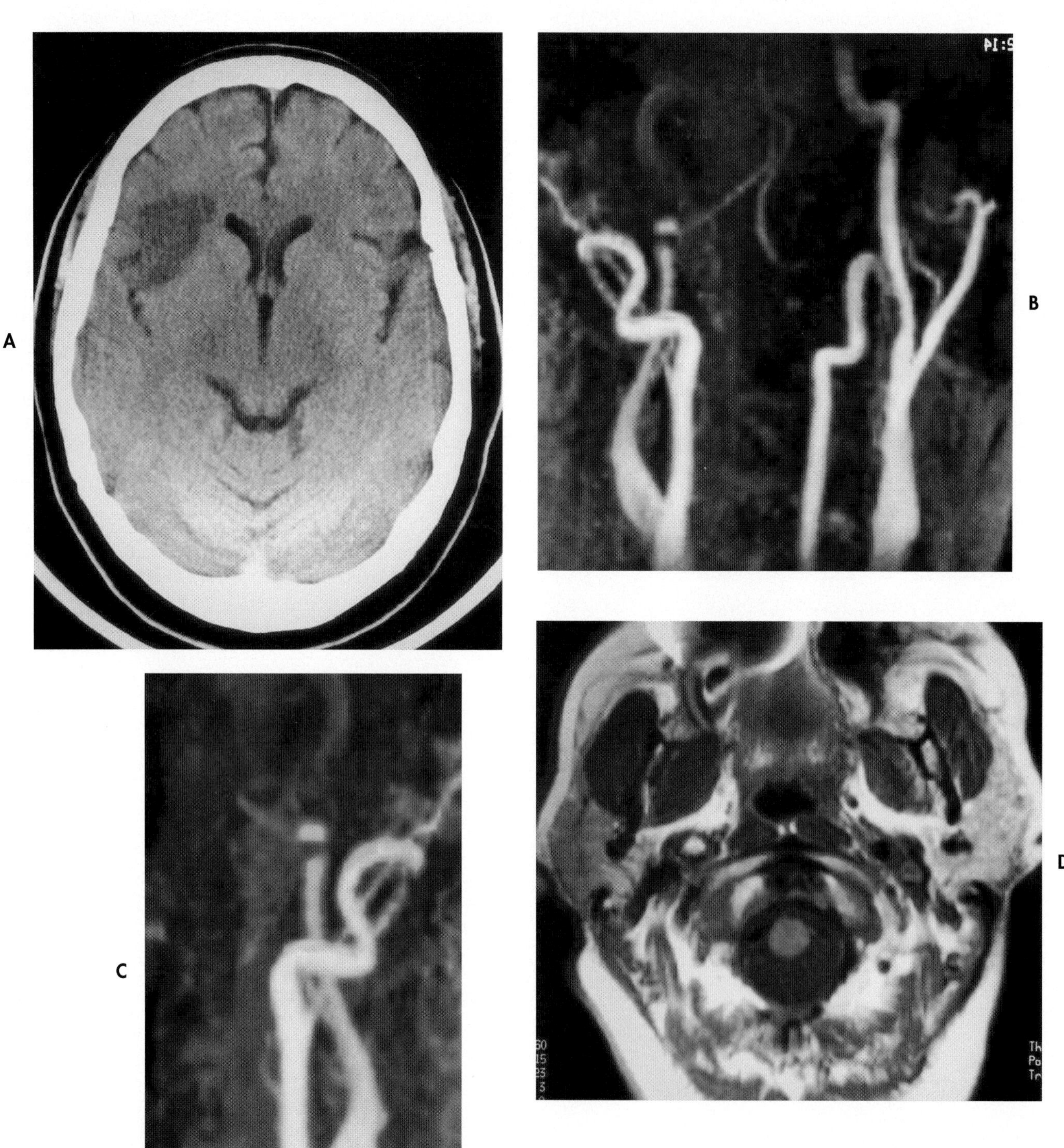

E

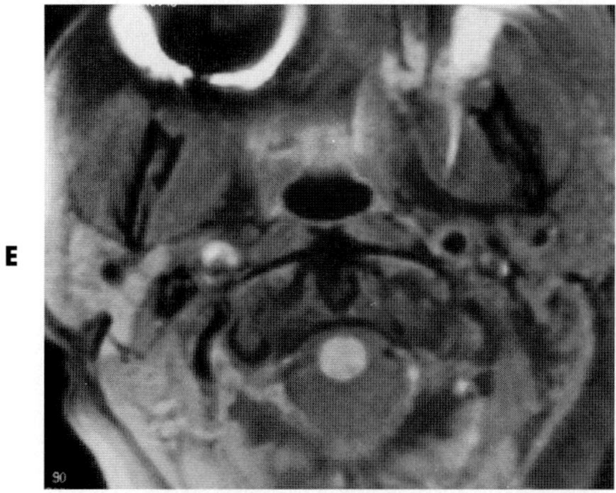

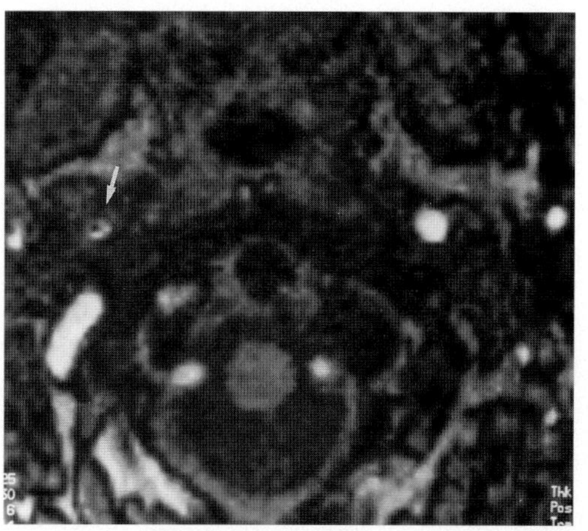

F

**Unenhanced computed tomographic scan of the brain (A) demonstrates an infarct involving the anterior portion of the right middle cerebral artery distribution. Anteroposterior maximum intensity projection (B) and targeted lateral maximum intensity projection views (C) of the three-dimensional time-of-flight MRA of the right carotid bifurcation demonstrate an apparent occlusion of the right internal carotid artery, which begins approximately halfway up the cervical segment. A rounded outpouching of signal intensity is seen at the distal portion of the visualized right internal carotid artery. There is also a subtle irregularity of the left internal carotid artery in its midportion along the medial wall. The vertebral arteries are normal in appearance, and the apparent cutoff relates to positioning of the maximum intensity projection volume. Conventional T1-weighted spin-echo (D) and T1-weighted axial with fat suppression images (E) demonstrate findings of carotid dissection on the right, with a large amount of high signal intensity methemoglobin along the anterior aspect of the right internal carotid artery. There continues to be a small amount of low signal intensity along the posterior margin of the internal carotid artery, which is consistent with a small patent residual lumen. Axial slice from the MRA data set just superior to the level of apparent occlusion of the internal carotid artery (F) shows a small focus of high signal intensity, which most likely represents a residual patent lumen *(arrow),* a structure not visible on the maximum intensity projection. Selective right common carotid artery injection (G) demonstrates a large focal defect involving the midportion of the right internal carotid artery, with associated wall irregularity, which represents focal dissection and intramural hematoma. A widely patent lumen of the right internal carotid artery is distal to the stenotic area.**

G

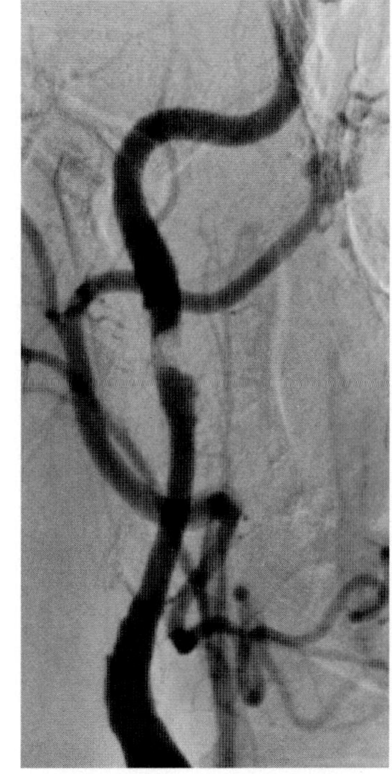

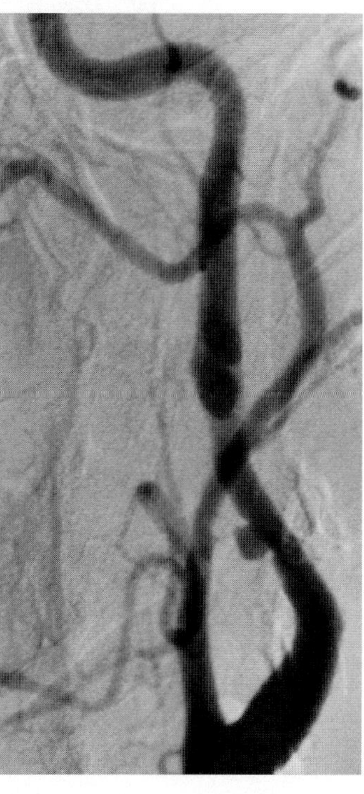

H

The appearance on the MRA reflects the visualization on the T1-weighted gradient-echo MRA sequence of the high signal intensity methemoglobin as well as of the high signal intensity flow in the inferior portion of the internal carotid artery. Lack of signal distal to the area of hematoma relates to slowed flow and turbulent flow secondary to the dissection-created stenosis. Oblique view of the left common carotid artery **(H)** demonstrates abnormal focal outpouching along the midportion of the internal carotid artery, which is consistent with an additional area of carotid dissection and pseudoaneurysm formation. Focal pseudoaneurysm involving the proximal internal carotid artery is not identified on the MRA sequence, probably because of slowed flow with saturation within the outpouching.

## CASE 187
## BILATERAL CAROTID DISSECTIONS

**History:** 42-year-old woman with a severe headache and, noted on examination, a neck bruit.

**Technique:** coronal volume, three-dimensional time-of-flight, 50/6/15, 256 × 128, 64 slices, 60-mm slab, 23-cm field of view (1/2 rectangular), 6:52.

A

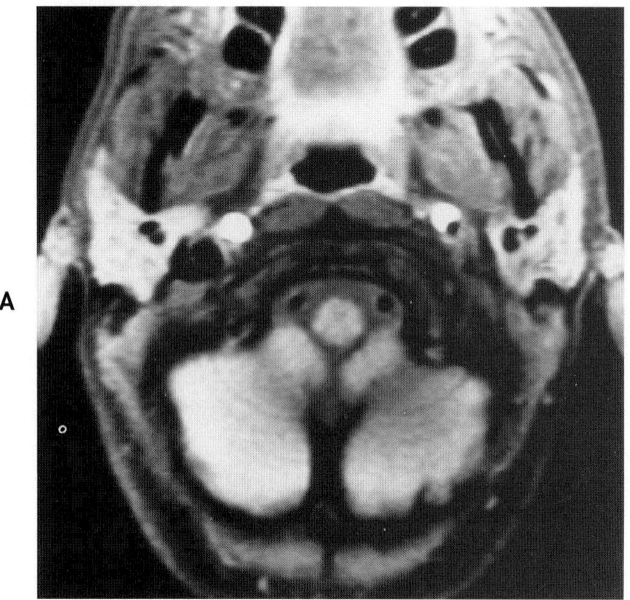

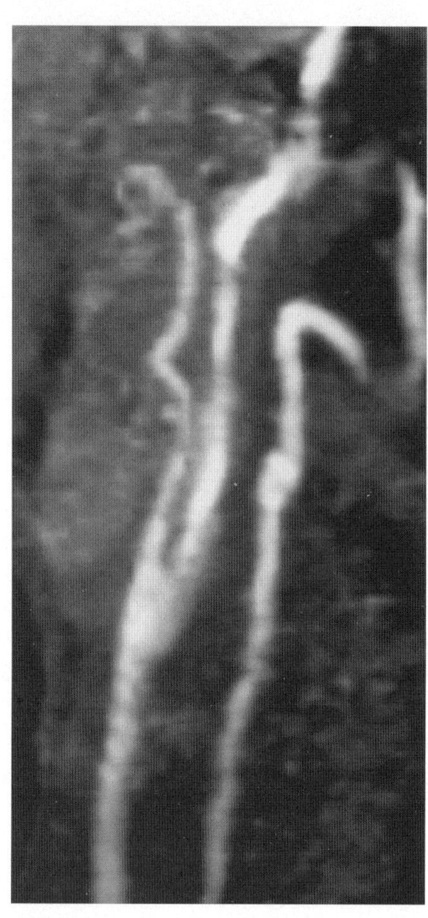

B

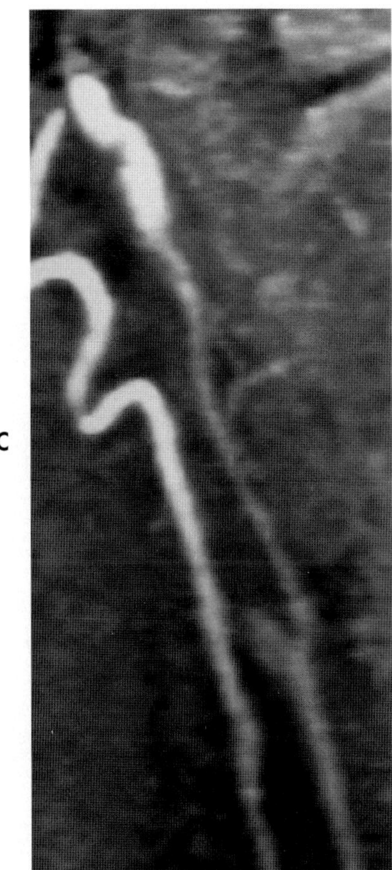

C

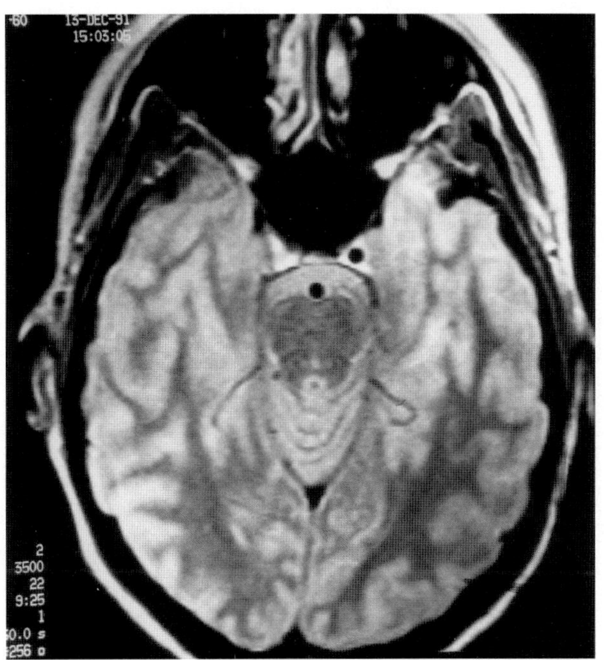

D

**Fat-saturated axial T1-weighted image (A) through the neck demonstrates a rounded area of high signal intensity (thrombus with methemoglobin) involving the region of the right internal carotid artery and no evidence of flow void to suggest a residual patent lumen. An additional focal area of abnormal increased signal intensity is present along the anterior wall of the left internal carotid artery, which is consistent with an additional area of dissection and intramural methemoglobin. Flow void is seen posteriorly, which represents the true patent lumen. Targeted lateral view from a maximum intensity projection demonstrates marked long segment of irregularity involving the left internal carotid artery (B). The abnormality starts distal to the carotid bifurcation and is not consistent with atherosclerotic disease in this young woman. On the right side, there is occlusion of the right internal carotid artery, with a patent external carotid artery (C). The high signal intensity involving the distal portion of the internal carotid distribution is the maximum intensity projection's identification of the methemoglobin within the false lumen. Flow abnormality is further demonstrated by the abnormal increased signal from the right carotid siphon on the spin density axial image (D).**

## CASE 188
## LEFT INTERNAL CAROTID DISSECTION

**History:** 44-year-old with left hemispheric transient ischemic attacks.

**Technique:** sagittal volume, three-dimensional time-of-flight, 80/7/40, 256 × 128, 64 slices, 60-mm slab, 20-cm field of view, 10:57.

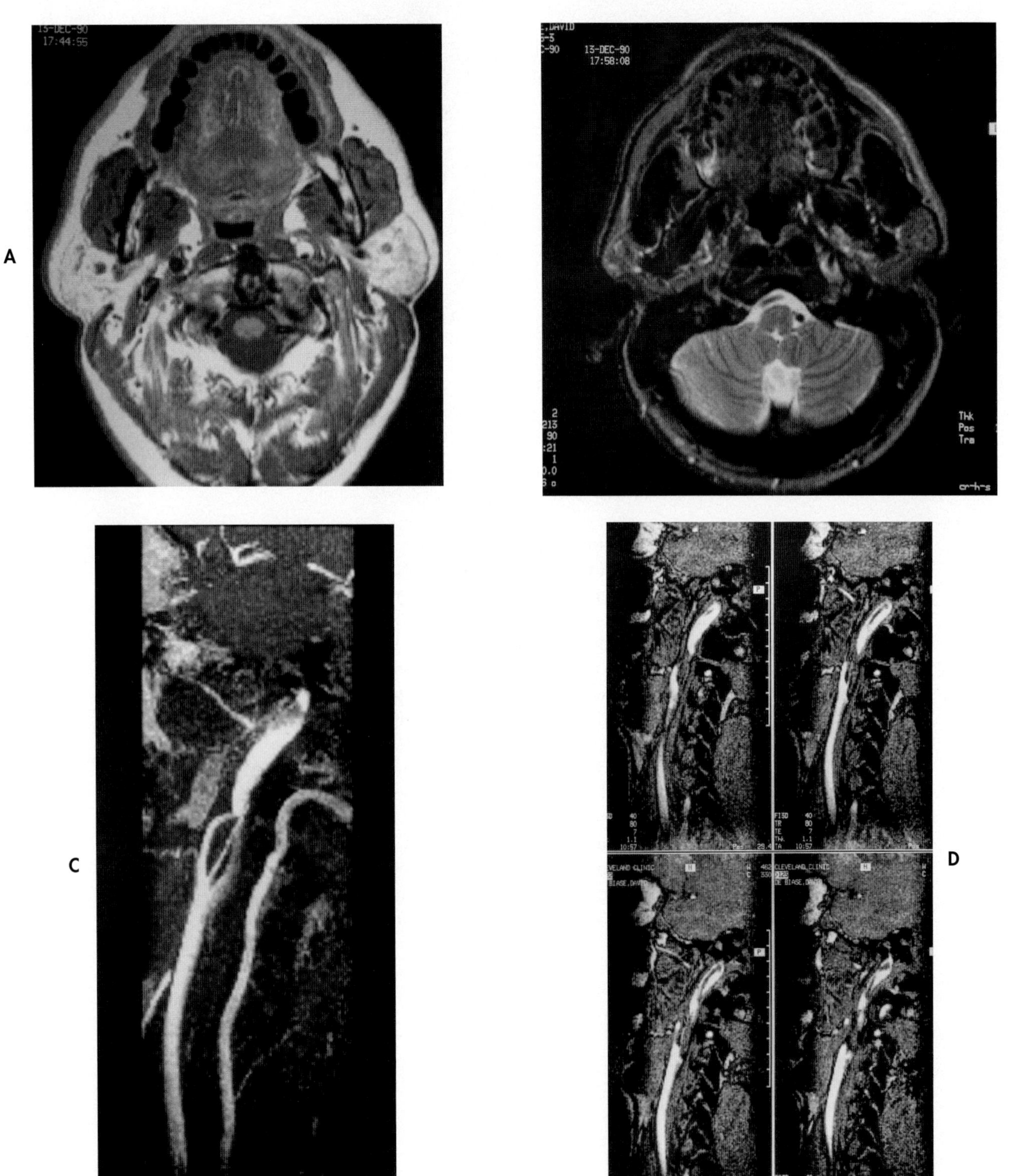

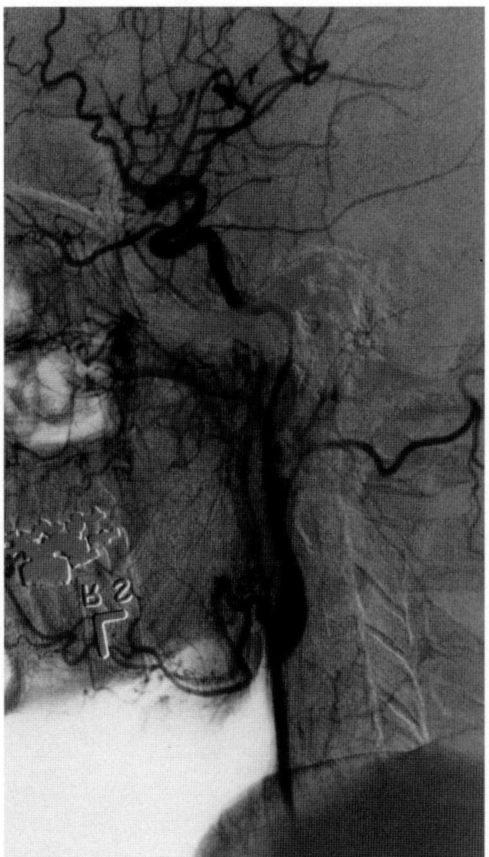

E

Axial T1- (A) and T2-weighted (B) spin-echo study through the neck demonstrates a rounded area of abnormally increased signal intensity along the medial and posterior aspect of the left internal carotid artery, which is consistent with intramural thrombus containing methemoglobin. A small residual flow void of the internal carotid artery is identified. MRA lateral maximum intensity projection view (C) demonstrates a smooth narrowing of the midportion of the left internal carotid artery, with a more distal ballooning of the high signal intensity up to the level of the petrous carotid artery. It is difficult to tell the nature of the abnormality on the maximum intensity projection views. Examination of the individual sagittal MRA slices (D) allows discrimination of the intimal flap as a line of low signal intensity outlined by high signal intensity on either side, which represents, in one instance, the methemoglobin within the false lumen and, on the other, the high signal intensity of the flowing residual patent carotid artery. Conventional angiographic lateral view of the left common carotid injection shows the smooth narrowing of the distal internal carotid artery, which is a classic sign of dissection (E).

## CASE 189
## LEFT CAROTID DISSECTION

**History:** 53-year-old with neck pain.

**Technique #1:** axial two-dimensional time-of-flight, 45/9/60, 256 × 128, one excitation, 1.5-mm slices with a total of 80 sections, tracking superior saturation pulse, 16-cm field of view, 7:40.

**Technique #2:** sagittal, two-dimensional phase contrast, 30/8/20, 512 × 256, eight excitations, 80-mm thick section, 24-cm field of view, 5 minutes.

A

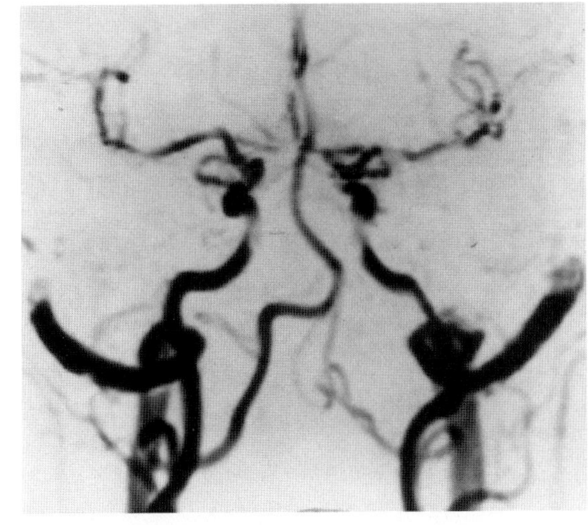

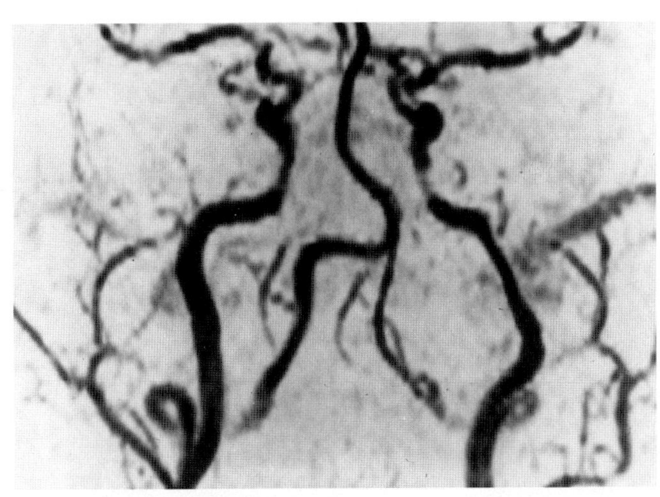

B

**Coronal two-dimensional phase-contrast "scout" study (A) demonstrates the narrowing of the left presellar internal carotid artery. This is further confirmed on the anteroposterior maximum intensity projection view of the axial two-dimensional time-of-flight sequence (B), with rather diffuse narrowing of the distal left internal carotid artery compared with the right. (Courtesy John Huston, Mayo Clinic, Rochester, Minn.)**

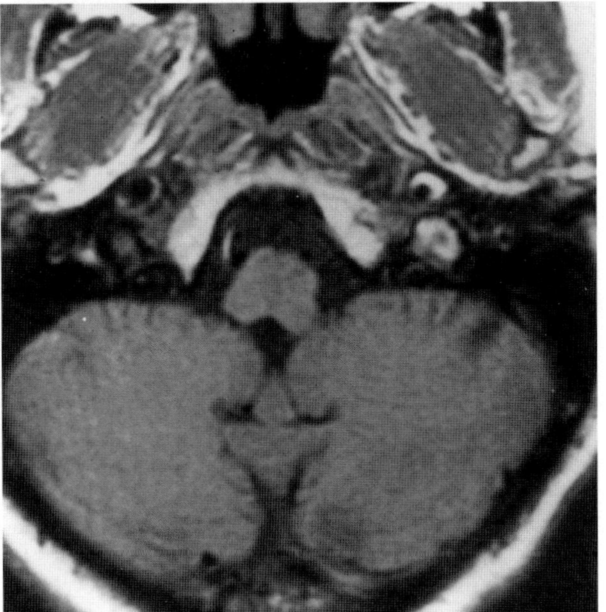

C

Although the phase-contrast and time-of-flight MRAs show nonspecific vessel narrowing, the diagnosis is quite easily made on a conventional T1-weighted axial spin-echo image through the skull base **(C),** which shows the circumferential methemoglobin as high signal intensity with the narrowed patent lumen, which in turn shows the flow void.

## CASE 190
## TRAUMATIC CAROTID DISSECTION

**History:** 22-year-old involved in a motor vehicle accident who has multiple facial fractures, cerebrospinal rhinorrhea, and left-sided hemiparesis.

**Technique:** axial volume, three-dimensional time-of-flight, 45/7/20, 256 × 256, 64 slices, 60-mm slab, 14-cm field of view, 12:20.

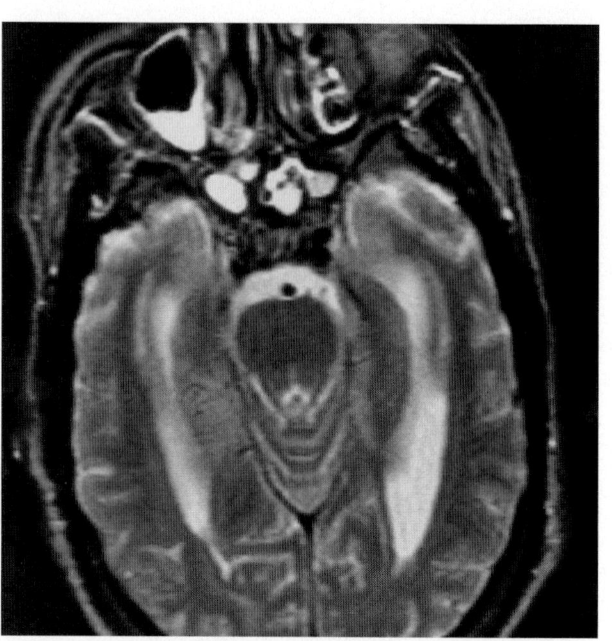

B

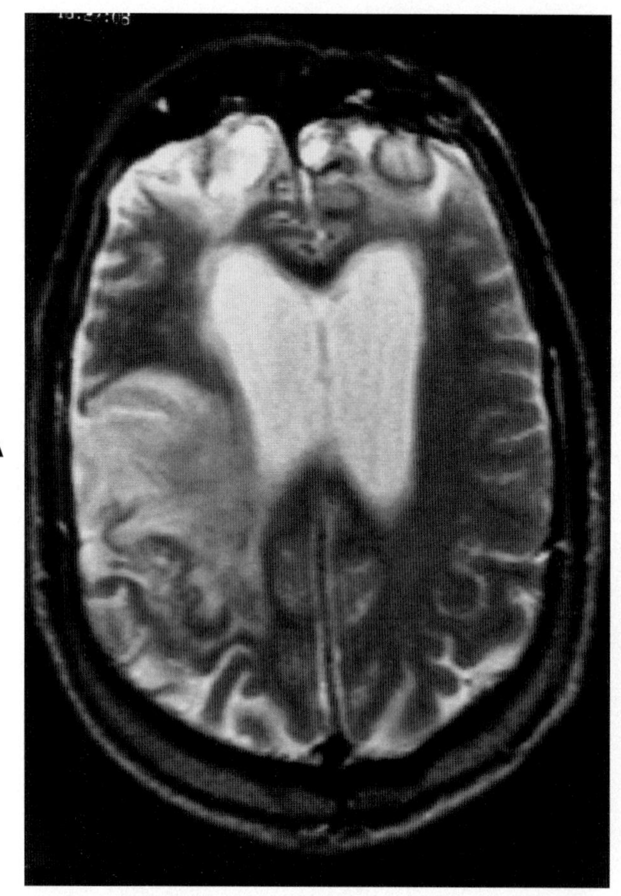

A

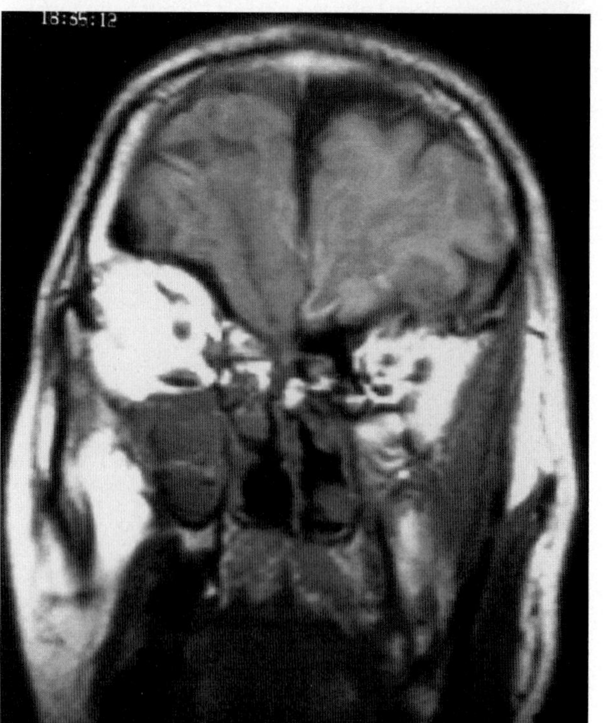

C

D 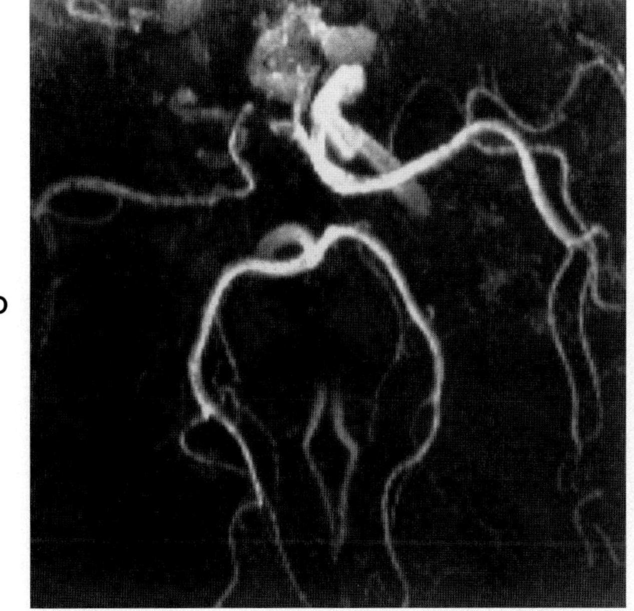

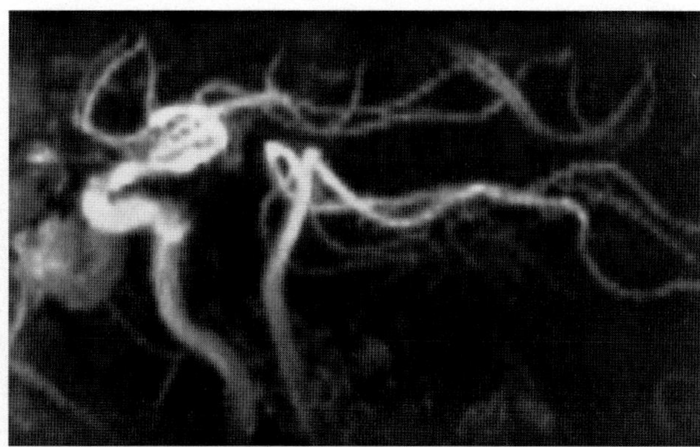 E

**T2-weighted spin-echo images through the levels of the lateral ventricles (A) and the brainstem (B) show a well-defined right hemispheric infarct and bifrontal contusions. There is absence of the usual flow void in the right carotid siphon. There is also abnormal increased signal in the sphenoid, ethmoid, and maxillary sinuses. The coronal T1-weighted image (C) shows a traumatic encephalocele involving the right cribriform plate and high signal intensity blood within the left maxillary sinus. Base (D) and lateral (E) views of the maximum intensity projection show a very attenuated right distal internal carotid artery, with a decreased caliber of the right middle cerebral artery.**

The findings represent a traumatic carotid dissection with decreased flow in the middle cerebral distribution (with saturation effects decreasing vessel caliber). The high signal intensity anterior to the carotid siphons on the maximum intensity projection is blood (methemoglobin) from the facial fractures within the sinuses.

## CASE 191
## RIGHT CAROTID DISSECTION

**History:** 34-year-old with an episode of right hemispheric transient ischemic attacks consisting of left arm numbness and weakness.

**Technique:** axial volume, three-dimensional time-of-flight, 45/7/20, 128 × 256, 128 slices, 140-mm slab, 24-cm field of view (1/2 rectangular), 12:20.

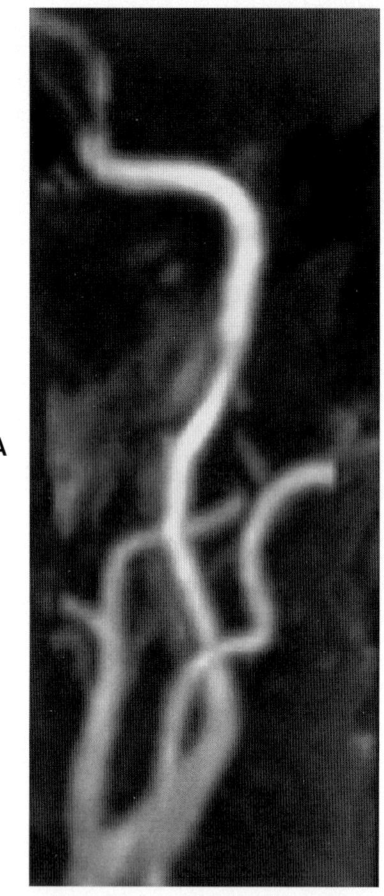

A

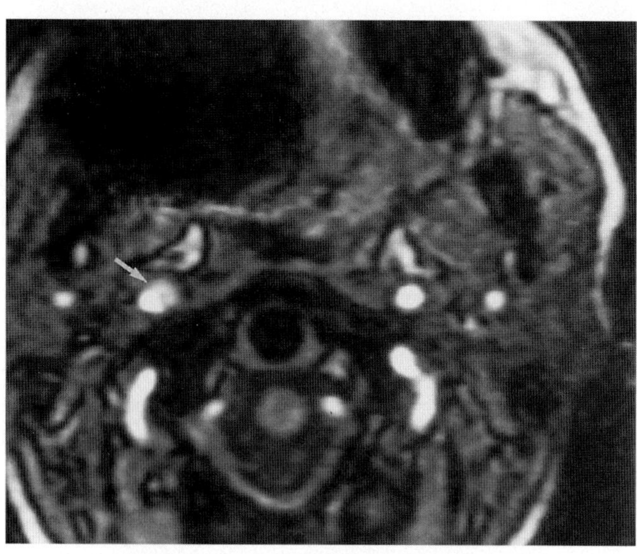

B

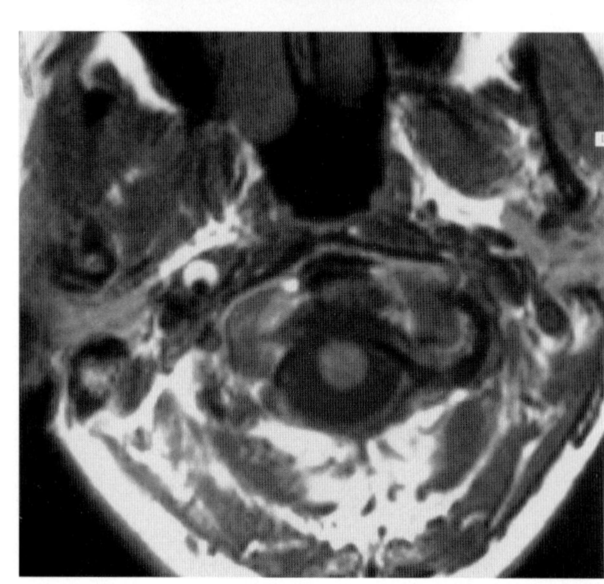

C

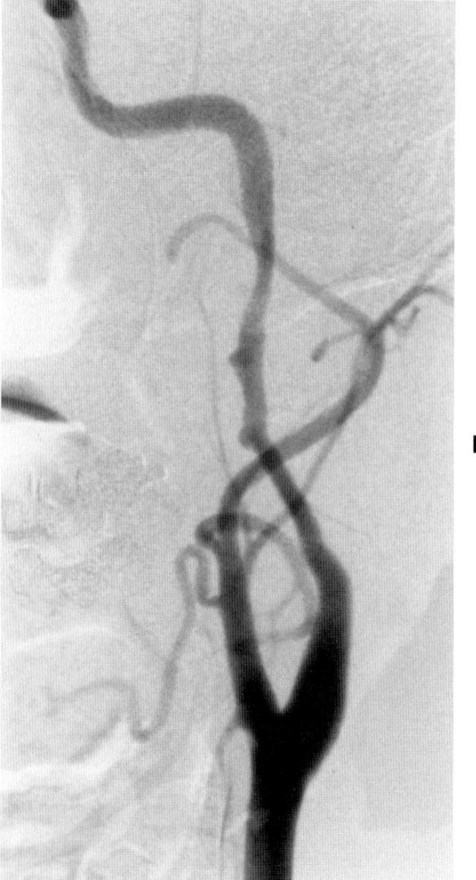

D

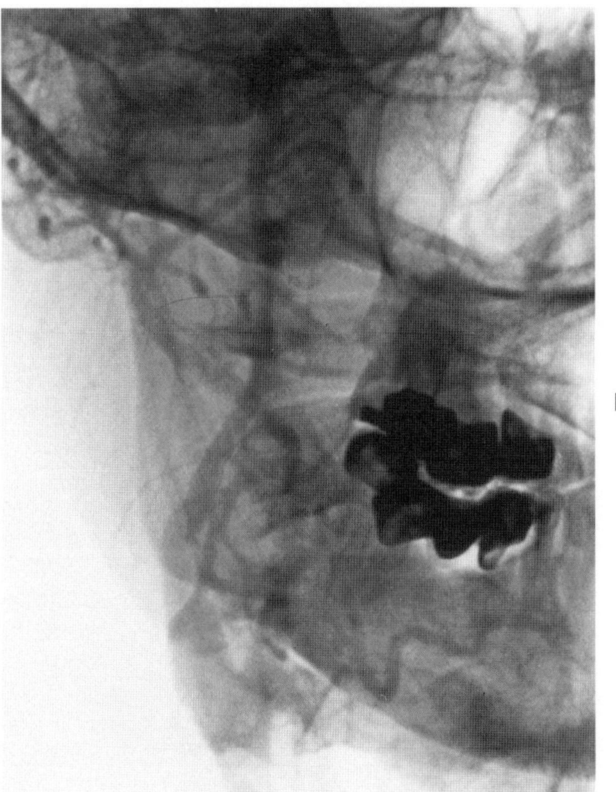


**Lateral maximum intensity projection view of the time-of-flight MRA (A) shows narrowing and irregularity of the cervical right internal carotid artery, with areas of faint increased signal in the periluminal region. Individual slice from the MRA data set (B) shows curvilinear increased signal in the anteromedial wall of the right internal carotid artery and associated narrowing, which represents a carotid dissection with an intimal hematoma *(arrow)*. The hematoma is further confirmed on the axial T1-weighted spin-echo MR (C) of the neck, in which the high signal methemoglobin is contrasted against the carotid flow void. A flow void is ensured in the carotid artery by use of an inferior saturation pulse. Conventional angiogram of the right carotid artery shows narrowing and irregularity typical for dissection (D).**

The fat-saturation T1-weighted sequence was uninterpretable in this case because of the adjacent metal artifact of dental fillings, as shown on the unsubtracted view from the conventional angiogram **(E).** The fat-saturation sequence is quite sensitive to local field inhomogeneities, which can occur at the chin/air or sinus interface and with implanted metal.

## CASE 192
## FIBROMUSCULAR DYSPLASIA WITH DISSECTION

**History:** 40-year-old with sudden onset of right extremity paresthesias.

**Technique:** axial two-dimensional time-of-flight, 46/9/60 degree flip angle, 256 × 128, one excitation, 1.5-mm thick sections with a total of 84 sections covering 126 mm, tracking superior saturation band, 20-cm field of view, 8:34.

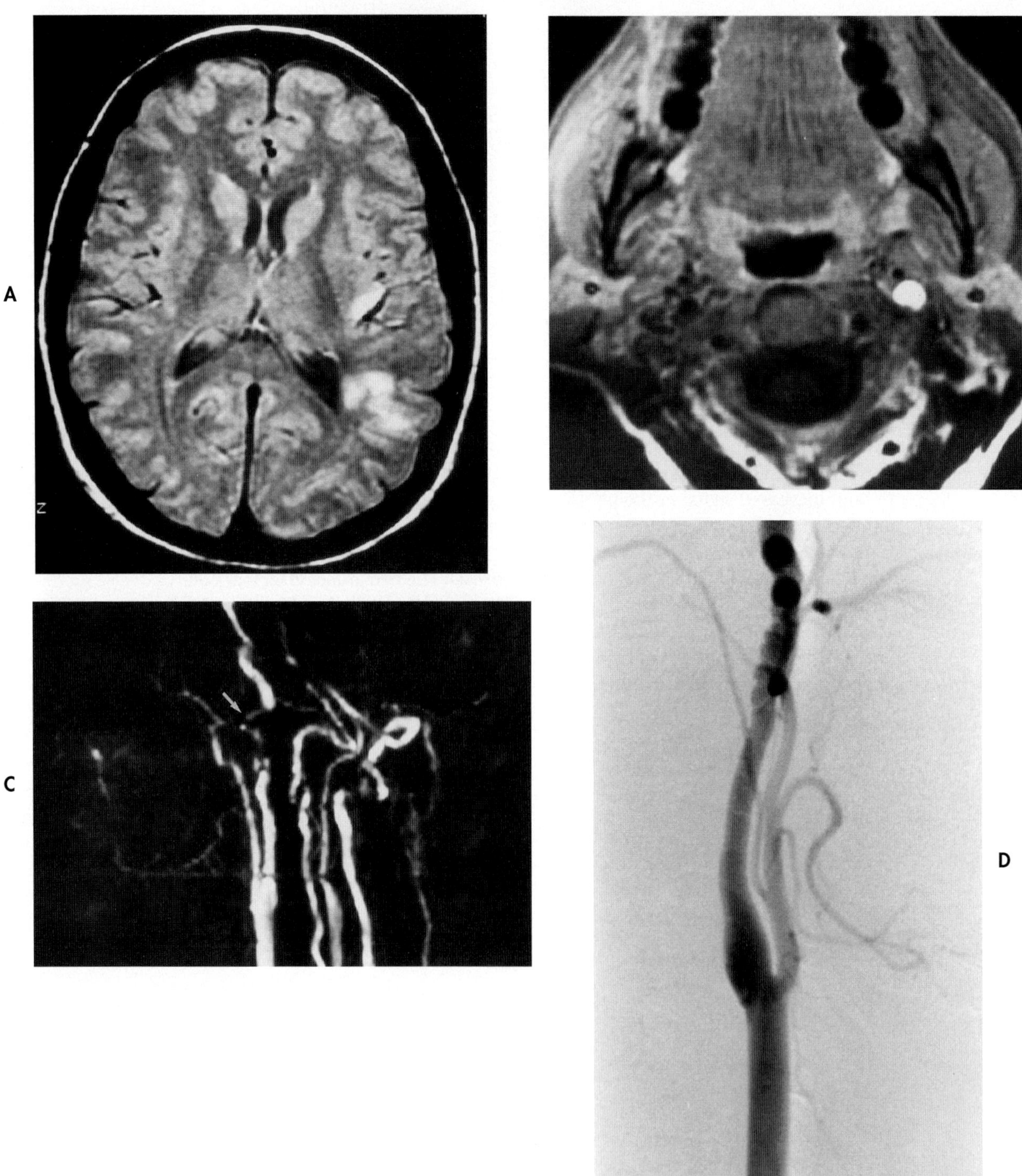

Axial spin-density image of the brain shows small infarcts involving the left middle cerebral distribution (A). Axial T1-weighted spin-echo image with fat saturation (B) shows abnormal increased signal from the left internal carotid artery related to methemoglobin within the dissected arterial wall. Left anterior oblique maximum intensity projection view of the two-dimensional time-of-flight MRA (C) shows occlusion of the left internal carotid artery and pronounced loss of signal and irregularity of the distal right internal carotid artery *(arrow)*. However, no abnormal signal is seen in the right internal carotid artery on the T1-weighted image to suggest right-sided dissection. Conventional angiographic lateral view of the right carotid bifurcation (D) shows typical findings of fibromuscular dysplasia but no significant lumen narrowing. Lateral conventional angiographic view of the left bifurcation (E) shows a classic tapering of the internal carotid lumen related to dissection.

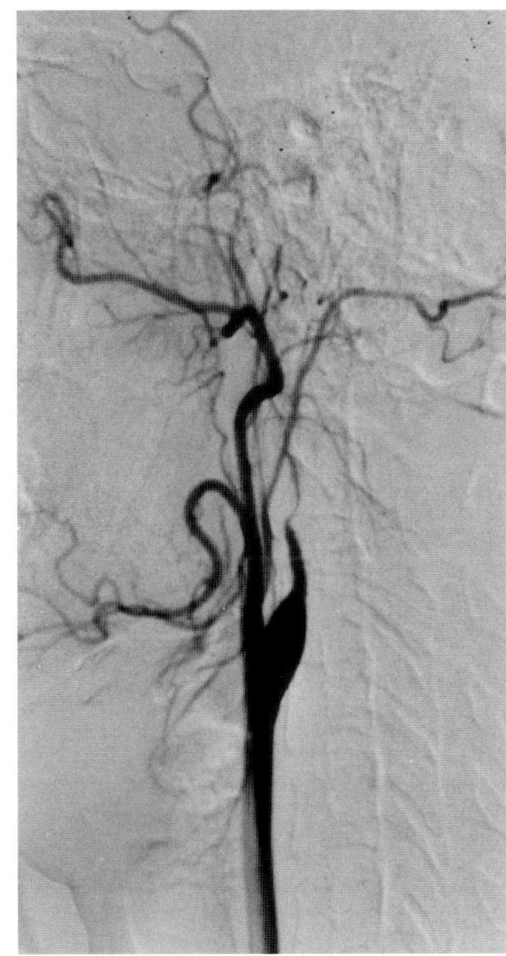

E

Fibromuscular dysplasia is an arteriopathy that affects medium and small arteries; the renal arteries are the most common sites. The cause of fibromuscular dysplasia is unknown. The cervical vessels (especially the internal carotids) are the second most common site of involvement; the C2 level is the most common location. Women are most commonly affected, usually in the fourth or fifth decades. The typical angiographic pattern, as shown in this case, are constrictions alternating with normal segments or dilated segments. This produces the so called stack-of-coins or string-of-beads appearance. Fibromuscular disease can be difficult to image by MRA because of the disturbed flow in the region of the disease. This disturbed flow causes spin dephasing, which produces signal loss. This may be particularly prominent in two-dimensional time-of-flight techniques, since they have a relatively large voxel size and longer echo times compared with three-dimensional techniques. As with a severe atherosclerotic stenosis, the loss of signal intensity at the diseased dysplasic segment is followed by reconstitution of signal downstream when more laminar flow is achieved. The string-of-beads appearance can be mimicked with normal vessels on two-dimensional time-of-flight MRA by a slight motion artifact between image slices.

## REFERENCES


Wesen CA, Elliott BM: Fibromuscular dysplasia of the carotid arteries, *Am J Surg* 151:448-451, 1986.

Heiserman JE, Drayer BP, Fram EK, Keller PJ: MR angiography of cervical fibromuscular dysplasia, *AJNR* 13:1454-1457, 1992.

Healton EB: *Fibromuscular dysplasia*. In Barnett HJM, ed: *Stroke* vol 2, New York, 1986, Livingstone.

# Technical Summary and Preferences

The following tables describe the preferred techniques for a variety of pathologies and regions.

| Aneurysms | Technical preference | Comments |
|---|---|---|
| *Rank* | | |
| Primary | 3D TOF axial volume (single or multiple slab) | Limited by slow flow in large aneurysms (saturation) |
| Secondary | 3D PC | Limited resolution, more susceptible to phase dispersion |
| Limited use | 2D PC | Evaluation of flow patterns with variable velocity encoding |
| Not recommended | 2D TOF | Limited resolution |

| Arteriovenous malformations | Technical preference | Comments |
|---|---|---|
| *Rank* | | |
| Primary | | |
| Arterial flow | 3D TOF, 3D PC (60-100 cm/s velocity encoding) | Limited to fast-flow component |
| Venous flow | 3D PC (with variable velocity encodings) | Limited by time constraints |
| Secondary | 2D TOF | Limited visualization of vessels with rapid flow |
| Secondary | 2D PC | Rapid assessment of flow velocities or venous drainage |

| Intracranial stenosis or occlusion | Technical preference | Comments |
|---|---|---|
| *Rank* | | |
| Primary | 3D TOF (multiple or single slab) | Limited usefulness for distal branches (i.e., M3 segments) |
| Secondary | 3D PC | Less resolution, overestimation of stenoses |
| Not recommended | 2D PC, 2D TOF | Limited resolution |

| Tumors and vascular loops | Technical preference | Comments |
|---|---|---|
| *Rank* | | |
| Primary | 3D TOF (multiple or single slab) | Background suppression (magnetization transfer) not recommended |
| Secondary | 3D PC | Visualization of vessel pathology but not of tumor per se (can use magnitude reconstruction) |
| Limited use | 2D PC, 2D TOF | Venous involvement |

*3D,* Three-dimensional; *TOF,* time-of-flight; *PC,* phase-contrast; *2D,* two-dimensional; *TR,* repetition time; *TE,* echo time; *FOV,* field of view; *FISP,* fast imaging with steady-state free precession; *GRASS,* gradient acquisition in steady state; *TONE,* tilted, optimized nonsaturating excitation.

| Venous disease | Technical preference | Comments |
|---|---|---|
| *Rank* | | |
| Primary | 3D PC | Limited by time constraints |
| | 2D TOF | |
| Secondary | 2D PC | Good for quick evaluation of slow flow |
| Not recommended | 3D TOF (multiple or single slab) | Not sensitive to slow flow because saturation or possible requirement of intravenous contrast administration |

| Cervical carotid arteries | Technical preference | Comments |
|---|---|---|
| *Rank* | | |
| Primary | 3D TOF (multiple or single slab) | Axial volume preferred because of improved flow-related enhancement |
| Secondary | 2D TOF | Good for slow-flow lesions |
| Limited use | 2D PC | Useful as "scout" (coronal or sagittal) |
| Not recommended | 3D PC | Examination time too long, suffers from dephasing |

| Technique 1.0 Tesla | Sequence | Orientation | TR | TE | Flip angle | Matrix | FOV (cm) | Thickness/slices | Saturation pulse | Comments |
|---|---|---|---|---|---|---|---|---|---|---|
| *Carotid artery* | | | | | | | | | | |
| Carotid MRA TOF | FISP/GRASS 3D | Axial | 40-45 | 10 | 20 | 128 × 256 (½ rectangular FOV) | 20 | 96 mm/64 | 50 mm superior | 1)TONE/ramp pulse<br>2)Single or multiple slabs |
| *Intracranial artery* | | | | | | | | | | |
| Arterial TOF | FISP/GRASS 3D | Axial | 40-45 | 10 | 20 | 256 × 256 | 14 | 60 mm/64 | 50 mm superior | 1)Magnetization transfer<br>2)TONE/ramp pulse<br>3)Single or multiple slabs |
| Venogram TOF | FLASH/spoiled GRASS 2D | Sagittal angled 12-15 degrees toward coronal plane | 32-40 | 10 | 10 | 256 × 256 | 25 | 3 mm (1 mm overlap)/45 | 50 mm inferior | Posterior-to-anterior direction (against flow) |

| Technique 1.5 Tesla | Sequence | Orientation | TR | TE | Flip angle | Matrix | FOV (cm) | Thickness/slices | Saturation pulse | Comments |
|---|---|---|---|---|---|---|---|---|---|---|
| *Carotids* | | | | | | | | | | |
| Carotid scout | 2D PC | Coronal | 25 | min | 30 | 192 × 256 | 28 | 80 mm/1 | — | Flow encoding all three directions |
| Carotid MRA TOF | 3D FISP/GRASS | Axial | 34 | 6.4 | 20 | 128 × 256 (½ rectangular FOV | 25 | 140 mm/128 | 50 mm superior | 1)TONE<br>2)Single or multiple slabs |
| Carotid MRA TOF | 2D FLASH/spoiled GRASS | Axial | 45 | min | 60 | 128 × 256 | 20 | 1.5 mm/1 or 2 sets of 60 slices | 50 mm superior or tracking | |

| Technique 1.5 Tesla | Sequence | Orientation | TR | TE | Flip angle | Matrix | FOV (cm) | Thickness/slices | Saturation pulse | Comments |
|---|---|---|---|---|---|---|---|---|---|---|
| *Intracranial* | | | | | | | | | | |
| Intracranial scout | 2D PC | Coronal | 25 | min | 30 | 192 × 256 | 25 | 60-80 mm/1 | — | Flow encoding all three directions |
| TOF arterial | 3D FISP/GRASS | Axial | 44 | 7 | 20 | 256 × 256 | 20 | 60 mm/64 | 80 mm superior | Magnetization transfer saturation/ TONE Single or multiple slabs |
| PC arterial | 3D | Axial | 25 | min | 20 | 128 × 256 | 20 | 60 mm/60 | — | 1)Flow encoding all three directions 2)Velocity encoding of 30-200 cm/s |
| Intracranial TOF venogram | 2D FLASH/spoiled GRASS | Sagittal angled 12-15 degrees toward coronal plane | 40 | 10 | 10 | 256 × 256 | 25 | 3 mm (1 mm overlap)/45 slices or to cover area of interest | 80 mm inferior | Posterior to anterior direction |
| Intracranial venogram PC | 2D | sagittal (superior sagittal sinus) axial (transverse sinus) | 25-35 | min | 30 | 192 × 256 | 25 | 60-80 mm/1 | — | Flow encoding all three directions |
| Intracranial venogram PC | 3D | axial | 25 | min | 20 | 128 × 256 | 20 | 60 mm/60 | — | 1)Flow encoding all three directions 2)Velocity encoding of 10-20 cm/s |

# INDEX


**A**

Absolute echo time, 316
Adenoma, pituitary, encasing internal carotid artery, 269
Adults, normal time-of-flight study in, 48-49
Aliasing, on phase-contrast MRA, 33
Anastomoses, transdural, with moyamoya disease, 255
Aneurysm clips, 97-99
Aneurysms, 79-161
  anterior communicating artery, 108-109, 112-113
    intracranial hemorrhage obscuring, 94-95
    with subarachnoid hemorrhage, 110-111
    thrombosed, 114-115
  atherosclerotic, 109
  basilar tip, 145, 146-147, 149
    left posterior parietal arteriovenous malformation with, 178-179
  berry (saccular), 109
  calcified
    posterior cerebral, 142-143
    posterior communicating artery, 126-127
  cavernous, left carotid, balloon occlusion with extracranial-intracranial bypass for, 132-133
  endarterectomy patch graft dilated by, 372
  false, 109
    from placement of targeted maximum intensity projection volume, 101
  fusiform (atherosclerotic), 109
  giant
    middle cerebral artery, 120-121
    partially thrombosed, 130-131
  intracranial, types of, 109
  large, ophthalmic artery, 137
  left carotid siphon, left posterior parietal arteriovenous malformation with, 178-179
  left middle cerebral bifurcation, 118-119
  left posterior communicating artery, infundibular dilatation with, 104-105
  middle cerebral artery bifurcation, 116, 117
  multiple, 138-139, 140-141
    and multiple extra aneurysms, 160-161
  multiple extra and intracranial, 160-161
  mycotic, 109
  neoplastic, 109
  ophthalmic artery, 135
    large, 137
  partially thrombosed
    giant, 130-131
    posterior inferior cerebellar, 154-155
  posterior cerebral, 150-151
    calcified and thrombosed, 142-143
  posterior cerebral loop mimic, 100
  posterior communicating artery, 123, 124-125
    calcified, 126-127
  right internal carotid artery, 128-129
  right posterior communicating artery, with right tuberculum sellae meningioma, 270-271
  saccular, 109
  technical preferences, 397
Aneurysms—cont'd
  three-dimensional time-of-flight MRA of
    limitations and pitfalls, 82-101, 104-105, 107
      summary, 79-80
    tortuous siphons in, 82-83
  thrombosed
    of anterior communicating artery, 114-115
    giant, 130-131
    posterior cerebral, 142-143
    posterior inferior cerebellar, 154-155
      with hemorrhage, 152-153
  traumatic, 109
  types of, 109
Angiographically occult vascular malformations, 173
Angiography; *see also* Magnetic resonance angiography
  conventional
    comparison with two-dimensional time-of-flight MRA, 369, 371
    severe carotid stenosis on MRA that directed, 356-357
  intraarterial, of carotid stenoses, comparison with three-dimensional time-of-flight MRAs, 361
Angioma
  cavernous, with venous angioma of posterior fossa, 172-173
  venous, 167
    with cavernous angioma of posterior fossa, 172-173
    left frontal, 168-169
    not on three-dimensional time-of-flight study, 166-167
Anterior cerebral artery, long common trunk (azygos), 51
Anterior clinoid, aerated, 103
Anterior communicating artery
  aneurysm of, 108-109, 112-113
    obscured by intracranial hemorrhage, 94-95
    with subarachnoid hemorrhage, 110-111
    thrombosed, 114-115
  left internal carotid artery occlusion with collateral flow via, 212-213
Arterial occlusion; *see* Occlusion
Arteriovenous malformations, 163
  basal ganglia, 186-187
  grading system, 181
  with hemorrhage, characteristics of, 179
  large frontal, 176-177
  left posterior parietal, with basilar tip and left carotid siphon aneurysms, 178-179
  right parietal, with thrombosed draining vein, 174-175
  right parietooccipital, 180 181
  right temporal lobe, 184-185
  right temporoparietal, 182-183
  technical preferences, 397
Artifacts
  3D imaging, 3
  mimicking stenosis and string sign, 332-333
  misregistration, in anterior limb of carotid siphons, 96
  motion
    affect on two-dimensional time-of-flight MRA, 345
    with severe right internal carotid stenosis, 324-325
    simulating focal occlusion of sagittal sinus, 295
  phase-contrast MRA, 9
  venetian blind, 17

Atherosclerosis
  differential diagnosis, 251
  phase-contrast MRA of, 204
  time-of-flight MRA of, 204
Atherosclerotic aneurysms, 109
Azygos anterior cerebral artery, 51

**B**

Background suppression
  for carotid time-of-flight MRA, 315-317
  comparison of techniques, 22-23
  magnetization transfer, 20-21
    disadvantages of, 265
    with high resolution and tilted, optimized nonsaturating excitation technique, 24-25
  with two-dimensional in-plane spatial saturation technique, 317
Bailey type IV cyst, 291
Balloon occlusion
  of carotid cavernous aneurysm, with extracranial-intracranial bypass, 132-133
  of carotid cavernous fistula, pseudoaneurysm of left cavernous carotid after, 134
Basal ganglia arteriovenous malformations, 186-187
Basilar artery
  dolichoectasia of, with incidental middle fossae meningioma, 158-159
  fenestration of, 68-69
  hypoplastic P1 segments bilaterally, 54-55
  occlusion of, 240-241
    with aberrant internal carotid artery, 242-243
    diagnosis of, 241
    prognosis for, 241
  stenosis of, 234-235, 238-239
    focal, 232-233
    multiple, 230-231
    with posterior circulation infarcts, 236-237
  thrombosis of, 244-245
    acute, prognosis for, 235
  vasculitis of, 248-249
Basilar artery loop, compressing seventh and eighth cranial nerves, 288-289
Basilar tip, 147
  aneurysm of, 145, 146-147, 149
    left posterior parietal arteriovenous malformation with, 178-179
  perforating arteries, 147
Berry (saccular) aneurysms, 109
Bipolar gradient, phase change of spins with, 9, 10
Black blood, 318
Blood
  black, 318
  bright, 318
Brainstem
  dorsal zone, 235
  exophytic glioma on, 278
  lateral zone, 235
  median zone, 235
  microvascular anatomic zones, 235
  paramedian zone, 235
Branchial pouch, second, cyst on, 291
Bright blood, 318
Bulk water, 21
Bypass; *see* Extracranial-intracranial bypass

**C**

Calcification
  of posterior cerebral aneurysm, 142-143
  of posterior communicating artery aneurysm, 126-127
Capillary telangiectasia, 163
Cardiac output, low, signal loss on time-of-flight MRA related to, 206
Carotid artery; *see also* Common carotid artery; External carotid artery; Internal carotid artery
  cavernous fistula
    classification, 191
    dural, 190-191
  cervical; *see* Carotid artery, dissection of
  dissection of
    bilateral, 384-385
    with pseudoaneurysms, 382-383
    technical preferences, 398
    traumatic, 390-391
  siphons
    anterior limb, misregistration artifacts in, 96
    left, left posterior parietal arteriovenous malformation with aneurysm of, 178-179
    signal loss, 205
  technique for, 399
  time-of-flight MRA of
    1.0 Tesla technique for, 399
    1.5 Tesla technique for, 399
    three-dimensional, variations, 28-29
    two-dimensional, 27
Carotid bifurcation, 313-372
  evaluation of
    current, 313-314
    MRA techniques for, 314-315
  flow separation in, 323
  left, stenosis of
    moderate, with severe right stenosis, 368-369
    severe, with decreased signal and intraluminal thrombus, 370-371
  MRA of
    black blood technique for, 318
    magnetization transfer contrast in, 317
    signal loss with, 322-323
  phase-contrast MRA of, 317-318
  right, stenosis of, severe, with moderate left stenosis, 368-369
  stenosis of
    severe
      with decreased intracranial signal, 214-215, 352-353, 354-355
      with string sign, 364-365
    severe bilateral, 362-363
      with multiplanar reformats, 366-367
  three-dimensional time-of-flight MRA of
    advantages of, 314
    background suppression for, 315-317
    coil selection for, 315
    disadvantages of, 314-315
    overestimation of stenosis with, 338-339
    pitfalls of, 322-323, 329, 330-331, 336-337, 338-339, 342-343
    radiofrequency pulse for, 315
    techniques for, 314
  two-dimensional time-of-flight MRA of
    disadvantages of, 314
    flow saturation from vascular loop with, 326-327
    motion artifact affects on, 345
    pitfalls of, 324-325, 326-327, 332-333, 335
    techniques for, 314
Carotid body tumors, 280-281
  angiographic findings of, 281
  classification of, 281
  clinical presentation of, 281
  manifestations of, 281
  treatment of, 281

Carotid bulb
flow separation at, 323
normal, signal loss with, 322-323
Carotid endarterectomy, efficacy, 313
Carotid scout MRA, 1.5 Tesla technique for, 399
Cavernous aneurysms, left carotid, balloon occlusion with extracranial-intracranial bypass for, 132-133
Cavernous angioma of posterior fossa with venous angioma, 172-173
Cavernous fistula
carotid, 190-191
left carotid, pseudoaneurysm after balloon occlusion of, 134
Cavernous malformations, 163
Cerebellar artery; *see also* Inferior cerebellar artery; Superior cerebellar artery
infarction of, 237
Cerebral artery. *see* Anterior cerebral artery, posterior; Middle cerebral artery; Posterior cerebral artery
Cerebral venous thrombosis, causes of, 293
Cerebritis, left sigmoid sinus thrombosis with, 308-309
Cerebrovascular disease
diagnosis of, 203
incidence of, 261
with sickle cell disease, 261
Cervical arteries; *see* Dissection
Chemodectomas, 281
Children
strokes in, 261
2-year-old, normal phase-contrast MRA in, 45
4-year-old, normal time-of-flight MRA in, 46-47
Cholesterol granuloma, petrous apex, 90-91
Chordoma, clival, 267
Circulatory breakthrough, 179
Clinoid; *see* Anterior clinoid, aerated
Clips
aneurysm, 97-99
endarterectomy, mimicking stenosis, 329
Clival chordoma, 267
Coil selection for three-dimensional carotid time-of-flight MRA, 315
Color ultrasound and comparison with two-dimensional time-of-flight MRA, 369
Common carotid artery
cavernous left, and pseudoaneurysm after balloon occlusion, 134
and severe stenosis with string sign, 364-365
Communicating artery; *see* Anterior communicating artery; Posterior communicating artery
Compensation gradients, advantages and disadvantages of, 9
Concha bullosa mucocele, 86-87
Congenital anomalies, 41-77
Coronal volume, advantages and disadvantages of, 351
Cranial nerves, seventh and eight, basilar artery loop compressing, 288-289
Cysts
Bailey type IV, 291
second branchial pouch, 290-291

**D**

Deep venous thrombosis, 306-307
findings, 307
signs of, 307
Dental fillings, sensitivity of fat-saturation sequences for, 393
Destructive interference on two-dimensional phase-contrast study, 209
Digital subtraction angiography of carotid stenoses, comparison with three-dimensional time-of-flight MRA, 361
Dissection, 373-395
bilateral carotid, 384-385
carotid, with pseudoaneurysms, 382-383
diagnosis of, 373
Dissection—cont'd
fibromuscular dysplasia with, 394-395
left carotid, 378-379, 389
left vertebral occlusion from, 380-381
MRA findings and, 373
MRA pitfalls and, 373-374
right carotid, 392-393
right internal carotid, 386-387
spin-echo evaluation of, 37
technical preferences and, 398
traumatic carotid, 390-391
vertebral artery, 381
left vertebral occlusion from, 380-381
Dolichoectasia
basilar, with incidental middle fossae meningioma, 158-159
with dilatation and thrombosis, 159
with dissection, 159
internal carotid, 66-67, 156-157
vertebrobasilar, 159
Dural fistula, 193, 194-195, 200-201
carotid cavernous, 190-191
not on time-of-flight MRA, 189
of ophthalmic artery, 197
Dural sinuses; *see also specific sinuses*
evaluation of, 293-294
two-dimensional time-of-flight MRA pitfalls, 295
Dyke-Davidoff-Masson syndrome, perinatal infarct with, 70-71
Dysplasia, fibromuscular, with dissection, 394-395

**E**

Echo time, 4
absolute, 316
cycling from in to out of phase, 4
effect on fat signal intensity, 4
field, 316
short, advantages and disadvantages of, 9
two-dimensional snapshot technique and, 317
ECST; *see* European Carotid Surgery Trial
Embolic infarction, 203
Embolus, tumor, carotid occlusion related to, 376
Empyema, subdural, left sigmoid sinus thrombosis with, 308-309
Encephalocele, occipital, 76-77
Endarterectomy, carotid, efficacy of, 313
Endarterectomy clip mimicking stenosis, 329
Endarterectomy patch graft, aneurysmally dilated, 372
Enhancement
flow-related, 3
paradoxical, 3
Entry-slice phenomenon, 3
European Carotid Surgery Trial (ECST), 313
External carotid artery, bilateral stenoses of, 358-359
severe, 362-363
Extracranial-intracranial bypass
balloon occlusion of cavernous aneurysm with, 132-133
superficial temporal artery to middle cerebral artery, 224-225

**F**

False aneurysms, 109
from placement of targeted maximum intensity projection volume, 101
False-positive MRA
for left carotid occlusion, 215
for stenosis in moyamoya disease, 208
Fat saturation
advantages of, 316-317
sequence sensitivity and, 393
Fat signal intensity, effect of echo time on, 4
Fenestration of basilar artery, 68-69

Fibromuscular dysplasia
  angiographic pattern, 395
  with dissection, 394-395
Field echo time, 316
First-order compensation, 6, 7
Fistula
  cavernous
    dural carotid, 190-191
    left carotid, pseudoaneurysm after balloon occlusion of, 134
  dural, 193, 194-195, 200-201
    cavernous carotid, 190-191
    not on time-of-flight MRA, 189
    of ophthalmic artery, 197
  petrosal sinus, 198-199
Flip angles
  high, advantages and disadvantages of, 9
  varied across volume, 19
Flow compensation, 6
  first-order, 6, 7
  second-order, 6, 7
  zero-order, 6
Flow direction, methods of determining, 213
Flow saturation from vascular loop, 326-327
Flow signal, 3-4
Flow supply, definition methods, 213
Flow-related enhancement, 3
Flow-sensitized gradient (bipolar gradient), phase change of spins with, 9, 10
Frontal lobe
  left, venous angioma of, 168-169
  right, large arteriovenous malformation in, 176-177
Frontal sinus mucocele, 88-89
Fusiform (atherosclerotic) aneurysms, 109

**G**

Gadolinium, intravenous
  disadvantages of, 265
  multiple overlapping slabs with, for vascular malformations, 163-164
  three-dimensional imaging after, 185
Generalized vasculitis, 161
Giant aneurysms, 131
  middle cerebral artery, 120-121
  partially thrombosed, 130-131
Glioma, exophytic brainstem, 278
Glomus jugulare tumors, 284-285
Glomus tympanicum tumors, 286-287
Glomus vagale tumors, 282-283
  angiographic findings of, 283
Gradient moment nulling, 6
Gradient motion refocusing, 6
Gradient-echo sequence, conventional, 1, 2
Gradients, 4-8
Grafts, aneurysmally dilated endarterectomy patch, 372
Granuloma, cholesterol, petrous apex, 90-91

**H**

Hematoma, subdural, 84-85
Hemifacial spasm, 289
Hemorrhage
  arteriovenous malformations with, characteristics of, 179
  intraplaque, 336-337
  obscuring anterior communicating artery aneurysm, 94-95
  parenchymal, venous angioma of posterior fossa with, 170-171
  subarachnoid
    anterior communicating aneurysm with, 110-111
    thrombosed posterior inferior cerebellar aneurysm with, 152-153
Hemorrhagic dissection, 373-395
  diagnosis of, 373
  MRA findings of, 373
  MRA pitfalls for, 373-374
Hemorrhagic plaque, 336-337
High resolution with magnetization transfer background suppression and tilted, optimized nonsaturating excitation technique, 24-25
Higher-order motion, 6
Hydranencephaly, 72-73
Hydration-layer water, 21
Hypoglossal artery, persistent, 60-61

**I**

Imaging time, 1
Infants, normal time-of-flight MRA in, 44
Infarction
  acute, middle cerebral, with peripheral vessel signal loss, 220-221
  cerebellar artery, 237
  embolic, 203
  left internal carotid occlusion with, 348-349
  perinatal, with Dyke-Davidoff-Masson syndrome, 70-71
  pontine lacunar, prognosis for, 235
  posterior circulation artery, with basilar artery stenosis, 236-237
  posterior inferior cerebellar, 237
  remote left posterior cerebral occlusion with, 227
  thrombotic, 203
Inferior cerebellar artery, posterior
  infarcts of, 237
  partially thrombosed aneurysm of, 154-155
  and thrombosed aneurysm with hemorrhage, 152-153
Infundibulum
  of internal carotid artery, 107
  of left posterior communicating artery, 105
    dilatation of, 104-105
Interference, destructive, on two-dimensional phase-contrast study, 209
Internal carotid artery
  aberrant, 64-65
    basilar occlusion with, 242-243
  dissection of, 373-395
    with fibromuscular dysplasia, 394-395
    schematic of appearances, 374
  distal, stenosis of, from vasculitis, 252-253
  dolichoectasia of, 66-67, 156-157
  hypoplastic, 62-63
  infundibulum of, 107
  left
    cavernous aneurysm of, balloon occlusion with extracranial-intracranial bypass for, 132-133
    dissection of, 378-379, 389
    distal, severe stenosis of, 216-217
    occlusion of, 346-347
      with collateral flow via anterior communicating artery, 212-213
      false-positive MRA for, 215
      with infarct, 348-349
      masked by collateral flow from right supraclinoid, 210-211
      related to tumor embolus, 376
      with right carotid stenosis, 350-351
  normal, 65
  occlusion of, with overlap on maximum intensity projection mimicking patent vessel, 330-331
  pituitary adenoma encasing, 269
  recanalized, mimicking string sign, 335

Internal carotid artery—cont'd
- right
  - aneurysm of, 128-129
  - dissection of, 386-387, 392-393
  - masking of left supraclinoid occlusion by collateral flow from, 210-211
  - occlusion of, 344-345
  - stenosis of
    - left internal carotid artery occlusion with, 350-351
    - motion artifact with, 324-325
- stenosis of
  - bilateral, 358-359, 362-363
  - multiple, 360-361
    - comparison between intraarterial angiography and three-dimensional time-of-flight MRAs, 361
  - with outpouching, 342-343
  - overestimation of, 247, 338-339
    - with two- vs three-dimensional time-of-flight techniques, 341
  - severe
    - bilateral, 362-363
    - with string sign, 364-365
    - that directed conventional angiographic views, 356-357

Intraarterial angiography, of carotid stenoses, comparison with three-dimensional time-of-flight MRAs, 361

Intracranial aneurysms; *see* Aneurysms; *specific arteries*

Intracranial atherosclerosis
- differential diagnosis, 251
- phase-contrast MRA of, 204
- time-of-flight MRA of, 204

Intracranial hemorrhage; *see* Hemorrhage

Intracranial MRA; *see* Magnetic resonance angiography

Intracranial occlusion; *see* Occlusion

Intracranial scout MRA; *see* Scout MRA

Intracranial stenosis; *see* Stenosis

Intracranial vascular malformations; *see* Vascular malformations

Intracranial vasculature, inphase vs opposed phase MRA of, 4, 5

Intraluminal thrombus, severe left carotid bifurcation stenosis with, 370-371

Intraplaque hemorrhage, 336-337

Intravenous gadolinium
- disadvantages of, 265
- multiple overlapping slabs with, for vascular malformations, 163-164
- three-dimensional imaging after, 185

**J**

Joint Study of Extracranial Arterial Occlusion, 313

Jugular foramen, meningioma of, 285

**K**

Kidney disease, polycystic, multiple aneurysms with, 138-139

**L**

Large vessel occlusive disease
- accuracy of MRA for, 203
- diagnosis of, 203
- sickle cell disease with, 260-261

**M**

Magnetic resonance angiography; *see also* Phase-contrast MRA; Scout MRA; Time-of-flight MRA
- accuracy of, for large vessel occlusive disease, 203
- basic principles of, 1-12
- for dissection, pitfalls of, 373-374
- false-positive
  - for left carotid occlusion, 215
  - for stenosis in moyamoya disease, 208

Magnetic resonance angiography—cont'd
- inphase vs opposed phase, 4, 5
- and perpendicular slice orientation, advantages and disadvantages of, 9
- and sequence parameters, advantages and disadvantages of, 9
- and spin-echo
  - conventional sequence and, 1, 2
  - evaluation of dissection with, 37
  - in sinus thrombosis, 293
- and spins, 3
- techniques for, 13-40
  - advantages and disadvantages of, 40
  - for carotid bifurcation evaluation, 314-315
  - general, 1-9
  - preferred, 397-400
- three-dimensional, 1-3; *see also* Three-dimensional phase-contrast MRA; Three-dimensional time-of-flight MRA
- two-dimensional in-plane spatial saturation technique for, background suppression with, 317
- two-dimensional snapshot technique for, for short echo time, 317

Magnetization transfer background suppression, 20-21
- disadvantages of, 265
- with high resolution and tilted, optimized nonsaturating excitation technique, 24-25

Magnetization transfer contrast, in carotid MRA, 317

Maximum intensity projection, 38-39
- internal carotid occlusion with overlap on, mimicking patent vessel, 330-331
- targeted volume, false aneurysm from placement of, 101

Melanoma metastasis with mass effect on middle cerebral artery, 277

Meningioma
- of jugular foramen, 285
- large, 274-275
  - posterior fossae, with occipital sinus, 276
- left tentorial and juxtasellar, 272-273
- middle fossae, incidental, with dolichoectasia of basilar artery, 158-159
- parasagittal, with superior sagittal sinus occlusion, 310
- recurrent, with superior sagittal sinus invasion, 311
- right occipital, 279
- right tuberculum sellae, with right posterior communicating artery aneurysm, 270-271
- sellar, 266

Methemoglobin, 336-337

Middle cerebral artery
- and acute infarct with peripheral vessel signal loss, 220-221
- acute occlusion of, 218-219
- and bifurcation aneurysm, 116, 117
- and giant aneurysm, 120-121
- left, and bifurcation aneurysm, 118-119
- and melanoma metastasis with mass effect on, 277
- stenosis of, 223
  - overestimation of, 207, 247
- superficial temporal artery bypass to, 224-225

Middle fossae meningioma, incidental, with dolichoectasia of basilar artery, 158-159

Misregistration artifacts, in anterior limb of carotid siphons, 96

Motion artifacts
- and effect on two-dimensional time-of-flight MRA, 345
- with severe right internal carotid stenosis, 324-325
- simulating focal occlusion of sagittal sinus, 295

Moyamoya disease, 254-255, 256-257
- description, 255
- disease process, 255
- early, vasculitis with, 246-247
- with false-positive results indicating stenosis, 208

Moyamoya disease—cont'd
MR findings of, 257
phase classification of, 257
sickle cell vasculopathy with, 259
transdural anastomoses with, 255
treatment of, 257
MRA; *see* Magnetic resonance angiography
Mucocele
concha bullosa, 86-87
frontal sinus, 88-89
Multiplanar reformatting, bilateral severe carotid stenoses with, 366-367
Multiple overlapping slabs technique; *see* Multiple overlapping thin-slab acquisition
Multiple overlapping thin-slab acquisition, 16-17
advantages and disadvantages of, 40
with intravenous gadolinium, for vascular malformations, 163-164
vs single-volume angiography, 17
Mycotic aneurysms, 109

**N**

NASCET; *see* North American Asymptomatic Carotid Endarterectomy Trial
Neoplasms; *see* Tumors
Neoplastic aneurysms, 109
Newborn
normal phase-contrast MRA in, 42-43
normal time-of-flight MRA in, 42-43
occipital encephalocele in, 76-77
Nonchromaffin paragangliomas, 281
North American Asymptomatic Carotid Endarterectomy Trial (NASCET), 313

**O**

Occipital regions
encephalocele in, 76-77
right, meningioma in, 279
right parietal, arteriovenous malformation in, 180-181
Occipital sinus, large posterior fossae meningioma with, 276
Occlusion, 203-264; *see also specific disease*
acute, middle cerebral artery, 218-219
angiographic findings, 293-294
basilar artery, 240-241
with aberrant internal carotid artery, 242-243
diagnosis of, 241
prognosis for, 241
classification of, 203
diagnosis of, 203, 293
focal, of sagittal sinus, motion artifact simulating, 295
internal carotid, with overlap on maximum intensity projection mimicking patent vessel, 330-331
large vessel
accuracy of MRA for, 203
diagnosis of, 203
sickle cell disease with, 260-261
left internal carotid, 346-347
with collateral flow via anterior communicating artery, 212-213
false-positive MRA for, 215
with infarct, 348-349
masked by collateral flow from right supraclinoid, 210-211
related to tumor embolus, 376
with right carotid stenosis, 350-351
left vertebral, from dissection, 380-381
phase-contrast MRA of, 203-204
remote left posterior cerebral artery, with infarct, 227
right internal carotid, 344-345
Occlusion—cont'd
superior sagittal sinus, parasagittal meningioma with, 310
technical preferences, 397
three-dimensional time-of-flight MRA of, 203-204
limitations of, 203
Ophthalmic artery
aneurysm of, 135
large, 137
dural fistula of, 197
Outpouching, carotid stenosis with, 342-343
Overestimation of carotid stenosis, 338-339
with two- vs three-dimensional time-of-flight techniques, 341
Overfolding, 25
Overlapping slabs; *see* Multiple overlapping thin-slab acquisition

**P**

Paradoxical enhancement, 3
Paragangliomas, nonchromaffin, 281
Parasagittal meningioma, with superior sagittal sinus occlusion, 310
Parenchymal hemorrhage, venous angioma of posterior fossa with, 170-171
Parietal lobe
left posterior, arteriovenous malformation in, with basilar tip and left carotid siphon aneurysms, 178-179
right, arteriovenous malformation in, 180-181, 182-183
with thrombosed draining vein, 174-175
Parietoccipital falx meningioma, recurrent, with invasion of superior sagittal sinus, 311
Parietoccipital regions, right, arteriovenous malformations in, 180-181
Perinatal infarct, with Dyke-Davidoff-Masson syndrome, 70-71
Petrosal sinus fistula, 198-199
Petrous apex cholesterol granuloma, 90-91
Phase change, 4
image production schematic, 11
of spins with bipolar gradient, 9, 10
Phase dispersion, 3
Phase-contrast MRA, 9-11
aliasing on, 33
artifacts, 9
of atherosclerotic disease, 204
of carotid bifurcation, 317-318
of intracranial stenosis and occlusion, 203-204
in newborn, 42-43
1.5 Tesla technique for, 400
three-dimensional
advantages and disadvantages of, 40
after gadolinium-dimeglumine pentaacetic acid, 185
technique for, 397, 398
of brain, 34-35
two-dimensional
advantages and disadvantages of, 40
destructive interference on, 209
to determine direction of flow, 213
and scout study of left carotid dissection, 389
technical preferences for, 397, 398
and technique for venous disease, 31
in 2-year-old child, 45
of vascular malformations, 164
venogram, 1.5 Tesla technique for, 400
venous applications of, 294
Pituitary gland
and adenoma encasing internal carotid artery, 269
posterior, 92-93
Plaque, hemorrhagic, 336-337
Polycystic kidney disease, multiple aneurysms with, 138-139
Pontine lacunar infarct, prognosis for, 235

Posterior cerebral artery
aneurysm of, 150-151
calcified and thrombosed, 142-143
of fetal origin, 52
and hypoplastic P1 segments bilaterally, 54-55
and infarcts, 236-237
and remote left, occlusion with infarct, 227
Posterior cerebral loop, mimicking aneurysm, 100
Posterior communicating artery
aneurysm of, 123, 124-125
calcified, 126-127
infundibular dilatation of, 105
left
infundibular dilatation with aneurysm, 104-105
junctional dilatation of, 105
right, aneurysm with right tuberculum sellae meningioma, 270-271
Posterior fossa
cavernous angioma of, 172-173
large meningioma of, 276
venous angioma of, 172-173
with hemorrhage, 170-171
Posterior inferior cerebellar artery, thrombosed aneurysm of, 154-155
with hemorrhage, 152-153
Posterior inferior cerebellar artery infarcts, 237
Protons, partially saturated, 3
Pseudoaneurysms
carotid dissections with, 382-383
left cavernous carotid, after balloon occlusion of carotid cavernous fistula, 134
Pseudobasilar tip, 249
Pulseless disease, 263

**R**

Radiofrequency pulse
fat saturation, advantages of, 316-317
for three-dimensional carotid time-of-flight MRA, 315
Radiosurgery, three-dimensional time-of-flight MRA followup, limitations of, 177
Ramp pulse technique, 19
Reformatting, multiplanar, bilateral severe carotid stenoses with, 366-367
Repetition time, long, advantages and disadvantages of, 9
Rete mirabile, 255

**S**

Saccular aneurysms, 109
Sagittal sinuses; *see also* Superior sagittal sinus
focal occlusion of, motion artifact simulating, 295
Saturation pulses; *see also* Fat saturation
tracking, flow saturation from vascular loop with, 326-327
Scout MRA
carotid, 1.5 Tesla technique for, 399
1.5 Tesla technique for, 400
two-dimensional phase-contrast, of left carotid dissection, 389
Second-order compensation, 6, 7
Sella turcica, meningioma on, 266, 270-271, 272-273
Sequence parameters, advantages and disadvantages of, 9
Sickle cell anemia, 203
with large vessel occlusive disease, 260-261
vasculopathy with moyamoya disease, 259
Sigmoid sinuses, left, thrombosis with subdural empyema and cerebritis, 308-309
Signal enhancement
flow-related, 3
paradoxical, 3
Signal intensity, fat, effect of echo time on, 4
Signal localizing gradients, 3
Signal loss
and carotid siphon, 205
guidelines for, 341
and normal carotid bulb, 322-323
peripheral vessel, acute middle cerebral artery infarct with, 220-221
related to low cardiac output, 206
severe carotid bifurcation stenosis with, 214-215, 352-353, 354-355, 370-371
Sinuses; *see also specific sinuses*
dural
evaluation of, 293-294
two-dimensional time-of-flight MRA of, pitfalls of, 295
occlusion of, diagnostic techniques for, 294
Siphons
carotid
and anterior limb misregistration artifacts, 96
left posterior parietal arteriovenous malformation with aneurysm of, 178-179
signal loss, 205
tortuous, 82-83
Skull base tumors, differential diagnosis for, 285
Slice orientation, perpendicular, advantages and disadvantages of, 9
Slices, overlapping; *see* Multiple overlapping thin-slab acquisition
Spasm, hemifacial, 289
Spin dephasing, 3
Spin rephasing, lack of, 6
Spin-echo MRA
conventional sequence for, 1, 2
evaluation of dissection with, 37
in sinus thrombosis, 293
Spins
fresh, 3
fully magnetized, 3
unsaturated, 3
Stack-of-coins appearance, 395
Stenosis, 203-264
artifact mimic, 332-333
basilar artery, 234-235, 238-239
with posterior circulation infarcts, 236-237
bilateral carotid, 358-359
carotid
with outpouching, 342-343
overestimation of, 247, 338-339
with two- vs three-dimensional time-of-flight techniques, 341
distal internal carotid, from vasculitis, 252-253
distal vertebral artery, 228-229
endarterectomy clip mimicking, 329
false-positive, in moyamoya disease, 208
middle cerebral artery, 223
overestimation of, 207, 247
moderate, left carotid bifurcation, with severe right stenosis, 368-369
multiple basilar, 230-231
multiple carotid, 360-361
comparison between intraarterial angiography and three-dimensional time-of-flight MRA of, 360-361
phase-contrast MRA of, 203-204
right carotid, left internal carotid artery occlusion with, 350-351
sensitivity of two-dimensional time-of-flight MRA for, 369
severe
bilateral carotid, 362-363
with multiplanar reformats, 366-367
carotid bifurcation
with decreased intracranial signal, 214-215, 352-353, 354-355

Stenosis—cont'd
severe—cont'd
carotid bifurcation—cont'd
with decreased signal and intraluminal thrombus, 370-371
with moderate left stenosis, 368-369
with string sign, 364-365
internal carotid, 216-217
directing conventional angiographic views, 356-357
motion artifact with, 324-325
string sign, 364-365
artifact mimic, 332-333
recanalized internal carotid mimic, 335
technical preferences for, 397
three-dimensional time-of-flight MRA of, 203-204
limitations, 203
String sign
artifact mimic, 332-333
recanalized internal carotid mimic, 335
severe carotid stenosis with, 364-365
String-of-beads appearance, 395
Strokes
in children, 261
vertebrobasilar, classification of, 235
Sturge-Weber syndrome, 74-75
Subarachnoid hemorrhage
anterior communicating artery aneurysm with, 110-111
thrombosed posterior inferior cerebellar artery aneurysm with, 152-153
Subclavian steal, Takayasu's arteritis with, 262-263
Subdural empyema, left sigmoid sinus thrombosis with, 308-309
Superficial temporal artery bypass to middle cerebral artery, 224-225
Superior cerebellar artery
duplicate, 53
infarcts, 237
Superior cerebellar artery syndrome, classic, 237
Superior sagittal sinus
and invasion by recurrent meningioma, 311
occlusion of, parasagittal meningioma with, 310
thrombosis of, 300-301, 303
subacute, 304-305

**T**

Takayasu's arteritis, 263, 264
chronic or burned-out stage of, 263
criteria for classification of, 263
differential diagnosis of, 263
prepulseless stage of, 263
stages of, 263
with subclavian steal, 262-263
types of, 263
TE; *see* Echo time
Telangiectasia, capillary, 163
Temporal artery, superficial, bypass to middle cerebral artery, 224-225
Temporal lobe, right, arteriovenous malformation in, 184-185
Temporoparietal regions, right, arteriovenous malformation in, 182-183
Tentorium, left, meningioma of, 272-273
Three-dimensional MRA, 1-3
advantages of, 1-3
artifacts, 3
problems of, 3
Three-dimensional phase-contrast MRA
advantages and disadvantages of, 40
after gadolinium-dimeglumine pentaacetic acid, 185
technique for, 34-35, 397, 398
Three-dimensional time-of-flight MRA
advantages and disadvantages of, 40
of aneurysms
limitations and pitfalls of, 82-101, 104-105, 107
summary of, 79-80
tortuous siphons in, 82-83
of atherosclerotic disease, 204
carotid
advantages of, 314
background suppression for, 315-317
coil selection for, 315
comparison with intraarterial angiography, 361
disadvantages of, 314-315
overestimation of stenosis with, 338-339, 341
pitfalls of, 322-323, 329, 330-331, 336-337, 338-339, 342-343
radiofrequency pulse and, 315
techniques for, 314
variations of, 28-29
dissection, pitfalls of, 373-374, 376-377
dural fistula not on, 189
to evaluate radiosurgery changes, limitations of, 177
after gadolinium-dimeglumine pentaacetic acid, 185
high resolution, and magnetization transfer background suppression and tilted, optimized nonsaturating excitation, 24-25
limitations of, 16
with magnetization transfer background suppression, 20-21
multiple overlapping slabs technique, 16-17
advantages and disadvantages of, 40
with intravenous gadolinium, for vascular malformations, 163-164
vs single-volume angiography, 17
of occlusion, 203-204
limitations of, 203
pitfalls of, 205, 206, 207, 208, 210-211
of posterior pituitary, 92-93
signal loss
and carotid siphon, 205
guidelines for, 341
with normal carotid bulb, 322-323
and peripheral vessel, acute middle cerebral artery infarct with, 220-221
related to low cardiac output, 206
severe carotid bifurcation stenosis with, 214-215
single-volume, vs multiple overlapping thin-slab acquisition, 17
of stenosis, 203-204
false-positive results in moyamoya disease, 208
limitations of, 203
overestimation, vs two-dimensional techniques, 341
pitfalls of, 205, 206, 207, 208, 210-211
technique for
generalized, 15
preferences for, 397, 398
with varying flip angle across volume, 19
of vascular malformations, 163-164
pitfalls of, 166-167, 174-175, 189
Thrombosed aneurysms
of anterior communicating artery, 114-115
giant, 130-131
of posterior cerebral artery, 142-143
of posterior inferior cerebellar artery, 154-155
with hemorrhage, 152-153
Thrombosed draining vein, right parietal arteriovenous malformation with, 174-175
Thrombosis
acute basilar, prognosis for, 235
angiographic findings of, 293-294
basilar artery, 244-245

Thombosis—cont'd
cerebral venous, causes of, 293
deep venous, 306-307
intraluminal, severe left carotid bifurcation stenosis with, 370-371
left sigmoid sinus, with subdural empyema and cerebritis, 308-309
left transverse sinus, 296-297, 298-299
diagnosis of, 299
superior sagittal sinus, 300-301, 303, 304-305
Thrombotic infarction, 203
Tilted, optimized nonsaturating excitation technique, 19
high resolution with magnetization transfer background suppression and, 24-25
Time-of-flight angiography, factors that influence, 3-4
Time-of-flight effects, 3
Time-of-flight MRA; *see also* Three-dimensional time-of-flight MRA; Two-dimensional time-of-flight MRA
in adult, 48-49
arterial
1.0 Tesla technique for, 399
1.5 Tesla technique for, 400
of atherosclerotic disease, 204
and background-suppression techniques, comparison of, 22-23
carotid
1.0 Tesla technique for, 399
1.5 Tesla technique of, 399
and dissection, pitfalls of, 373-374, 376-377
in 4-year-old child, 46-47
in infant, 44
in newborn, 42-43
and signal loss
guidelines for, 341
related to low cardiac output, 206
of vascular malformations, 163-164
venogram
1.0 Tesla technique for, 399
1.5 Tesla technique for, 400
Toddlers; *see* Children
TOF effects; *see* Time-of-flight effects
Top-of-the-basilar syndrome, 235
Tortuous siphons, 82-83
TR; *see* Repetition time
Tracking saturation pulse, flow saturation from vascular loop with, 326-327
Transdural anastomoses, with moyamoya disease, 255
Transverse sinuses, left, thrombosis of, 296-297, 298-299
diagnosis of, 299
Traumatic aneurysms, 109
Traumatic carotid dissection, 390-391
Trigeminal artery, persistent, 56-57, 59
Tuberculum sellae, meningioma on, 266, 272-273
with right posterior communicating artery aneurysm, 270-271
Tumor embolus, carotid occlusion related to, 376
Tumors, 265-291; *see also specific tumors*
of carotid body, 280-281
of glomus jugulare, 284-285
of glomus tympanicum, 286-287
of glomus vagale, 282-283
MRA of, 265
and preoperative evaluation, 265
of skull base, 285
technical preferences for, 397
Two-dimensional in-plane spatial saturation technique, background suppression with, 317
Two-dimensional phase-contrast MRA
advantages and disadvantages of, 40
destructive interference on, 209
Two-dimensional phase-contrast MRA—cont'd
to determine direction of flow, 213
scout study of left carotid dissection, 389
technical preferences for, 397, 398
technique for venous disease, 31
Two-dimensional snapshot technique for short echo time, 317
Two-dimensional time-of-flight MRA
advantages and disadvantages of, 40
carotid, 27
background suppression technique for, 317
and comparison with color ultrasound, 369
and comparison with conventional angiography, 369, 371
disadvantages of, 314
flow saturation from vascular loop with, 326-327
motion artifact affects on, 345
overestimation of stenosis with, 341
pitfalls of, 324-325, 326-327, 332-333, 335
techniques for, 314
dissection, pitfalls of, 373-374, 376-377
of dural sinuses, 294
pitfalls of, 295
and motion artifacts
with severe right internal carotid stenosis, 324-325
simulating focal occlusion of sagittal sinus, 295
of right internal carotid artery occlusion, 344-345
and signal loss, guidelines for, 341
of stenosis
overestimation, vs three-dimensional techniques, 341
sensitivity, 369
technical preferences for, 397, 398
and technique for venous disease, 30
tracking saturation pulse, flow saturation from vascular loop with, 326-327
of vascular malformations, 163-164
Tympanicum tumors, glomus, 286-287


**U**


Ultrasound, color, comparison with two-dimensional time-of-flight MRA, 369


**V**


Vagale tumors, glomus, 282-283
Varices, 163
Vascular anatomy, 41-77
Vascular compression of seventh and eighth cranial nerves by basilar artery loop, 288-289
Vascular loops, 265-291
basilar artery, compressing seventh and eighth cranial nerves, 288-289
flow saturation from, 326-327
posterior cerebral, mimicking aneurysm, 100
technical preferences for, 397
Vascular malformations, 163-201; *see also* Arteriovenous malformations; Venous disease
angiographically occult, 173
classification of, 163
identification of, 163
phase-contrast MRA of, 164
three-dimensional time-of-flight MRA of, 163-164
pitfalls of, 166-167, 174-175, 189
time-of-flight MRA of, 163-164
two-dimensional time-of-flight MRA of, 163-164
Vasculitis, 251
basilar artery, 248-249
differential diagnosis of, 251
distal internal carotid stenosis from, 252-253
with early moyamoya disease, 246-247
generalized, 161

Vasoocclusive disease; *see also* Occlusion; *specific disease*
diagnosis of, 203
large vessel
accuracy of MRA for, 203
diagnosis of, 203
sickle cell disease with, 260-261
Vault moyamoya, 255
Velocity change across voxels, 8-9
Venetian blind artifact, 17
Venous anatomy, normal, 50-51
Venous angioma, 167
left frontal, 168-169
not on three-dimensional time-of-flight study, 166-167
of posterior fossa
with cavernous angioma, 172-173
with hemorrhage, 170-171
Venous disease, 163, 292-311; *see also* Vascular malformations
technical preferences for, 398
two-dimensional phase-contrast technique for, 31
two-dimensional time-of-flight technique for, 30
Venous occlusion; *see* Occlusion
Venous sinuses; *see also specific sinuses*
dural
evaluation of, 293-294
two-dimensional time-of-flight MRA of, pitfalls of, 295
Venous thrombosis; *see also* Thrombosis
cerebral, causes of, 293
deep, 306-307
Vertebral artery
dissection of, 381
left vertebral occlusion from, 380-381
distal, stenosis of, 228-229
left, occlusion of, from dissection, 380-381
Vertebrobasilar dolichoectasia, 159
Vertebrobasilar stroke
classification of, 235
multizone, 235
prognosis for, 235
single-zone, 235
top-of-the-basilar, 235
Voxels
small size of, advantages and disadvantages of, 9
velocity change across, 8-9

**W**

Wrap-around, 25

**Z**

Zero-order compensation, 6